TWEL EDITION

TEXAS AND FEDERAL
PHARMACY
& DRUG LAW

FRED S. BRINKLEY, JR., R.Ph., MBA

GARY G. CACCIATORE, Pharm.D., JD

Published by Pharmacy Regulatory Advisors

For additional copies, supplements, or new editions, please contact:

info@txpharmacylaw.com

© 2020 by Fred S. Brinkley, Jr., and Gary G. Cacciatore. All rights reserved.

No part of this publication may be reproduced, stored in a database or retrieval system, or transmitted in any form or by any means electronic, mechanical, photocopying, recording, or otherwise without written permission of the publisher.

VIOLATION OF COPYRIGHT WILL RESULT IN LEGAL ACTION INCLUDING CIVIL AND/OR CRIMINAL PENALTIES.

The consent of the publisher does not extend to copying for general distribution, for promoting, for creating new works, or for resale. Specific permission must be obtained in writing from Pharmacy Regulatory Advisors.

Trademark Notice: Product or corporate names may be trademarks or registered trademarks and are used only for identification and explanation, without intent to infringe.

ISBN: 978-0-578-58207-8

Texas and Federal Pharmacy and Drug Law
12th Edition

Table of Contents

Preface	xii
About the Authors	xiii
Glossary	xiv

CHAPTER A
Federal Food, Drug, and Cosmetic Act (FDCA) and Other Federal Laws and Regulations

Introduction and History	A.1
Definitions (FDCA)	A.9
Prohibited Acts (Section 301)—Violations of the FDCA	A.10
Adulterated Drugs (Section 501)	A.11
Misbranded Drugs (Section 502)	A.11
Over-the-Counter (OTC) Drug Regulations	A.11
Drug and Device Recall Classifications and FDA Enforcement	A.16
Advertising and Promotion of Prescription Drugs	A.16
Consumer Medication Information	A.17
Risk Evaluation and Mitigation Strategies (REMS)	A.18
New Drugs	A.20
National Drug Code (NDC) Number	A.22
Current Good Manufacturing Practices (CGMPs)	A.22
Information on Medication Use During Pregnancy and Breastfeeding	A.22
FDA Orange Book	A.23
FDA Purple Book	A.23
Dietary Supplements and Medical Foods	A.23
Medical Devices	A.25
Other Federal Laws and Regulations	A.30
Federal Hazardous Substances Act of 1966	A.30
Federal Hazard Communication Standard	A.31
Poison Prevention Packaging Act of 1970 (PPPA)	A.31
Omnibus Budget Reconciliation Act of 1990 (OBRA-90)	A.34
Delivering Prescriptions by U.S. Mail or Common Carrier	A.34
Tamper-Resistant Prescription Requirements	A.35
Federal Alcohol Regulations	A.35
Health Insurance Portability and Accountability Act of 1996 (HIPAA)	A.36
Chapter A Highlights	A.44

CHAPTER B
Controlled Substance Laws and Regulations
Federal Controlled Substances Act (FCSA) and Texas Controlled Substances Act (TCSA)

Introduction to the Federal Controlled Substances Act (FCSA)	B.1
Structure and Functions of DEA	B.3

Enforcement of TCSA and Rules..B.3
Drug Classifications Under the FCSA and TCSA..B.3
Scheduling of Controlled Substances..B.5
Determining the Schedule of Compounded Controlled Substances.................................B.5
Registration—How Entities and Persons are Regulated Under the FCSA........................B.7
Ordering Schedule II Controlled Substances...B.12
Ordering Schedule III–V Controlled Substances...B.16
Distributions of Controlled Substances by a Pharmacy to Another Registrant, Transfer Upon Sale, and
    Other Miscellaneous Distributions..B.16
Storage, Security, and Theft or Loss of Controlled Substances......................................B.19
Disposal and Destruction of Controlled Substances (21 CFR 1317.01–1317.95)..........B.23
Inspections...B.25
Records...B.26
Controlled Substance Prescriptions...B.28
Schedule II Prescriptions...B.37
Schedule III, IV, and V Prescriptions..B.44
Texas Prescription Program for Controlled Substances (Texas Prescription Monitoring Program).............B.47
Methadone and Treatment of Narcotic Dependence...B.50
State and Federal Methamphetamine Controls...B.51
Online Resources..B.53
Summary of Major Differences Between Federal Controlled Substances Act (FCSA) and Texas Controlled
    Substances Act (TCSA) and Texas Pharmacy Act and Rules......................................B.55
Chapter B Highlights..B.57

CHAPTER C
CHAPTER 483 TEXAS HEALTH and SAFETY CODE
Texas Dangerous Drug Act (TDDA)
and Related Texas Laws and Rules

Section 483.001	Definitions and Practice Issues	C.1
Section 483.002	Rules	C.3
Section 483.003	Department of State Health Services Hearings Regarding Certain Drugs	C.3
Section 483.004	Commissioner of State Health Services	C.3
Section 483.021	Determination by Pharmacist on Request to Dispense Certain Drugs	C.3
Section 483.022	Practitioner's Designation of Agent; Practitioner's Responsibilities	C.4
Section 483.023	Retention of Prescriptions	C.4
Section 483.024	Records of a Drug Acquisition or Disposal	C.4
Section 483.025	Inspections and Inventories	C.4
Section 483.041	Possession of Dangerous Drugs	C.4
Section 483.042	Delivery (Sale) or Offer to Deliver a Drug	C.5
Section 483.043	Manufacture of a Dangerous Drug	C.6
Section 483.045	Forging or Altering Prescriptions	C.6
Section 483.046	Failure to Retain a Prescription	C.6
Section 483.047	Refilling a Prescription Without Authorization (Emergency Refills)	C.6
Section 483.048	Unauthorized Communication of Prescription	C.6
Section 483.049	Failure to Maintain Records	C.6
Section 483.050	Refusal to Permit Inspection	C.6
Section 483.073	Search Warrant	C.6
Section 483.074	Seizure and Destruction	C.7
Section 483.101	Definitions (Subchapter E—Opioid Antagonists)	C.7
Section 483.102	Prescription for an Opioid Antagonist; Standing Order From a Prescriber	C.7

Section 483.103   Dispensing of Opioid Antagonist by a Pharmacist...C.7
Board of Pharmacy Rule 295.14 Dispensing of Opioid Antagonist by a Pharmacist C.8
Section 483.104   Distribution of Opioid Antagonist; Standing Order C.8
Section 483.105   Possession of Opioid Antagonist...C.8
Section 483.106   Administration of Opioid Antagonist C.8
Prescriptive Authority for Advanced Practice Registered Nurses and Physician Assistants.....................C.9
Limited Independent Prescriptive Authority of Therapeutic Optometrists and
   Optometric Glaucoma Specialists...C.11
Drugs That May be Prescribed by Optometrists..C.13
Over-the-Counter Sales of Dextromethorphan C.14
Possession and Administration of Certain Dangerous Drugs by Home and
   Community Support Services Agencies..C.15
Texas Food, Drug, and Cosmetic Act—Subtitle M Drug Donation Program C.16
TDSHS RULE 229.22 Donation of Drugs to Charitable Medical Clinics C.17
Texas Food, Drug, and Cosmetic Act—Subtitle A Donation of Prescription Drugs................................C.19
Medical Gases (Oxygen)..C.20
Quick Reference Guide—Prescriptions Which May Be Dispensed in Texas C.21
Chapter C Highlights C.22

Chapter D
Texas Pharmacy Act (TPA)
(and Selected Board of Pharmacy Rules)

Chapter 551 General Provisions...D.1
Chapter 552 State Board of Pharmacy..D.6
Chapter 553 Executive Director and Other Board Personnel D.9
Chapter 554 Board Powers and Duties; Rulemaking Authority..D.10
   Board of Pharmacy Rule 291.27 Pharmacy Residency Programs..D.11
   *Board of Pharmacy Rule 291.23 Pilot or Demonstration Research Projects for Innovative Applications
      in the Practice of Pharmacy* D.13
   *Board of Pharmacy Rule 295.15 Administration of Immunizations or Vaccinations by a Pharmacist Under
      Written Protocol of a Physician*..D.16
Chapter 557 Pharmacist Interns..D.18
Chapter 558 License to Practice Pharmacy D.19
   Board of Pharmacy Rule 281.12 Criminal History Evaluation Letter D.19
   Board of Pharmacy Rule 283.7 Examination Requirements D.21
   Board of Pharmacy Rule 283.11 Examination Retake Requirements...D.22
   Board of Pharmacy Rule 283.2 Internship—Definitions..D.23
   Board of Pharmacy Rule 283.3 Educational and Age Requirements..D.25
   Board of Pharmacy Rule 283.4 Internship Requirements..D.25
   Board of Pharmacy Rule 283.5 Pharmacist Intern Duties D.30
   Board of Pharmacy Rule 283.6 Preceptor Requirements and Ratio of Preceptors to Pharmacist Interns.........D.30
   Board of Pharmacy Rule 283.8 Reciprocity Requirements D.32
   *Board of Pharmacy Rule 283.9 Fee Requirements for Licensure by Examination, Score Transfer,
      and Reciprocity*..D.33
   *Board of Pharmacy Rule 283.12 Licenses for Military Service Members, Military Veterans,
      and Military Spouses*...D.33
   Board of Pharmacy Rule 295.6 Emergency Temporary Pharmacist License..D.34
Chapter 559 Renewal of License to Practice Pharmacy (Pharmacists) D.35
   Board of Pharmacy Rule 295.5 Pharmacist License or Renewal Fees D.36
   *Board of Pharmacy Rule 283.10 Requirements for Application for a Pharmacist License
      Which Has Expired*...D.37

Board of Pharmacy Rule 295.8 Continuing Education Requirements D.39
Board of Pharmacy Rule 295.9 Inactive Status (License) D.45
Chapter 560 Licensing of Pharmacies D.46
Board of Pharmacy Rule 291.1 Pharmacy License Application D.50
Board of Pharmacy Rule 291.6 Pharmacy License Fees D.50
Board of Pharmacy Rule 291.22 Petition to Establish an Additional Class of Pharmacy D.51
Board of Pharmacy Rule 291.127 Emergency Remote Pharmacy License D.52
Chapter 561 Renewal of a Pharmacy License D.53
Board of Pharmacy Rule 291.14 Pharmacy License Renewal D.54
Chapter 562 Practice by a License Holder (Pharmacist), SUBCHAPTER A. Prescription and Substitution Requirements D.55
Board of Pharmacy Rule 291.33(c)(4)(A)(B) Substitution of a Dosage Form Permitted D.59
Chapter 309 Board of Pharmacy Generic Substitution Rules D.60
Board of Pharmacy Rule 309.1 Objective D.60
Board of Pharmacy Rule 309.2 Definitions D.60
Board of Pharmacy Rule 309.3 Generic Substitution Requirements D.61
Board of Pharmacy Rule 309.4 Patient Notification D.64
Board of Pharmacy Rule 309.6 Records D.64
Board of Pharmacy Rule 309.7 Dispensing Responsibilities D.65
Board of Pharmacy Rule 309.8 Advertising of Generic Drugs by Pharmacies D.66
Board of Pharmacy Rule 295.1 Change of Address and/or Name D.66
Board of Pharmacy Rule 295.2 Change of Employment D.66
Board of Pharmacy Rule 295.16 Administration of Epinephrine by a Pharmacist D.68
Introduction to Remote Pharmacy Services Laws and Rules D.72
Summary of Board of Pharmacy Rule 291.121(b) Remote Pharmacy Services Using an Emergency Medication Kit D.73
Summary of Board of Pharmacy Rule 291.121(a) Remote Pharmacy Services Using Automated Pharmacy Systems (primarily used in nursing homes) D.74
Summary of TPA Section 562.110 and Board of Pharmacy Rule 291.121(c) Remote Pharmacy Services Using Telepharmacy Systems D.76
Summary of Board of Pharmacy Rule 291.121(d) Remote Pharmacy Services Using Automated Storage and Delivery Systems D.78
Chapter 563 Prescription Requirements; Delegation of Administration and Provision of Dangerous Drugs D.80
Chapter 564 Program to Aid Impaired Pharmacists and Pharmacy Students: Pharmacy Peer Review D.82
Chapter 568 Pharmacy Technicians and Pharmacy Technician Trainees D.84
Board of Pharmacy Rule 291.32(d)(3)(B) Ratio of Onsite Pharmacists to Pharmacy Technicians and Pharmacy Technician Trainees D.85
Board of Pharmacy Rules—Chapter 297 Pharmacy Technicians and Pharmacy Technician Trainees D.86
297.1 Purpose D.86
297.2 Definitions D.86
297.3 Registration Requirements D.86
297.4 Fees D.88
297.5 Pharmacy Technician Trainees D.88
297.6 Pharmacy Technician and Pharmacy Technician Trainee Training D.88
297.7 Exemption from Pharmacy Technician Certification Requirements D.90
297.8 Continuing Education Requirements D.90
297.9 Notifications D.95
297.10 Registration for Military Service Members, Military Veterans, and Military Spouses D.95
297.11 Temporary Emergency Registration D.95
Chapter 569 Reporting Requirements for Professional Liability Insurers D.96
Board of Pharmacy Rule 281.18 Reporting Professional Liability Claims D.97
Chapter D Highlights D.100

Chapter E
Miscellaneous Texas Pharmacy and Drug Laws and Rules
General Rules for Pharmacists
Chapter 295

Board of Pharmacy Rule 295.3 Responsibility of a Pharmacist E.1
Board of Pharmacy Rule 295.4 Sharing Money Received for Prescriptions (Kickbacks) E.1
Board of Pharmacy Rule 295.12 Pharmacist Certification Programs E.1
Board of Pharmacy Rule 295.13 Drug Therapy Management by a Pharmacist Under the Written Protocol of a Physician E.2
All Classes of Pharmacy—Chapter 291 .... E.6
Board of Pharmacy Rule 291.1 Pharmacy License Application E.6
Board of Pharmacy Rule 291.3 Required Notifications E.6
Summary Chart of Major Notifications Required by TSBP E.10
Board of Pharmacy Rule 291.5 Closing a Pharmacy E.10
Board of Pharmacy Rule 291.7 Prescription Drug Recalls E.12
Board of Pharmacy Rule 291.8 Return of Prescription Drugs E.12
Board of Pharmacy Rule 291.9 Prescription Pick Up Locations E.14
Board of Pharmacy Rule 291.10 Pharmacy Balance Registration/Inspection E.14
Board of Pharmacy Rule 291.15 Storage of Drugs E.15
Board of Pharmacy Rule 291.16 Samples E.15
Board of Pharmacy Rule 291.17 Inventory Requirements E.16
Board of Pharmacy Rule 291.24 Pharmacy Residency Programs E.18
Board of Pharmacy Rule 291.27 Confidentiality E.18
Board of Pharmacy Rule 291.28 Patient Access to Confidential Records E.19
Board of Pharmacy Rule 291.29 Professional Responsibility of Pharmacists E.20
Board of Pharmacy Rule 291.125 Centralized Prescription Dispensing E.23
Board of Pharmacy Rule 291.123 Centralized Prescription Drug or Medication Order Processing E.24
Board of Pharmacy Rule 291.129 Satellite Pharmacy E.25
Destruction and Disposal of Dangerous Drugs and Controlled Substances—Chapter 303 .... E.30
Board of Pharmacy Rule 303.1 Destruction of Dispensed Drugs E.30
Board of Pharmacy Rule 303.2 Destruction of Stock Prescription Drugs E.33
Board of Pharmacy Rule 303.3 Records E.33
Confidentiality of Certain Information Regarding the Execution of a Convict E.33
Medication Synchronization E.33
Chapter E Highlights E.34

Chapter F
Complaints, Inspections, Disciplinary Actions, and Procedures

Chapter 555 Public Interest Information and Complaint Procedures F.1
Board of Pharmacy Rule 291.3(h)(1) Notification to Consumers Regarding Filing a Complaint (For Licensed Pharmacies) F.2
Board of Pharmacy Rule 295.11 Notification to Consumers Regarding Filing a Complaint (For Licensed Pharmacists) F.3
TSBP Complaint Process F.4
Chapter 556 Administrative Inspections and Warrants, SUBCHAPTER A. General Provisions F.6
SUBCHAPTER B. Inspections F.6
Board of Pharmacy Rule 291.18 Time Limit for Filing a Complaint F.7
Board of Pharmacy Rule 291.19 Administrative Actions as a Result of a Compliance Inspection F.7
SUBCHAPTER C. Warrants F.8

Chapter 565 Disciplinary Actions and Procedures; Reinstatement of License,
   SUBCHAPTER A. Grounds for Discipline of an Applicant or a License Holder F.8
  Board of Pharmacy Rule 281.7.A. Unprofessional Conduct F.9
  Board of Pharmacy Rule 281.7.B. Gross Immorality F.12
  Board of Pharmacy Rule 281.7.C. Fraud, Deceit, or Misrepresentation F.12
  Board of Pharmacy Rule 291.11 Operation of a Pharmacy F.14
  Board of Pharmacy Rule 281.8 Grounds for Discipline for a Pharmacy License F.15
Chapter 568 Pharmacy Technicians (Selected Disciplinary Provisions) F.16
  Board of Pharmacy Rule 281.9 Grounds for Discipline for a Pharmacy Technician or
    a Pharmacy Technician Trainee F.16
SUBCHAPTER B. Disciplinary Actions and Procedures F.19
  Board of Pharmacy Rule 281.61 Definitions of Discipline Authorized F.19
  Board of Pharmacy Rule 281.6 Mental or Physical Examination F.20
  Board of Pharmacy Rule 281.23 Subpoenas F.23
  Board of Pharmacy Rule 281.68 Remedial Plan F.24
  Board of Pharmacy Rule 281.31 Burden of Proof F.25
  Board of Pharmacy Rule 281.12 Rules Governing Cooperating Practitioners F.26
SUBCHAPTER C. Petition for Reinstatement of a License or Removal of a Restriction F.26
  Board of Pharmacy Rule 281.66 Application for the Reissuance or Removal of Restrictions
    of a License or Registration F.26
Chapter 566 Penalties and Enforcement Provisions F.28
SUBCHAPTER A. Administrative Penalty (Fine) F.28
SUBCHAPTER B. Injunctive Relief F.29
SUBCHAPTER C. Civil Penalty F.30
SUBCHAPTER D. Criminal Penalties F.30
  Summary of Texas Pharmacy Administrative Practice and Rules of Procedure F.31
Chapter 281 (Board Rules 281.1–281.68) F.31
TSBP Disciplinary Process F.32
  Board of Pharmacy Rule 281.60 General Guidance F.34
  Board of Pharmacy Rule 281.62 Aggravating and Mitigating Factors F.35
  Board of Pharmacy Rule 281.63 Considerations for Criminal Offenses F.36
  Board of Pharmacy Rule 281.64 Sanctions for Applicants with Criminal Offenses F.36
  Board of Pharmacy Rule 281.65 Schedule of Administrative Penalties
    (Fines for Pharmacies, Pharmacists, and Pharmacy Technicians) F.37
  Board of Pharmacy Rule 281.67 Sanctions for Out-of-State Disciplinary Actions F.37
Chapter F Highlights F.38

Chapter G
Community Pharmacy (Class A) Rules

Board of Pharmacy Rule 291.31 Definitions G.1
Board of Pharmacy Rule 291.32 Personnel G.5
  Pharmacist-in-Charge (PIC) G.5
  Owner G.6
  Pharmacists (applies to pharmacists-in-charge and staff pharmacists) G.6
  Pharmacy Technicians and Pharmacy Technician Trainees G.8
Class A Pharmacy Technician/Trainee Duties G.10
Board of Pharmacy Rule 291.33 Operational Standards G.11
  Licensing Requirements G.11
  Environment G.12
  Prescription Dispensing and Delivery G.15
  Prescription Containers G.20

Labeling	G.20
Returning Undelivered Medication to Stock	G.22
Label Requirements for Dispensed Prescriptions	G.23
Equipment and Supplies	G.24
Library	G.24
Drugs	G.24
Prepacking of Drugs (only for internal distribution by the pharmacy)	G.24
Customized Patient Medication Packages	G.25
Automated Devices and Systems in a Pharmacy	G.27
Questions and Answers on Automation in Class A (Community) Pharmacies	G.30
Questions and Answers on Automated Counting Devices	G.31
Questions and Answers on Automated Pharmacy Dispensing Systems	G.31
Questions and Answers on Automated Checking Devices	G.32
Board of Pharmacy Rule 291.34 Records	G.33
Maintenance of Records	G.33
Prescriptions	G.33
Patient Medication Records (PMR)	G.42
Prescription Drug Order Records Maintained in a Manual System	G.43
Records Maintained in a Data Processing System (computer system)	G.43
Limitation to One Type of Recordkeeping System	G.46
Transfer of Prescription Drug Order Information	G.46
Distribution of Prescription Drugs to Another Registrant	G.48
Other Records	G.49
Permission to Maintain Central Records	G.49
Ownership of Pharmacy Records	G.50
Documentation of Consultation With a Prescriber	G.50
Board of Pharmacy Rule 291.36 Pharmacies Compounding Sterile Preparations (Class A–S)	G.50
Records Pharmacists Should be Able to Locate in a Class A Pharmacy	G.51
Chapter G Highlights	G.52

Chapter H
Compounding Laws and Rules

History of Compounding Regulation	H.1
Texas Pharmacy Act Compounding Provisions (Chapter 562 Subchapter D)	H.3
TSBP Rule on Nonsterile Compounding	H.5
Board of Pharmacy Rule 291.131 Pharmacies Compounding Nonsterile Preparations	H.5
Purpose	H.5
Definitions	H.5
Personnel	H.6
Operational Standards	H.7
Records	H.14
Office Use Compounding and Distribution of Compounded Preparations	H.15
Recall Procedures	H.18
TSBP Rule on Sterile Compounding	H.18
Board of Pharmacy Rule 291.133 Pharmacies Compounding Sterile Preparations	H.19
Purpose	H.19
Definitions	H.19
Personnel	H.24
Operational Standards	H.32
Records	H.59
Office Use Compounding and Distribution of Sterile Compounded Preparations	H.61
Recall Procedures	H.64

USP Chapter 800 Hazardous Drugs—Handling in Healthcare Settings (Review and Summary) H.64
Chapter H Highlights H.70

Chapter I
Institutional Pharmacy (Class C) Rules

Definition from Pharmacy Practice Act... I.1
 Board of Pharmacy Rule 291.71 Purpose I.1
 Board of Pharmacy Rule 291.72 Definitions I.1
 Board of Pharmacy Rule 291.73 Personnel I.4
  Requirements for Pharmacist Services I.4
  Pharmacist-in-charge (PIC) I.4
  Consultant Pharmacist I.6
  Pharmacists... I.6
  Pharmacy Technicians and Pharmacy Technician Trainees I.7
  Owner... I.11
  Identification of Pharmacy Personnel.. I.11
  Ratios I.11
Class C (Institutional) Pharmacy Technician/Trainee Duties I.11
 Board of Pharmacy Rule 291.74 Operational Standards... I.13
  Licensing Requirements I.13
  Environment... I.15
  Equipment and Supplies I.15
  Library I.15
  Absence of a Pharmacist I.16
  Drugs I.17
  Pharmaceutical Care Services I.21
  Emergency Rooms (ER).. I.22
  Radiology Departments... I.23
  Automated Devices and Systems I.23
Questions and Answers on Automation in Class C (Institutional) Pharmacies I.27
Questions and Answers on Automated Compounding or Counting Devices I.28
Questions and Answers on Automated Medication Supply Systems I.28
Questions and Answers on Automated Checking Devices I.30
 Board of Pharmacy Rule 291.75 Records I.31
Records That Pharmacists Should Be Able to Locate in a Class C Pharmacy............................... I.34
 Board of Pharmacy Rule 291.77 Pharmacies Compounding Sterile Preparations (Class C-S).............. I.34
Rules for Class C Pharmacies Located in a Freestanding Ambulatory Surgical Center...................... I.36
 Board of Pharmacy Rule 291.76 Class C Pharmacies Located in a
  Freestanding Ambulatory Surgical Center (ASC) I.36
Chapter I Highlights I.40

Chapter J
Other Classes of Pharmacies

Nuclear Pharmacy (Class B) Rules J.1
 Board of Pharmacy Rule 291.51 Purpose J.1
 Board of Pharmacy Rule 291.52 Definitions J.1
 Board of Pharmacy Rule 291.53 Personnel J.1
 Board of Pharmacy Rule 291.54 Operational Standards... J.5
  Licensing Requirements J.5
  Environment... J.6

    Prescription Dispensing and Delivery J.6
    Equipment J.7
    Library J.7
    Radiopharmaceuticals and/or Radioactive Materials J.8
  Board of Pharmacy Rule 291.55 Records J.8
    Policy and Procedure Manual J.8
    Prescription J.8
Clinic Pharmacy (Class D) Rules J.9
  Board of Pharmacy Rule 291.91 Definitions J.9
  Board of Pharmacy Rule 291.92 Personnel J.10
  Board of Pharmacy Rule 291.93 Operational Standards J.11
  Board of Pharmacy Rule 291.94 Records J.18
Nonresident Pharmacies (Class E) Statutes and Rules (Primarily Out-of-State Mail Service Pharmacies
    or Out-of-State Internet Pharmacies) J.20
  Section 556.0551   Inspection of a Licensed Nonresident Pharmacy J.20
  Section 560.052   Qualifications J.20
  Section 561.0031   Additional Renewal Requirement for a Class E Pharmacy J.21
  Board of Pharmacy Rule 291.14 Pharmacy License Renewal J.22
  Section 565.003   Additional Grounds for Discipline Regarding an Applicant for or a Holder
       of a Nonresident Pharmacy License J.22
  Section 565.053   Discipline of a Nonresident Pharmacy; Notice to Resident State J.22
  Section 565.054   Service of Process on a Nonresident Pharmacy J.22
  Board of Pharmacy Rule 291.101 Purpose J.22
  Board of Pharmacy Rule 291.102 Definitions J.23
  Board of Pharmacy Rule 291.103 Personnel J.24
  Board of Pharmacy Rule 291.104 Operational Standards J.24
  Board of Pharmacy Rule 291.105 Records J.29
  Board of Pharmacy Rule 291.106 Pharmacies Compounding Sterile Preparations (Class E-S) J.30
Freestanding Emergency Medical Care Facility Pharmacy (Class F) Rules (FEMCF) J.31
  *Board of Pharmacy Rule 291.151 Pharmacies Located in a Freestanding Emergency Medical Care Facility
    (Class F)* J.31
    Purpose J.31
    Definitions J.32
    Personnel J.33
    Operational Standards J.36
    Records J.43
Central Prescription Drug or Medication Order Processing Pharmacy (Class G) Rule J.47
  *Board of Pharmacy Rule 291.153 Central Prescription Drug or Medication Order Processing Pharmacy
    (Class G)* J.47
    Purpose J.47
    Definitions J.47
    Personnel J.48
    Operational Standards J.51
    Records J.52
Limited Prescription Delivery Pharmacy (Class H) Rule J.53
  Board of Pharmacy Rule 291.155 Limited Prescription Delivery Pharmacy (Class H) J.53
    Purpose J.53
    Definitions J.53
    Personnel J.53
    Operational Standards J.54
    Records J.56
Chapter J Highlights J.57

Preface

Texas and Federal Pharmacy and Drug Law (originally published as *The Guide to Texas and Federal Pharmacy and Drug Law*) is now in its 12th edition and is a comprehensive book designed to assist pharmacists, pharmacy students, attorneys, and other interested parties in understanding the laws and rules that affect the practice of pharmacy in Texas. Chapters A and B also discuss some of the federal laws that impact the practice of pharmacy, but the primary focus of the book is on Texas pharmacy and drug law. Our goal is to provide a practical book that can be used both in the classroom and by pharmacists and attorneys who have questions concerning the practice of pharmacy in Texas. The book also serves as an excellent study guide for those preparing to take the Multistate Pharmacy Jurisprudence Exam® for Texas.

Where possible, we have attempted to bring together sections of the Texas State Board of Pharmacy rules with the relevant portions of the law to which they apply. We believe that this makes it easier to understand the law and the rules on a given subject without having to refer between the law and the rules.

While many provisions in the book are taken verbatim from the applicable law or rule, we have also taken the liberty to delete, modify, and/or edit certain sections to make the information clearer to the reader. We have not changed the meaning of any section of the law or rules, but in certain places we have edited the language to make it more understandable for students and pharmacists. We have also added notes throughout the book to clarify the meaning of certain sections. Because of this, the reader should not rely upon the language in this book as the official law or rule language and should consult official sources such as the Texas State Board of Pharmacy's website for the definitive and current language of a particular law or rule. In addition, while every attempt is made to make this material as accurate as possible, the information herein should not be construed as legal advice. The reader is encouraged to consult a qualified attorney for legal advice.

The authors would like to thank the Texas State Board of Pharmacy for its assistance with this book and for the use of excerpts from the *State Board of Pharmacy Newsletter* and *Texas Pharmacy Laws and Regulations*. The authors also would like to thank E. Paul Holder from Texas A&M Rangel College of Pharmacy for his contributions to Chapter H, Kurt Wehrs for his guidance in the publication of this book, and Debra Smith for her invaluable editing assistance.

Fred S. Brinkley, Jr.	Gary G. Cacciatore	January 2020
Austin, Texas	Houston, Texas	

This publication is designed to provide accurate and authoritative information regarding the subject matter covered. It is sold with the understanding that neither the publisher nor the authors are engaged in rendering legal, accounting, or other professional services. If legal advice or other expert assistance is required, the services of a competent professional person should be sought.

From a Declaration of Principles jointly adopted by a Committee of the American Bar Association and a Committee of Publishers.

About the Authors

Fred S. Brinkley, Jr., R.Ph., M.B.A.

Fred S. Brinkley, Jr., is a native of San Antonio and resides in Austin, Texas. Mr. Brinkley received the B.S. in pharmacy from The University of Texas at Austin (UT), attended Drake University's Graduate School of Public Administration, and received his M.B.A. from UT Austin. He recently retired from coordinating and teaching the pharmacy law course at the UT College of Pharmacy after 30 years. He continues to practice as a pharmacy regulatory consultant.

Mr. Brinkley began his career as a community pharmacist in San Antonio and subsequently served as a professional service representative for E.R. Squibb & Sons, Inc. From 1969 to 1972, he held a joint appointment as Director of Public Affairs of the Texas Pharmacy Association (TPA) and Assistant to the Dean of the UT College of Pharmacy. He also served as Director of the National Drug Abuse Education Training Center in San Antonio, a cooperative effort of the UT College of Pharmacy and the UT Medical School at San Antonio.

In 1972, Mr. Brinkley accepted an appointment as Director of the Iowa Drug Abuse Authority, an independent executive agency located within the Iowa Governor's office. He served in this position until 1976 before accepting an appointment as Executive Director of the Texas State Board of Pharmacy, a position he held for two decades. In 1997, Mr. Brinkley accepted a position as Vice President of Professional Affairs for Medco Health Solutions and remained in this position until he retired in 2009.

He has served as a member of the American Pharmaceutical Association (APhA) Advisory Committee on Pharmaceutical Care, as a member of the Editorial Advisory Board of the APhA's *Pharmacy Today*, and as a member-at-large of the United States Pharmacopeial Convention. Mr. Brinkley received the 1993 William J. Sheffield Outstanding Alumnus Award and the 2005 Legend of Pharmacy Award from the UT Austin College of Pharmacy Alumni Association and was honored by TPA as "2000 Pharmacist of the Year." He also served as President of the UT College of Pharmacy Alumni Association, as well as Chairman of the UT College of Pharmacy Advisory Council.

Mr. Brinkley was appointed by Governor Rick Perry as the pharmacist member of the Texas Statewide Health Coordinating Council in 2010. He served as Vice Chairman of the Council until he completed his term of office in 2015.

Gary G. Cacciatore, Pharm.D., J.D.

Gary Cacciatore serves as Associate Regulatory Counsel and Vice President of Regulatory Affairs for Cardinal Health, Inc., a global, integrated healthcare services and products company, providing customized solutions for hospitals, health systems, pharmacies, ambulatory surgery centers, clinical laboratories, and physician offices worldwide.

Dr. Cacciatore is responsible for interactions with state and federal regulatory agencies and for advising and representing the company on healthcare legal and regulatory matters. He has worked with, advised, and represented the company before several regulatory agencies including state boards of pharmacy, departments of health, and other state regulatory bodies. He has also advised and represented the company on matters before federal agencies such as the Food and Drug Administration, Drug Enforcement Administration, and U.S. Customs.

Prior to joining Cardinal Health, Dr. Cacciatore was an Assistant Professor at the University of Houston College of Pharmacy and the University of Houston Law Center where he taught courses in pharmacy law and ethics, drug information, and food and drug law. He is well published in the area of pharmacy law and formerly served as an editor for *Pharmacy Law Digest*. Dr. Cacciatore is a frequent lecturer on pharmacy law issues and has served as a consultant to various groups on legal issues in pharmacy practice. He currently serves as an Adjunct Associate Professor at the University of Houston College of Pharmacy.

Dr. Cacciatore received his Doctor of Pharmacy degree with high honors from the University of Florida College of Pharmacy and his Doctor of Jurisprudence degree with honors from the University of Houston Law Center.

Dr. Cacciatore is admitted to the bar in Texas and is a registered pharmacist in Texas and Florida. He is a member of numerous local, state, and national pharmacy and legal organizations and is a Past President of the American Society for Pharmacy Law (ASPL). In 2015, Dr. Cacciatore received the Joseph L. Fink III Founders Award from ASPL for sustained and outstanding contributions to the professions of pharmacy and law. Most recently he received the University of Florida College of Pharmacy's Outstanding Alumnus Award for 2020.

Texas and Federal Pharmacy and Drug Law Glossary

Class A Pharmacy	Community Pharmacy
Class B Pharmacy	Nuclear Pharmacy
Class C Pharmacy	Institutional Pharmacy
Class D Pharmacy	Clinic Pharmacy
Class E Pharmacy	Nonresident Pharmacy
Class F Pharmacy	Freestanding Emergency Medical Care Facility Pharmacy
Class G Pharmacy	Central Prescription Drug or Medication Order Processing Pharmacy
Class H Pharmacy	Limited Prescription Delivery Pharmacy

APRN	Advanced Practice Registered Nurse
ACPE	Accreditation Council for Pharmacy Education
CBD	Cannabidiol
CE	Continuing Education
CFR	Code of Federal Regulations
CGMP	Current Good Manufacturing Practices
CS	Controlled Substance
CSA	Controlled Substances Act
DEA	Drug Enforcement Administration
DPS	Department of Public Safety (Texas)
DUR	Drug Utilization Review
FDA	Food and Drug Administration
FDAMA	Food and Drug Administration Modernization Act of 1997
FDCA	Food, Drug, and Cosmetic Act
FCSA	Federal Controlled Substances Act
HCSA	Home and Community Support Agency
HIPAA	Health Insurance Portability and Accountability Act
LTCF	Long Term Care Facility
LVN	Licensed Vocational Nurse
MPJE	Multistate Pharmacy Jurisprudence Examination
NABP	National Association of Boards of Pharmacy
NAPLEX	North American Pharmacist Licensure Examination
NDC	National Drug Code
OBRA 90	Omnibus Budget Reconciliation Act of 1990
OTC	Over-the-Counter
PA	Physician Assistant
PMP	Prescription Monitoring Program
PDMA	Prescription Drug Marketing Act
PIC	Pharmacist-in-Charge
PPI	Patient Package Insert
PPPA	Poison Prevention Packaging Act
REMS	Risk Evaluation and Mitigation Strategies
TCSA	Texas Controlled Substances Act
TDDA	Texas Dangerous Drug Act
TDSHS	Texas Department of State Health Services
TMB	Texas Medical Board
TPA	Texas Pharmacy Act
TSBP	Texas State Board of Pharmacy

CHAPTER A

Federal Food, Drug, and Cosmetic Act (FDCA)
and
Other Federal Laws and Regulations

CHAPTER A

Federal Food, Drug, and Cosmetic Act (FDCA) and Other Federal Laws and Regulations

I. **Introduction and History**

The Food, Drug, and Cosmetic Act (FDCA) is designed to protect the public health by requiring that only safe, effective, and properly labeled drugs and devices be introduced into interstate commerce and to assure that food and cosmetics are safe and properly labeled. The Food and Drug Administration (FDA), which is part of the U.S. Department of Health and Human Services (HHS), is part of the executive branch of the federal government, has the authority to make regulations, and administers and enforces the Act.

A. Legislative History of the FDCA
1. 1906—Pure Food and Drug Act
   a. Prohibited interstate commerce of misbranded and adulterated foods, drinks, and drugs.
   b. Administered by the Department of Agriculture.
   c. Only required that drugs meet standards of purity and strength.
   d. No information had to be submitted to the government before putting a product on the market and there was no efficacy requirement.
   e. The government had to prove an intent to defraud before a product could be removed.
   f. Many products were allowed on the market with false or fraudulent claims.
2. 1938—Federal Food, Drug, and Cosmetic Act (FDCA)
   a. Passed in response to the Elixir Sulfanilamide tragedy in which 107 people died when diethylene glycol was used as a solvent in the elixir.
   b. Extended coverage of the Act to cosmetics and devices.
   c. Required predistribution clearance for the safety of new drugs through a New Drug Application (NDA) process.
   d. Eliminated the requirement to prove intent to defraud in drug misbranding cases.
   e. Created the FDA as we know it today.
   f. Authorized factory inspections by FDA.
   g. Added injunction procedures by FDA.
3. 1951—Durham-Humphrey Amendments
   a. Basic provision required that drugs which cannot be used safely without medical supervision must be dispensed only pursuant to a prescription order issued by a qualified practitioner.
   b. Provided which drugs must be administered or dispensed on prescription only basis.
      (1) Essentially created the over-the-counter (OTC) and prescription drug categories.
      (2) Provided how prescription drugs must be dispensed.
         (a) Upon a written prescription issued by a licensed practitioner.
         (b) Upon an oral prescription by such practitioner which is promptly reduced to writing and filled by a pharmacist.
         (c) By refilling a written or oral prescription if authorized by the practitioner either in the original prescription or by a subsequent oral order.
         (d) By administration or dispensing directly by the practitioner.

(3) Drugs dispensed on prescription are exempted from most of the manufacturer's labeling requirements discussed under "Misbranded Drugs" if the label of the prescription container has:
  (a) Name and address of dispenser (pharmacy).
  (b) Serial number (prescription number) of prescription.
  (c) Date of the prescription or filling.
  (d) Name of prescriber.
  (e) Name of patient.
  (f) Directions for use and cautionary statements, if any, contained in the prescription.

4. 1962—Kefauver-Harris Amendments
In response to the discovery of birth defects caused by the drug thalidomide, Congress passed the Kefauver-Harris Amendments which:
  a. Required new drug products to be proven safe and effective for claimed use.
  b. Increased safety requirements and required more clinical investigations.
  c. Increased and strengthened inspection authority of the FDA.
  d. Established Good Manufacturing Practices (GMP).

5. 1965—Drug Abuse Control Amendments
  a. Controlled use of depressants, stimulants, and hallucinogens.
  b. Precursor to the Federal Controlled Substances Act of 1970. (*See Chapter B in this book.*)

6. 1976—Medical Device Amendment
  a. Assured the safety and effectiveness of medical devices and certain diagnostic and laboratory products.
  b. Upgraded regulatory authority over such devices by the FDA.

7. 1983—Orphan Drug Act
  a. Amended the FDCA to provide incentives for manufacturers to deliver and market drugs or biological products intended for a rare disease or medical condition occurring in the U.S.
  b. Extended the patent life of such drugs to enhance profitability.

8. 1984—Drug Price Competition and Patent Restoration Act (Hatch-Waxman Act)
  a. Purpose of the Act was to reduce healthcare costs.
  b. Codified FDA's authority to accept abbreviated new drug applications (ANDAs) for generic versions of "pioneer" drug products first approved after 1962.
  c. Streamlined the approval of generic drugs by eliminating duplicate and unnecessary testing and required no clinical testing for safety or efficacy; however, required the generic drug to be bioequivalent to the pioneer drug.
  d. Created a patent litigation framework where a generic manufacturer can challenge a brand manufacturer's patents in federal court without risking liability for patent infringement damages.
  e. Provided an incentive to generic manufacturers to challenge patents for brand name pharmaceuticals by providing a 180-day market exclusivity period for the first marketed generic.
  f. Gave brand name pharmaceutical companies a 5-year exclusivity period during which generic manufacturers cannot submit FDA applications for new generic versions of the brand name pharmaceutical and restoring some of the patent term lost due to the lengthy FDA regulatory approval process.

9. 1988—Prescription Drug Marketing Act of 1987 (PDMA)
  a. The PDMA became law in 1988 and amended the Federal Food, Drug, and Cosmetic Act to reduce the potential public health risks that may

result from diversion of prescription drugs from legitimate commercial channels. The PDMA bans the reimportation of prescription human drugs produced in the United States except when reimported by the manufacturer or, after FDA approval, for emergency use. It also bans the sale, trade, or purchase of drug samples and the trafficking in and counterfeiting of drug coupons (forms that may be redeemed for a prescription drug at no cost or reduced cost). The PDMA requires that all requests for drug samples be made in writing by licensed practitioners. It also requires that drug samples be properly stored and handled and that certain recordkeeping be followed. The PDMA also bans, with certain specific exceptions, the resale of prescription drugs purchased by hospitals or healthcare facilities. In addition, the resale of prescription drugs donated or supplied to charitable institutions is prohibited. The PDMA originally addressed prescription drug wholesaling and the provision of a drug "pedigree" or statement of prior sales of a drug, but these requirements have been superseded by the Drug Supply Chain Security Act of 2013. *See section 15.b. below.*

  b. Summary of PDMA

    (1) Bans reimportation of prescription drugs produced in the U.S.

Note: The Medicine Equity and Drug Safety (MEDS) Act of 2000 and the Medicare Prescription Drug Improvement and Modernization Act of 2003 both have provisions that modified this part of the PDMA and would allow importation of drugs under specific conditions. However, one of those conditions is that the Secretary of HHS must certify to Congress that such imports do not threaten the health and safety of the American public and provide cost savings. To date, HHS has not provided such certification. Several states have passed laws to allow drug importation from Canada, but they must also receive HHS approval before those programs can go into effect.

    (2) Bans the sale, trade, or purchase of prescription drug samples.

    (3) Mandates storage, handling, and recordkeeping requirements for prescription drug samples.

    (4) Prohibits with certain exceptions the resale of prescription drugs purchased by hospitals or healthcare facilities.

    (5) Establishes criminal and civil penalties for violations of the Act.

  c. PDMA and Texas Laws/Rules on Prescription Drug Samples

    (1) Authority of Advanced Practice Registered Nurses (APRNs) and Physician Assistants (PAs) concerning prescription drug samples.

The PDMA allows manufacturers to provide prescription samples upon the written (i.e., signed) request of a practitioner. In Texas, an APRN or PA may also sign the request for samples, receive samples from the manufacturer, and distribute samples to patients.

    (2) Texas State Board of Pharmacy Rule 291.16 is in compliance with the PDMA. This rule prohibits a pharmacy from selling, purchasing, trading, or possessing prescription drug samples unless the pharmacy meets all of the following conditions:

      (a) The pharmacy is owned by a charitable organization described in the Internal Revenue Code of 1986 or by a city, state, or county government;

      (b) The pharmacy is a part of a healthcare entity which provides health care primarily to indigent or low-income patients at no or reduced cost;

      (c) The samples are for dispensing or provision at no charge to patients of such a healthcare entity; and

(d) The samples are possessed in compliance with the federal Prescription Drug Marketing Act of 1987.

If a pharmacy does not meet all of the exemptions and is in possession of prescription drug samples, the drugs must be properly disposed of immediately. Since sale or offer to sell, purchase, or trade of prescription drug samples is prohibited, the drugs must be properly destroyed in compliance with Board rules. Pharmacies may possess and dispense prescription drugs which have been provided by the manufacturer as starter prescriptions or as replacement for outdated drugs. In addition, a pharmacy may possess and dispense prescription drugs which have been provided by a manufacturer in replacement for such manufacturer's drugs that were dispensed pursuant to written starter prescriptions from practitioners. The PDMA does not apply to OTC drugs; therefore, a pharmacy may be in possession of sample OTC drugs.

10. 1992—Prescription Drug User Fee Act (PDUFA)

PDUFA authorized FDA to assess fees on manufacturers seeking approval of drugs or biologicals. Sponsors of each drug or biological application must pay application fees, establishment fees for each facility, and product fees for each product. Since its passage, PDUFA has become a major supplemental source of funding for FDA. Many of the later amendments to the Food, Drug, and Cosmetic Act have been passed to continue these fees by reauthorizing PDUFA.

11. 1997—FDA Modernization Act (FDAMA)
    a. Reauthorized user fees.
    b. Replaced prescription legend "Caution: Federal law prohibits dispensing without a prescription" with "Rx only."
    c. Eliminated requirement that certain substances be labeled "Warning—May be habit forming."
    d. Clarified conditions under which a pharmacist may compound prescription drugs. This part of the law was subsequently invalidated in a Supreme Court case and has since been replaced by the provisions in the Compounding Quality Act in 2013.

12. 2007—Food and Drug Administration Amendments Act (FDAAA)
    a. Reauthorized user fees for drug and medical device approvals.
    b. Reauthorized the law that increases information about new and existing drug safety and efficacy in pediatrics and extends requirements to medical devices.
    c. Established the Reagan-Udall Foundation, an independent 501(c)(3) organization to advance the mission of the FDA to modernize product development, accelerate innovation, and enhance product safety.
    d. Established new conflict of interest policies for FDA Advisory Committees.
    e. Expanded the clinical trials registry beyond studies for serious and life-threatening diseases to include all trials beyond Phase I. *See www.clinicaltrials.gov.*
    f. Enhanced FDA's authority for post-marketing safety of drugs.
    g. Established Risk Evaluation and Management Strategies (REMs) for certain drugs and biologics.
    h. Requires a "toll-free" number to be distributed with new and refilled prescription drugs for reporting adverse drug effects. This required labeling is referred to as the "side effects statement." The statement is not required for OTC products if their product packaging already contains a toll-free number for reporting complaints to the manufacturer or distributor. For prescription drugs, the statement must include *"Call your doctor for medical advice about side effects. You may report side effects to*

the FDA at 1-800-FDA-1088." Pharmacists and other authorized dispensers may distribute this statement in one of five ways:
   (1) On a sticker attached to the unit package, vial, or container of the drug product.
   (2) On a preprinted pharmacy prescription vial cap.
   (3) On a separate sheet of paper.
   (4) In a consumer medication information sheet.
   (5) In the appropriate FDA-approved Medication Guide.
13. 2009—Biologics Price Competition and Innovation Act
    a. Creates an abbreviated approval pathway for biological products that are shown to be "biosimilar" and thus "interchangeable" with an FDA licensed biological product. This pathway is similar to the ANDA process for generic drugs.
    b. Biosimilarity means that the biological product is highly similar to the U.S.-licensed reference biological product notwithstanding minor differences in clinically inactive components. Also, it means there are no clinically meaningful differences between the biologic product and the reference product in terms of the safety, purity, and potency of the product.
    c. Interchangeability means that the biologic product is biosimilar to the U.S.-licensed reference biological product and can be expected to produce the same clinical result as the reference product in any given patient. For a biological product that is administered more than once to an individual, the risk of safety or diminished efficacy of alternating or switching between use of the biological product and the reference product will not be greater than the risk of using the reference product without such alternation or switch. Interchangeable biological products may be substituted at the pharmacy level without the intervention of a healthcare provider.
    d. FDA's *Lists of Licensed Biological Products with Reference Product Exclusivity and Biosimilarity or Interchangeability Evaluations* or The Purple Book allows users to see whether a particular biological product has been determined by the FDA to be biosimilar to or interchangeable with a reference biological product and can be viewed on the FDA's website.
14. 2012—FDA Safety and Innovation Act (FDASIA)
    a. Reauthorized user fees for drug and medical devices and added user fees for generic drugs and biosimilar biological products.
    b. Allowed FDA to designate a new drug as a "breakthrough therapy" to expedite the development and review of the drug.
    c. Gave FDA new authority to address the globalization of the pharmaceutical supply chain including funds to increase the number of inspections of foreign facilities and to strengthen partnerships with foreign regulators.
    d. Required FDA to develop a unique device identification (UDI) system for medical devices.
15. 2013—The Drug Quality and Security Act (DQSA)
    These amendments to the FDCA addressed two primary topics: large scale compounding by pharmacies and the establishment of a framework for a uniform track and trace system for prescription drugs throughout the supply chain.
    a. Title 1—Compounding Quality Act
       (1) Passed in response to an outbreak of fungal meningitis in over 20 states in the fall of 2012 that was traced to a contaminated injectable steroid produced by the New England Compounding Center.

Notes

This outbreak resulted in the death of over 60 patients and over 750 cases of infection.

(2) Under Section 503A of the FDCA, compounding pharmacies that meet certain requirements are exempt from FDA requirements for premarket approval, adequate directions for use labeling, and for complying with current good manufacturing regulations. Among those requirements is one requiring that the drug is compounded in a pharmacy based on receipt of a valid patient-specific prescription. The Compounding Quality Act maintains these exemptions for these "503A pharmacies" but establishes a new Section 503B to the FDCA that allows facilities that are compounding sterile pharmaceuticals without a patient-specific prescription to register with the FDA as an "Outsourcing Facility."

(3) Outsourcing facilities that meet the Act's requirements are exempt from the premarket approval requirements for new drugs (FDCA Section 505), adequate directions for use requirements (FDCA Section 502(f)(1)), and drug track and trace provisions (FDCA Section 582).

Note: Outsourcing facilities are not exempt from good manufacturing practices.

(4) Outsourcing facilities do not have to be licensed pharmacies unless they are also compounding or dispensing patient-specific prescriptions. However, they must:

(a) Have a licensed pharmacist who provides direct oversight over the drugs compounded;

(b) Compound only drugs from bulk ingredients that appear on a list developed by the Secretary of HHS. This list is being developed through notices published in the Federal Register following a 60-day comment period and must take into consideration clinical need;

Note: FDA issued an Interim Policy on Compounding Using Bulk Drug Substances under Section 503B of the Federal Food, Drug, and Cosmetic Act that explains the process FDA is using to develop this list. See the compounding section of FDA's website for more information.

(c) Register as an outsourcing facility. The FDA website provides a list of the names of each outsourcing facility along with the state where the facility is located, whether the facility compounds from bulk drug substances, and whether drugs compounded from bulk are sterile or nonsterile;

(d) Report to the Secretary of HHS upon registering, and every six months thereafter, the drugs sold in the previous six months;

(e) Be inspected by FDA according to a risk-based inspection schedule and pay annual fees to support it;

(f) Report serious adverse event experiences within 15 days and conduct a follow-up investigation and reporting similar to current drug manufacturers; and

(g) Label products with a statement identifying them as a compounded drug and other specified information about the drug.

(5) The Act also deleted the advertising and promotion restrictions in the compounding provisions of the FDCA that were found to be unconstitutional.

(6) FDA is developing regulations and issuing guidance documents with more specific requirements. For updates on FDA's implementation

of the Compounding Quality Act including guidance documents, see the compounding section of FDA's website.

Note: For more information on outsourcing facilities and the distinction between compounding and manufacturing, see Chapter H in this book.

b. Title 2—Drug Supply Chain Security Act (Track and Trace)
  (1) Provides a uniform national framework for an electronic track and trace system for prescription drugs as they move through the supply chain and sets national standards for states to license drug wholesaler distributors.
  (2) The Drug Supply Chain Security Act preempts all state laws and regulations for tracing drugs through the supply chain including recordkeeping and pedigree requirements. It also preempts state laws and regulations and requirements regarding wholesale distributor licensure that are inconsistent with, less stringent than, directly related to, or covered by the standards established by the Act.
  (3) Traceability
    (a) Applies to prescription drugs for human use in finished dosage form.
    (b) Certain products are exempted including blood and blood components, radioactive drugs, imaging drugs, certain intravenous products for fluid replacement, dialysis solutions, medical gases, legally compounded drugs, medical convenience kits containing drugs, certain combination products, sterile water, and products for irrigation.
    (c) Involves transfers of product where a change of ownership occurs but excludes intracompany distribution, distribution among hospitals under common control, public health emergencies, product sample distribution, minimal quantities by a licensed pharmacy to a licensed practitioner, certain activities by charitable organizations, and distributions pursuant to a merger or sale.
    (d) All trading partners in the supply chain must be authorized. This means that manufacturers must have a valid FDA registration, wholesale distributors must have a valid state or federal license and comply with all reporting requirements, and pharmacies must have a valid state license.
    (e) Manufacturers are required to provide "Transaction Data" for each product sold, and pharmacies are required to receive transaction data and pass this information along if they further distribute the product.
    (f) Transaction Data includes Transaction Information, Transaction History, and a Transaction Statement.
      (i) Transaction Information includes the product's name, strength, and dosage form; NDC number; container size and number of containers; date of transaction; and name and address of the person from whom ownership is being transferred and to which ownership is being transferred.
      (ii) Transaction History is a paper or electronic statement that includes prior transaction information for each prior transaction back to the manufacturer.
      (iii) Transaction Statement is a paper or electronic statement by the seller that the seller is authorized (licensed), received the product from an authorized (licensed) person, received the

Transaction Information and Transaction History from the prior owner if required, did not knowingly ship a suspect or illegitimate product, has systems and processes to comply with verification requirements, and did not knowingly provide false transaction information.

(g) Dispensers (including pharmacies) are required to:
  (i) Receive lot-level Transaction Histories, Transaction Information, and Transaction Statements on every prescription product they purchase;
  (ii) Be able to retrieve, analyze, and provide Transaction Histories, Transaction Information, and Transaction Statements within two business days during suspect product investigations and recalls;
  (iii) Quarantine and investigate any product identified as suspect and notify FDA and supply chain partners (*see (h) below*); and
  (iv) Retain product compliance documentation for six years.

(h) Pharmacies must investigate and properly handle suspect and illegitimate products.
  (i) Suspect products are products that one has reason to believe are potentially counterfeit, diverted, stolen, subject of a fraudulent transaction, intentionally adulterated, or appear otherwise unfit for distribution such that would result in serious adverse health consequences or death to humans. Pharmacists should look for things such as altered product information, missing information on the label, bubbling on the label, no "Rx only" symbol, missing or wrong package inserts, damaged or broken seals, open packages, lot numbers or expiration dates that do not match the outer/inner container, and foreign language.
  (ii) Illegitimate products are products for which credible evidence shows that the product is counterfeit, diverted, stolen, subject of a fraudulent transaction, intentionally adulterated, or appears otherwise unfit for distribution such that it would result in serious adverse health consequences or death to humans.
  (iii) If a product is illegitimate, pharmacies should notify FDA using Form FDA 3911 and notify trading partners within 24 hours about a suspect illegitimate product. Pharmacies should also work with the manufacturer to take steps to prevent the illegitimate product from reaching patients.

(i) Pharmacies that are "distributing" (distributing is defined as providing a drug to anyone other than the consumer/patient) as compared to "dispensing" (dispensing is defined as providing advice to the patient/consumer) are required to have a wholesale distribution license and will have to pass DSCSA transaction data with that distribution. The only exceptions to having a distribution license and passing transaction data are as follows:
  (i) When the distribution is between two entities that are affiliated or under common ownership;
  (ii) When a dispenser is providing product to another dispenser on a patient-specific basis;
  (iii) When a dispenser is distributing under emergency medical reasons; or

(iv) When a dispenser is distributing "minimal quantities" to a licensed practitioner for office use.
(j) Manufacturers are required to serialize product by attaching a "Product Identifier" to each individual package and homogenous case. A product identifier is a standardized graphic that carries the product's standardized numerical identifier, lot number, and expiration date in both human and machine-readable format. This means each individual package has a unique serial number. FDA requires a 2D barcode as the product identifier.
(k) Wholesale distributors may only accept products that contain a product identifier and must verify products before redistributing returned products.
(l) Starting in 2020, pharmacies may only accept products that contain a product identifier.
(m) Starting in 2023, supply chain members will be required to electronically track and trace products at the individual package level using the product identifier.

(4) Wholesale licensing standards
   (a) Updates the standards for licensing of wholesale drug distributors originally found in the PDMA including facility requirements, recordkeeping, furnishing of a bond or other security, background checks of facility managers or designated representatives, personnel qualifications, and facility inspections.
   (b) The FDA will issue regulations further detailing these standards.

II. Definitions (FDCA)

A. **Biological Products**—Biological products include a wide range of products such as vaccines, blood and blood components, allergenics, somatic cells, gene therapy, tissues, and recombinant therapeutic proteins. Biologics can be composed of sugars, proteins, nucleic acids, or complex combinations of these substances or may be living entities such as cells and tissues. Biologics are isolated from a variety of natural sources such as human, animal, or microorganism and may be produced by biotechnology methods and other cutting-edge technologies. Gene-based and cellular biologics, for example, often are at the forefront of biomedical research and may be used to treat a variety of medical conditions for which no other treatments are available. Although biological products are approved for marketing under the Public Health Service Act, most biologics also meet the definition of a "drug" and are subject to regulation by FDA's Center for Biologics Evaluation and Research (CBER).

B. **Drug** [Section 201(g)]
   1. Articles recognized in an official compendium—U.S. Pharmacopeia/National Formulary (USP/NF).
   2. Articles intended for use in the diagnosis, cure, mitigation, treatment, or prevention of disease in human or animal.
   3. Articles (other than food) intended to affect the structure or any function of the body of human or animal (i.e., if the substance alters the biological or chemical function of the body).
   4. Articles intended for use as a component of the above.

C. **Cosmetic** [Section 201(i)]—Articles intended to be rubbed, poured, etc., into or on the body for the purpose of cleansing, beautifying, or altering the appearance of the body.

D. **Medical device** [Section 201(h)]—An instrument, apparatus, etc., intended for use in the diagnosis, cure, mitigation, treatment, or prevention of disease in human or animal. Also intended to affect the structure or any function of the body of human or animal which does not achieve its intended purpose through chemical or biological action within or on the body.

 E. **Types of Drugs Covered Under the FDCA**
  1. Prescription—Human and Animals
   a. A drug which is habit-forming, toxic, or potentially harmful or the New Drug Application (NDA) limits its use to physician supervision.
   b. Previously, it was required that the label for human drugs contain the federal legend, "Caution: Federal law prohibits dispensing without a prescription." FDAMA changed the labeling requirement so that the label must now provide at minimum the symbol "Rx only." Since the previous legend does not include the "Rx only" symbol, it would not satisfy the new requirement.
   c. Veterinary products are required to be labeled, "Caution: Federal law restricts this drug to use by or on the order of a licensed veterinarian."
   d. Certain products in the same drug class may be either prescription or nonprescription depending on the product. For example, most insulin products are nonprescription; however, certain newer insulin products such as Lantus® and Humalog® are prescription only products.
  2. Over-the-Counter (OTC)
   a. Defined as drugs recognized among experts to be safe and effective for self-use (self-administration).
   b. Must be labeled with directions for the layperson that indicate their safe and effective use.
   c. An OTC drug may be approved for marketing by:
    (1) Filing a New Drug Application (NDA) or Abbreviated New Drug Application (ANDA) or
    (2) Marketing the product in compliance with the requirements of an OTC monograph which sets forth the requirements for the active ingredients, labeling, and other general requirements.
  3. Controlled Substances
   a. Are drugs which have a high abuse potential with psychological or physical dependency liability.
   b. Have additional controls which are regulated under the Federal Controlled Substances Act and administered by the DEA and individual states. (*See Chapter B.*)
 F. **Label**—Display of written, printed, or graphic matter on the immediate container.
 G. **Labeling**—All labels and other written, printed, or graphic matter (1) upon the article or container or (2) accompanying such article (package insert). Labeling also includes the label on the product and any advertising as well as representations made by a detail person (manufacturer's representative).

III. Prohibited Acts (Section 301)—Violations of the FDCA
 A. The adulteration or misbranding of any drug in interstate commerce.
 B. The introduction into interstate commerce of any drug that is adulterated or misbranded.
 C. The receipt in interstate commerce of any drug that is adulterated or misbranded and the delivery of it.
 D. The alteration, mutilation, removal, etc., of the labeling of a drug or the doing of any other act while the drug is held for sale which results in the drug being adulterated or misbranded.
 E. Failure to keep adequate records.
 F. Refusal to permit entry to FDA inspectors to inspect and verify records.

IV. Adulterated Drugs (Section 501)
A drug is adulterated if:
A. It contains any filthy, putrid, or decomposed substance.
B. It has been prepared, packed, or held under unsanitary conditions where it may have been contaminated.
C. The methods of manufacture do not conform with Current Good Manufacturing Practices (CGMPs).
D. The container is composed of any poisonous or deleterious substance which may contaminate the drug.
E. It contains an unsafe color additive.
F. It purports to be a drug in an official compendium, and its strength differs from or its quality or purity falls below the compendium standards, unless the difference is plainly stated on the label.
G. It is not in a compendium, and its strength differs from or its quality falls below that which it represents.
H. It is mixed or packed with any substance which reduces its strength or quality or the drug has been substituted wholly or in part.

V. Misbranded Drugs (Section 502)
A drug is misbranded if:
A. The labeling is false or misleading in any particular way.
B. It is a prescription drug, and the manufacturer's labeling fails to contain the following information:
   1. The name and address of the manufacturer, packer, or distributor.
   2. An accurate statement of the quantity (e.g., Number: 100 tablets).
   3. The generic name of the drug, if any, and the proprietary name.
   4. A statement of the quantity of the ingredients (e.g., 0.25 mg per tablet).
   5. Adequate information for use (intended for healthcare professionals).
   6. Adequate warnings against use where dangerous.
   7. Expiration date.
   8. Any other information required (e.g., certain products, including opioids and benzodiazepines, require "black boxed warnings" to alert healthcare professionals about essential information regarding the product).

   Note: Prescription drugs that are correctly dispensed to a patient pursuant to a valid prescription from a practitioner are generally exempt from the manufacturer's labeling requirements.
C. A pharmacist fills a prescription without authorization of the practitioner.
D. It is an over-the-counter drug and fails to contain all required information. (*See OTC labeling below.*)
E. It is a drug liable to deterioration unless it is packaged and labeled accordingly.
F. The container is made, formed, or filled as to be misleading.
G. The drug is an exact imitation of another drug or offered for sale under the name of another drug.
H. It is dangerous to health when used in the dosage or manner suggested in the labeling.
I. Its packaging or labeling is in violation of the Poison Prevention Packaging Act (PPPA).

VI. Over-the-Counter (OTC) Drug Regulations
A. The FDA OTC Review
   1. The OTC drug review was established to evaluate the safety and effectiveness of OTC drug products marketed in the United States before May 11, 1972. It is a three-phase public rulemaking process (each phase requiring

a Federal Register publication) resulting in the establishment of standards (monographs) for an OTC therapeutic drug category.
2. Phase 1—The first phase was accomplished by advisory review panels. The panels were charged with reviewing the ingredients in nonprescription drug products to determine whether these ingredients could be generally recognized as safe and effective for use in self-treatment. The panels were also charged with reviewing claims and recommending appropriate labeling, including therapeutic indications, dosage instructions, warnings about side effects of the drugs, and preventing misuse. According to the terms of the review, the panels classified ingredients in three categories as follows:
   a. Category I: generally recognized as safe and effective for the claimed therapeutic indication;
   b. Category II: not generally recognized as safe and effective or unacceptable indications;
   c. Category III: insufficient data available to permit final classification.
3. Phase 2—The second phase of the OTC drug review was the agency's review of ingredients in each class of drugs based on the panel's findings, on public comment, and on new data that may have become available. The agency then publishes its conclusions in the Federal Register in the form of a tentative final monograph. After publication of the tentative final monograph, a period of time is allotted for objections to the agency's proposal or for requests to be submitted for a hearing before the Commissioner of the FDA.
4. Phase 3—The publication of final regulations in the form of drug monographs is the third and last phase of the review process. The monographs establish conditions under which certain OTC drug products are generally recognized as safe and effective.

B. OTC Drug Approval
1. OTC Monographs—FDA develops and publishes OTC drug monographs for over 80 therapeutic classes. OTC monographs are published in the Federal Register and can be found in Section 300 of Chapter 21 of the Code of Federal Regulations. An OTC drug monograph contains the acceptable active ingredients and labeling requirements for a particular therapeutic class (e.g., analgesics). Once a final monograph is implemented, companies can make and market an OTC product without the need for FDA pre-approval. Manufacturers may petition FDA to change a final monograph to include additional ingredients or to modify labeling. Products that do not conform to a monograph must go through the new drug approval process.
2. New Drug Application—An OTC drug that does not conform to an FDA OTC Monograph must go through pre-approval by FDA including filing of a New Drug Application (NDA) or Abbreviated New Drug Application (ANDA). This process is the same used for prescription drugs.

C. OTC Drug Labeling
1. For OTC drugs, the label and labeling are directed at the consumer. OTC labeling helps assure that the drug will be safe for self-administration, so the labeling must contain adequate directions for use, dosage, and precautionary statements. This labeling is different from prescription drug labeling (including the package label and package insert) which is directed at the health professional. Prescription drug labeling must contain adequate information for use by the health professional.
2. OTC drug labels must contain the following:
   a. A principal display panel including a statement of identity of the product.
   b. The name and address of the manufacturer, packer, or distributor.
   c. Net quantity of contents.

d. Cautions and warnings needed to protect user.
e. Adequate directions for safe and effective use (for layperson).
f. Content and format of OTC product labeling in "Drug Facts" panel format (*see 21 CFR 201.66 for details and example*).
    (1) Active ingredients
    (2) Purpose
    (3) Use(s)—indications
    (4) Warnings
    (5) Directions
    (6) Other information
    (7) Inactive ingredients
    (8) Questions? followed by telephone number
3. OTC drugs marketed without an approved application (primarily OTC monograph drugs) must include a domestic address or domestic phone number through which the manufacturer, packer, or distributor identified on the label can receive reports of serious adverse events associated with the use of the product.
4. Content Labeling
    a. FDA requires content labeling for OTC drugs containing levels of calcium, magnesium, sodium, or potassium that might be harmful to persons with certain underlying medical conditions. Under the rules, oral OTC drugs must state the exact amount of a particular ingredient in each dose if they contain:
        (1) 5 mg or more of sodium in a single dose (21 CFR 201.64(a))
        (2) 20 mg or more of calcium in a single dose (21 CFR 201.70(a))
        (3) 8 mg or more of magnesium in a single dose (21 CFR 201.71(a))
        (4) 5 mg or more of potassium in a single dose (21 CFR 201.72(a))
    b. The rules also require warnings to alert customers on restricted diets to consult with their physician before using oral products that contain maximum daily doses of:
        (1) More than 140 mg of sodium (21 CFR 201.64(c))
        (2) More than 3.2 grams of calcium (21 CFR 201.70(c))
        (3) More than 600 mg of magnesium (21 CFR 201.71(c))
        (4) More than 975 mg of potassium (21 CFR 201.72(c))

D. Special Warning Requirements for OTC Products in FDCA
1. FD&C Yellow No. 5 (tartrazine) and No. 6 (21 CFR 201.20)—Must disclose presence and provide warning in "precautions" section of the label that may cause allergic reaction in certain susceptible persons.
2. Aspartame (21 CFR 201.21)—Must contain warning in "precautions" section of the labeling to the following effect: Phenylketonurics: Contains phenylalanine __ mg per __ (dosage unit).
3. Sulfites (21 CFR 201.22)—Prescription drugs containing sulfites (often used as preservative) must contain an allergy warning in the "warnings" section of the labeling.
4. Mineral Oil (21 CFR 201.302)—Requires warning to only be taken at bedtime and not be used in infants unless under advice of a physician. Label also cannot encourage use during pregnancy.
5. Wintergreen Oil (methyl salicylate) (21 CFR 201.303 and 201.314(g)(1)) Any drug containing more than 5% methyl salicylate (often used as flavoring agent) must include warning that use other than directed may be dangerous and that the article should be kept out of reach of children.
6. Isoproterenol Inhalation Preparations (21 CFR 201.305)—Requires a warning not to exceed dose prescribed and to contact physician if difficulty in breathing persists.

7. Potassium Salt Preparations for Oral Ingestions (21 CFR 201.306)—Requires a warning regarding nonspecific small-bowel lesions consisting of stenosis, with or without ulceration, associated with the administration of enteric-coated thiazides with potassium salts. Warning must state that coated potassium-containing formulations should be administered only when indicated and should be discontinued immediately if abdominal pain, distention, nausea, vomiting, or gastrointestinal bleeding occurs. In addition, coated potassium tablets should be used only when adequate dietary supplementation is not practicable. (Although the warning statement includes references to enteric-coated potassium salt preparations, it applies to any capsule or coated tablet of a potassium salt intended for oral ingestion without prior dilution with an adequate volume of liquid to preclude gastrointestinal injury.)
8. Sodium Phosphates (21 CFR 201.307)—Limits the amount of sodium phosphates oral solution to not more than 90 ml per OTC container. Also requires specific warnings.
9. Ipecac Syrup (21 CFR 201.308)
    a. The following statement (boxed and in red letters) must appear: "For emergency use to cause vomiting in poisoning. Before using, call physician, the poison prevention center, or hospital emergency room immediately for advice."
    b. The following warning must appear: "Warning: Keep out of reach of children. Do not use in unconscious persons."
    c. The dosage of the medication must appear. The usual dosage is 1 tablespoon (15 ml) in individuals over one year of age.
    d. It may only be sold in 1 oz. (30 ml) containers.
    e. Note difference between the fluid extract and the syrup. Fluid extract is 14 times as potent as the syrup.
10. Phenacetin (acetophenetidin) (21 CFR 201.309)—Must contain warning about possible kidney damage when taken in large amounts or for a long period of time.
11. Salicylates (21 CFR 201.314)—Aspirin and other salicylate drugs must have special warnings for use in children including a warning regarding Reye's syndrome. Retail containers of 1¼ grain (pediatric) aspirin tablets cannot be distributed in retail containers containing more than 36 tablets.
12. OTC Drugs for Minor Sore Throat (21 CFR 201.315)—Lozenges or troches containing a local anesthetic, chewing gum containing aspirin, various mouthwashes and gargles, and other articles sold over the counter for the relief of minor irritations of the mouth or throat may be labeled, "For the temporary relief of minor sore throats," provided this wording is immediately followed in the labeling with a warning statement in prominent type stating essentially: "Warning—Severe or persistent sore throat or sore throat accompanied by high fever, headache, nausea, and vomiting may be serious. Consult physician promptly. Do not use more than 2 days or administer to children under 3 years of age unless directed by physician."
13. Alcohol Warning (21 CFR 201.322)—Internal analgesics and antipyretics including acetaminophen, aspirin, ibuprofen, naproxen, ketoprofen, etc., are required to have a warning for persons consuming three or more alcoholic beverages per day and to consult with a doctor before taking.
14. OTC Pain Relievers (21 CFR 301.326)
    a. Acetaminophen
        (1) The ingredient acetaminophen must be prominently identified on the product's principal display panel of the immediate container and the outer carton (if applicable). This wording is intended to help

consumers identify the active ingredient and reduce the number of consumers inadvertently exposed to multiple products containing acetaminophen.
- (2) The product label must contain warnings that highlight the potential for liver toxicity and warn consumers against using more than the recommended dose of acetaminophen, using more than one product (over-the-counter or prescription) containing acetaminophen, and taking acetaminophen with moderate amounts of alcohol.
- (3) The product label must contain a warning not to use acetaminophen with any other drug containing acetaminophen and to ask a doctor or pharmacist if persons are not sure whether a drug contains acetaminophen, a warning to ask a doctor before use if persons have liver disease, and a warning to ask a doctor or pharmacist before use if persons are taking the blood thinning drug warfarin.

b. Nonsteroidal Anti-Inflammatory Drugs (NSAIDs)
- (1) The term "NSAID" must be prominently identified on the product's principal display panel of the immediate container and the outer carton (if applicable). This wording is intended to help consumers identify that the active ingredient of the product is a NSAID ingredient.
- (2) The product label must contain a "Stomach bleeding warning" which highlights the potential for stomach bleeding in persons over age 60, in persons who have had prior ulcers or bleeding, in persons who take a blood thinner, when taking more than one product containing a NSAID, when taken with moderate amounts of alcohol, and when taking for a longer time than directed.
- (3) The product label must contain warnings to ask a doctor before use if persons are at increased risk for stomach bleeding problems and to stop use and ask a doctor if specific signs of stomach bleeding occur.

E. Packaging and Repackaging of OTC Drugs
1. Tamper-Evident Packaging
   a. Manufacturers and packagers of OTC drugs (except dermatological, dentifrice, insulin, or lozenge products) for retail sale must package products in a tamper-evident package, if this product is accessible to the public while held for sale. A tamper-evident package is a package having one or more indicators or barriers to entry which, if breached or missing, can reasonably be expected to provide visible evidence to consumers that tampering has occurred. To reduce the likelihood of successful tampering and to increase the likelihood that consumers will discover if a product has been tampered with, the package is required to be distinctive by design or by the use of one or more indicators or barriers to entry that employ an identifying characteristic (e.g., a pattern, name, registered trademark, logo, or picture).
   b. In addition to the tamper-evident packaging requirement, any two-piece, hard gelatin capsule must be sealed using an acceptable tamper-evident technology.
   c. To alert consumers to the specific tamper-evident feature(s) used, each retail package of an OTC drug product is required to bear a statement that identifies all tamper-evident feature(s) and any capsule sealing technologies. This information must be prominently placed on the package.
2. Repackaging of OTC Products
The repackaging and resale of any OTC drug product, including repackaging by a pharmacist, is subject to the same CGMP and labeling requirements of a manufacturer.

F. Filling and Refilling OTC Drugs Pursuant to a Prescription
   1. Prescribers will sometimes write prescriptions for OTC drugs for patients for a variety of reasons including reimbursement purposes such as flexible spending account qualification.
   2. FDA OTC labeling requirements are not necessary for OTC drugs filled pursuant to a prescription since the prescription label satisfies the FDA labeling requirements.
   3. If an OTC drug is filled as a prescription (i.e., in a prescription bottle with a label), it is deemed a prescription drug, and it must be labeled with the prescriber's directions for use. The prescription must also be valid and in date. Once the prescription has expired, the pharmacist cannot refill it, but nothing precludes a pharmacist from selling the same OTC product in its original packaging to the patient.
   4. If an OTC prescription calls for a dosage different than the recommended dose on the OTC labeling, it must be filled as a prescription, and refill instructions of the prescriber must be followed.

VII. Drug and Device Recall Classifications and FDA Enforcement
A. Recall Classifications
   1. Class I exists where there is a reasonable possibility that the use of or exposure to a violative product will cause serious adverse effects on health or death.
   2. Class II exists where the use of or exposure to a violative product may cause temporary or medically reversible adverse effects on health or where the probability of serious adverse effects on health is remote.
   3. Class III exists where the use of or exposure to a violative product is not likely to cause adverse health consequences.
B. FDA Enforcement (Regulatory Action)
   There are three basic forms of regulatory action FDA can impose.
   1. Injunction or restraining order from a court—A civil procedure.
   2. Seizure or embargo—A civil procedure.
   3. Regulatory letter—Administrative action by FDA.
      FDA cannot technically order a recall for most drugs, but manufacturers or distributors generally will conduct a drug recall at the request of the FDA or upon their own initiative. FDA does have the authority to order a recall of controlled substance drugs, devices, biological products, tobacco products, and foods (including dietary supplements). If FDA determines there is a reasonable probability that a controlled substance drug, device, biological product, tobacco product, or food intended for human use would cause serious, adverse health consequences or death (i.e., a Class I recall), FDA may issue an order requiring the appropriate person (including the manufacturers, importers, distributors, or retailers of the device):
      a. To immediately cease distribution of such product.
      b. To immediately notify health professionals and product user facilities of the order and to instruct such professionals and facilities to cease use of such product.
   4. In addition to regulatory action, FDA can pursue criminal action in federal court for certain violations of the Act.

VIII. Advertising and Promotion of Prescription Drugs
A. Prescription drug advertising is regulated by FDA.
B. Over-the-counter (OTC) advertising is regulated by the Federal Trade Commission (FTC).
C. Advertising by Pharmacists—The advertising of prescription drug prices is considered reminder advertising under FDA regulations (21 CFR 200.200). However,

such advertising is exempt from FDA advertising regulations provided that the following conditions are met:
1. The only purpose of the advertising is to provide information on price, not information on the drug's safety, efficacy, or indications for use.
2. The advertising contains the proprietary name of the drug (if any), the generic name of the drug, the drug's strength, the dosage form, and the price charged for a specific quantity of the drug.
3. The advertising may include other information such as the availability of professional or other types of services as long as it is not misleading.
4. The price stated in the advertising shall include all charges to the consumer; mailing fees and delivery fees, if any, may be stated separately.

IX. Consumer Medication Information
A. Patient Package Inserts (PPIs). The FDA requires that pharmacists provide PPIs with:
1. Oral contraceptives (21 CFR 310.501)
2. Estrogen containing products (21 CFR 310.515)
B. How Patient Package Insert Requirements Affect the Pharmacist
1. It is required that the manufacturer of the affected drug provide the pharmacist with a sufficient number of PPIs to provide one to each patient to whom the drug is dispensed. Sample forms of PPIs are provided by the FDA, and the manufacturer is obligated to provide a PPI in Spanish upon the request of the distributor or dispenser.
2. The pharmacist is required to provide the PPI to the patient upon dispensing of the drug that is subject to the PPI requirements. This requirement applies to both new and refill prescriptions. Special rules apply to the hospitalized or institutionalized patient. The PPI may be provided as detailed above, or it may be provided before the administration of the first dose and once every 30 days thereafter. Outpatient prescriptions dispensed by hospitals are subject to the same requirements as those dispensed by the community pharmacist. PPIs do not need to be provided to patients undergoing emergency treatment. Failure to provide a PPI would cause the drug to be misbranded.
C. Medication Guides (MedGuides) (*See 21 CFR 208.*)
1. FDA requires Medication Guides be provided to patients when certain products are dispensed. FDA requires Medication Guides for products that the agency has determined pose a serious and significant public health concern and that one or more of the following circumstances exist:
    a. Patient labeling could help prevent serious adverse effects.
    b. The product has serious risks relevant to its benefits of which the patient should be aware of because such information could affect the patient's decisions to use or continue to use the product.
    c. Patient adherence to directions is crucial to the drug's effectiveness.
2. Medication Guides are required as part of the labeling for certain drugs, drug classes, and biologicals and are often an important component of Risk Evaluation and Mitigation Strategies (REMs). (*See Section X below.*)
3. Medication Guides must be written in a standard format and in language suitable for patients. Manufacturers must obtain FDA approval before distributing Medication Guides and are responsible for ensuring that a sufficient number of Medication Guides are provided to pharmacies.
4. FDA maintains a searchable Medication Guide database on its website, and there are over 1000 products that require a Medication Guide.
5. Medication Guides are required to be provided when these products are dispensed for outpatient use and are required for both new and refilled prescriptions. Many manufacturers include the Medication Guide at the bottom

of the package insert for the drug, but most pharmacy computer systems also print the Medication Guides for the products that need them at the time of dispensing.
6. Although not generally required for inpatients, when drugs and biologicals requiring a Medication Guide are provided to a healthcare professional where they will be administered in an outpatient setting (such as a clinic, infusion center, emergency department, or outpatient surgery center), FDA requires a Medication Guide be provided the first time the drug is administered. *See FDA Guidance—Medication Guides issued November 2011.*
7. Some of the drugs, drug classes, and biologicals requiring Medication Guides include:
    a. Accutane® (isotretinion)
    b. Antidepressants in children and teenagers
    c. Coumadin® (warfarin sodium)
    d. Epogen® (epoetin alfa)
    e. Forteo® (teriparatide, rDNA origin)
    f. Lindane® shampoo and lotion
    g. Lotronex® (alosetron hydrochloride) Coumadin®
    h. Nolvadex® (tamoxifen)
    i. Non-Steroidal Anti-Inflammatory Drugs (NSAIDs)
    j. Remicade® (infliximab)
    k. Trizivir® (abacavir sulfate, lamivudine, and zidovudine)
    l. Opioid analgesics and cough products
    m. Benzodiazepines
D. PPI and Medication Guides vs. Patient Information Sheets
The PPI and Medication Guide requirements are federal requirements for specific drugs or drug classes and should not be confused with the written patient information sheets required as part of the patient counseling requirements of federal OBRA-90 and TSBP rules.

X. **Risk Evaluation and Mitigation Strategies (REMS)**
A. A Risk Evaluation and Mitigation Strategy (REMS) is a strategy to manage a known or potential serious risk associated with a drug, drug class, or biological product. FDA requires REMS if FDA finds that it is necessary to ensure that the benefits of the drug, drug class, or biological product outweigh the risks of the product. A REMS can include a Medication Guide, a Patient Package Insert, a communication plan, elements to assure safe use, and an implementation system. It must also include a timetable for assessment of the REMS.
B. Elements to assure safe use may include:
    1. Special training, experience, or certification of healthcare practitioners prescribing the drugs;
    2. Special certification for pharmacies, practitioners, or healthcare settings that dispense the drug;
    3. Dispensing drugs to patients only in certain healthcare settings such as hospitals;
    4. Dispensing drugs to patients with evidence or other documentation of safe use conditions such as laboratory test results;
    5. Monitoring patients using the drug; or
    6. Enrolling each patient using the drug in a registry.
C. REMS may include other elements to minimize risk such as a Medication Guide, a Patient Package Insert (PPI), or an education/communication plan for healthcare providers or patients.
D. A complete list of products with approved REMS can be found on the FDA's website and may include an entire drug class that includes many products such as the Opioid Analgesic REMS. A summary of some REMS is provided below.

1. Accutane (Isotretinoin) iPLEDGE Program
   a. The FDA's iPLEDGE program is aimed at preventing use of isotretinoin during pregnancy.
   b. Only wholesalers registered in iPLEDGE can obtain isotretinoin from manufacturers. Only pharmacies registered in iPLEDGE can receive isotretinoin from registered wholesalers. Unregistered wholesalers and pharmacies must return unused isotretinoin.
   c. Program Requirements
      (1) Only doctors registered in iPLEDGE can prescribe isotretinoin. Doctors registered with iPLEDGE must agree to assume the responsibility for pregnancy counseling of female patients of childbearing potential. Prescribers must obtain and enter into the iPLEDGE system negative test results for those female patients of childbearing potential prior to prescribing isotretinoin.
      (2) Only patients registered in iPLEDGE can be prescribed isotretinoin. In addition to registering with iPLEDGE, patients must comply with a number of key requirements that include completing an informed consent form, obtaining counseling about the risks and requirements for safe use of the drug, and, for women of childbearing potential, complying with required pregnancy testing and use of contraception.
      (3) Only pharmacies registered in iPLEDGE can dispense isotretinoin. To register in iPLEDGE, a pharmacy must select a Responsible Site Pharmacist who must obtain iPLEDGE program information and registration materials via the Internet (*www.ipledgeprogram.com*) or telephone (1-866-495-0654) and sign and return the completed registration form. To activate registration, the Responsible Site Pharmacist must access the iPLEDGE program via the internet (*www.ipledgeprogram.com*) or telephone (1-866-495-0654) and attest to the following points:
         (a) I know the risk and severity of fetal injury/birth defects from isotretinoin.
         (b) I will train all pharmacists on the iPLEDGE program requirements.
         (c) I will comply and seek to ensure that all pharmacists comply with iPLEDGE program requirements.
         (d) I will obtain isotretinoin from iPLEDGE registered wholesalers.
         (e) I will return to the manufacturer (or delegate) any unused product.
         (f) I will not fill isotretinoin for any party other than a qualified patient.
      (4) To dispense isotretinoin, pharmacists must obtain authorization from iPLEDGE via the Internet (*www.ipledgeprogram.com*) or telephone (1-866-495-0654) signifying the patient is registered, has received counseling and education, and is not pregnant.
      (5) Prescriptions must be picked up within seven days of a pregnancy test (not necessarily the date the prescription was written). With the exception of the initial prescription, if a prescription is not filled within seven days of a pregnancy test, the patient is allowed to get another test and then fill the prescription. If a prescription is not picked up within the seven-day window, it must be "reversed" by accessing the iPLEDGE system via phone.
      (6) A maximum 30-day supply may be dispensed.
      (7) Blister packages may not be broken.
      (8) No refills are allowed.

Notes

2. Clozaril®
   a. Clozaril® (clozapine) is used to treat schizophrenia but requires monitoring for potentially fatal adverse reaction of agranulocytosis.
   b. Previously, each manufacturer of clozapine had its own REMs and patient registry. Now all programs have been consolidated into a single REMS called the Clozapine REMS Program.
   c. Practitioners and pharmacies must be certified in the program. Details can be found at *http://www.clozapinerems.com*.
3. Lotronex®
   a. After being withdrawn from the market, Lotronex® (alosetron hydrochloride) was reintroduced on the market in 2002 under restricted conditions of use.
   b. Lotronex® is indicated only for women with severe diarrhea-predominant irritable bowel syndrome (IBS) who have failed to respond to conventional therapy and whose IBS symptoms are chronic (generally lasting six months or longer).
   c. Prescribing Program for Lotronex® is part of a Risk Management Program and requires a Prescribing Program Sticker to be affixed to all prescriptions for Lotronex® (original and subsequent prescriptions).
   d. Telephone, facsimile, or electronic prescriptions for Lotronex® are not valid.
   e. Prescriptions must be dispensed in the original Retail Pack which includes a Medication Guide, package insert, and follow-up survey enrollment form for patients.
4. Opioid Analgesic REMS
   a. The goal of the Opioid Analgesic REMS is to educate prescribers and other healthcare providers (including pharmacists and nurses) on the treatment and monitoring of patients with pain.
   b. Requires manufacturers of opioid drugs to provide education for healthcare providers who participate in the treatment and monitoring of pain including pharmacists.
   c. Requires manufacturers of opioid products to provide information for healthcare providers to use when counseling patients about the risks of opioid analgesic use and a Medication Guide for patients.
   d. More information can be found at *https://opioidanalgesicrems.com*.

XI. New Drugs
   A. Definitions
      1. A drug is a "new drug" if:
         a. It contains a new chemical substance for medical use.
         b. It is an established drug offered in a new dosage form.
         c. It is an established drug offered with new medical claims.
         d. It is an established drug offered at new dosage levels.
         e. It is an established drug packed in a new or novel packaging material.
      2. A drug is an "approved drug" if:
         a. A New Drug Application (NDA) has been approved by the FDA.
         b. A drug that was in use prior to the effective date of the 1938 FDCA is not subject to the NDA requirements (drug efficacy) if the drug is distributed and promoted in accordance with labeling and established use as it then existed.
            (1) The number of drugs in the pre-1938 era is very small (e.g., aspirin and digitalis).
            (2) Due to labeling and use requirements being as they existed in the pre-1938 era, these drugs are vulnerable to misbranding.

3. Approved Use of Drugs
   The approved use of a drug is the prescribing or administering of a drug within the limits of the required dosage and route of administration, therapeutic indications, precautions, warnings, and contraindications (i.e., to prescribe or administer a drug within the limits of the package insert information).
B. Approved Drugs for Unapproved Uses ("unlabeled use" or "off label use")
   1. From time to time, a physician may prescribe an approved drug for an unapproved or "unlabeled" use (i.e., prescribes the drug outside of the limits of the package insert information).
   2. Pharmacist's Liability
      Presuming the prescription is labeled correctly and the pharmacist uses good professional judgment, the exposure to liability should be minimal. The physician has the primary liability. However, if something goes wrong, the pharmacist could have secondary liability.
   3. General negligence laws should be followed.
   4. Keep in mind "corresponding responsibility" relative to controlled substance prescriptions.
   5. Manufacturers generally cannot promote an approved drug for an unapproved use through literature, advertisements, salespersons, seminars, etc.
      a. There are some exceptions to this law as the 1997 FDA Modernization Act does allow manufacturers to distribute literature containing unlabeled use information under certain conditions.
      b. Recent FDA Guidance allows manufacturers to provide certain types of information to payors, formulary committees, and similar entities regarding unapproved products and unapproved uses of their approved products.
      c. The FDA's authority to restrict off-label promotion has been challenged in the courts, and some court decisions have found that manufacturers' truthful and non-misleading communications about drugs, including off label uses, are permissible and constitutionally protected as commercial free speech. A full discussion of the legal issues in this area is beyond the scope of this book.
C. FDA Classification System for New Drugs
   1. Therapeutic Classification
      a. Type P—(Priority review drug) A drug that appears to represent an advance over available therapy.
      b. Type S—(Standard review drug) A drug that appears to have therapeutic qualities similar to those of an already marketed drug.
      c. Type O—(Orphan drug) The drug treats a rare disease affecting fewer than 200,000 Americans.
   2. Chemical Classification
      a. Type 1—New molecular entity.
      b. Type 2—New active ingredient (new salt, new noncovalent derivative, and new ester).
      c. Type 3—New dosage form.
      d. Type 4—New combination.
      e. Type 5—New formulation or new manufacturer.
      f. Type 6—New indication (no longer used).
      g. Type 7—Drug already marketed without an approved NDA.
      h. Type 8—OTC (over-the-counter) switch.
      i. Type 9—New indication submitted as distinct NDA, consolidated with original NDA after approval.
      j. Type 10—New indication submitted as distinct NDA and not consolidated.

XII. National Drug Code (NDC) Number

A. An NDC number is an FDA standard for uniquely identifying drugs.

B. The NDC for each listed drug in the United States is a unique 10-digit, 3-segment number. The 3 segments of an NDC include the labeler code, product code, and package code. The first segment, the labeler code, is a unique 4- or 5-digit number assigned by FDA that identifies the manufacturer, repacker, relabeler, or private label distributor of the drug. The second segment, the product code, identifies a specific strength, dosage form, and formulation of a drug manufactured, repackaged, relabeled, or distributed by the labeler. The third segment, the package code, identifies package sizes and types. The NDC for a given drug is currently in one of the following configurations (with each number representing the number of digits in that segment): 4-4-2, 5-3-2, or 5-4-1.

Example of 4-4-2 configuration:
Valium® 2mg Roche 100-count bottle
NDC: 0140 0004 01
Roche Valium® 2mg 100-count bottle

C. Assignment of the NDC number does not necessarily mean the product has an approved NDA. It also is not a determination that a product is a drug nor does it denote that a product is covered by or eligible for reimbursement by Medicare, Medicaid, or other payers.

D. The NDC is not required to be on the manufacturer's label. However, because it is used to facilitate automated processing of drug data by government agencies, drug manufacturers and wholesalers, third party administrators, etc., most manufacturers include it on a drug's label.

E. The FDA maintains a list of NDC numbers for prescription drugs and insulin products called the National Drug Code Directory that can be searched and accessed on the FDA's website.

F. The FDA has proposed to standardize the NDC format configurations and move to an 11-digit number, but these proposals have not been finalized.

XIII. Current Good Manufacturing Practices (CGMPs)

A. FDA's CGMP regulations apply to a pharmacy only if it is engaged in manufacturing, repackaging, and/or relabeling drugs beyond the usual conduct of dispensing and selling at retail.

B. Situations in pharmacy practice that may require the pharmacy to register with FDA and comply with FDA regulations, inspections, and CGMPs are these:
1. A pharmacy in hospital "A" repackages drug products for its own use as well as that for hospitals "B" and "C."
   Note: Texas law allows a hospital pharmacy to repackage drug products for distribution to other hospital pharmacies under common ownership as part of the practice of pharmacy.
2. A pharmacy chain repackages and relabels quantities of drug products from the manufacturer's original commercial containers for shipment to the individual stores.
3. Similar repackaging and relabeling conducted by individual pharmacies as members of an informal buying group (co-op).
4. If the pharmacy actually manufactures a drug product.

C. A pharmacy that repackages drugs for sale or distribution to other pharmacies or facilities not under common ownership must also be registered by the Texas Department of State Health Services (Drug and Medical Device Division) as a distributor.

XIV. Information on Medication Use During Pregnancy and Breastfeeding

A. Previously, FDA used product letter categories (A, B, C, D, and X) to classify the risk of using prescription drugs during pregnancy.

B. That system was replaced with the following that are part of the manufacturer's required labeling:
1. Pregnancy—Provides information relevant to the use of the drug in pregnant women, such as dosing and potential risks to the developing fetus, and will require information about whether there is a registry that collects and maintains data on how pregnant women are affected when they take the drug.
2. Lactation—Provides information about using the drug while breastfeeding such as the amount of the drug in breast milk and potential effects on the breastfeeding child.
3. Females and Males of Reproductive Potential—Includes information about pregnancy testing, contraception, and fertility as it relates to the drug.

XV. **FDA Orange Book**
A. The official name of this publication is *Approved Drug Products with Therapeutic Equivalence Evaluations.*
B. It serves as the primary source for determining generic equivalency of drugs.
C. It uses a two-letter coding system to indicate equivalency with the first letter being the key:
1. A = Drug products that the FDA considers to be pharmaceutically equivalent (having the same active ingredient) and therapeutically equivalent (providing the same therapeutic effect, identical in duration and intensity).
2. B = Drug products that the FDA considers NOT to be pharmaceutically equivalent and therapeutically equivalent.
D. Products with no known or suspected bioequivalence issues:
1. AA—conventional dosage forms
2. AN—solutions and powders for aerosolization
3. AO—injectable oil solutions
4. AP—injectable aqueous solutions
5. AT—topical products
E. Products with actual or potential bioequivalence problems where adequate scientific evidence has established bioequivalence are given a rating of AB.
F. The Orange Book can be searched electronically on the FDA's website.

XVI. **FDA Purple Book**
A. The official name of this publication is *Lists of Licensed Biological Products with Reference Product Exclusivity and Biosimilarity or Interchangeability Evaluations.*
B. It serves as the primary source for determining which products are considered biosimilar to a referenced biological product, as well as whether FDA considers a biosimilar product to be interchangeable with a reference product.
C. A biosimilar product is a biological product that is approved based on a showing that it is highly similar to an FDA-approved biological product, known as a reference product, and has no clinically meaningful differences in terms of safety and effectiveness from the reference product. Only minor differences in clinically inactive components are allowable in biosimilar products.
D. An interchangeable biological product is biosimilar to an FDA-approved reference product and meets additional standards for interchangeability. An interchangeable biological product may be substituted for the reference product by a pharmacist without the intervention of the healthcare provider who prescribed the reference product.
Note: Not all biosimilar products are considered interchangeable.

XVII. **Dietary Supplements and Medical Foods**
A. The Food, Drug, and Cosmetic Act defines a "dietary supplement" as:
1. A product (other than tobacco) intended to supplement the diet that bears or contains one or more of the following dietary ingredients: a vitamin; a

mineral; an herb or other botanical; an amino acid; a dietary substance for use by human to supplement the diet by increasing the total dietary intake; or a concentrate, metabolite, constituent, extract, or combination of any ingredient above;
2. A product intended for ingestion in tablet, capsule, powder, softgel, gelcap, or liquid form; or if not intended for ingestion in such a form, is not represented as a conventional food and is not represented for use as a sole item of a meal or of the diet; and
3. A product labeled as a dietary supplement.

B. The Dietary Supplement and Health Education Act of 1994 (DSHEA)
1. The Act makes dietary supplement manufacturers responsible for determining that the dietary supplements they manufacture or distribute are safe and that any representations or claims made about them are substantiated by adequate evidence to show that they are not false or misleading.
2. Dietary supplements do not need approval from FDA before they are marketed. Except in the case of a new dietary ingredient where premarket review for safety data and other information is required by law, companies do not have to provide FDA with the evidence they rely on to substantiate safety or effectiveness before or after they market the products.
3. A manufacturer or distributor must notify FDA if it intends to market a dietary supplement in the U.S. that contains a "new dietary ingredient." The manufacturer (and distributor) must demonstrate to FDA why the ingredient is reasonably expected to be safe for use in a dietary supplement, unless it has been recognized as a food substance and is present in the food supply.
4. The Act places the burden on the FDA to prove that a dietary supplement is unsafe before it can be removed from the market.
5. Dietary supplements cannot make claims that they treat, prevent, or cure a specific disease or condition. This claim would make them an unapproved drug. However, under DSHEA, manufacturers may make three types of claims for their dietary supplement products: health claims, structure/function claims, and nutrient content claims. Some of these claims describe the link between a food substance and a disease or a health-related condition, the intended benefits of using the product, or the amount of a nutrient or dietary substance in a product. Different requirements generally apply to each type of claim.
    a. Structure/function claims may include that the product affects the normal structure or function of the body and claims for common, minor symptoms often associated with life stages, but not claims to prevent, treat, cure, mitigate or diagnose a disease. *See FDA Final Rule 21 CFR 101.93(f) and (g).*
    b. Products making such claims must include the following disclaimer: "This statement has not been evaluated by the Food and Drug Administration. This product is not intended to diagnose, treat, cure, or prevent any disease." Manufacturers must also notify FDA within 30 days of marketing a product with such statements.

C. Current Good Manufacturing Practices (CGMPs) for Dietary Supplements
1. Dietary supplement manufacturers must abide by Current Good Manufacturing Practices (CGMPs) to ensure that dietary supplements are manufactured consistently as to the identity of the dietary ingredients, purity, quality, strength, and composition of the product.
2. The requirements include provisions related to:
    a. The design and construction of physical plants that facilitate maintenance.
    b. Cleaning,

c. Proper manufacturing operations.
d. Quality control procedures.
e. Testing final product or incoming and in-process materials.
f. Handling consumer complaints.
g. Maintaining records.
D. The Dietary Supplement and Nonprescription Drug Consumer Protection Act of 2006
1. This Act requires dietary supplement manufacturers, packers, or distributors to report serious adverse effects to the FDA.
2. A "serious adverse event" is an adverse event that:
a. Results in death, a life-threatening experience, inpatient hospitalization, a persistent or significant disability or incapacity, or a congenital anomaly or birth defect or
b. Requires based on reasonable medical judgment a medical or surgical intervention to prevent an outcome described above.
3. A "serious adverse event report" is a report that must be submitted to FDA on MedWatch Form 3500A when a manufacturer, packer, or distributor of a dietary supplement receives any report of a serious adverse event associated with the use of the dietary supplement in the United States.
4. The manufacturer, packer, or distributor whose name (pursuant to Section 403(e)(1) of the FD&C Act) appears on the label of a dietary supplement marketed in the United States is required to submit to FDA all serious adverse event reports associated with use of the dietary supplement in the United States.
5. Serious adverse event reports received through the address or phone number on the label of a dietary supplement, as well as all follow-up reports of new medical information received by the responsible person within one year after the initial report, must be submitted to FDA no later than 15 business days after the report is received by the responsible person.
E. Medical Foods
1. The Food, Drug, and Cosmetic Act defines a medical food as "a food which is formulated to be consumed or administered enterally under the supervision of a physician and which is intended for the specific dietary management of a disease or condition for which distinctive nutritional requirements, based on recognized scientific principles, are established by medical evaluation."
2. Medical foods are not drugs; therefore, they are not subject to any regulatory requirements that specifically apply to drugs.
3. Medical foods are not required to be dispensed on a prescription. The requirement for a written or oral prescription under the FDCA only applies to the dispensing of prescription drug products.
4. Although some medical foods are labeled "Rx only," FDA Guidance documents make clear that the use of the symbol "Rx only" in the labeling of a medical food is inappropriate and would cause the product to be misbranded. FDA permits medical food manufacturers to use language to communicate that physician supervision is required by using a phrase such as "must be used under the supervision of a physician."

XVIII. **Medical Devices**
A. Devices Regulated by FDA
1. A device is an instrument, apparatus, implement, machine, contrivance, implant, in vitro reagent, or other similar or related articles, including any component, part, or accessory, which is:
a. Recognized in the USP or NF;

b. Intended for use in the diagnosis of disease or other conditions or in the cure, mitigation, treatment, or prevention of disease in humans or animals; or
c. Intended to affect the structure or any function of the body of humans or animals and does not achieve its desired action by chemical means or by being metabolized by the body.

2. Classification of Devices
   a. Class I—Controls
   Class I devices are those intended for human use for which controls that are authorized under the Medical Device Act (MDA) are sufficient to provide reasonable assurance of their safety and efficacy. Class I devices are those devices which insufficient information exists to determine that controls under the Act are sufficient to provide reasonable assurance of their safety and efficacy. However, because the devices are not purported to support or sustain human life or to be used substantially in preventing impairment of human health and do not present a potential unreasonable risk of illness or injury, they are regulated by controls authorized by the MDA (i.e., FDA controls over adulteration, misbranding, and manufacturing procedures are sufficient to assure the safety and efficacy of a device with a low potential risk of causing illness or injury.). Some examples of Class I devices are needles, scissors, stethoscopes, toothbrushes, tongue depressors, ice bags, and eye pads.
   b. Class II—Controls and Performance Standards
   Class II devices are those intended for human use and those for which controls alone (such as Class I) are insufficient to provide reasonable assurance of safety and efficacy. There is sufficient information about Class II devices to establish performance standards that provide such assurance (i.e., controls alone will not assure safety and efficacy, but controls in addition to a performance standard will). Some examples of Class II devices are insulin syringes, thermometers, diagnostic reagents, tampons, blood pressure gauges, and electric heating pads.
   c. Class III—Controls, Performance Standards, and Premarket Approval
   Class III devices are those intended for human use that are purported to be supportive or sustaining of human life or of substantial importance in preventing impairment of human health. Class III devices present a potential unreasonable risk of illness or injury and are subject to premarket approval to provide reasonable assurance of safety and efficacy. Some examples of Class III devices are pacemakers, intraocular lenses, replacement heart valves, insulin pumps, and breast implants.
   d. Sale of Prescription Devices
   Certain devices may be sold only to or on the prescription or other order of a practitioner. The label of the device, other than surgical instruments, bears the statement "Caution: Federal law restricts this device to sale by or on the order of a _____." with the blank to be filled with the word "physician," "dentist," or "veterinarian." Although prescription drug products have been able to use the "Rx only" designation on labels, this symbol statement was technically not allowed on prescription medical devices. However, since 2000, FDA has informally allowed it by exercising enforcement discretion. In September 2016, FDA finalized a rule to formally allow medical device manufacturers to use the symbol statement "Rx only" on these products.
   e. Medical devices are subject to the Current Good Manufacturing Practice (CGMP) requirements set forth in the Quality System (QS) regulation (21 CFR 820). They require that domestic or foreign manufacturers

have a quality system for the design, manufacture, packaging, labeling, storage, installation, and servicing of finished medical devices intended for commercial distribution in the United States. The regulation requires that various specifications and controls be established for devices; that devices be designed under a quality system to meet these specifications; that devices be manufactured under a quality system; that finished devices meet these specifications; that devices be correctly installed, checked and serviced; that quality data be analyzed to identify and correct quality problems; and that complaints be processed.
- f. In September 2013, FDA finalized a rule requiring a Unique Device Identifier (UDI) on medical device labels and packaging unless a specific exemption is met. The UDI requirement is intended to reduce medical errors, simplify the integration of device use information into data systems, and provide for more rapid adverse event information for medical devices and more rapid and efficient recalls. The UDI requirements are being phased in over several years, starting September 24, 2013 through September 24, 2020, depending on the device classification. For more information, see the FDA's UDI webpage.

A complete explanation of the regulatory requirements for medical devices is beyond the scope of this book, but the following sections provide a summary of the major amendments to the FDCA relating to medical device regulation.

B. Medical Device Amendments of 1976 (amended the FDCA)
1. Intended to provide reasonable assurance of the safety and effectiveness of medical devices.
2. Created the three-class, risk-based classification system for all medical devices described above.
3. Established the regulatory pathways for new medical devices (devices that were not on the market prior to May 28, 1976, or had been significantly modified) to get to market by:
   a   Premarket Approval (PMA) and
   b. Premarket notification (510(k)).
4. Created the regulatory pathway for new investigational medical devices to be studied in patients (Investigational Device Exemption (IDE)).
5. Established several key postmarket requirements: registration of establishments and listing of devices with the FDA, Good Manufacturing Practices (GMPs), and reporting of adverse events involving medical devices.
6. Authorized the FDA to ban devices.

C. Safe Medical Device Act of 1990
1. Required a "device user facility" (hospital, ambulatory surgical center, nursing home, home healthcare agency, or outpatient diagnostic or treatment facility which is not a physician's office) to report to the FDA when the facility becomes aware that a device probably caused or contributed to:
   a. The death of a facility's patient or
   b. The serious illness or injury to a facility's patient.
2. Required a manufacturer of the following types of devices to adopt a method of device tracking which would ensure that patients who receive devices can be notified if necessary.
   a. A device the failure of which would likely cause serious adverse health consequences and which is:
      (1) A permanently implantable device or
      (2) A life sustaining or life supporting device used outside a "device facility user."
   b. Any other device designated by FDA.

3. Required a manufacturer to conduct postmarket surveillance of any device introduced into interstate commerce after January 1, 1991, that is:
   a. A permanent implant, the failure of which may cause serious, adverse health consequences or death;
   b. Intended for a use in supporting or sustaining human life; or
   c. Potentially presents a serious risk to human health.
4. Defined "substantial equivalence" as the standard for marketing a device through the 510(k) program.
5. Modified procedures for the establishment, amendment, or revocation of performance standards.
6. Created the Humanitarian Use Device (HUD)/Humanitarian Device Exemption (HDE) programs to encourage development of devices targeting rare diseases.

D. Medical Device Amendments of 1992
   1. These amendments required device distributors to maintain records and provide information to help the FDA or the manufacturer locate a patient in the event of a device recall or patient notification.
   2. The FDA defines a "final distributor" as any person who distributes a traced device intended for use by a single patient over the useful life of the device. The term includes but is not limited to licensed practitioners, retail pharmacies, hospitals, and other types of device user facilities. A "multiple distributor" is any device user facility (including hospitals, rental companies, or any other entity) that distributes a life-sustaining or life-supporting device intended for use by more than one patient over the useful life of the device.
   3. The three categories of devices requiring tracking are these:
      a. Life-supporting or life-sustaining devices that are used outside a device user facility if the failure of these devices would be likely to have serious adverse health consequences.
         Examples: Breathing frequency (apnea) monitors, DC-defibrillator, and paddles.
      b. Permanently implantable devices if the failure of these devices would be reasonably likely to have serious adverse health consequences.
         Examples: Replacement heart valves and implantable infusion pumps.
      c. Any other devices designated by the FDA as those which must be tracked.

E. Food and Drug Administration Modernization Act (FDAMA) of 1997
   1. Created the "least burdensome" provisions for premarket review.
   2. Created the option of accredited third parties to conduct initial premarket reviews for certain devices.
   3. Permitted the use of data from studies of earlier versions of a device in premarket submissions for new versions of the device.
   4. Provided for expanded access to investigational devices.
   5. Established the De Novo program through which novel low-to-moderate risk devices could be classified into Class I or II instead of automatically classifying them into Class III.

F. Medical Device User Fee and Modernization Act (MDUFMA) of 2002
   1. Granted FDA the authority to collect user fees for select medical device premarket submissions to help the FDA improve efficiency, quality, and predictability of medical device submission reviews.
   2. Enacted the Small Business Determination program to permit reduced premarket approval fees for qualifying small businesses.
   3. Created FDA performance goals for decisions on certain premarket submissions.
   4. Established new regulatory requirements for "reprocessed" devices.
   5. Authorized electronic registration of medical device firms.
   6. Established the Office of Combination Products.

G. Food and Drug Administration Amendments Act (FDAAA) of 2007
   1. Reauthorized the medical device user fee (MDUFA II) including improvements to premarket review times.
   2. Required that all registration and listing be performed electronically.
   3. Required FDA to establish a unique device identification (UDI) system for medical devices to require device labels to bear a unique identifier.
H. Food and Drug Administration Safety and Innovation Act (FDASIA) of 2012
   1. Reauthorized the medical device user fee program (MDUFA III) including improvements to premarket review times and added shared outcome goals with industry.
   2. Created direct De Novo pathway, permitting the classification of novel, low-to-moderate risk devices into Class I or II (rather than Class III) without first having to submit a 510(k).
   3. Changed the standards associated with disapproval of an Investigational Device Exemption.
   4. Permitted FDA to work with foreign governments to harmonize regulatory requirements.
   5. Required FDA to provide a Substantive Summary when requested by the holder of the submission for significant decisions.
   6. Expanded the application of the "least burdensome" principles in premarket reviews.
I. 21st Century Cures Act of 2016
   1. Mandated the creation or revision of policies and processes intended to speed patient access to new medical devices including:
      a. Codifying into law the FDA's expedited review program for breakthrough devices;
      b. Expanding the application of the "least burdensome" principles in premarket reviews;
      c. Streamlining processes for exempting devices from the premarket notification (510(k)) requirement;
      d. Increasing the population estimate required to qualify for Humanitarian Use Device (HUD) designation from "fewer than 4,000" to "not more than 8,000" patients in the U.S. per year;
      e. Permitting the use of Central Institutional Review Board (CIRB) oversight rather than requiring only local Institutional Review Boards (IRBs) for Investigational Device Exemption and Humanitarian Device Exemption activities;
      f. Requiring the FDA to revise the regulation of combination products; and
      g. Codifying into law a process for submitting requests for recognition/nonrecognition of a standard.
   2. Clarified how certain digital health products can be regulated by defining the categories of medical software that can and cannot be regulated as devices.
J. Food and Drug Administration Reauthorization Act (FDARA) of 2017
   1. Reauthorized the medical device user fee program (MDUFA IV), including improvements to premarket review times and investments in strategic initiatives like the National Evaluation System for health Technology (NEST) and patient input.
   2. Authorized risk-based inspection scheduling for device establishments and prescribed other process improvements related to device establishment inspections.
   3. Decoupled accessory classification from classification of the parent device.
   4. Required FDA to conduct at least one pilot project to explore how real-world evidence can improve post market surveillance.

Other Federal Laws and Regulations

I. **Federal Hazardous Substances Act of 1966**
   (Administered and enforced by the Consumer Product Safety Commission (CPSC))
   A. Intent and Purpose
      The intent of this Act was that all hazardous substances be regulated regardless of their packaging and wrapping. The purpose was to protect the consumer, especially children, from household and non-household substances.
      1. Hazardous items that could not be labeled safely for household use were banned from interstate commerce.
      2. The sale of toys and other children's articles containing hazardous substances was banned.
   B. Definitions
      1. **Hazardous substance**—A substance or a mixture of substances that can cause injury or illness through handling and that can cause potential danger, especially to children, if misused.
      2. **Toxic substance**—Any substance (other than radioactive substances) which has the capacity to produce personal injury or illness to a human through ingestion, inhalation, or absorption through any bodily surface.
      3. **Highly toxic**—One in which a single oral dose of 50 mg or less per kilogram body weight would kill half or more of the white rats to which it is fed.
   C. Labeling Requirements
      The label on the immediate package of a hazardous product and any outer wrapping or container that might cover up the label on the package must have the following information in English:
      1. The name and business address of the manufacturer, packer, distributor, or seller;
      2. The common or usual or chemical name of each hazardous ingredient;
      3. The signal word "Danger" for products that are corrosive, extremely flammable, or highly toxic;
      4. The signal word "Caution" or "Warning" for all other hazardous products;
      5. An affirmative statement of the principal hazard or hazards that the product presents (e.g., "Flammable," "Harmful if Swallowed," "Causes Burns," "Vapor Harmful," etc.);
      6. Precautionary statements telling users what they must do or what actions they must avoid to protect themselves;
      7. Where it is appropriate, instructions for first aid treatment to perform if the product injures someone;
      8. The word "Poison" for a product that is highly toxic, in addition to the signal word "Danger";
      9. Instructions for consumers to follow to protect themselves if a product requires special care in handling or storage; and
      10. The statement "Keep out of the reach of children." If a hazardous product such as a plant does not have a package, it still must have a hang tag that contains the required precautionary information. This information must also be printed in any literature that accompanies the product and contains instructions for use.
   D. The Act deals primarily with household items such as bleach, cleaning fluids, antifreeze, drainpipe cleaners, and muriatic acid.
   E. Sale of Items in Pharmacies
      The pharmacist should sell the products in the original manufacturer's container or label properly.

II. Federal Hazard Communication Standard
(Administered and enforced by the Occupational and Safety Health Administration (OSHA))
- A. OSHA requires all employers (including pharmacies) that deal with hazardous materials to meet the Hazard Communication Standard. *See 29 CFR 1910.1200.*
- B. The standard requires chemical manufacturers and importers to classify the hazards of chemicals they produce or import and to prepare appropriate labels and Safety Data Sheets (SDS), which were formerly known as Material Safety Data Sheets (MSDS).
- C. Pharmacies are required to have a written Hazard Communication Plan.
- D. The plan must include a list of hazardous chemicals in the workplace, must ensure all such products are appropriately labeled and have a Safety Data Sheet, and must include training for all workers on the hazards of chemicals, appropriate protective measures, and where and how to obtain additional information. *Note: Additional details can be found in OSHA's publication entitled Small Entity Compliance Guide for Employers that Use Hazardous Chemicals.*
- E. Drugs in solid, final dosage form for administration to patients are exempt from these requirements, but hazardous chemicals or products not in solid, final dosage form for administration (such as liquid products used in compounding) may be covered. Generally, a pharmacy may rely on the manufacturer to determine if a product is considered hazardous.

III. Poison Prevention Packaging Act of 1970 (PPPA)
(Administered and enforced by the Consumer Product Safety Commission (CPSC))
- A. Purpose
  The primary purpose of the Act was to extend to prescription and nonprescription drugs special packaging requirements known as "child-resistant containers." Other household substances are also included (those under the Federal Hazardous Substances Act).
- B. Requirements
  Packaging must meet a test by children. A package fails if more than 20% of the child test group can open the package AFTER DEMONSTRATION and/or if more than 10% of the ADULTS tested cannot open the package. Usually a time period of 10 minutes is used for the children and 5 minutes for adults. Regulations effective in 1998 require that packaging also meets new senior testing requirements to ensure that the packaging is not too difficult for senior citizens to open. Unit-dose packaging also must meet PPPA standards but is evaluated somewhat differently. A test failure is defined as the ability of one child to open more than eight individual units or the number of units representing a toxic amount, whichever is less.

  A child-resistant container (CRC) made of plastic or any component made of plastic CANNOT be reused according to the Act, since wear of the components may limit the package's ability to be child resistant. If a prescription container is reused (i.e., when refilling a prescription), the pharmacy has violated both PPPA and TSBP rules. Unless specifically exempted, ALL drugs (over-the-counter or prescription) produced by a manufacturer must be sold in child-resistant containers meeting the requirements if the containers will be sold or dispensed to the consumer.

  Note: These are child-resistant standards and are required and enforced by CPSC. The standards for tamper-evident packaging for OTC drugs are required and enforced by FDA. See the OTC Drug Regulation section in this chapter.

Notes

    C. Exemptions to Child-Resistant Container Requirement
       1. Patient/Physician Request
          a. A non-child resistant container can be used at the request of the physician or patient.
          b. A blanket request for all prescriptions may be obtained from the patient BUT NOT FROM THE DOCTOR. It is good practice to verify this with the patient yearly.
          c. The law doesn't require a written request, but all requests should be documented.
          d. The pharmacist may initiate the request for a non-CRC container, but it must be the patient's decision.
       2. Bulk containers shipped to manufacturers, wholesalers, and pharmacies (not intended for household use).
       3. Drugs distributed to institutionalized patients provided the drugs are administered to patients by institution (hospital) employees.
       4. One package size designed for elderly patients of an over-the-counter drug as long as it is labeled: THIS PACKAGE IS FOR HOUSEHOLDS WITHOUT YOUNG CHILDREN.
    D. Drugs Covered Under the Poison Prevention Packaging Act and Drug Exemptions from the Act
       1. Prescription drugs—Any drug for human use that is in a dosage form for oral administration and that is required by federal law to be dispensed only by or upon an oral or written prescription of a practitioner licensed by law to administer such drugs.
       Exemptions:
          a. Sublingual dosage forms of nitroglycerin.
          b. Sublingual and chewable forms of isosorbide dinitrate in dosage strengths of 10 mg or less.
          c. Erythromycin ethylsuccinate granules for oral suspension and oral suspensions in packages containing no more than 8 g or the equivalent of erythromycin.
          d. Erythromycin ethylsuccinate tablets in packages containing no more than the equivalent of 16 g erythromycin.
          e. Anhydrous cholestyramine in powder form.
          f. Potassium supplements in unit-dose forms, including individually wrapped effervescent tablets, unit-dose vials of liquid potassium, and powdered potassium in unit-dose packets containing no more than 50 mEq per unit dose.
          g. Sodium fluoride drug preparations, including liquid and tablet forms, containing no more than 264 mg of sodium fluoride per package.
          h. Betamethasone tablets packaged in manufacturers' dispenser packages containing no more than 12.6 mg betamethasone.
          i. Mebendazole in tablet form in packages containing no more than 600 mg of the drug.
          j. Methylprednisolone in tablet form in packages containing no more than 84 mg of the drug.
          k. Colestipol in powder form in packages containing no more than 5 g of the drug.
          l. Pancrelipase preparations in tablet, capsule, or powder form.
          m. Medically administered oral contraceptives in manufacturers' mnemonic (memory aid) dispenser packages which rely solely upon the activity of one or more progestogen or estrogen substances.
          n. Prednisone in tablet form when dispensed in packages containing no more than 105 mg of the drug.

o. Conjugated estrogen tablets when dispensed in mnemonic dispenser packages containing no more than 26.5 mg of the drug.
p. Norethindrone acetate tablets in mnemonic dispenser packages containing no more than 50 mg of the drug.
q. Medroxyprogesterone acetate tablets.
r. Sacrosidase (sucrose) preparations in a solution of glycerol and water.
s. Hormone replacement therapy products that rely solely upon the activity of one or more progestogen or estrogen substances.

2. Aspirin—Any aspirin-containing preparation for human use in dosage form intended for oral administration.
Exemptions: Aspirin-containing effervescent tablets, other than those intended for pediatric use, provided that the tablet contains less than 10% aspirin, the tablet has an oral median lethal dose greater than 5 g/kg of body weight, and the tablet when placed in water releases at least 85 ml of carbon dioxide per grain of aspirin. In addition, unflavored aspirin-containing preparations in powder form that are packaged in unit doses, providing that these are intended for uses other than pediatric. They must contain no other substance subject to special packaging requirements and not more than 13 grains of aspirin per unit dose.

3. Methyl salicylate (oil of wintergreen)—Liquid preparations containing more than 5% by weight of methyl salicylate unless packaged in pressurized spray containers.

4. Controlled drugs—Any preparation for human use in a dosage form intended for oral administration that consists in whole or in part of any substance subject to control under the Federal Controlled Substances Act.

5. Methyl alcohol (methanol)—Household substances in liquid form containing 4% or more by weight of methyl alcohol unless packaged in a pressurized spray container.

6. Iron-containing drugs—With the exception of animal feeds used as vehicles for the administration of drugs, noninjectable animal and human drugs providing iron for therapeutic or prophylactic purposes, which contain a total amount of elemental iron equivalent to 250 mg.

7. Dietary supplements containing iron—With the exception of those preparations in which iron is present solely as a colorant, dietary supplements that contain an equivalent of 250 mg or more of elemental iron in a single package.

8. Acetaminophen—Preparations for human use in a dosage form intended for oral administration and containing more than 1 g of acetaminophen in a single package.
Exemptions:
a. Acetaminophen-containing effervescent tablets or granules containing less than 10% acetaminophen with a median lethal dose greater than 5 g/kg of body weight and that release at least 85 ml of carbon dioxide per grain of acetaminophen when placed in water.
b. Unflavored acetaminophen-containing preparations in powder form, other than those intended for pediatric use, that are packaged in unit doses with no more than 13 grains of acetaminophen per unit dose and that contain no other substance subject to the special packaging requirements.

9. Diphenhydramine HCl—Preparations for human use in oral dosage forms containing more than the equivalent of 66 mg of diphenhydramine base in a single package.

10. Ibuprofen—Preparations for human use in oral dosage forms containing 1 gram or more of ibuprofen in a single package.

Copyright © 2020 Fred S. Brinkley, Jr., and Gary G. Cacciatore

11. Loperamide—Preparations for human use in oral dosage forms containing more than 0.045 mg of loperamide in a single package.
12. Lidocaine—Products containing more than 5 mg of lidocaine in a single package (includes all dosage forms including creams, sprays, and transdermal patches).
13. Dibucaine—Products containing more than 0.5 mg of dibucaine in a single package (includes all dosage forms including creams, sprays, and transdermal patches).
14. Naproxen—Preparations for human use in oral dosage forms containing 250 mg or more of naproxen in a single package.
15. Ketoprofen—Preparations for human use in oral dosage forms containing more than 50 mg of ketoprofen in a single package.
16. Fluoride—Products containing more than 50 mg of elemental fluoride and more than 0.5% fluoride in a single package.
17. Minoxidil—Preparations for human use containing more than 14 mg of minoxidil in a single package (includes topical products that must continue to meet requirements once applicator is installed by consumer).
18. Imidazolines—Products containing 0.08 mg or more in a single package. Imidazoline is a drug class that includes tetrahydrozoline, naphazoline, oxymetazoline, and xylometazoline often found in ophthalmic and nasal products.
19. Any drug switched from Rx to OTC status.

IV. Omnibus Budget Reconciliation Act of 1990 (OBRA-90)
   A. Intent and Purpose
   OBRA-90 provides for expansion of Medicare and Medicaid programs which are funded by the federal government. Most of the provisions relating to the practice of pharmacy are contained within the amendments to the Medicaid program which is administered by state governments.
   B. Impact on Pharmacy Practice
   OBRA-90 has a number of provisions that substantially impact the practicing pharmacist. Even though the requirements of OBRA-90 only apply to Medicaid patients, the majority of states (including Texas) have expanded these requirements to apply to all patients receiving pharmaceutical services. These services include mandatory prospective drug use review and patient counseling. Texas has specific and detailed rules governing these services. (*See Chapter G on Class A Rules, Prescription, Dispensing, and Delivery in this book.*)

V. Delivering Prescriptions by U.S. Mail or Common Carrier
   A. Delivery by Mail (postal regulations administered by the U.S. Postal Service)
   General postal regulations do not allow dangerous substances to be mailed; however, there are exceptions for prescription drugs.
   1. Noncontrolled—Prescriptions containing noncontrolled substances (dangerous drugs) may be mailed by the physician or pharmacist to the ultimate user provided that the medications are not alcoholic beverages, poisons, or flammable substances. However, highly toxic substances may be sent by a manufacturer to the pharmacist or physician.
   2. Controlled substances (narcotic/nonnarcotic in Schedule II–V) may be mailed under the following requirements.
      a. The prescription container must be labeled in compliance with prescription labeling rules.
      b. The outer wrapper or container in which the prescription is placed must be free of markings that would indicate the nature of the contents (i.e., including the name of the pharmacy as part of the return address on the

mailing package as that may alert individuals that drugs may be in the package).
     c. No markings of any kind may be placed on the package to indicate the nature of contents.
   3. Mailing controlled substances to other registrants
      Provided controlled substances are placed in a plain outer container or securely overwrapped in plain paper, a pharmacy may mail controlled substances to other registrants (practitioners, distributors, DEA registered drug disposal firms, or DEA).
  B. Delivery by Common Carrier
     Any prescription drug may be delivered from a pharmacy to a patient by common carrier such as United Parcel Service (UPS) or FedEx. This includes all schedules of controlled substances (narcotic and nonnarcotic) and dangerous drugs. Common carriers are not affected nor are they subject to postal regulations.

VI. Tamper-Resistant Prescription Requirements (Administered by Centers for Medicare and Medicaid Services—part of HHS)
  A. All written prescriptions for Medicaid recipients must be on paper with at least one tamper-resistant feature as outlined by CMS and defined by the states.
  B. These same prescriptions must be on paper that meets all three baseline characteristics of tamper-resistant pads. CMS has outlined the three baseline characteristics as those that:
   1. Prevent unauthorized copying of a completed or blank prescription form;
   2. Prevent the erasure or modification of information written on the prescription by the prescriber; and
   3. Prevent the use of counterfeit prescription forms.
  C. The tamper-resistant requirement does not apply to electronic prescriptions, prescriptions transmitted to the pharmacy by telephone or fax, and orders for drugs in institutional settings (including hospitals and nursing homes) where drug orders are written into a medical record and then the order is given by medical staff directly to the pharmacy. The requirement also does not apply when a managed care entity pays for the prescription.
  D. A pharmacy may fill prescriptions on an emergency basis so long as the pharmacy obtains a compliant prescription in writing or by telephone, fax, or electronic prescription within 72 hours.
  E. For more information see www.cms.hhs.gov/center/intergovernmental.asp.

VII. Federal Alcohol Regulations
(Administered by the Alcohol and Tobacco Tax and Trade Bureau (TTB) which is under the Department of Treasury)
Note: The 2003 Homeland Security Act split the functions of the Bureau of Alcohol, Tobacco, and Firearms (ATF), which had the tax and trade functions and the Tax-Free Alcohol requirements, and moved them to the TTB. The law enforcement functions now are under the Bureau of Alcohol, Tobacco, Firearms, and Explosives (ATFE). This bureau is under the U.S. Department of Justice.
  A. Tax-free Alcohol
   1. Ethyl alcohol or ethanol having a proof of 190 degrees or more when withdrawn from the bonded premises of a distilled spirits plant free of tax is known as tax-free alcohol.
   2. Tax-free alcohol may be procured and used for authorized purposes by:
     a. Federal, state, and local government agencies.
     b. Colleges and universities.
     c. Laboratories used for scientific research.

d. Hospitals, sanitariums, blood banks, or pathological laboratories engaged exclusively in making analyses or tests for hospitals or sanitariums.
e. Charitable, non-profit clinics.
3. Tax-free alcohol may be used for scientific, medicinal, and mechanical purposes and in the treatment of patients.
4. Tax-free alcohol may not be used for beverage purposes or in any food product.
5. Tax-free alcohol may not be sold.
6. Tax-free alcohol may not be given to doctors for use in their private practice by hospitals even if the doctor has an office in the hospital.
7. An Industrial Alcohol User Permit must be applied for and significant recordkeeping and storage requirements must be met.
8. If only small quantities will be used for compounding or for patient use (e.g., brandy at bedtime), it is often easier to purchase the alcohol from a licensed retail dealer.
9. A community pharmacy selling alcohol in the form of a beverage must obtain a retail dealer's stamp.

B. Denatured Alcohol
1. Specially denatured alcohol is ethyl alcohol with the addition of denaturants such as benzene and methyl alcohol and may be used in the production of external-use medicines and products not intended for human consumption.
2. Regulations and formulas concerning the use of denatured alcohol can be found at 27 CFR Part 20.

VIII. Health Insurance Portability and Accountability Act of 1996 (HIPAA)

The Health Insurance Portability and Accountability Act of 1996 (HIPAA) was a massive bill dealing with a broad range of topics. The "portability" section was aimed at making health insurance more "portable" by making it easier for people to continue their health insurance coverage when leaving a job. Title II of the Act contained the Administrative Simplification provisions which were intended to improve the efficiency and effectiveness of the healthcare system by standardizing the electronic data interchange of certain administrative and financial transactions while protecting the security and privacy of transmitted information. The Act and its subsequent regulations have had a tremendous impact on how patient information is handled by healthcare entities including pharmacies. The major provisions can be found in three sets of regulations—the HIPAA Transactions and Code Set Regulations, the HIPAA Privacy Regulations, and the HIPAA Security Regulations. The Health Information Technology for Economic and Clinical Health (HITECH) Act, enacted as part of the American Recovery and Reinvestment Act of 2009, made significant modifications to HIPAA including expanding the reach of HIPAA to business associates and imposing a nationwide security breach notification requirement for entities that possess electronic protected health information. A summary of the major provisions under HIPAA and the HITECH Act is provided below.

A. HIPAA Transactions and Code Set Regulations
1. Adopts standards for eight electronic transactions and code sets to be used for those transactions.
2. If a pharmacy conducts an electronic transaction with another covered entity or business associate, the transaction must be conducted as a standard transaction using the designated code sets.
3. Retail pharmacy drug claim standard is the National Council for Prescription Drug Programs (NCPDP) standard.

B. Covered Entities and HIPAA Privacy Regulations
1. Covered entities are defined in the HIPAA rules as health plans, healthcare clearinghouses, and healthcare providers who electronically transmit

any health information in connection with transactions for which HHS has adopted standards. Pharmacies are a "covered entity" under the Act and must be in compliance with the regulations.
2. Notice and Acknowledgment
   a. Pharmacies must provide patients with a "Notice of Privacy Practices" and make a good faith effort to obtain a written acknowledgment of receipt of the Notice from the patient.
   b. The Notice must be provided upon first service delivery to the patient.
   c. The Privacy Rule requires mandatory provisions in the Notice.
3. Use and Disclosure of Protected Health Information (PHI)
   a. Protected Health Information (PHI) is the HIPAA term for patient-identifiable information.
   b. Pharmacies may use and disclose PHI to provide treatment, for payment, and for healthcare operations without authorization from the patient.
   c. Pharmacies may also use and disclose PHI for certain governmental functions without authorization from the patient. This includes uses and disclosures for public health activities such as reporting adverse events to FDA, to health oversight agencies such as boards of pharmacies or state drug monitoring programs, and to law enforcement agencies.
   d. Other uses and disclosures such as for marketing purposes require a signed authorization from the patient. If the covered entity receives remuneration for the marketing, the authorization form must expressly inform the patient of such. Refill reminder programs and face-to-face communications regarding alternative drugs or health products are considered part of treatment and not marketing.
4. Business Associates (BAs)
   a. Persons or entities, other than members of a pharmacy's workforce, who perform a function or service on behalf of the pharmacy that requires the use or disclosure of PHI are called "business associates."
   b. Pharmacies are required to enter into business associate contracts with these BAs, which require the BAs to meet many of the same requirements for protecting PHI as a covered entity under HIPAA.
   c. Examples of BAs would include collection agencies, external auditors, outside attorneys handling a case that requires the use or disclosure of PHI, and software vendors who have access to computer systems containing PHI to provide updates or repairs. Pharmacy Benefit Managers (PBMs) are generally considered business associates of the health plans and not the pharmacy.
   d. The HIPAA Privacy Rule provides suggested language for a BA contract.
5. Patient Rights
   a. Access
      (1) Patients have a right to inspect and obtain a copy of their PHI.
      (2) Pharmacies must comply within 30 days of a request, but they may extend the time by no more than 30 additional days with notification to the individual of the reason for the delay.
      Note: TSBP Rule 291.28 requires pharmacies to reply to a request from a patient for a copy of his or her confidential information within 15 days. See Chapter E in this book.
      (3) Under certain limited circumstances, pharmacies may deny a patient's request to inspect or obtain a copy of his or her PHI.
   b. Amendment
      (1) Patients have a right to amend their PHI or records containing PHI that are maintained by a pharmacy.

Notes

(2) Pharmacies must comply within 60 days of receiving a request, but they may extend the time by no more than 30 additional days with notification to the individual of the reason for the delay.

(3) Under certain limited circumstances, pharmacies may deny a patient's request to amend his or her PHI, but they must provide in writing the basis for the denial and allow the patient to submit a statement that explains the patient's disagreement with the denial.

   c. Accounting

(1) Patients have a right to an accounting of disclosures of PHI made by the pharmacy in the six years prior to the date on which the accounting is requested.

(2) Detailed requirements for this accounting can be found at 164.528(b)(2) of the HIPAA Privacy Rules.

(3) Pharmacies do not have to provide an accounting of disclosures if the disclosure is for treatment, payment, or healthcare operations made pursuant to an authorization, an incidental disclosure for national security or intelligence purposes, to correctional facilities or law enforcement authorities, part of a limited data set, or if made prior to April 14, 2003. The HITECH Act eliminates the exemption for disclosures made for treatment, payment, or healthcare operations for covered entities that maintain electronic health records. However, the rule implementing this requirement has yet to be finalized. (*See HITECH Act below.*)

(4) Disclosures to health oversight agencies such as state-controlled substance agencies or boards of pharmacy are not considered part of healthcare operations and must be included in an accounting.

6. Minimum Necessary Standard

   a. When using and disclosing PHI, a pharmacy must make reasonable efforts to limit PHI to the minimum necessary to accomplish the intended purpose.

   b. The minimum necessary standard does not apply to disclosures to healthcare providers for treatment purposes. These disclosures would include prescription transfers or providing prescription information to physicians.

   c. The minimum necessary standard does not apply to disclosures for which the patient has signed an authorization.

   d. The minimum necessary standard does apply to disclosures for payment.

7. Administrative Requirements

   a. Pharmacies must establish policies and procedures to protect from accidental or intentional uses and disclosures of PHI through the use of appropriate administrative, technical, and physical safeguards to protect the privacy of PHI.

   b. Pharmacies must train all employees on privacy policies and impose sanctions on employees for any violations of privacy policies.

8. Incidental Disclosures

   a. Unintended "incidental" disclosures are not a violation of the Privacy Rule as long as reasonable safeguards are in place.

   b. Examples: Sales representatives or janitorial service members accidentally see PHI during the normal course of their jobs; a customer overhears counseling that is performed in a private area in a discreet manner.

9. Privacy Official and Contact Person

   a. Pharmacies must designate a Privacy Official who is responsible for development and implementation of HIPAA-related policies and procedures and compliance.

b. Pharmacies must also designate a contact person to receive complaints. This person may also be the Privacy Official.
  10. Enforcement and Penalties
   a. HIPAA is enforced by the U.S. Department of Health and Human Services (HHS) Office for Civil Rights (OCR).
   b. If the entity did not know (or by exercise of reasonable diligence would not have known), the penalty is at least $100 per violation, not to exceed $25,000 per calendar year for all violations of an identical requirement or prohibition.
   c. If a violation is due to reasonable cause and not to willful neglect, the penalty is at least $1,000 per violation, not to exceed $100,000 per calendar year for all violations of an identical requirement or prohibition.
   d. If a violation is due to willful neglect and the failure to comply is corrected within 30 days of when the entity knew or should have known that the failure to comply occurred, the entity is subject to a penalty of $10,000 per violation, not to exceed $250,000 per calendar year for all violations of an identical requirement or prohibition.
   e. If a violation is due to willful neglect and the violation is not corrected within 30 days, the entity is subject to a penalty of at least $50,000 per violation, not to exceed $1.5 million per calendar year for all violations of an identical requirement or prohibition.
  11. State Law Preemption—State privacy laws that are more stringent than the federal privacy laws must be adhered to.
 C. HIPAA Security Regulations
  1. Applies to information in electronic form only.
  2. Sets standards for administrative, physical, and technical safeguards to protect the confidentiality, integrity, and availability of electronic PHI.
  3. Requires pharmacies to implement basic safeguards to protect electronic PHI from unauthorized access, alteration, deletion, and transmission.
  4. Required or Addressable Standards
   a. Required standards are mandatory and must be met by all covered entities.
   b. Addressable does not mean optional. Addressable standards may be met in a variety of ways:
    (1) If the standard is determined to be reasonable and appropriate, it must be implemented.
    (2) If the standard is determined to be inappropriate and/or unreasonable but the standard can be met by implementing an alternative safeguard, the covered entity may implement an alternative measure.
    (3) If the standard is simply not applicable to a covered entity, a decision can be made not to implement the addressable specification as long as that decision and the rationale behind it is documented.
  5. Administrative Safeguards
   a. Security Management Process—Includes required standards relating to risk analysis, risk management, sanction policy, and information system activity review (internal audit).
   b. Assigned Security Responsibility—A required standard for covered entities to have an assigned individual to be responsible for compliance with the Security Rule.
   c. Workforce Security—Includes addressable standards for authorization and supervision of workforce, workforce clearance procedures, and termination procedures.
   d. Information Access Management—Includes required and addressable standards establishing policies for defining levels of access for personnel

authorized to access PHI and how that access is granted, modified, and terminated.
- e. Security Awareness/Training—Includes addressable standards for security training of workforce including periodic security reminders, virus protection, log-in monitoring, and password management.
- f. Security Incident Procedures—Includes required standards on addressing and reporting of security incidents.
- g. Contingency Plan—Includes required standards to have a data backup plan, a disaster recovery plan, and an emergency mode operation plan.
- h. Evaluation—Includes required standards to periodically conduct an evaluation of security safeguards and document compliance with policies and the HIPAA Security Rule.

6. Physical Safeguards
    - a. Facility Access Controls—Addressable standards to limit physical access to electronic information systems.
    - b. Workstation Use—Addressable standards to document policies and procedures on workstation use to maximize security.
    - c. Workstation Security—Required standard to put in place physical safeguards to restrict access to information on workstations.
    - d. Device and Media Controls—Required and addressable standards that govern the receipt and removal of hardware or electronic media containing PHI into and out of a facility and movement within the facility, including disposal, media reuse, accountability, and storage.

7. Technical Safeguards
    - a. Access Control—Required and addressable standards to only allow access to PHI to persons or programs granted access rights. Includes unique user IDs, emergency access procedures, automatic logoff, encryption, and decryption.
    - b. Audit Control—Required standard for the implementation of hardware, software, and/or procedural mechanisms to record and examine activity in information systems.
    - c. Integrity—Addressable standard requiring the implementation of policies and procedures to protect electronic PHI from improper alteration or destruction.
    - d. Person or Entity Authentication—Required standard to implement procedures to verify that a person or entity seeking access to an electronic PHI is the one claimed.
    - e. Transmission Security—Addressable standard regarding technical security measures to guard against unauthorized access to electronic PHI being transmitted over an electronic communications network.

8. Business Associate Contracts—Requires covered entities to modify business associate contracts to require business associates to implement administrative, physical, and technical safeguards to protect the confidentiality, integrity, and availability of electronic PHI.

D. HITECH Act Provisions
1. The HITECH Act makes the Administrative, Physical, and Technical Safeguards of the HIPAA Security Rule directly applicable to Business Associates.
2. Breach Notification
    - a. Covered entities, including pharmacies, must notify individuals of a breach of their "unsecured" PHI within 60 calendar days after the breach is discovered.
    - b. BAs are required to report any breaches of unsecured PHI to the covered entity and provide the identities of each affected individual.

- c. A "breach" is defined as unauthorized acquisition, access, use, or disclosure of PHI that compromises its security or privacy. It does not include instances in which there has been an inadvertent disclosure from an authorized individual to another person authorized to access PHI within the same organization. A breach also does not include instances in which the covered entity or BA has a good faith belief that the PHI is not further acquired, accessed, retained, used, or disclosed.
- d. For breaches affecting fewer than 500 individuals, covered entities must maintain a log of these breaches and notify HHS of these breaches annually.
- e. If more than 500 individuals are affected, the Secretary of HHS and prominent local media must be notified in addition to the affected individuals within 60 days after the breach is discovered.

3. Accounting of Disclosures

The HITECH Act eliminates the exception for an accounting of disclosures made for treatment, payment, or healthcare operations for entities that maintain electronic health records (EHRs). Covered entities maintaining EHRs must produce, upon an individual's request, an accounting of all disclosures of the individual's PHI, including disclosures made for treatment, payment, and healthcare operations over a three-year period.

Note: This requirement has been controversial. As of the date of this book's publication, the rule to implement this change has yet to be finalized, so this requirement is not in effect.

4. Penalties and Enforcement
   - a. The HITECH Act makes the civil and criminal penalties for violations of HIPAA or the HITECH Act applicable to business associates in addition to covered entities.
   - b. The penalties for violations of HIPAA or the HITECH Act now include a tiered penalty structure based on the organization's knowledge of the violation as outlined in B.10.
   - c. The HITECH Act also provides for enforcement by the Attorney General of each state to enjoin further violations or obtain damages on behalf of the residents of the state in an amount equal to $100 per violation for a maximum of $25,000 per year.

E. Texas Privacy Laws (Texas HIPAA)

Note: Although this is not a federal law, it is included here for readers since the Texas privacy laws are more stringent in many regards than the federal HIPAA laws.

1. Texas laws significantly expand the definition of a covered entity to any person/entity who:
   - a. For commercial, financial, or professional gain, monetary fees, or dues, or on a cooperative, nonprofit, or pro bono basis, engages in whole or in part and with real or constructive knowledge in the practice of assembling, collecting, analyzing, using, evaluating, storing, or transmitting protected health information;
   - b. Comes into possession of protected health information;
   - c. Obtains or stores protected health information; or
   - d. Is an employee, agent, or contractor of a person described by 1.a.–c. above insofar as the employee, agent, or contractor creates, receives, obtains, maintains, uses, or transmits protected health information.

2. Restrictions on Use and Disclosure of PHI
   - a. Texas law prohibits the sale of PHI, except for treatment, payment, healthcare operations, performing an insurance function, or as otherwise allowed by state or federal law. This provision is consistent with HIPAA as amended by the HITECH Act.

b. Covered entities must provide notice to and obtain authorization from patients for the electronic disclosure of their PHI, except in instances for treatment, payment, or healthcare operations, for performance of an insurance function, or as otherwise allowed by state or federal law. The Texas Attorney General will adopt a standard for authorization of such disclosures consistent with both HIPAA and the Texas Privacy Law.
c. Covered entities must provide notice to patients of their policies on their website or other prominent place where patients will see the notice.
3. More Stringent Training Requirements
    a. Covered entities must provide ongoing training to their employees regarding state and federal law concerning PHI.
    b. The training must be customized to the covered entity's particular course of business and each employee's scope of employment.
    c. The covered entity must train a new employee no later than the 60th day after the employee is hired, and the training must be repeated at least once every two years.
    d. All covered entities must maintain paper or electronic records documenting each employee's attendance at training programs.
4. Provision of Electronic Health Records (EHRs)
    a. Covered entities must provide patients with a copy of their EHRs in electronic format within 15 business days of receiving a written request. *Note: This is the same as the TSBP rule for any request for a copy of confidential information regardless of the format.*
    b. The Texas Health and Human Services Commission is required to recommend a standard format for the release of EHRs that is consistent with federal law.
5. Increased Penalties
    a. The Texas Attorney General may institute penalties against covered entities that violate state laws regarding electronic disclosure of PHI.
    b. Penalties for privacy violations include a maximum of $5,000 per negligent violation, a maximum of $25,000 per knowing or intentional violation, and a maximum of $250,000 if the use or disclosure is for financial gain.
    c. The maximum annual civil penalty that may be assessed for a pattern or practice of violations is increased to $1.5 million. In addition, a healthcare provider's Texas professional or institutional license may be revoked for repeated violations of the Texas Privacy Law.
    d. It is a state felony if an individual, without the consent of the patient, accesses, reads, scans, stores, or transfers PHI via a scanning device or electronic payment card.
6. Enforcement
    a. The Texas Health and Human Services Commission, Texas Health Services Authority, Texas Department of Insurance, and the Texas Attorney General's office have authority to audit compliance with the Texas Privacy Law.
    b. The complaint system and information website is set up by the Attorney General's office.
    c. The Texas Health Services Authority develops standards for the electronic sharing of PHI in compliance with HIPAA to ensure the secure maintenance and disclosure of records.
7. Breach Notification Requirements for All Texas Businesses
    a. The Texas Business and Commerce Code also requires that any organization that conducts business in Texas and handles PHI provides notification to Texas residents if their PHI is wrongfully disclosed.

b. This notification requirement is consistent with the requirement in the HITECH Act that subjects vendors of personal health records and their service providers to the same security breach notification requirements as HIPAA covered entities.
c. Any business that fails to make the required notification is subject to state penalties not exceeding $250,000 for a single breach.

Notes

CHAPTER A HIGHLIGHTS
Federal Food, Drug, and Cosmetic Act (FDCA)

1. The FDCA was passed in 1938 following the sulfanilamide tragedy involving diethylene glycol. It is designed to protect the public health by requiring that only safe, effective, and properly labeled drugs and devices be introduced into interstate commerce and to assure that food and cosmetics are safe and properly labeled.
2. Some Major Amendments to the FDCA
    a. The Durham-Humphrey amendments to the FDCA established the two classes of drugs—prescription drugs and over-the-counter drugs.
    b. The Prescription Drug Marketing Act (PDMA) prohibits pharmacies, with a few exceptions, from selling, purchasing, trading, or possessing prescription drug samples.
    c. The Compounding Quality Act (part of the Drug Quality and Security Act) still allows traditional compounding to be regulated by the states under Section 503(a) of the FDCA but establishes a new Section 503(b) under the FDCA that allows facilities that compound sterile pharmaceuticals to register with FDA as "outsourcing facilities."
    d. The Drug Supply Chain Security Act (part of the Drug Quality and Security Act) sets up a national framework for an electronic track and trace system for prescription drugs. The law will be phased in over a 10-year time period.
3. Adulteration of a drug means there are problems with the cleanliness, purity, or strength of the drug.
4. Misbranding of a drug means there are problems with the drug's labeling.
5. The following elements are required on prescription drug labels:
Note: These elements are for a container from a manufacturer and are not the label requirements when dispensing pursuant to a prescription.
    a. The name and address of the manufacturer, packer, or distributor.
    b. An accurate statement of the quantity (i.e., Number: 100 tablets).
    c. The generic name of the drug, if any, and the proprietary name.
    d. A statement of the quantity of the ingredients (i.e., 0.25 mg per tablet).
    e. Adequate information for use (intended for healthcare professionals).
    f. Adequate warnings against use where dangerous.
    g. Expiration date.
    h. Any other information required (e.g., certain products require "black boxed warnings" to alert healthcare professionals about essential information regarding the product).
6. The following elements are required on OTC drug labels:
    a. A principal display panel including a statement of identity of the product.
    b. The name and address of the manufacturer, packer, or distributor.
    c. Net quantity of contents.
    d. Cautions and warnings needed to protect user.
    e. Adequate directions for safe and effective use (for layperson).
    f. Content and format of OTC product labeling in "Drug Facts" panel format (*see 21 CFR 201.66 for details and example*).
        (1) Active ingredients
        (2) Purpose
        (3) Use(s)—indications
        (4) Warnings
        (5) Directions
        (6) Other information
        (7) Inactive ingredients
        (8) Questions? followed by telephone number

7. The FDCA requires Patient Package Inserts (PPIs) be given to patients (including inpatients) for oral contraceptives and estrogen products. PPIs are different from Medication Guides and from general drug information provided by pharmacies as part of patient counseling requirements.
8. Medication Guides are required for over 1000 drugs and biological products and are part of a product's required labeling. They must be provided to patients when certain drugs and biologicals are dispensed. In addition, if the drug or biological product is administered in an outpatient setting, they must be provided the first time the drug is administered.
9. Risk Evaluation and Mitigation Strategies (REMS) are strategies FDA uses to manage serious risks with a drug and generally include elements to assure safe use such as special training or certification of prescribers or pharmacists, restricted dispensing, or documentation requirements prior to dispensing.
10. Dietary supplements and medical foods are not regulated as drugs. They are subject to specific regulatory requirements.
11. FDA has the legal authority to order recalls for medical devices, biological products, and foods (including dietary supplements) but not drugs except for controlled substances.

Poison Prevention Packaging Act (PPPA)

1. The PPPA is administered by the Consumer Product Safety Commission (CPSC).
2. The PPPA requires child-resistant containers on all prescription drugs and certain over-the-counter drugs unless an exemption applies.
3. It is important to know all the exemptions and how they apply.

Health Insurance Portability and Accountability Act (HIPAA) and Texas Privacy Laws

1. Most pharmacies are covered entities under HIPAA.
2. Covered entities must provide patients a Notice of Privacy Practices upon first service delivery, have a designated Privacy Official, be able to prove an accounting of disclosures of protected health information (PHI), conduct employee training, and have policies and procedures.
3. Covered entities may use and disclose PHI to provide treatment and payment and for healthcare operations without authorization from the patient. Most other uses and disclosures require authorization from the patient unless an exception applies.
4. Covered entities are required to have business associate agreements with persons or entities performing a function on their behalf that requires the use or disclosure of PHI.
5. Under the HITECH Act, covered entities must notify patients of a breach of unsecured PHI within 60 days and notify HHS and local media if the breach involves more than 500 individuals.
6. Texas privacy laws, among other requirements, have a broader definition of a covered entity, a requirement that covered entities provide patients with information in electronic health records within 15 days (as opposed to 30 days under HIPAA), and more stringent training requirements. The Texas breach notifications are also more extensive as they require any entity that handles PHI (not just HIPAA covered entities and business associates) to provide notification to Texas residents if their PHI is wrongfully disclosed.

CHAPTER B

Controlled Substance Laws and Regulations

Federal Controlled Substances Act (FCSA)

Administered by the Drug Enforcement Administration (DEA)

and

Texas Controlled Substances Act (TCSA)

Administered by the Texas State Board of Pharmacy (TSBP)

(as it relates to pharmacy practice)

CHAPTER B

Controlled Substance Laws and Regulations
Federal Controlled Substances Act (FCSA)
Administered by the Drug Enforcement Administration (DEA)
and
Texas Controlled Substances Act (TCSA)
Administered by the Texas State Board of Pharmacy (TSBP)
(as it relates to pharmacy practice)

Note: Throughout this chapter, unless otherwise noted, requirements listed as part of the FCSA are the same under the TCSA.

I. **Introduction to the Federal Controlled Substances Act (FCSA)**
   A. Statutory Authority
   The Federal Controlled Substances Act (FCSA) is part of Title II of the Federal Comprehensive Drug Abuse Prevention and Control Act of 1970 (Public Law 91-513) and includes these three titles:
   Title I—Rehabilitation Programs for Drug Abusers.
   Title II—Federal Controlled Substances Act (21 U.S.C. 801 et. seq;).
   Title III—Controlled Substances Import and Export Act.
   B. Regulatory Authority
   Title 21, Code of Federal Regulations, Part 1300 to end, implements the Federal Controlled Substances Act.
   C. History
   The Drug Enforcement Administration (DEA), an agency of the Department of Justice, is the lead federal law enforcement agency charged with the responsibility for combating controlled substance abuse. The DEA was established on July 1, 1973. It resulted from the merger of the Bureau of Narcotics and Dangerous Drugs (BNDD), the Office for Drug Abuse Law Enforcement, the Office of National Narcotic Intelligence, those elements of the Bureau of Customs which had drug investigative responsibilities, and those functions of the Office of Science and Technology which were drug enforcement related. The DEA was established to control more effectively narcotic and dangerous drug abuse through enforcement and prevention.

   Since 1914, Congress has enacted more than 50 pieces of legislation relating to control and diversion of drugs. The FCSA became effective May 1, 1971. It collected and combined most of these diverse laws into one piece of legislation. The law is designed to improve the administration and regulation of manufacturing, distribution, and dispensing of controlled substances by providing a "closed" system of legitimate handlers of these drugs. Such a closed system is intended to help reduce the widespread diversion of these drugs out of legitimate channels into the illicit market.

   The Federal Controlled Substances Act differs substantially from earlier drug control laws in its approach to controlling access to regulated substances. Control is achieved through federal registration of all persons in the legitimate chain of manufacturing, distributing, and dispensing of controlled drugs, except the ultimate user. However, even ultimate users are affected by the Act since it sets forth conditions under which the users may possess controlled drugs. In contrast, its predecessor, the Harrison Narcotic Act, exerted control over narcotic drugs by imposition of a tax. It should also be noted that the Harrison Narcotic Act was only concerned with narcotic drugs, while the FCSA covers both narcotic and nonnarcotic, stimulant, depressant, and hallucinogenic drugs.

D. Federal Versus State Drug Controls

Since federal drug control laws or regulations may vary from state drug control laws, the practicing pharmacist must learn certain basic principles to know how to comply with the law. These precepts are summarized as follows:

1. A pharmacist is responsible to the same degree for compliance with both federal and state laws and regulations governing the practice of pharmacy.
2. A state drug control law or regulation may be more stringent than its federal counterpart (e.g., Texas official prescription form for Schedule II drugs and controlled substance inventory requirements (TSBP)).
3. A pharmacist must comply with a state drug control law or regulation when it is stricter than the federal law or when there is no similar prohibition or requirement under the federal law.
4. If a federal drug control law or regulation is more stringent than the comparable state law or regulation, the federal requirement must be followed.
5. Summary—The more stringent law or regulation is to be followed in all cases unless the two cannot consistently stand together. If that is the case, then the state law must yield to the federal.
6. Medical and Recreational Marijuana—A number of states have passed laws legalizing the use and or selling of marijuana for medical purposes, and some states have legalized recreational use of marijuana. However, marijuana remains a Schedule I controlled substance under federal law. Based on the principles above, use of marijuana for medical or recreational purposes, even if allowed under state law, would be a violation of federal law. Whether the federal government enforces those laws is a separate issue and often depends on the enforcement priorities of DEA and the presidential administration.
7. Cannabidiol (CBD)
   a. The 2018 Farm Bill removed hemp from the Federal Controlled Substances Act. A similar 2019 bill in Texas did the same thing under the Texas Controlled Substances Act.
   b. Hemp is defined as the plant Cannabis Sativa L. and any part of that plant. This includes the seeds of the plant and all derivatives, extracts, cannabinoids, isomers, acids, salts, and salts of isomer, whether growing or not with a delta-9 tetrahydrocannabinol (THC) concentration of not more than 0.3% on a dry weight basis.
   c. Prior to passage of the 2018 Farm Bill, FDA approved Epodiolex® (cannabidiol oral solution), and DEA subsequently placed it and all FDA-approved cannabidiol products containing no more than 0.1% THC into Schedule V. This has resulted in the awkward situation that the FDA-approved CBD product containing no more than 0.1% THC is a Schedule V controlled substance and non-FDA approved products derived from hemp that are less than 0.3% THC are not scheduled at all.
   d. There are many products on the market containing CBD. Pharmacists should proceed cautiously in dealing with these products to ensure that they meet the strict definition of hemp because marijuana-derived CBD and CBD that is greater than 0.3% THC remain Schedule I controlled substances.
   e. The Texas Compassionate Use Act allows certain physicians on a registry created by the Texas Department of Public Safety (DPS) to prescribe

low-THC cannabis to patients who have been diagnosed with intractable epilepsy, a seizure disorder, multiple sclerosis, spasticity, amyotrophic lateral sclerosis, autism, terminal cancer, or an incurable neurodegenerative disease. DPS has licensed three dispensing organizations to cultivate, process, and dispense low-THC cannabis to prescribed patients. Only those three organizations may dispense these products. (*See DPS website for more information.*)

II. **Structure and Functions of DEA**
   A. DEA is an agency under the authority of the U. S. Department of Justice.
   B. DEA implements the Federal Controlled Substances Act through regulations.
   C. The DEA Office of Diversion Control is tasked with preventing, detecting, and investigating the diversion of controlled pharmaceuticals and listed chemicals from legitimate sources (e.g., pharmacies) while ensuring an adequate and uninterrupted supply for legitimate medical, commercial, and scientific needs. DEA primarily inspects manufacturers and wholesalers but can inspect pharmacies.
   D. DEA also investigates and enforces illegal activities with controlled substances including criminal enforcement on the interstate (national) and international level.

III. **Enforcement of TCSA and Rules**
   A. There is a shared responsibility between the Texas Department of Public Safety (DPS) and the Texas State Board of Pharmacy (TSBP) for enforcement of the TCSA. Since September 1, 2016, there is no longer a state controlled substance registration requirement through DPS, so DPS will likely only be involved in criminal enforcement matters. Violations of the TCSA may be enforced by TSBP by taking disciplinary action against the license of a pharmacist, pharmacy, or registration of a pharmacy technician or trainee. TSBP has the authority under the Texas Pharmacy Act to enforce all laws relating to the practice of pharmacy as they relate to pharmacists and pharmacies (e.g., Federal Controlled Substances Act, Texas Controlled Substances Act, U.S. Food, Drug, and Cosmetic Act, and Texas Food, Drug, and Cosmetic Act).
   B. Both DPS and TSBP have authority to promulgate rules under specific sections of the TCSA. The legislation that eliminated the DPS controlled substance registration requirement for pharmacies also transferred operation of the Prescription Monitoring Program (PMP) from DPS to TSBP, effective September 1, 2016, and gave TSBP the authority to adopt rules to administer Sections 481.073, 481.074, 481.075, 481.076, and 481.0761 of the TCSA. These are the sections of the TCSA dealing with prescriptions and the Prescription Monitoring Program (PMP).

IV. **Drug Classifications Under the FCSA and TCSA**
   A. Schedule I (C-I) Drugs
      1. Drugs having no accepted medical use in the U.S. and a high abuse potential.
      2. Include opiates and derivatives such as heroin and dihydromorphine; hallucinogens such as marijuana, lysergic acid diethylamide (LSD), MDMA (Ecstasy), peyote, mescaline; and depressants such as methaqualone.
   B. Schedule II (C-II) Drugs
      1. Drugs having a currently accepted medical use and a high abuse potential.
      2. Abuse of the drugs or other substances may lead to severe physical or psychological dependence.
      3. Include opium and other narcotics as single active ingredients, such as morphine, codeine, dihydrocodeine, hydrocodone, oxycodone, methadone, meperidine, hydromorphone, fentanyl, and cocaine; some narcotic combination products such as hydrocodone with acetaminophen (Vicodin®),

oxycodone with acetaminophen (Percocet®), and oxycodone with aspirin (Percodan®); stimulants such as amphetamine, methamphetamine, phenmetrazine, and methylphenidate; and depressants such as pentobarbital (oral), secobarbital (oral), amobarbital (oral), glutethimide, and phencyclidine.

Note: The term "narcotic" refers to drugs that are derivatives of opium, poppy straw, cocaine, or ecgonine. While all narcotics are controlled substances, not all controlled substances are narcotics.

C. Schedule III (C-III) Drugs
1. Drugs having a currently accepted medical use and an abuse potential less than those in Schedule I and II.
2. Abuse of the drugs or other substances may lead to moderate or low physical dependence or high psychological dependence.
3. Include some narcotic Schedule II drugs, but in combination with another ingredient such as aspirin with codeine; acetaminophen with codeine; suppository forms of amobarbital, secobarbital, or pentobarbital; stimulants such as chlorphentermine, phendimetrazine, and benzphetamine; and anabolic steroids, including testosterone; ketamine; and paregoric. They also include Fiorinal®, a combination of butalbital, aspirin, and caffeine.

Note: While Fiorinal® is a Schedule III controlled substance, Fioricet®, a combination of butalbital, acetaminophen, and caffeine, is an exempt prescription drug product (see F. below) and is not labeled as a controlled substance.

4. Use of Anabolic Steroids in Texas
   a. These drugs may be dispensed, prescribed, delivered, or administered by a practitioner for a valid medical purpose and in the course of professional practice.
   b. These drugs may be dispensed or delivered by a pharmacist pursuant to a prescription of a practitioner for a valid medical purpose and in the course of professional practice.
   c. Bodybuilding, muscle enhancement, or increasing muscle bulk or strength through the use of anabolic steroids by a person who is in good health is not a valid medical purpose.
   d. The provisions of the Texas Controlled Substances Act relating to the possession and distribution of anabolic steroids do not apply to the use of anabolic steroids that are administered to livestock or poultry.

D. Schedule IV (C-IV) Drugs
1. Drugs having a currently accepted medical use and an abuse potential less than those in Schedule III.
2. Abuse may lead to limited physical or psychological dependence relative to Schedule III.
3. Include narcotics such as propoxyphene and products with no more than 1mg of difenoxin and no less than 25 micrograms of atropine sulfate per dosage unit (Motofen®); mixed opioid agonist-antagonists such as pentazocine and butorphanol; benzodiazepines such as alprazolam, diazepam, lorazepam, and barbiturates such as phenobarbital; sleep aids such as eszopiclone (Lunesta®); stimulants used for weight loss such as diethylpropion and phentermine; the muscle relaxant carisoprodol (Soma®); and the pain reliever tramadol.

E. Schedule V (C-V) Drugs
1. Drugs having a currently accepted medical use and an abuse potential less than those in Schedule IV.
2. Abuse of the drug or other substance may lead to limited physical or psychological dependence relative to Schedule IV.
3. Include antitussive products containing codeine (Robitussin AC®); antidiarrheal products containing opium, diphenoxlate, and atropine (Lomotil®);

FDA-approved cannabidiol products containing no more than 0.1% THC (Epodiolex®); and pregabalin (Lyrica®) for neuropathic pain.
F. Exempted Prescription Drug Products
1. Manufacturers may apply to DEA to exempt a product or chemical from certain provisions of the Controlled Substances Act (labeling and inventory) if the product or chemical is not likely to be abused. These products may still be considered controlled substances for certain criminal violations even though they are not labeled as controlled substances.
2. Exempted prescription drug preparations include nonnarcotic products containing small amounts of phenobarbital, butalbital, chlordiazepoxide, or meprobamate.
3. The DEA Exempt Prescription Product List can be found at *http://www.deadiversion.usdoj.gov/schedules/exempt/exempt_rx_list.pdf*.
G. Scheduled Listed Chemicals
1. Scheduled Listed Chemicals include products containing ephedrine, pseudoephedrine, or phenylpropanolamine that may be marketed or distributed lawfully in the United States under the Food, Drug, and Cosmetic Act as nonprescription drugs.
2. These products are subject to certain sales limitations and other restrictions. (*See Section XXI. of this chapter.*)

V. Scheduling of Controlled Substances
A. FCSA
The U.S. Attorney General, as head of the Department of Justice, may add, delete, or reschedule substances and often consults with the Director of DEA. However, the Attorney General must also obtain a scientific and medical evaluation and recommendation from the Secretary of the U.S. Department of Health and Human Services. This function is usually delegated by HHS to the FDA.
B. TCSA
1. The Commissioner of the Texas Department of State Health Services may add, delete, or reschedule substances with the approval of the Texas Board of Health.
2. The Commissioner cannot add any substance to the schedules if the substance has been deleted from the schedules by the Texas legislature.
3. The Commissioner cannot delete any substance to the schedules if the substance was added by the Texas legislature.
4. The Commissioner cannot reschedule a substance if the substance has been placed in a schedule by the Texas legislature.
5. If a controlled substance is added, deleted, or rescheduled under the FCSA, it will be included or removed from that schedule in Texas unless the Commissioner objects to the inclusion or deletion.

VI. Determining the Schedule of Compounded Controlled Substances
A. DEA allows pharmacists to compound narcotic controlled substances in Schedules II–V so long as the concentration of the final solution, compound, or mixture is not greater than 20%. If a pharmacy is compounding narcotics that are greater than 20%, this activity may be considered manufacturing by DEA and would require a DEA registration as a manufacturer. (*See chart of coincident activities allowed at 21 CFR 1301.13.*) DEA does not permit a pharmacist to compound a controlled substance for "office use."
B. If a compounded prescription contains narcotics in an amount greater than the maximum allowed for Schedule V, the prescription then becomes a Schedule III. It will never be a Schedule IV.
C. If the concentration exceeds the maximum allowable for Schedule III, it becomes a Schedule II.

D. Codeine Example
   1. Schedule V maximum:
      a. Is 200 mg/100 ml or 2 mg/ml or 2 mg/gm. If any amount of codeine is added to a C-V cough syrup (Robitussin AC®), the product becomes a Schedule III.
   2. Schedule III maximum:
      a. Is 1.8 gm (1800 mg)/100 ml or 18 mg/ml
      b. Dosage Unit—90 mg/dosage unit
      If Schedule III limit is exceeded, the product is a Schedule II.
E. The narcotics must be compounded with other nonnarcotic, active ingredients in recognized therapeutic amounts (e.g., compounding codeine with cherry syrup would be classified as a Schedule II because cherry syrup is not therapeutic and codeine could be "recovered" in its pure form).
F. Any "straight" narcotic, regardless of strength or concentration, is a Schedule II (i.e., 30 mg codeine tablet or opium powder).
G. A Schedule II narcotic not included in the following table will remain a Schedule II regardless of concentration (e.g., meperidine (Demerol®) or hydromorphone (Dilaudid®)).

SCHEDULE III
Maximum Allowable Limits Under Federal Law

narcotic substance	limit: concentration	limit/dosage unit
Codeine	1.8 gm/100 ml	90 mg
Morphine	50 mg/100 ml or 100 gm	
Opium	500 mg/100 ml or 100 gm	25 mg
Ethylmorphine	300 mg/100 ml	15 mg
Dihydrocodeine	1.8 gm/100 ml	90 mg
Dihydrocodeinone	300 mg/100 ml	15 mg

SCHEDULE V
Maximum Allowable Limits Under Federal Law

narcotic substance	limit: concentration	limit/dosage unit
Codeine	200 mg/100 ml or 100 gm	
Dihydrocodeine	100 mg/100 ml or 100 gm	
Ethylmorphine	100 mg/100 ml or 100 gm	
Opium	100 mg/100 ml or 100 gm	
Lomotil:		
Diphenoxylate &		2.5 mg
Atropine combo		not less than 25 mcg
Difenoxin &		0.5 mg
Atropine		25 mcg

H. Examples
Most Schedule V drugs having codeine contain 2 mg of codeine/ml. The maximum allowable limit for Schedule V codeine-containing compounds is 200 mg/100 ml (or 2 mg/ml). Most of the listed Schedule V drugs containing codeine meet the absolute maximum for Schedule V. If even 1 mg/ml is added to any of these products, it has exceeded the maximum allowable limit for Schedule V. However, to exceed the Schedule III limits (18 mg/1 ml), codeine in excess of 16 mg/ml must be added to the Schedule V codeine-containing syrup.

Rx #1			Rx #2		
Cheracol®	120 ml	(240 mg Codeine)	Cheracol®	120 ml	(240mg Codeine)
Codeine	800 mg	(800 mg Codeine)	Codeine	2000 mg	(2000 mg Codeine)
		1040 mg Codeine/120 ml			2240 mg Codeine/120 ml
		or 8.66 mg/ml			or 18.66 mg/ml

<u>Rx #1</u> The prescription contains 1040 mg/120 ml. This does not exceed the Schedule III limits (18 mg/ml). It does exceed the Schedule V limits (2 mg/ml). Therefore, it is a Schedule III prescription.

<u>Rx #2</u> The prescription contains 2240 mg/120 cc. This exceeds the Schedule III limits (18 mg/ml). Therefore, it is a Schedule II prescription.

    I. Texas Law
        1. Although the Texas concentrations for codeine-containing products are the same as federal law, the TCSA requires that any product containing codeine or dihydrocodeine (even if it is a Schedule V) be dispensed only pursuant to a prescription. Products such as Robitussin AC® and Cheracol®, which can often be purchased without a prescription in some states, require a prescription in Texas.
        2. The maximum concentration for Schedule V opium products in Texas is stricter (50 mg/100 ml) than the federal law (100 mg/100 ml).
Note: The Schedule V opium limit under the TCSA is 50 mg/100 ml or half the concentration under federal law. This stricter requirement means that the Schedule V commercially available products containing opium cannot be purchased without a prescription in Texas. They are Schedule III under Texas law and require a prescription.
    J. Summary
A prescription calling for compounding a Schedule V narcotic-containing product and adding more narcotic to it will be in Schedule III or Schedule II depending on the amount of narcotic added.
Note: The narcotic substances listed must be compounded in combination with one or more therapeutic ingredients in recognized therapeutic amounts. Cherry syrup, simple syrup, etc., do not contain therapeutic ingredients. To place a narcotic substance in one of these vehicles is like placing the drug in water. The law views this as having a prescription for a straight narcotic (codeine, morphine, etc.) which is classified as a Schedule II drug.

VII. Registration—How Entities and Persons are Regulated Under the FCSA
    A. Closed System of Distribution
        1. The Federal Controlled Substances Act and DEA regulations create a closed system for the manufacturing, distributing, and dispensing of controlled substances.
        2. Only persons or entities that are registered with the DEA or who are specifically exempted may engage in these activities.
        3. Texas does not have a state-controlled substance registration.
    B. Classification of Registrants (independent activities)
        1. Manufacturers
        2. Distributors
        3. Reverse distributors
        4. Dispensers—Include practitioners, hospitals/clinics, retail pharmacies, central fill pharmacies, and teaching institutions. However, pharmacists are not considered dispensers unless state law grants them prescriptive authority for controlled substances which Texas does not.
        5. Researchers—Schedule I
        6. Researchers—Schedule II–V
        7. Narcotic treatment programs
        8. Chemical analysts

9. Importers
10. Exporters
C. Dispenser Registrations
   1. The definition of dispense under the FCSA includes not only dispensing of controlled substances but also prescribing and administering controlled substances. Dispenser registrations include:
      a. Pharmacies—Licensed by the state to dispense controlled substances to patients pursuant to a lawful prescription of an individual practitioner. *Note: Pharmacies are considered practitioners under the FCSA but are not institutional or individual practitioners.*
      b. Institutional Practitioners—Hospitals or other facilities authorized to dispense controlled substances but do not include pharmacies.
      c. Individual Practitioners—Physicians, dentists, veterinarians, podiatrists, or other practitioners who are authorized to prescribe, dispense, or administer controlled substances. However, pharmacists, pharmacies, or institutional practitioners are not included.
   2. For individual practitioners (physicians, dentists, etc.), hospitals/clinics, pharmacies, and teaching institutions, the first letter of the DEA number is an "A," "B," or "F" (or "G" for Department of Defense personal service contractors). The second letter of the prefix will be the first letter of the practitioner's last name ("B" for Dr. Brown) for individual practitioners or the first letter of a pharmacy's or hospital's name ("C" for Crestview Pharmacy).
   3. Mid-Level Practitioners
      a. DEA issues registrations that begin with the letter "M" to mid-level practitioners.
      b. Mid-level practitioners are individual practitioners (other than physicians, dentists, veterinarians, or podiatrists) who are authorized (by state law) to dispense (includes prescribe and administer) controlled substances.
      c. Examples of mid-level practitioners include physician assistants (PAs), advanced practice registered nurses (APRNs), nurse anesthetists, ambulance services, animal shelters, or veterinary euthanasia technicians.
      d. The second letter of a mid-level practitioner registration corresponds to the first letter of the mid-level practitioner's last name or the facility name.
D. Separate Registrations for Separate Locations
   1. A separate registration is required for each general physical location where controlled substances are manufactured, distributed, imported, exported, or dispensed.
   2. Each pharmacy must have its own DEA registration regardless of whether it is owned by the same person or company. An exception is a satellite pharmacy within a hospital.
   3. A hospital that owns a facility such as a clinic or ambulatory surgical center that is at a different physical location must obtain a separate DEA registration for those facilities, and all transfers of controlled substances between the hospital and those facilities must follow DEA requirements. DEA will sometimes issue a campus registration that may include multiple buildings, but this is done on a case-by-case basis.
   4. Hospital Registration—Only one registration is needed for a hospital and the hospital's pharmacy. If the pharmacy obtains a separate registration from the hospital, all drug distributions would be registrant (pharmacy) to registrant (hospital), requiring DEA Form 222 (C-II) or invoices (C-III-V). As a result, most hospitals have one DEA registration as a hospital/clinic for the entire facility.
   5. Individual practitioners who register at one location but practice at other locations within the same state are not required to register for any other location in that state at which they only prescribe controlled substances.

    a. If, however, they maintain supplies of controlled substances, administer controlled substances, or directly dispense them at another location, they must register for that location as well.
    b. If they practice in more than one state, a separate DEA registration is required for each state.
E. Certificate of Registration (DEA Form 223)
    1. This form contains the name, address, and registration number of the registrant; activity authorized (e.g., dispensing or manufacturing); schedules of controlled substances authorized to handle; fee paid; and expiration date.
    2. The certificate shall be maintained at the pharmacy in a readily retrievable manner and be available for inspection authorized by a federal or state agent. However, it does not have to be displayed.
F. Confirmation of Registrant's DEA Number
    1. Add 1st, 3rd, and 5th digits.
    2. Add 2nd, 4th, and 6th digits and multiply the sum by 2.
    3. Add the sum of A and B above, and the last digit of the sum should correspond to the last digit of the DEA number.
    4. Example:
       DEA #: AB1234563
       $1+3+5 = 9$
       $(2+4+6) \times 2 = 24$
       TOTAL $= 33$

       The last digit in the total is "3" which corresponds to the last digit in the DEA number: AB1234563.
    5. The first letter of the prefix of a DEA number is an "A" if the registrant is a pharmacy or practitioner (MD, DDS, etc.) if registered before 6/1/85; the first prefix letter will be a "B" or "F" if registered after 6/1/85.
    6. The second letter of the DEA registration should also match the first letter of the practitioner's last name.
G. Persons Exempt From DEA Registration Requirements
    1. The agent or employee of a registrant, if such agent or employee is acting in the usual course of business or employment. Examples are a pharmacist, pharmacy technician, nurse, or delivery person. If a pharmacist is not acting in the usual course of business (i.e., agent), the pharmacist cannot possess controlled substances.
    2. An individual practitioner (physician, dentist, veterinarian, or podiatrist) who is an employee of another practitioner (other than a mid-level practitioner) registered to dispense controlled substances may, when acting in the normal course of business or employment, administer or dispense controlled substances but may not issue a prescription.
    3. An individual practitioner who is an agent or employee of a hospital or other institution may, when acting in the normal course of business or employment, administer, dispense, or prescribe controlled substances under the registration of the hospital or other institution which is registered without being registered himself or herself provided that:
        a. Such dispensing, administering, or prescribing is done in the usual course of his or her professional practice;
        b. Such individual practitioner is authorized or permitted to do so by the jurisdiction in which he or she is practicing;
        c. The hospital or other institution by which he or she is employed has verified that the individual practitioner is permitted to dispense, administer, or prescribe drugs in the jurisdiction;
        d. Such individual is acting only within the scope of his or her employment in the hospital or institution;
        e. The hospital or other institution authorizes the individual practitioner to administer, dispense, or prescribe under the hospital registration and

Notes

designates a specific internal code number for each individual practitioner so authorized. The code number shall consist of letters, numbers, or a combination thereof and shall be a suffix to the institution's DEA registration number preceded by a hyphen (e.g., AP0123456-10 or AP 0123456-A12); and
- f. A current list of internal codes and the corresponding individual practitioners is kept by the hospital or other institution and is made available at all times to law enforcement agencies upon request for the purpose of verifying the authority of the prescribing individual practitioner.
4. Officials of the U.S. Army, Navy, Marine Corps, Air Force, Coast Guard, Public Health Service, or Bureau of Prisons acting in the course of official duties. (*See 21 CFR 1301.23.*) The prescription will have:
    a. The branch of service (e.g., "U.S. Army") and service identification number or
    b. The name of the agency (e.g., "U.S. Public Health Service") and social security number of the practitioner.

    Note: Because these military and federal practitioners are exempt from DEA registration requirements, their Schedule III–V prescriptions can be filled off base. However, any Schedule II prescriptions they write can only be filled on base unless they have obtained official prescription forms from the Texas State Board of Pharmacy. The Board requires a valid DEA number from the practitioner to order official prescription forms. This exemption does not apply to private practitioners who contract with the military to provide health services.
5. Federal and state law enforcement officials such as U.S. Customs Service, FDA, and TSBP officials. (*See 21 CFR 1301.24.*)
6. Oceans vessels and certain air carriers. (*See 21 CFR 1301.25.*)
7. Individuals possessing a lawfully obtained controlled substance for personal use or for administration to an animal accompanying him or her may enter or exit the United States without being registered provided certain conditions are met. (*See 21 CFR 1301.26.*)

H. Application for Registration and Renewal of Registration
1. DEA registrations are issued contingent upon meeting state requirements and obtaining appropriate state licenses.
2. For a pharmacy, one must first obtain a pharmacy license from the state board of pharmacy.
3. DEA has online registration applications on its website. Application forms for registration differ depending on the type of activity.
    a. DEA Form 224—For dispensers including retail pharmacies, hospitals/clinics, practitioners, mid-level practitioners, and teaching institutions. The renewal form is DEA Form 224a.
    b. DEA Form 225—For manufacturers, distributors, researchers, analytical laboratories, importers, and exporters. The renewal form is DEA Form 225a.
    c. DEA Form 363—For narcotic treatment facilities. The renewal form is DEA Form 363a.
4. To expedite registration, an affidavit attesting that a new pharmacy license has been issued by a board of pharmacy may be submitted with DEA Form 224. (*See 21 CFR 1301.17.*)
5. If the registration is defective, DEA will return it for completion.
6. Although not required for dispenser registrations, recently some DEA offices have been conducting preregistration inspections before issuing pharmacies new DEA registrations.
7. Initial registrations for dispensers are valid for a period of at least 28 months but not more than 39 months.

8. The DEA registration period for dispensers (pharmacies, practitioners, etc.) is for a three-year period. The DEA registration period for other activities (manufacturing, distributing, etc.) is for a one-year period.
9. A renewal registration form is mailed to the pharmacy within 60 days of expiration.
10. If the renewal application is not received 45 days prior to expiration, the pharmacy must contact DEA in writing.
11. DEA Policy on Renewal of Registrations
    a. If a renewal application is submitted in a timely manner prior to expiration, the registrant may continue operations authorized by the registration beyond the expiration date until final action is taken on the application.
    b. DEA allows the reinstatement of an expired registration for one calendar month after the expiration date. If the registration is not renewed within that calendar month, an application for a new DEA registration will be required.
    c. Regardless of whether a registration is reinstated within the calendar month after expiration, federal law prohibits the handling of controlled substances or List 1 chemicals for any period of time under an expired registration.
12. Both initial registrations and renewals may be completed online at *http://www.deadiversion.usdoj.gov/*.
13. Registration applications must be signed (or electronically signed) by the applicant if for an individual (e.g., a physician); by a partner if it is for a partnership; or by an officer if it is for a corporation, corporate division, association, trust, or other entity. The applicant can authorize another individual to sign an application by filling out a Power of Attorney granting that individual the authority to sign applications and renewals and filing that Power of Attorney with the DEA Registration Unit. See 21 CFR 1301.13(j).

I. Grounds for Denial, Revocation, or Suspension of DEA Registration
DEA may deny, revoke, or suspend a DEA registration if the registrant:
1. Materially falsified any application filed under the FCSA.
2. Has been convicted of a felony under the FCSA or any other federal or state law relating to controlled substances.
3. Had his or her state controlled substance registration suspended, revoked, or denied.
4. Has been excluded (or directed to be excluded) from participation in any federal healthcare program (Medicare/Medicaid).
5. Has committed such an act which would render the registration inconsistent with the public interest. In determining the public interest, the following factors shall be considered:
    a. The recommendation of the appropriate state licensing board or professional disciplinary authority.
    b. The applicant's experience in dispensing or in conducting research with respect to controlled substances.
    c. The applicant's conviction record under federal or state laws relating to the manufacture, distribution, or dispensing of controlled substances.
    d. Compliance with applicable state, federal, or local laws relating to controlled substances.
    e. Such other conducts which may threaten the public health and safety.

J. Termination of Registration (without transferring business activities to another person)
1. A DEA registration terminates if the registrant dies, ceases legal existence, or ceases business or professional practice.
2. A registrant desiring to discontinue business activities altogether with respect to controlled substances (without transferring such business activities to

another person) shall return for cancellation his or her registration certificate and any unexecuted order forms to the Registration Unit of DEA. Any controlled substances must be disposed of in accordance with 21 CFR 1307.21.

K. Temporary Use of Registration

If the new owner has not yet obtained a DEA registration, DEA does permit the new owner to continue the business of the pharmacy under the previous owner's registration provided the following requirements are met:

1. The new owner must expeditiously apply for an appropriate DEA and state registration.
2. The previous owner executes a Power of Attorney to the new owner that provides for the following:
   a. The previous owner agrees to allow the controlled substance activities of the pharmacy to be carried out under his or her DEA registration;
   b. The previous owner agrees to allow the new owner to carry out the controlled substance activities of the pharmacy, including the ordering of controlled substances, as an agent of the previous owner;
   c. The previous owner acknowledges as the registrant that he or she will be held accountable for any violations of controlled substance laws which may occur;
   d. The new owner must notify the appropriate local DEA office of the proposed use of the previous owner's DEA registration, and, if requested, furnish a copy of the Power of Attorney; and
   e. The previous owner agrees that the controlled substance activities of the pharmacy may be carried out under his or her DEA registration and shall remain in effect for no more than 45 days after the purchase date. *Note: Some DEA offices allow the Power of Attorney to be for more than 45 days. Check with your local DEA office to confirm requirements.*

VIII. Ordering Schedule II Controlled Substances

A. Electronic Orders for Schedule II Controlled Substances
   1. The Controlled Substances Ordering System (CSOS) allows for electronic orders of Schedule II controlled substances.
   2. The CSOS uses a public key infrastructure (PKI) to allow electronic orders based on digital certificates issued by the DEA Certification Authority. These digital certificates serve as an electronic equivalent to DEA Form 222. Each CSOS certificate is issued to only one individual person. This person, called a CSOS Subscriber, is an individual who enrolled in the CSOS program with DEA and whose name appears in the digital certificate. A digital signature using a CSOS certificate is required when submitting an electronic order for controlled substances. Only the individual subscriber whose name appears in the certificate is authorized to perform this digital signature.
   3. All CSOS applications must be audited by an independent third party auditor prior to use and any time changes are made to the software to ensure that the software is in compliance with DEA regulations.
   4. A DEA registrant must appoint a CSOS coordinator who will serve as that registrant's recognized agent regarding issues pertaining to issuance of, revocation of, and changes to digital certificates issued under that registrant's DEA registration.
   5. Use of the electronic ordering is optional; registrants may continue to order using DEA Form 222 as outlined below.

B. Obtaining DEA Form 222 for Manual Orders of Schedule II Controlled Substances
   1. Any person with an active registration that is authorized to order Schedule II controlled substances may obtain a DEA Form 222 which will be supplied at any time after a DEA registration is granted.

2. DEA Form 222 may be requested through a DEA secured network connection or by contacting any Division Office or the Registration Section of DEA.
3. Each request must include the name, address, and registration number of the registrant and the number of forms desired.
4. DEA Form 222 will have an order form number (i.e., serial number) and will be preprinted with the name, address, and registration number of the registrant. Any errors on the form should be reported to the local Division Office or the Registration Section of DEA.

C. Power of Attorney (POA) to Sign DEA Form 222
1. A registrant may execute a Power of Attorney authorizing other individuals to sign DEA Form 222 to purchase Schedule II drugs.
2. The Power of Attorney must be signed (or electronically signed) by the registrant if the registrant is an individual, a partner if the registrant is a partnership, or by an officer if the registrant is a corporation, corporate division, association, trust, or other entity. It also must be signed (or electronically signed) by the person being authorized to execute DEA Form 222 and two witnesses. *Note: Previously DEA allowed the person who signed the last registration application or renewal to issue a POA to allow other individuals to sign DEA Form 222. That provision was removed by DEA effective October 30, 2019. This means that if the registrant authorized another individual to sign the registration application or renewal as allowed under H.13. above, that person may not issue a POA to others to allow them to sign DEA Form 222. That POA must be issued by the registrant (i.e., the individual, partner, or officer).*
3. The Power of Attorney must be maintained in the pharmacy and be available for inspection.
4. A Power of Attorney may be revoked at any time by executing a Notice of Revocation.
5. A sample Power of Attorney form and Notice of Revocation form are provided below and can also be found at 21 CFR 1305.05(c) as well as in the *DEA Pharmacist's Manual*.

Sample Power of Attorney for DEA Forms 222 and Electronic Orders

_____ (Name of registrant)
_____(Address of registrant)
_____ (DEA registration number)

I, _____ (name of person granting power), the undersigned, who is authorized to sign the current application for registration of the above named registrant under the Controlled Substances Act or Controlled Substances Import and Export Act, have made, constituted, and appointed, and by these presents, do make, constitute, and appoint _____ (name of attorney-in-fact), my true and lawful attorney for me in my name, place, and stead, to execute applications for books of official order forms and to sign such order forms in requisition for schedule I and II controlled substances, in accordance with Section 308 of the Controlled Substances Act (21 U.S.C. 828) and part 1305 of Title 21 of the Code of Federal Regulations. I hereby ratify and confirm all that said attorney shall lawfully do or cause to be done by virtue hereof.

_____
(Signature of person granting power)

I, _____ (name of attorney-in-fact), hereby affirm that I am the person named herein as attorney-in-fact and that the signature affixed hereto is my signature.

_____
(Signature of attorney-in-fact)

Witnesses:
1. _____
2. _____

Signed and dated on the ____ day of _____ in the year _____ at _____.

> **Sample Notice of Revocation**
>
> The foregoing power of attorney is hereby revoked by the undersigned, who is authorized to sign the current application for registration of the above-named registrant under the Controlled Substances Act. Written notice of this revocation has been given to the attorney-in-fact _____ this same day.
>
> _____
> (Signature of person revoking power)
>
> Witnesses:
>
> 1. _____
>
> 2. _____
>
> Signed and dated on the ____ day of _____ in the year _____ at _____.

D. Single Copy DEA Form 222
  1. Effective October 30, 2019, DEA finalized new rules to transition from triplicate (3 copy) DEA Form 222 to single copy DEA Form 222 with additional security features. There is a two-year transition period during which existing triplicate DEA Form 222 can continue to be used.
  2. The new single forms contain 20 order lines per form rather than 10 order lines on the triplicate forms.
  3. The purchaser filling out a single copy DEA Form 222 must make a copy of the original form for its records and submit the original form to the supplier. The copy may be retained in paper or electronic form.
  4. The supplier may only fill an order from the original form and not from a copy. The supplier, if possible and if the supplier desires to do so, must record on the original form its DEA registration number, the number of containers furnished for each ordered item, and the date the products are shipped to the purchaser.
  5. Most suppliers (e.g., wholesalers) are required to report the acquisition and disposition of Schedule II and certain Schedule III and IV controlled substances to DEA's Automation of Reports and Consolidated Orders System (ARCOS) under 21 CFR 1304.339(c). A supplier who reports transactions to ARCOS is not required to send a copy of the original DEA Form 222 to the DEA. However, if a supplier is not required to report transactions to ARCOS (e.g., a pharmacy or practitioner acting as a supplier under the 5% rule), it must submit a copy of the original DEA Form 222 to DEA either by mail or by email to *DEA.Orderforms@usdoj.gov* when acting as a supplier.
  6. When the product has been received, the purchaser must record the number of containers received and the date received for each item on the copy of the DEA Form 222 it made when ordering the product.
  7. Registrants may continue to use existing triplicate DEA Form 222 using the procedures outlined below until October 30, 2021.
E. Triplicate DEA Form 222
  1. Existing triplicate DEA Form 222 may continue to be used until October 30, 2021.
  2. Triplicate DEA Form 222 contains 10 order lines per form.
  3. Purchaser fills out the name and address of the supplier, date ordered, and products ordered. Only one product per line may be ordered although multiple packages of each product can be ordered.
  4. The total number of lines needs to be completed, and the form must be signed.

5. The form may only be signed by the registrant (individual, partner, or officer) or an individual who has a written Power of Attorney to sign the form issued by the registrant.
6. Triplicate DEA Form 222 Copies
   a. Copies 1 and 2 go to the supplier and may not be separated.
   b. Purchaser retains copy 3 for its records.
   c. Supplier indicates the number of packages shipped and date shipped on each line, sends copy 2 to DEA, and retains copy 1 for its records.
7. Upon receipt of the product, the purchaser records on the retained copy 3 the number of packages received and the date received for each line. Texas rules also require a pharmacist to verify that controlled substances listed on a supplier's invoice were actually received by recording on the invoice his or her initials and the actual date of receipt. Once the order is complete, copy 3 should be filed separately or attached to the Schedule II invoices that are initialed by the pharmacist.

F. Examples of Errors Which May Result in a DEA Form 222 Not Being Accepted by a Wholesaler (or a pharmacy selling controlled substances to a practitioner or another pharmacy)
   1. Entering the number of items ordered instead of the number of lines completed.
   2. Using Roman Numerals in the "NO. OF LINES COMPLETED" box.
   3. Leaving the "NO. OF LINES COMPLETED" box blank.
   4. Having DEA Form 222 which is incomplete, illegible, improperly prepared, or improperly executed.
   5. Having a person who does not have Power of Attorney sign DEA Form 222.
   6. Forms showing any alterations, erasures, or changes of any kind.
   7. Forms showing any alteration to the preprinted information on DEA Form 222.
   8. Forms which are illegible or unable to identify the customer, customer's registration number, items specified, or quantities or forms that are improperly executed.
   9. Forms with a calendar date older than sixty (60) days.

G. Preprinted Information on DEA Form 222
   1. Name, address, and DEA number of pharmacy.
   2. Serial number of order form and date issued by DEA.
   3. Schedules authorized to be dispensed: 2 (narcotic), 2N (nonnarcotic), 3, 3N, 4, 5. (Particular schedules are sometimes limited by DEA.)

H. Executed DEA Form 222 used by a pharmacy to order Schedule II controlled substances may be handled for a drug distribution center by common or contract drivers as long as the forms are in sealed envelopes. In addition, DEA Form 222 may be sent via facsimile (fax) by the pharmacy to a distribution center to expedite the filling process and/or via fax on behalf of a customer by an employee driver or other employee to a distribution center to facilitate the filling process. DEA Form 222 sent via fax can be filled at a distribution center from the fax. However, filled Schedule II orders may not be released until the original DEA Form 222 is received at the distribution center and is compared by an employee of the DEA registrant filling the Schedule II controlled substance order to the fax of the DEA Form 222 previously received by the drug distribution center.

I. Partial Filling by Supplier—Partial fills of an order are permitted if the supplier sends the balance within 60 days.

J. Order Forms Sent by Pharmacy to Supplier That Are Lost
   1. Execute another DEA Form 222 and include a statement to the supplier containing:
      a. Serial number of lost form.
      b. Date of order.
      c. List of unreceived drugs.

2. Send supplier a new order form with the above statement.
3. If using a triplicate DEA Form 222, file copy 3 of the replacement order form and statement with copy 3 of the original order form that was lost. If using a single DEA Form 222, file the copy of the replacement order form and statement with the copy of the original form that was lost.
K. Lost or Stolen Used or Unused Forms
Notify the registration unit of DEA in Washington immediately.
L. If the registrant discontinues business, send all unused forms and the DEA registration certificate to the appropriate DEA divisional office by registered mail.

IX. **Ordering Schedule III–V Controlled Substances**
A. There are no special ordering forms for purchasing Schedule III–V controlled substances. They can be ordered like any other prescription drug.
B. The pharmacy must maintain a readily retrievable record of the receipt of any Schedule III–V controlled substances. This record is usually the supplier's invoice. Readily retrievable means the record is kept or maintained in such a manner that it can be separated from all other records in a reasonable time and/or that it is identified by an asterisk, redline, or some other identifiable manner which makes it easily distinguishable from all other records.
C. Schedule III–V invoices must contain:
1. Name of controlled substance.
2. Dosage form and strength.
3. Number of units or volume in each container (e.g., 100-tablet bottle).
4. Quantity received (number of containers).
5. Date of actual receipt.
6. Name, address, and DEA registration number of the registrant from which controlled substances were received.

Note: TSBP rules require all controlled substance invoices to be initialed by a pharmacist and to indicate the actual date of receipt.

X. **Distributions of Controlled Substances by a Pharmacy to Another Registrant, Transfer Upon Sale, and Other Miscellaneous Distributions**
A. Although a pharmacy's DEA registration is as a dispenser, DEA permits pharmacies to distribute controlled substances without having to obtain a separate DEA registration as a distributor under the conditions below.
1. Transferee (purchaser) must be registered with DEA for the schedule(s) of drugs being transferred.
2. The 5% Rule—A pharmacy does not have to register as a distributor with DEA as long as total quantities of the controlled substances distributed during a 12-month period in which the pharmacy is registered do not exceed 5% of the total quantity of all controlled substances dispensed and distributed during that same 12-month period. An example would be a pharmacy that dispenses and distributes a total of 10,000 doses (i.e., tablets, capsules, teaspoons, etc.) of all controlled substances (not just CII drugs). This pharmacy would be allowed to transfer 500 doses without being registered as a distributor.
3. Schedule II Transfers—Transferee (purchasing pharmacy or doctor) must execute and send a DEA Form 222 to the transferring (selling) pharmacy (supplier or distributor).
4. Schedule III, IV, and V Transfers
   a. Provide original commercial invoice from transferring pharmacy to purchasing registrant containing:
      (1) Date of transfer.
      (2) Number or volume of units (i.e., 50 tablets; 120 ml).
      (3) Number of commercial containers.
      (4) Name, strength, and dosage form.

SAMPLE TRIPLICATE DEA FORM 222

Notes

See Reverse of PURCHASER'S Copy for Instructions	No order form may be issued for Schedules I and II substances unless a completed application form has been received (21 CFR 1305.04).	OMB Approval No. 1117-0010
TO: (Name of Supplier) ① **Cardinal Health**	STREET ADDRESS **667 Vista Dr.**	
CITY and STATE **Houston, Texas** — DATE ② **6/15/20**	TO BE FILLED IN BY SUPPLIER — SUPPLIER'S DEA REGISTRATION NO.	

Line No.	③ TO BE FILLED IN BY PURCHASER			National Drug Code ⑤	④ Packages Shipped	Date Shipped
	No. of Package	Size of Package	Name of Item			
1	1	500	PERCODAN		1	6/18/20
2	6	100	RITALIN 10MG TABLETS		6	6/18/20
3	6	20 ML	DEMEROL HCL, 100 MG/ML		6	6/18/20
etc.						

▲ LAST LINE ⑥ COMPLETED (MUST BE 10 or LESS)	SIGNATURE OF PURCHASER OR HIS ATTORNEY OR AGENT ⑦
Date Issued — DEA Registration No.	(Name and Address of Registrant) (NOTE: THE NAME AND ADDRESS APPEARING IN THIS BLOCK MUST BE EXACTLY THE SAME AS THE NAME AND ADDRESS ON THE DEA FORM 223 – CONTROLLED SUBSTANCE REGISTRATION)
Schedules ⑧ 2, 2N, 3, 3N, 4, 5	**Main Street Pharmacy** ⑨ **3820 Twin Creeks Drive**
Registered as a — Form No.	

Note: DEA Form 222 shall be prepared by use of a typewriter, pen, or indelible pencil (lead pencil is not acceptable).

1. The name and address of the supplier from whom the controlled substances are being ordered shall be entered on the form. Only one supplier may be listed on any one form.
2. No order form shall be valid more than 60 days after its execution by the purchaser.
3. Each item shall consist of the name of the drug ordered, the dosage form, the strength of the controlled substance, the number of units or volume in each commercial container, or the quantity or volume of each bulk container. If the controlled substance is not in pure form, the name and quantity per unit of the controlled substance is necessary.
4. The purchaser shall record on copy 3 of the order form the number of commercial or bulk containers furnished on each item and the dates on which the containers are received by the purchaser. (TSBP rules also require the pharmacist receiving the drugs for the pharmacy to enter his or her initials.)
5. The NDC number of the item may be included at the discretion of the purchaser.
6. The number of lines completed needs to be entered, not the number of items ordered.
7. The person signing must have Power of Attorney (POA) to sign DEA Form 222. The POA must be maintained on file at the pharmacy.
8. Schedule 2, 2N, 3, 3N, 4, and 5 are defined by DEA as follows:
   - 2 = Schedule II Narcotic
   - 2N = Schedule II Nonnarcotic
   - 3 = Schedule III Narcotic
   - 3N = Schedule III Nonnarcotic
   - 4 = Schedule IV
   - 5 = Schedule V

   This denotes which schedules the registrant can possess, administer, or dispense.
9. The address imprinted on the order form is the ONLY address to which drugs may be delivered. If a pharmacy or practitioner moves to a different address, no drugs may be delivered (or stored) at the new location until the registrant obtains a new DEA Form 222 imprinted with the new address.

(5) Name, address, and DEA registration number of the transferring pharmacy.
(6) Name, address, and DEA registration number of the pharmacy or practitioner to whom the controlled substances are transferred.
  b. A copy of the invoice should be retained by the supplier or distributor (pharmacy) and the original retained by the recipient (physician, wholesaler, transferee, or receiving pharmacy).
B. Transfer of Controlled Substances Upon Sale of a Pharmacy (21 CFR 1301.52(d))
  Note: This rule allows transfer of controlled substances upon the sale of a pharmacy without regard to the 5% rule above.
  1. Any pharmacy desiring to discontinue business activities altogether with respect to controlled substances (by transferring such business activities to another person) shall submit in person or by registered or certified mail (return receipt requested) to the nearest DEA Registration Field Office the following information:
     a. The name, address, registration number, and authorized business activity of the pharmacy discontinuing the business (registrant-transferor);
     b. The name, address, registration number, and authorized business activity of the person acquiring the pharmacy (registrant-transferee);
     c. Whether the business activities will be continued at the location registered by the person discontinuing business or moved to another location (if the latter, the address of the new location should be listed); and
     d. The date on which the transfer of controlled substances will occur.
  2. Unless the registrant-transferor is informed by DEA before the date on which the transfer was stated to occur that the transfer may not occur, the pharmacy may distribute (without being registered to distribute) substances in its possession to the pharmacy acquiring the business in accordance with the following:
     a. On the date of transfer of the controlled substances, a complete inventory of all controlled substances being transferred shall be taken in accordance with 21 CFR 1304.11. This inventory shall serve as the final inventory of the registrant-transferor and the initial inventory of the registrant-transferee, and a copy of the inventory shall be included in the records of each person. It is not necessary to file a copy of the inventory with the DEA unless requested by the Special Agent in Charge. Transfers of any substances listed in Schedule II shall require the use of a DEA Form 222.
     b. On the date of transfer of the controlled substances, all records required to be kept by the registrant-transferor with reference to the controlled substances being transferred under 21 CFR 1304 shall be transferred to the registrant-transferee. Responsibility for the accuracy of records prior to the date of transfer remains with the transferor, but responsibility for custody and maintenance shall be upon the transferee.
C. Distribution of Controlled Substances to Ambulances or EMS Units (not affiliated with a hospital)
  1. The Protecting Patient Access to Emergency Medications Act of 2017 amended the FCSA to allow DEA registrations for EMS agencies, approved the use of standing orders from a medical director or authorizing medical professional for administration of controlled substances by EMS personnel, and established requirements for the maintenance and administration of controlled substances used by EMS agencies.
  2. An EMS Agency may have a single registration per state instead of separate registrations for each location.
  3. Storage of the controlled substances must be at a registered agency or in a designated vehicle from the agency.

4. A hospital may provide controlled substances to a registered emergency medical services agency for purposes of restocking an emergency medical services vehicle following an emergency response, and without the use of DEA Forms 222 for Schedule II controlled substances provided all of the following conditions are satisfied:
    a. The registered or designated location of the agency where the vehicle is primarily situated maintains a record of such receipt.
    b. The hospital maintains a record of such delivery to the agency.
    c. If the vehicle is primarily situated at a designated location, such location notifies the registered location of the agency within 72 hours of the vehicle receiving the controlled substances.
D. Distribution of Controlled Substances to Hospital-Owned Ambulances
    1. If the ambulance is owned and operated by a hospital, the ambulance may be considered a department of the hospital. Controlled substances may be distributed to the ambulance on a "proof-of-use" form or other internal distribution record in the same manner as controlled drugs are distributed as floor stock, and a separate DEA registration for the EMS service is not required.
    2. If Schedule II drugs are distributed by the hospital pharmacy to the ambulance, recordkeeping must comply with TSBP rules pertaining to inpatient records. The records would be maintained in the ambulance and returned to the pharmacy when all stocks are used.
E. Distribution of Controlled Substances to Other Mobile Emergency Care Units
    The above procedures apply to helicopters, airplanes, or other mobile emergency care units which transport patients for treatment.
F. Return of Controlled Substances to Supplier (also considered a distribution of controlled substances)
    1. Schedule II
        a. The wholesaler or distributor issues DEA Form 222 to the pharmacy.
            (1) If using a triplicate DEA Form 222, the wholesaler or distributor keeps copy 3 of the DEA Form 222 and provides the pharmacy with copies 1 and 2.
            (2) If using the single copy DEA Form 222, the wholesaler or distributor makes a copy of the original DEA Form 222 and sends the original to the pharmacy.
        b. The date of shipment (return) is recorded by the pharmacy on copies 1 and 2 if using a triplicate DEA Form 222 or on the original if using a single DEA Form 222.
        c. The pharmacy then sends a copy of DEA Form 222 to the DEA by the end of the month that the order was completely filled.
            (1) If using a triplicate DEA Form 222, the pharmacy retains copy 1 and sends copy 2 to the DEA.
            (2) If using a single copy DEA Form 222, the pharmacy must make a copy of the original DEA Form 222 and send the copy to DEA either by mail or email.
    2. Schedule IIIs, IVs, and Vs—The pharmacy handles returns just like dangerous drugs (credit memo, etc., from wholesaler) but must maintain an "invoice" as a record of the return.
G. Transfer of Controlled Substances to a DEA Registered Disposal Firm ("Reverse Distributor") for Destruction
    See Section XIII. of this chapter.

XI. Storage, Security, and Theft or Loss of Controlled Substances
A. Storage of Controlled Substances in a Pharmacy
    1. Acceptable—Storage of controlled substances in a secure cabinet that is locked.

2. Acceptable—Storage of controlled substances by dispersal throughout the noncontrolled drug stock to deter theft.
3. Unacceptable—Storage of all controlled substances on one unsecured shelf.
4. Although many pharmacies store Schedule II controlled substances (or all controlled substances) in a secure locked cabinet, there is no requirement to do so in a Class A (community) pharmacy.
5. Class C (institutional), Class C-S (institutional which prepares sterile products), Class C-ASC (Ambulatory Surgical Centers), and Class F-FEMCF (Freestanding Emergency Medical Care Facility) pharmacies are required by TSBP rules to have locked storage for Schedule II controlled substances.

B. Theft or Significant Loss of Controlled Substances
DEA 21 CFR 1301.76(b) requires pharmacies to report a theft or significant loss of controlled substances.
Note: Any theft must be reported, but only "significant" losses. (See 6. below.)
1. DEA requires the initial notification to be in writing and within one business day of discovery. (*See 5. below.*) TSBP rules require notification immediately upon discovery.
2. Complete DEA Form 106—Provide a copy to:
   a. Drug Enforcement Administration (DEA);
   b. Texas State Board of Pharmacy (TSBP requirement); and
   c. Local police (recommended by DEA).
3. Although a paper version is still available, DEA recommends DEA Form 106 be filled out online at the Office of Diversion Control's website (*www.deadiversion.usdoj.gov*).
4. DEA Form 106 must include:
   a. Name and address of the registrant (pharmacy).
   b. DEA registration number.
   c. Date of theft.
   d. Name and telephone number of local police department notified.
   e. Type of theft (break-in, employee, etc.).
   f. Listing of symbols or cost code used by pharmacy in marking containers (if any).
   g. Listing of controlled substances missing from theft or significant loss.
   h. The NDC number of the missing products is required when using the online version of DEA Form 106. Using the NDC number allows the online system to auto-populate the information for name of product, dosage form, strength, and quantity per container.
5. While filing a DEA Form 106 is not immediately necessary if the registrant needs time to investigate the facts surrounding a theft or significant loss, a registrant must provide in writing initial notification of the event within one business day of discovery. This notification may be a short statement provided by fax or other means, but it must be in writing. If the investigation of a theft or significant loss lasts longer than two months, registrants should provide updates to DEA. This initial notification as well as updates should also be sent to TSBP.
6. Factors to Consider in Determining If a Loss is Significant
   a. The actual quantity of controlled substances lost in relation to the type of business.
   b. The specific controlled substance lost.
   c. Whether the loss of the controlled substances can be associated with access to those controlled substances by specific individuals or whether the loss can be attributed to unique activities that may take place involving the controlled substances.
   d. A pattern of losses over a specific time period, whether the losses appear to be random, and the results of efforts taken to resolve the losses.

e. Whether the specific controlled substances are likely candidates for diversion.
   f. Local trends and other indicators of the diversion potential of the missing controlled substances.

   Note: If a registrant is in doubt as to whether the loss is significant, DEA advises the registrant to err on the side of caution in alerting the appropriate law enforcement authorities.

   7. Breakage or Spillage of Controlled Substances
   Breakage of controlled substances does not constitute a "loss" of controlled substances. When there is breakage, damage, spillage, or some other form of destruction, any recoverable controlled substances must be disposed of according to DEA requirements. Damaged goods may be disposed of through shipment to a "reverse distributor" or by a DEA approved process. The DEA recommends that any registrant seeking to dispose of controlled substances first contact the nearest DEA Diversion Field Office for disposal instructions. If the breakage or spillage is not recoverable, the registrant must document the circumstances of the breakage in his or her inventory records. Two individuals who witnessed the breakage must sign the inventory records indicating what they witnessed. The submission of DEA Form 41 titled "Registrants Inventory of Drugs Surrendered" is not required for nonrecoverable controlled substances.

C. DEA Rule and Policy on Convicted Felons and Impaired Pharmacists (21 CFR 1301.76)
   1. The registrant (pharmacy, practitioner, etc.) shall not employ as an agent or employee who has access to controlled substances any person who has been convicted of a felony offense relating to controlled substances or who at any time had an application for registration (i.e., for a pharmacy) denied, revoked, or surrendered for cause.
   2. "For cause" means a surrender in lieu of or as a consequence of any federal or state administrative, civil, or criminal action resulting from an investigation of the individual's handling of controlled substances.
   3. DEA Waiver Policy
   An exception to the rule occurs if a pharmacy is granted a waiver of the DEA rule. The employer (pharmacy) and not the employee (pharmacist or pharmacy technician) may apply for the DEA waiver. The waiver applies to only one individual employee and one specific pharmacy. If the employee changes place of employment, then the employee's new pharmacy must obtain another waiver. The following is information from DEA about the agency's current procedures for handling waiver applications.
      a. DEA generally does not grant a waiver request for pharmacists convicted of felonies involving drug trafficking except under unusual circumstances.
      b. Waivers for pharmacists who have been convicted of felonies that involve diversion of controlled substances and who have used alcohol or drug impairment as a defense will be considered on a case-by-case basis. DEA encourages impaired pharmacists to seek treatment. Once they are "rehabilitated," DEA may grant them waivers.
      c. DEA has not yet specified how long a recovering pharmacist (who was convicted of a felony involving diversion of controlled substances) must wait for a waiver. However, DEA says that, in general, pharmacists with older convictions have a better chance of getting waivers than those with recent convictions. DEA has never granted a waiver request in less than three years from the date the pharmacist was convicted. (DEA may deny a waiver even though the pharmacist's state board of pharmacy has removed any restrictions from the pharmacist's license.)
      d. DEA advises recovering pharmacists with felony convictions not to lie about convictions on any employment application. Even if the pharmacist

lied only on the preliminary job application and explained the conviction during the interview, the employer's request for a DEA waiver will be denied. DEA considers lying on an application for employment convincing evidence that the impaired pharmacist has not been successful in his or her recovery program.
    e. Recovering pharmacists who have no felony convictions do not require waivers, but they should seek treatment to forestall DEA involvement.

D. Employee Screening Procedures for Non-Practitioners (including pharmacies) (21 CFR 1301.90)
  1. It is the position of DEA that the obtaining of certain information by non-practitioners is vital to fairly assess the likelihood of an employee committing a drug security breach. The need to know this information is a matter of business necessity, essential to overall controlled substances security. In this regard, conviction of crimes and unauthorized use of controlled substances are activities that are proper subjects for inquiry. It is, therefore, assumed that the following questions will become a part of an employer's comprehensive employee screening program:
      a. Within the past five years, have you been convicted of a felony or within the past two years have you been convicted of any misdemeanor or are you presently formally charged with committing a criminal offense? (Do not include any traffic violations, juvenile offenses, or military convictions except by general court martial.) If the answer is yes, furnish details of conviction, offense, location, date, and sentence.
      b. In the past three years, have you ever knowingly used any narcotics, amphetamines, or barbiturates other than those prescribed to you by a physician? If the answer is yes, furnish details.
  2. Advice—An authorization in writing that allows inquiries to be made of courts and law enforcement agencies for possible pending charges or convictions must be executed by a person who is allowed to work in an area where access to controlled substances clearly exists. A person must be advised that any false information or omission of information will jeopardize his or her position with respect to employment. The application for employment should inform a person that information furnished or recovered as a result of any inquiry will not necessarily preclude employment but will be considered as part of an overall evaluation of the person's qualifications. The maintaining of fair employment practices, the protection of the person's right of privacy, and the assurance that the results of such inquiries will be treated by the employer in confidence will be explained to the employee.

E. Employee Responsibility to Report Drug Diversion (21 CFR 1301.91)
  1. Reports of drug diversion by fellow employees are not only a necessary part of an overall employee security program but also serve the public interest at large.
  2. It is the position of DEA that an employee who has knowledge of drug diversion from his or her employer by a fellow employee has an obligation to report such information to a responsible security official of the employer.
  3. The employer shall treat such information as confidential and shall take all reasonable steps to protect the confidentiality of the information and the identity of the employee furnishing the information.
  4. Failure to report information of drug diversion will be considered in determining the feasibility of continuing to allow an employee to work in a drug security area.
  5. The employer shall inform all employees concerning this policy.
  Note: The employer, as a DEA registrant, would be required to report any diversion under the DEA theft and loss rule.

XII. Disposal and Destruction of Controlled Substances (21 CFR 1317.01—1317.95)

A. Disposal of Stock Controlled Substances by Pharmacies
Pharmacies may dispose of controlled substances in one of the following manners:
1. Onsite Destruction
   a. Onsite destruction of controlled substances must be done using DEA Form 41 which now requires recording the method by which the drugs were destroyed and two signatures of employees who witnessed the destruction.
   b. Destruction must be done in compliance with all federal, state, and local laws and must render the controlled substances non-retrievable. Non-retrievable is defined as "to permanently alter any controlled substance's physical and/or chemical condition or state through irreversible means in order to render the controlled substance unavailable and unusable for all practical purposes."

   Note: The above procedure is difficult to execute. In addition to the difficulty of complying with other laws such as EPA laws, DEA has stated that methods such as mixing controlled substances with items such as kitty litter or coffee grounds and depositing in the garbage do not meet the non-retrievable standard. For these reasons, most pharmacies do not participate in onsite destruction.

   c. Any request for onsite destruction should be made to the DEA Special Agent in Charge (SAC) as follows:
      (1) The request shall be made by submitting one copy of DEA Form 41 to the SAC in the practitioner's area. DEA Form 41 shall list the controlled substance or substances which the registrant desires to dispose.
      (2) The SAC shall instruct the registrant to dispose of the controlled substance in one of the following ways:
         (a) By transfer to a registrant authorized to transport or destroy the substance;
         (b) By delivery to an agent of the DEA or to the nearest office of the DEA; or
         (c) By destruction in the presence of an agent of the DEA or other authorized person.
      (3) If a pharmacy is required regularly to dispose of controlled substances, the SAC may authorize the pharmacy to dispose of such substances using onsite destruction with DEA Form 41 without prior application in each instance. This may be done on the condition that the pharmacy keeps records of such disposals and files periodic reports with the SAC summarizing the disposals. The SAC may place such conditions as he or she deems proper on the pharmacy's procedures regarding the disposal of controlled substances.
2. Delivery to a DEA Registered Reverse Distributor
   a. This method of disposal is preferred and is simply a transfer from one DEA registrant (the pharmacy) to another DEA registrant (the reverse distributor).
   b. Because this is a transfer between registrants, a DEA Form 41 is not required. Instead the transfer must be documented by an invoice for Schedule III–V drugs and a DEA Form 222 for Schedule II drugs.
3. Returns or recalls may be delivered to:
   a. The registered person from whom it was obtained (e.g., wholesaler);
   b. The registered manufacturer of the drug; or
   c. Another registrant authorized by the manufacturer to accept returns or recalls on the manufacturer's behalf.

Notes

Note: These returns or recalls are also transfers between registrants and require an invoice or DEA Form 222.

B. Disposal of Controlled Substances Collected From Ultimate Users and Other Non-Registrants

This DEA rule allows a number of ways for ultimate users including patients, the personal representative of the patient in the event of the patient's death, and long term care facilities to dispose of unwanted controlled substances. These proposed collection methods are voluntary. A pharmacy or hospital is not required to serve as a collector. The methods include:

1. Authorized Collectors and Collection Receptacles
   a. Pharmacies and hospitals with an onsite pharmacy may amend their DEA registrations to be designated as an "Authorized Collector" and may also operate collection receptacles at long term care facilities.
   b. Collectors may allow ultimate users to deposit controlled substances into collection receptacles at the registered location (or at an authorized LTCF).
   c. The controlled substances may be commingled with noncontrolled substances.
   d. The deposited substances may not be counted, sorted, inventoried, or individually handled. This means that the pharmacist should not be handling these controlled substances on the patient's behalf. Patients must be the ones who place the controlled substances into the collection receptacles.
   e. LTCF staff may dispose of a patient's controlled substances into an authorized collection receptacle. Disposal into a collection receptacle must occur within three business days after the discontinuation of use by the patient.
   f. Collection receptacles must be in the immediate proximity (where they can be seen) from where controlled substances are stored (i.e., the pharmacy).
   g. Collection receptacles must be securely fastened to a permanent structure, locked, and securely constructed with a permanent outer container and a removable inner container.
   h. The inner liner must be waterproof, tamper-evident, removable, and able to be sealed immediately upon removal with no emptying or touching the contents or ability to view the contents. The inner liner also must have a permanent unique identification number that allows tracking.
   i. The inner liner must be removed by or under the supervision of at least two employees of the Authorized Collector.
   j. Sealed inner liners may not be opened, x-rayed, analyzed, or otherwise penetrated.
   k. Collectors can either destroy the collected drugs onsite, transfer the collected drugs for final disposal to a DEA registered reverse distributor, or contact the DEA Special Agent in Charge for assistance.
   Note: Most pharmacies do not have the capability to destroy collected drugs onsite.
   l. Texas law requires that pharmacies that dispense Schedule II controlled substances that are not authorized collectors and are not regularly accepting controlled substances for destruction are required to provide patients a notification on the safe disposal of controlled substances. *See Chapter G in this book.*
2. Mail-Back Programs
   a. Pharmacies and other authorized collectors may also conduct a mail-back program to allow patients to return unwanted controlled substances for destruction.

        b. Packages used in mail-back programs must:
            (1) Be nondescript and shall not have any markings or other information that might indicate that the package contains controlled substances;
            (2) Be waterproof, tamper-evident, tear-resistant, and sealable;
            (3) Be preaddressed with and delivered to the collector's registered address;
            (4) Include prepaid shipping costs;
            (5) Have a unique identification number to enable tracking; and
            (6) Include instructions for the user.
        c. A collector that conducts a mail-back program may only accept packages that the collector made available. If the collector receives a package that the collector did not make available, the collector must notify DEA within three business days of receipt.
    3. Collection Events
        a. Only law enforcement agencies can operate drug take-back events.
        b. Pharmacies and other entities may partner or co-sponsor such events with law enforcement.
C. Disposal of Controlled Substances of a Hospice Patient by Employees of the Hospice
    1. Federal legislation passed in late 2018 authorizes an employee of a qualified hospice program to handle controlled substances for the purposes of destruction that were lawfully dispensed to a person receiving hospice care.
    2. If the disposal is necessary because of the death of the hospice patient or the controlled substance has expired, a properly trained physician, physician assistant, nurse, or other employee licensed to perform medical or nursing services may handle and destroy the drugs.
    3. If the disposal is necessary because the plan of care has changed, the DEA registered physician of the person receiving hospice care must handle and destroy the drugs.
    4. The controlled substances must be destroyed onsite and in accordance with all federal, state, and local laws.
    5. Records of the destruction must be made in the patient's clinical record.
    Note: DEA is expected to provide further guidance and/or rules on these provisions.
D. Waste of Controlled Substances
    1. The disposal and destruction rules above apply to a pharmacy's inventory (A. above) and to controlled substances from patients (B. and C. above) but not to pharmaceutical waste.
    2. In a "Dear Practitioner" letter posted on DEA's website on October 17, 2014, DEA states: "... once a controlled substance has been dispensed by an institutional practitioner on the basis of an order for immediate administration to a patient at the registered location, the substance is no longer in the practitioner's inventory." For example, after a prefilled syringe or a single-dose vial or syringe is administered to the patient, any remaining substance in the syringe or vial is not required to be destroyed in accordance with DEA rules. However, the remaining substance should be destroyed in accordance with applicable federal, state, tribal, and local laws or regulations.
    3. Texas Class C pharmacy rules require records of waste of controlled substances to be witnessed and cosigned electronically or manually by another individual. (*See TSBP Rule 291.75.*)

XIII. Inspections
A. Controlled Premises
    1. Places where original or other records or documents required under FCSA are kept.

2. Places where persons registered under FCSA dispense controlled substances (i.e., pharmacies).
B. DEA can inspect and copy any record, report, or other document required under the FCSA.
C. DEA can inspect the pharmacy with regard to controlled substances.
D. DEA can inspect the inventory of controlled substances and obtain samples.
E. DEA may not inspect the following records without consent of the registrant:
1. Financial data.
2. Sales data.
3. Pricing data.

XIV. Records
A. Inventories
1. Initial inventory is required on the day or date the pharmacy opens for business.
2. Inventory of a newly scheduled drug or drug moved from one schedule to another must be made on the effective date of scheduling.
3. Biennial Inventory (must be maintained in the pharmacy for two years).
   a. Federal—FCSA requires inventory every two years on any date as long as within two years of the previous inventory (no longer required to be within six months of the previous inventory).
   b. Texas—TCSA also requires inventory every two years.
   c. Texas—TSBP rules require pharmacies to take an annual inventory of all controlled substances.
4. Count Requirements
   a. Exact count (or measure if liquid) necessary for all Schedule IIs.
   b. Estimate on Schedule IIIs, IVs, and Vs permitted unless container holds more than 1000 tablets or capsules. An exact count is necessary if container has been opened.
5. Inventory Format Requirements
   a. Name, address, and DEA number of the pharmacy.
   b. Date and time (opening or closing of business) when inventory taken.
   c. Signature of the pharmacist taking the inventory.
   d. Inventory maintained on file in the pharmacy for at least two years.
   e. List inventory of Schedule IIs must be separate from the inventory of Schedule III–V substances.
   f. Drugs in stock for commercial containers.
      (1) Name of drug.
      (2) Dosage form.
      (3) Number of units or volume.
      (4) Number of containers.
   g. Drugs in stock for compounding or awaiting disposal (destruction or return for credit).
      (1) Name of drug.
      (2) Total quantity.
      (3) Reason for being maintained.
6. Other Texas Inventory Requirements (*See Chapter E in this book.*)
   a. TSBP requires controlled substance inventories (other than initial inventories and change of pharmacist-in-charge inventories) to be signed by the pharmacist-in-charge and notarized within three days of the day the inventory is completed, excluding Saturdays, Sundays, and federal holidays.
   b. Although many pharmacies maintain a perpetual inventory of Schedule II controlled substances or all controlled substances, the FCSA,

TCSA, or TSBP does not require this type of inventory in most pharmacies. A perpetual inventory is only required in Texas by TSBP for:
- (1) Schedule II controlled substances in Class C (institutional) pharmacies.
- (2) All controlled substances stored at a remote location under the Remote Pharmacy Rules. (*See Chapter D in this book.*)
- (3) All controlled substances in Class C Ambulatory Surgical Centers (ASCs). (*See Chapter I in this book.*)
- (4) All controlled substances in Class F (Freestanding Emergency Medical Facility) pharmacies. (*See Chapter J in this book.*)

B. Record of Receipts
  1. Schedule IIs
     a. Copy 3 of DEA Form 222—Indicate date and number of containers received on DEA Form 222.
     b. TSBP rules also require the initials of the receiving pharmacist.
  2. Schedules III, IV, and V—Supplier's Invoice
     a. Must be readily retrievable on a separate invoice and filed separately or identified by an asterisk, redline, or some other identifiable manner such that it is easily distinguishable from all other records.
     b. Invoices must contain:
        (1) Name of controlled substance.
        (2) Dosage form and strength.
        (3) Number of units or volume in each container (e.g., 100-tablet bottle).
        (4) Quantity received (number of containers).
        (5) Date of actual receipt.
        (6) Name, address, and DEA registration number from which controlled substances were received.
        (7) TSBP rules also require the initials of the receiving pharmacist.
     c. Files of receipts.
        (1) Separate file for Schedule IIs.
        (2) File for Schedule IIIs, IVs, and Vs usually with commercial invoices.

C. Prescription Files—FCSA and TCSA both permit three methods of maintaining hard copies of controlled substance prescriptions in files as listed below. However, TSBP rules only permit one method of three separate files.
  1. Three Separate Files
     (Only method allowed by TSBP rules)
     a. File #1—Schedule II.
     b. File #2—Schedule III, IV, and V.
     c. File #3—Dangerous drugs and OTC drugs.
  2. Two Separate Files
     a. File #1—Schedule IIs only.
     b. File #2—Schedule III–V, dangerous drugs, and OTC drugs. Controlled substance prescriptions have to be stamped with red ink in the lower right corner of the prescription with a "C" (not less than 1 inch in height) so as to be readily retrievable from noncontrolled substances.
  3. Two Separate Files
     a. File #1—Schedule II–V with IIIs, IVs, and Vs stamped with red "C" so as to be readily retrievable from IIs.
     b. File #2—All dangerous drugs and OTC drugs.

  Note: If a pharmacy maintains records in a data processing system for prescriptions which permits identification by prescription number and retrieval of original documents by prescriber's name, patient's name, drug dispensed, and date filled, then the requirement to mark the hardcopy prescription with a red "C" is waived.

  4. These requirements apply to written prescriptions and verbal prescriptions that are reduced to writing by a pharmacist only. If a controlled substance

prescription is transmitted electronically, DEA requires that those electronic prescriptions be maintained electronically.

   D. Inpatient Distribution Records (Hospitals)
1. Medication orders (for individual patients).
2. "Proof-of-use" sheets for drugs that are administered to patients from floor stock.
3. Medication profile sheets (transcribed from a medication order).
4. Discharge, outpatient clinic, and emergency room prescriptions maintained as described in C. (Prescription Files) above.

   E. Central Recordkeeping—Invoices and financial data for controlled substances may be maintained at a central location provided:
1. Prior to the initiation of central recordkeeping, the pharmacy submits written notification by registered or certified mail to the divisional director of the Drug Enforcement Administration as required by Title 21, Code of Federal Regulations, 1304.04(a). Unless the registrant is informed by the divisional director of the DEA that permission to keep central records is denied, the pharmacy may maintain central records commencing 14 days after receipt of notification by the divisional director. (A copy of the notification to DEA must be sent to TSBP.)
2. The pharmacy maintains a copy of the notification to DEA.
3. The records to be maintained at the central recordkeeping location shall not include executed (used) DEA Forms 222, prescriptions, or controlled substance inventories. These documents shall be maintained at the pharmacy.

   F. Computerization of Prescription Information

A pharmacy is permitted to use a data processing system as an alternative method for the storage and retrieval of prescription order refill information for controlled substances in Schedules III, IV, and V. The computerized system must provide immediate retrieval (via CRT display or hardcopy printout) of original prescription order information for those prescription orders which are currently authorized for refilling. The information which must be readily retrievable from this type of system must include, but is not limited to, data such as the original prescription number, date of issuance of the prescription order by the physician, and full name and address of the patient; the physician's name and DEA registration number; the name, strength, dosage form, and quantity of the controlled substance prescribed; and the total number of refills authorized by the prescribing physician.

In addition, the system must provide immediate retrieval of the current refill history for Schedule III or IV controlled substance prescription orders that have been authorized for refill during the past six months and backup documentation to show that the refill information is correct. The backup documentation must be stored in a separate file at the pharmacy and be maintained for a two-year period from the dispensing date. Section 1306.22 of the Code of Federal Regulations (DEA) details specific requirements for a computerized recordkeeping system. These DEA requirements are incorporated in TSBP Rule 291.34E.

XV. Controlled Substance Prescriptions
   A. Persons Entitled to Prescribe Controlled Substances or Communicate Controlled Substance Prescriptions (determined by state law)
1. Practitioners—Must be registered with DEA.
   a. Physicians (MD or DO).
   b. Dentists.
   c. Podiatrists.
   d. Veterinarians.

  e. Optometric Glaucoma Specialists (limited authority). (*See Chapter C in this book.*)
 2. Mid-Level Practitioners—Must be registered with DEA.
  a. Practitioners other than a physician, dentist, veterinarian, or podiatrist who are authorized by state law to prescribe controlled substances.
  b. Examples may include nurse practitioners, nurse midwives, clinical nurse specialists, and physician assistants.
  c. Texas law allows in-state advanced practice registered nurses and physician assistants to prescribe controlled substances in Schedules III–V (and in certain practice settings Schedule II controlled substances) with some restrictions. (*See Chapter C in this book.*)
 3. Designated Agent
  a. An employee or agent of the practitioner is allowed to communicate a prescription to the pharmacist over the phone but is not allowed to authorize a prescription.
  b. Employees of a practitioner such as a physician assistant, nurse, or receptionist may be a designated agent.
  c. For several years DEA took issue with the ability of nurses or other persons at long term care facilities and other locations to communicate controlled substance prescriptions to pharmacies since they were not employees of the practitioner. In October 2010, DEA published a statement of policy specifying that a non-employee agent of the prescriber may perform the following activities:
   (1) Prepare a controlled substance prescription for the prescriber's signature.
   (2) Verbally communicate a C-III, C-IV, or C-V prescription to a pharmacy.
   (3) Transmit by facsimile a C-II prescription to a pharmacy if the patient is enrolled in hospice care or is a resident of a LTCF, in which case the faxed prescription serves as the original.
 Note: The policy does not permit any agent of the prescriber (employee or non-employee) to verbally communicate emergency C-II prescriptions to a pharmacist. It also states that for non-employees of the prescriber to qualify as an agent of the prescriber, there must be a formal written appointment of the agent by the prescriber. DEA provides a sample written appointment of agent in the federal register notice of this statement of policy. See 75 F.R. 61653 October 6, 2010.

B. Mandatory Electronic Prescriptions for Controlled Substances
 1. The Texas Legislature passed legislation in 2019 that mandates that prescriptions for controlled substances be issued electronically starting January 1, 2021. There are many exceptions to this requirement, and rules will need to be adopted by TSBP to implement this legislation. The information below is a summary of the parts of the the legislation (HB 2174) related to this requirement.
 2. Exceptions
  a. Written prescriptions may be valid if written on a Texas Official Prescription Form for the following:
   (1) Prescriptions written by veterinarians;
   (2) In circumstances in which electronic prescribing is not available due to temporary technological or electronic failure as prescribed by Board rule;
   (3) By a practitioner to be dispensed by a pharmacy located outside this state as prescribed by Board rule;

(4) When the prescriber and dispenser are in the same location or under the same license;
(5) In circumstances in which necessary elements are not supported by the most recently implemented national data standard that facilitates electronic prescribing;
(6) For a drug for which the United States Food and Drug Administration requires additional information in the prescription that is not possible with electronic prescribing;
(7) For a non-patient specific prescription pursuant to a standing order, approved protocol for drug therapy, collaborative drug management, or comprehensive medication management, in response to a public health emergency or in other circumstances in which the practitioner may issue a non-patient specific prescription;
(8) For a drug under a research protocol;
(9) By a practitioner who has received a waiver under Section 481.0756 of the Texas Controlled Substances Act from the requirement to use electronic prescribing;
(10) Under circumstances in which the practitioner has the present ability to submit an electronic prescription but reasonably determines that it would be impractical for the patient to obtain the drugs prescribed under the provisions for electronic prescriptions in a timely manner and that a delay would adversely impact the patient's medical condition; and
(11) A medication order written for a patient who is admitted to a hospital at the time the order is written and filled.

b. Emergency verbal prescriptions
(1) In an emergency as defined by Board rule, a pharmacist may fill a controlled substance prescription based on a verbal prescription.
(2) A designated agent of the prescriber may communicate the emergency verbal prescription.
Note: Although the Texas Controlled Substances Act appears to permit a designated agent to provide a verbal prescription for a Schedule II controlled substance in an emergency, DEA's position is that an emergency verbal Schedule II controlled substance prescription may not be provided by a designated agent. The order must come from the prescribing practitioner. See 75 Fed. Reg. 193 (Oct. 6, 2010).
(3) No later than the seventh day after an emergency verbal prescription was authorized by a practitioner, the practitioner shall cause an electronic prescription to be delivered to the dispensing pharmacy.

c. A dispensing pharmacist who receives a controlled substance prescription in a manner other than electronically is not required to verify that the prescription is exempt from the requirement that it be submitted electronically. The pharmacist may dispense a controlled substance pursuant to an otherwise valid written or verbal prescription.

3. Until the mandatory electronic prescription requirements go into effect, pharmacists should continue to follow existing rules for written, verbal, and electronic controlled substances including requirements for emergency verbal Schedule II prescriptions.

C. Manner of Issuance of Written Controlled Substance Prescriptions
1. Prescriptions may be prepared by the practitioner or his or her agent, but the prescription must be manually signed by the practitioner the same way he or she would sign a legal document. (TSBP rules require all written prescriptions to be manually signed by the practitioner; no rubber stamps are allowed.)

2. All prescriptions shall be dated and signed on the day the prescription is issued and bear:
   a. The full name and address of the patient.
   b. The drug name, strength, and dosage form.
   c. The quantity prescribed.
   d. The name, address, and DEA number of the practitioner.
   e. If for a Schedule II prescription to be filled at a later date, the earliest date on which a pharmacy may fill a prescription.
   f. Additional requirements for controlled substance prescriptions in Texas:
      (1) The quantity prescribed must be written numerically and as a word (e.g., Vicodin #20 (twenty)). If the quantity is not written as a word, the pharmacist should call to verify the quantity.
          Note: This is not required for electronic prescriptions.
      (2) Date of birth or age of the patient.
      (3) The practitioner's telephone number at the practitioner's usual place of business.
      (4) The intended use of the drug unless the practitioner determines the furnishing of this information is not in the best interest of the patient (required for all prescriptions in Texas, not just controlled substances).
3. Changing Information or Information Omitted From a Written Prescription
   a. Dual responsibility—Responsibility for the completeness of the prescription rests with both the prescriber and the pharmacist.
   b. The pharmacist may make informational changes or additions such as changing or adding the patient's address upon verification. Most other changes require contacting the prescribing practitioner.
   c. Schedule II prescriptions
      (1) A pharmacist may not change the following items on a Schedule II prescription:
          (a) Name of the patient.
          (b) Name of the drug.
          (c) Name of the prescribing physician.
          (d) Date of the prescription.
      (2) Any other item such as drug strength, dosage form, quantity, or directions for use may be changed provided the pharmacist:
          (a) Contacts the prescribing practitioner and receives verbal permission for the change and
          (b) Documents on the prescription that the change was authorized, the name or initials of the individual granting the authorization, and the pharmacist's initials.
   d. Schedule III–V written prescriptions—A pharmacist may add or change the patient's address upon verification without contacting the prescriber. As with Schedule II controlled substances, a pharmacist may add or change the dosage form, drug strength, drug quantity, directions for use, or issue date only after consultation with and agreement of the prescribing practitioner. Such consultations and corresponding changes should be noted by the pharmacist on the prescription. While DEA guidance suggests that a pharmacist may not change the name of the patient, name of the drug, name of the prescribing physician, and date on any controlled substance prescription, this is not an issue for Schedule III–V prescriptions. If a pharmacist needs to change the name of the patient, name of the drug prescribed, name of the prescribing practitioner, or the date on a Schedule III–V prescription, the pharmacist can

take a new verbal prescription from the prescriber rather than "changing" the original written prescription.
            e. Controlled substance prescriptions cannot be postdated; however, the FCSA and TCSA allow practitioners to issue multiple prescriptions for Schedule II drugs at one time under certain conditions. (*See Section XVI. in this chapter.*)
        4. Pharmacist Preparation of Prescription for Practitioner's Signature
            a. DEA does not allow pharmacists to prepopulate a controlled substance prescription with all required information and then fax or electronically send the prescription to a practitioner to be signed.
            b. This practice was commonly done when patients no longer had refills of prescriptions. However, in 2012 DEA clarified that a pharmacist cannot do this because he or she is not an agent of the practitioner.
            c. A pharmacist can communicate to a prescriber that a new prescription is needed, and this can be done via telephone, email, fax, etc. However, the pharmacist should not prepare the prescription for signature by the prescriber unless the pharmacy has been designated as an agent of the practitioner.
    D. Oral (Verbal) Prescriptions
        1. Controlled substance prescriptions for Schedule III, IV, or V drugs may be communicated to a pharmacist by a practitioner or his or her agent.
        2. Controlled substance prescriptions for Schedule II drugs generally cannot be communicated verbally except in the case of an emergency. (*See Section XVI. of this chapter.*)
        3. Rules for designated agents under Texas Controlled Substance Rules
            a. A practitioner may not designate as an agent another practitioner who is not a registrant.
            b. A designated agent must be:
                (1) A registered nurse licensed in Texas;
                (2) A vocational nurse licensed in Texas;
                (3) A physician assistant licensed in Texas; or
                (4) An employee located in the designating practitioner's office who is a member of the healthcare staff of the office.
            c. A practitioner shall maintain in the practitioner's usual place of business a current written list of persons designated as agents, and the practitioner shall provide the current list to all pharmacists who request it.
        4. DEA requires non-employee agents of practitioners who will communicate controlled substance prescriptions to be designated in writing. (*See A.3.c. above.*)
    E. Electronic Controlled Substance Prescriptions
        1. DEA issued an interim final rule effective June 1, 2010 that authorized electronic prescribing of controlled substances.
        2. The purpose of this rule was to prevent one person from granting access to an electronic prescription prescribing application or pharmacy application.
        3. Computer-generated prescriptions that are printed or faxed are not considered electronic prescriptions.
        4. Prescriber Requirements
            a. Must receive authentication credentials or digital signatures by federally recognized private credential service providers, credential authorities, or internal institutional credentialing authorities.
            b. Must receive permission to access electronic prescribing application using logical access controls involving two individuals, one of whom is a DEA registrant.

c. Once a prescriber has received appropriate credentials and has been granted access, the prescriber must sign the prescription using a two-factor authentication method. Prescribers must select from two of the following:
   (1) Something you have (hard token that is separate from the computer);
   (2) Something you know (user ID and password or PIN); or
   (3) Something you are (biometrics).
d. Agents may not be given access to the system or use two-factor authentication to sign prescriptions. However, agents can enter prescription information for later approval and authentication by prescribers.

5. Transmission of Electronic Controlled Substance Prescriptions
   a. Pharmacies may change the prescription to allow generic substitution.
   b. The prescription is not required to contain the patient's address when approved by the prescriber but must be added prior to transmission to the pharmacy.
   c. Other non-DEA required information may be added after approval but before transmission.
   d. Intermediaries may make formatting changes after transmission.

6. Pharmacy Requirements
   a. A pharmacy cannot process electronic prescriptions for controlled substances until its pharmacy application provider obtains a third-party audit or certification review that determines the application complies with DEA's requirements and the application provider gives the audit/certification report to the pharmacy.
   b. The system must be able to digitally sign and archive the controlled substance prescription or import and archive the record that the last intermediary signed.
   c. The system must electronically accept and store all of the information that DEA requires be annotated to document the dispensing of a prescription.
   d. The system must allow the pharmacy to limit access for the annotation, alteration, or deletion of controlled substance prescriptions to specific individuals or roles.
   e. The system must have an internal audit trail that documents whenever a prescription is received, altered, annotated, or deleted.
   f. The pharmacy must conduct an internal audit daily that identifies any potential security problems, and the system must generate a report for review by the pharmacy if a problem is identified.
   g. Pharmacy records must be backed up daily.
   h. Electronic prescription records must be kept electronically. No hard copy is required to be kept.

7. Audit Requirements—Prescriber and pharmacy systems must be audited by a third party for compliance with DEA requirements every two years or whenever the application is altered in a way that could affect its functionalities.

8. Guidance From DEA Website
   a. If a pharmacist receives a written prescription that was originally transmitted electronically, the pharmacist must check the pharmacy records to ensure that the electronic version was not received and the prescription dispensed. If both prescriptions were received, the pharmacist must mark one as void. The pharmacy is responsible for verifying that no controlled substances were dispensed pursuant to the electronic prescription prior to filling the written prescription.
   b. If a pharmacist receives a written prescription that indicates it was originally transmitted electronically to another pharmacy, the pharmacist

must check with the other pharmacy to determine whether the prescription was received electronically and dispensed. If the pharmacy that received the original electronic prescription had not dispensed the prescription, that pharmacy must mark the electronic version as void or cancelled. If the pharmacy that received the original electronic prescription dispensed the prescription, the pharmacy with the written prescription must not dispense the prescription and must mark the written prescription as void.
   9. The TCSA allows electronic controlled substance prescriptions as long as all DEA requirements are met.
   10. A comprehensive opioid bill passed by Congress in 2018 requires electronic prescriptions for all controlled substances for Medicare and Medicaid patients by 2021. There are several exceptions in the law where an electronic prescription will not be required. Texas law will require this for all controlled substance prescriptions effective January 1, 2021. *See B. above.*
F. Pharmacist Responsibilities—The "Corresponding Responsibility"
   1. For a controlled substance prescription to be valid, it must be issued for a legitimate medical purpose by an individual practitioner acting in the usual course of his or her professional practice.
   2. The responsibility for the proper prescribing and dispensing of controlled substances is upon the prescribing practitioner, and a corresponding responsibility rests with the pharmacist who fills the prescription.
   3. Under the "corresponding responsibility" doctrine, a pharmacist that fills an invalid controlled substance prescription that the pharmacist knows to be invalid has violated the FCSA, TCSA, and Texas Pharmacy Act. The knowledge requirement has been interpreted in case law to mean that a pharmacist either knew or should have known that the prescription was invalid. A pharmacist cannot simply claim that he or she had no knowledge that a prescription was invalid if a reasonable and prudent pharmacist would have known the prescription was invalid.
   4. "Red Flags"—Through enforcement actions, DEA and TSBP have identified a number of "red flags" that may alert a pharmacist to do further investigation as to the legitimacy of controlled substance prescriptions. TSBP Rule 291.29 on Professional Responsibility of Pharmacists includes many "red flags" related to controlled substance prescriptions. (*See Chapter E in this book.*) These include but are not limited to the following:
      a. Substantially identical prescriptions for the same controlled substances, potentially paired with other drugs, for numerous persons indicating a lack of individual drug therapy in prescriptions issued by the practitioner;
      b. Prescriptions by a prescriber that are routinely for controlled substances commonly known to be abused drugs, including opioids, benzodiazepines, muscle relaxants, psychostimulants, and/or cough syrups containing codeine, or any combination of these drugs;
      c. Prescriptions for controlled substances by a prescriber that contain non-specific or no diagnoses or lack the intended use of the drug;
      d. Prescriptions for controlled substances for the highest strength of the drug and/or for large quantities (e.g., monthly supply), indicating a lack of individual drug therapy in prescriptions issued by the practitioner;
      e. The controlled substance(s) or the quantity of the controlled substance(s) prescribed is/are inconsistent with the practitioner's area of medical practice;
      f. The Texas Prescription Monitoring Program indicates the person presenting the prescriptions is obtaining similar drugs from multiple

practitioners and/or that the person is being dispensed similar drugs at multiple pharmacies;
    g. Multiple persons with the same address present substantially similar controlled substance prescriptions from the same practitioner;
    h. Persons consistently pay for controlled substance prescriptions with cash or cash equivalents more often than through insurance; and
    i. Persons presenting controlled substance prescriptions are doing so in such a manner that varies from the manner in which persons routinely seek pharmacy services (e.g., persons arriving in the same vehicle with prescriptions from the same practitioner; one person seeking to pick up prescriptions for multiple others; and drugs referenced by street names).

G. Examples of Invalid Controlled Substance Prescriptions
1. A forged prescription issued by a person not licensed to prescribe.
2. A prescription issued for a narcotic-dependent person for the purpose of continuing his or her dependency.
3. A prescription issued for a fictitious person.
4. A prescription for a physician's office use (not written for a patient).
5. A prescription issued not in the usual course of the prescriber's medical practice (e.g., dentist prescribing hydrocodone for kidney stones).
6. A prescription issued for other than a legitimate medical purpose (e.g., amphetamines to keep a person awake such as truck drivers; anabolic steroids for athletic performance). (*See also TSBP Rule 291.29 in Chapter E of this book.*)

H. Self-Prescribing and Prescribing Controlled Substances for Family Members
1. DEA rules do not specifically address this practice, but all controlled substance prescriptions must be issued for a legitimate medical purpose and in the usual course of professional practice.
2. Texas Medical Board rules are stricter and state that it is grounds for discipline if a physician self-prescribes or prescribes dangerous drugs or controlled substances for family members or others where there is a close personal relationship without taking an adequate history, performing a proper physical examination, or maintaining records. There is an exception if the controlled substance prescription is for immediate use only (limited to a 72-hour supply). (*See Chapter C in this book.*)

I. Ryan Haight Online Pharmacy Consumer Protection Act of 2008 (Amendment to the FCSA)

The intent of this legislation was to address problems with Internet-based prescribing of controlled substance prescriptions and dispensing of such prescriptions by pharmacies. The bill includes the following provisions:
1. Bans delivery, distribution, or dispensing of controlled substances over the Internet without a "valid prescription."
2. A "valid prescription" is defined as a prescription that is issued for a legitimate medical purpose in the usual course of medical practice by a practitioner who has conducted at least one in-person medical evaluation of the patient.
3. Allows a "covering physician" to write a valid prescription at the request of a practitioner who has made an in-person or telemedicine examination within the previous 24 months and is temporarily unavailable to evaluate the patient.
4. In addition to the covering physician exception, the Act provides exceptions to the in-person medical evaluation for telemedicine, but the exceptions are narrow and haven't been useful to telemedicine practitioners. As part of a comprehensive opioid bill passed by Congress in late 2018, DEA is required

to issue regulations to provide a special DEA registration for telemedicine practitioners which may allow more controlled substance prescriptions issued via telemedicine to be valid.
5. Requires an online pharmacy to provide a 30-day notification to the U.S. Attorney General and state boards of pharmacy in any state where the online pharmacy plans to offer to sell, distribute, or dispense controlled substances.
6. Allows the attorney general of each state to bring a civil action in a federal district court to enjoin the actions of an online pharmacy or person which/who is operating in violation of the Act.
7. Creates website design requirements for online pharmacies.
8. Increases penalties for any unlawful distributors and dispensers of controlled substances, not just online pharmacies.

J. Dispensing Controlled Substances in Texas
   1. Delivering Controlled Substances (TCSA 481.074(m) and (n))
      a. A pharmacist may permit the delivery of a controlled substance to the person or address of the person authorized on the prescription to receive the controlled substance:
         (1) By an authorized delivery person;
         (2) By a person known to the pharmacist, a pharmacist intern, or the authorized delivery person; or
         (3) By mail.
      b. If a pharmacist permits delivery of a controlled substance under this Act, the pharmacist shall retain a record of:
         (1) The name of the authorized delivery person if delivery is made by that person;
         (2) The name of the person known to the pharmacist, pharmacist intern, or delivery person if delivery is made by that person; or
         (3) The mailing address to which the delivery was made if delivery is made by mail.
      c. A pharmacist may permit the delivery of a controlled substance to a person not known to the pharmacist, pharmacy intern, or the authorized delivery person without first requiring the identification of the person to whom the controlled substance is delivered if the pharmacist determines that an emergency exists and the controlled substance is needed for the immediate well-being of the patient. The pharmacist must maintain a record of the name, address, and date of birth or age of the person to whom the controlled substance is delivered.

   Note: J.1. above appears to require an identification of a patient when delivering controlled substances if the person is not known to the pharmacist but c. above provides an exception even when the pharmacist does not know the patient. While many pharmacies require identification of all patients when picking up controlled substance prescriptions, this is generally a best practice issue and is not specifically required by federal or Texas law. Pharmacists should use professional judgment when dispensing controlled substances to ensure that the prescriptions are being dispensed for legitimate medical purposes and to the correct patient.

   2. Prescriptions From Out-of-State Practitioners (not practitioners in Mexico or Canada)
      a. Schedule II—Texas pharmacies can only fill Schedule II controlled substances from a practitioner in another state if:
         (1) A share of the pharmacy's business involves the dispensing, delivery, or mailing of controlled substances;
         (2) The prescription is issued by a prescribing practitioner in the ordinary course of practice; and

(3) The prescription is filled in compliance with a written plan providing the manner in which the pharmacy may fill a Schedule II prescription issued by an out-of-state practitioner. The plan must be approved by TSBP.
   b. Schedule III–V—Texas pharmacies can fill Schedule III–V prescriptions from out-of-state practitioners pursuant to valid written, oral, faxed, or electronically (computer to computer) communicated prescriptions. However, Schedule III–V controlled substance prescriptions from out-of-state nurse practitioners or physician assistants are not valid in Texas and cannot be filled by Texas pharmacies.

XVI. Schedule II Prescriptions

Note: Several of the requirements below will no longer be applicable once the Texas requirements for mandatory electronic prescriptions go into effect. These changes are scheduled to occur on January 1, 2021. In the interim or in case that date gets postponed, pharmacists need to know the requirements for written, faxed, and verbal Schedule II prescriptions. Also, since there are several exceptions to mandatory electronic controlled substance prescriptions, the requirements for the Texas Official Prescription Form will still be in effect.

A. Written Schedule II Prescriptions
   1. Schedule II prescriptions may generally only be dispensed pursuant to a written prescription.
   2. Texas requires Schedule II prescriptions to be written on a Texas Official Prescription Form. (*See I. below.*)
B. Faxed Schedule II Prescriptions
   Faxed prescriptions for Schedule II drugs are generally treated the same as oral prescriptions and are, therefore, not valid for Schedule II prescriptions. However, the DEA and Texas allow faxed prescriptions to serve as the original prescription in the three limited situations below:
   1. Prescriptions faxed by a practitioner or practitioner's agent for a Schedule II narcotic controlled substance to be compounded for the direct administration to a patient by parenteral, intravenous, intramuscular, subcutaneous, or intraspinal infusion. (*See 21 C.F.R. 1306.11(e).*)
   Note: This provision is only for narcotic Schedule II controlled substances.
   2. Prescriptions faxed by a practitioner or practitioner's agent for a Schedule II controlled substance for a resident of a long term care facility. (*See 21 C.F.R. 1306.11(f).*)
   3. Prescriptions faxed by a practitioner or practitioner's agent for a Schedule II narcotic controlled substance for a patient enrolled in a hospice care program certified and/or paid for by Medicare or licensed by the state. (*See 21 C.F.R. 1306.11(g).*)
      a. This provision is only for narcotic Schedule II controlled substances.
      b. The practitioner or practitioner's agent must note on the prescription that the patient is a hospice patient.
      c. The patient need not be in a hospice facility and may be in a home-based program as long as he or she is enrolled in a hospice program.
C. Electronic Schedule II Prescriptions
   1. Schedule II prescriptions may be transmitted electronically so long as DEA requirements outlined in Section XV.E. of this chapter are met.
   2. A comprehensive opioid bill passed by Congress in 2018 will require electronic prescriptions for all controlled substances (including Schedule IIs) for Medicare and Medicaid patients by 2021. There are several exceptions in the law where an electronic prescription will not be required. Texas law

will require this for all controlled substance prescriptions (also with several exceptions) effective January 1, 2021.
- D. Emergency Verbal Prescriptions for Schedule II Drugs
  1. An "emergency situation" occurs when:
     a. Immediate administration of the controlled substance is necessary for the proper treatment of the intended ultimate user;
     b. No appropriate alternative treatment is available including the administration of a drug which is not a Schedule II; and
     c. It is not reasonably possible for the practitioner to provide a written prescription to be presented to the person dispensing the substance prior to the dispensing.
  2. Restrictions/Requirements of Emergency Dispensing of Schedule IIs
     a. The communication must be directly from the prescribing practitioner (not from an agent of the practitioner).
     b. The quantity of the drug dispensed is limited to an amount adequate to treat the patient during the emergency period.
     c. The verbal emergency prescription must be immediately reduced to writing by the pharmacist containing this information:
        (1) Full name, address, and age the of the patient;
        (2) Full name, address, and DEA number of the practitioner;
        (3) Date the verbal prescription was communicated to the pharmacist; and
        (4) Drug name, strength, quantity, and directions for use.
     d. The pharmacist should make a good faith effort to verify the identity of the prescriber if not known. The pharmacist should use the prescriber's DEA number and call the prescriber to verify the prescription.
     e. The practitioner must deliver a written prescription (Official Prescription Form in Texas) or a valid electronic prescription for the emergency quantity within seven days. A written prescription may be delivered in person or by mail. If mailed, it must be postmarked within a seven-day period. The prescription must have written on its face "Authorization for Emergency Dispensing."
     f. The pharmacist shall notify the nearest DEA office if the prescribing practitioner fails to deliver a written prescription. Failure of the pharmacist to notify DEA voids the pharmacist's authority to dispense the Schedule II drug without a written prescription of the practitioner. If the written prescription isn't received, both the pharmacist and practitioner have violated the Act.
     g. Upon receiving a written prescription, the pharmacist attaches the oral emergency prescription to the written prescription and files both in the Schedule II file.
     h. Upon receiving an electronic prescription, the pharmacist shall annotate the electronic prescription record with the original authorization and date of the emergency verbal or telephonically communicated prescription.
- E. Refills and Multiple Prescriptions for Schedule II Drugs
  1. Refills of Schedule II prescriptions are not permitted under any circumstances.
  2. Multiple Prescriptions for Schedule II Drugs
     a. DEA and Texas permit an individual practitioner to issue multiple prescriptions on the same day authorizing the patient to receive up to a 90-day supply of a Schedule II controlled substance provided the following conditions are met:
        (1) The individual practitioner properly determines there is a legitimate medical purpose for the patient to be prescribed the controlled substance, and the individual practitioner is acting in the usual course of professional practice;

(2) The individual practitioner writes instructions on each prescription or electronic prescription (other than the first prescription if the practitioner intends for that prescription to be filled immediately) indicating the earliest date on which a pharmacy may fill the prescription;

(3) The individual practitioner concludes that providing the patient with multiple prescriptions in this manner does not create an undue risk of diversion or abuse;

(4) The issuance of multiple prescriptions as described in this section is permissible under applicable state laws;

(5) The individual practitioner complies fully with all other applicable requirements under the FCSA, TCSA, and TPA; and

(6) Where a Schedule II prescription has been issued indicating that the prescription shall not be filled until a certain date, a pharmacist may not fill the prescription before that date.

    b. This 90-day limit for a Schedule II only applies when the prescriber is issuing multiple prescriptions for a Schedule II substance on the same day with instructions that some of the prescriptions are not to be filled until a later date. On a single prescription, there is no 90-day supply limit. Insurance plans may limit the amount that may be filled on a single prescription, and pharmacists should exercise caution in filling a Schedule II prescription for more than a 90-day supply. However, a single prescription for a Schedule II controlled substance may be legally written and filled for more than a 90-day supply.

F. Partial Filling of Schedule II Prescriptions
1. 72-Hour Rule
If a pharmacist is unable to fill the entire quantity called for on a Schedule II controlled substance prescription, a partial quantity may be provided so long as the remaining quantity is provided within 72 hours. If the remaining quantity is not or cannot be provided, the pharmacist must notify the prescribing practitioner.
2. 30-Day Rule
Both federal and Texas law allow partial fills of Schedule II controlled substances issued in writing or electronically (but not for emergency verbal prescriptions) to be dispensed for up to 30 days after the date the prescription was issued if such a request is made by the patient or the practitioner who wrote the prescription, and the total quantity dispensed in all partial fills does not exceed the total quantity prescribed. At the time of this book's publication, DEA had not yet modified its rules to implement this law.
3. 60-Day Rule—Patients in Long Term Care Facilities (LCTFs) and Terminally Ill Patients
    a. A prescription for a Schedule II controlled substance for a patient in a long term care facility (LTCF) or for a hospice patient with a medical diagnosis documenting a terminal illness may be filled in partial quantities for up to 60 days from the date the prescription was issued.
    b. How does the partial fill rule for LTCF or terminally ill patients work with the Texas requirement that Schedule II controlled substance prescriptions be filled within 21 days after the date issued? In this situation, the initial partial filling must occur within 21 days after the date the prescription was issued. Subsequently, the pharmacist would have 60 days to fill the remaining quantity of the prescription with partial fills. However, the partial fills must be completed within 60 days of the date when the prescription was issued, not the date of the initial partial fill.
    c. If there is any question whether a hospice patient may be classified as having a terminal illness, the pharmacist must contact the practitioner prior

to partially filling the prescription. Both the pharmacist and the practitioner have a corresponding responsibility to ensure that the controlled substance is for a terminally ill hospice patient or an LTCF patient.
- d. The pharmacist must record on the prescription (or electronic record if an electronic prescription) whether the patient is "a terminally ill hospice patient" or an "LTCF patient." A prescription that is partially filled and does not contain the notation "terminally ill" or "LTCF patient" shall be deemed to have been filled in violation of the Federal Controlled Substances Act.
- e. For each partial filling, the dispensing pharmacist shall record on the back of the prescription or electronic record (or on another appropriate record uniformly maintained and readily retrievable) the date of the partial filling, quantity dispensed, remaining quantity authorized to be dispensed, and the identification of the dispensing pharmacist. Prior to any subsequent partial filling, the pharmacist needs to determine that the additional partial filling is necessary.
- f. Information pertaining to current Schedule II prescriptions for patients in a LTCF or for hospice patients with a medical diagnosis documenting a terminal illness may be maintained in a computerized system.

G. Time Limit for Filling Schedule II Prescriptions
1. FCSA—There is no time limit for filling a single Schedule II prescription under the FCSA.
2. TCSA—The time limit in Texas for filling a Schedule II prescription is as follows:
    a. A Schedule II prescription must be filled within 21 days after the date issued. The day after a prescription is issued is considered day one (i.e., a prescription issued on February 1 must be filled by February 22).
    Note: The date issued is the date written or the date electronically prescribed.
    b. A Schedule II prescription issued to be filled at a later date must be filled within 21 days after the first date authorized to be filled rather than 21 days from the date issued. For example, if a Schedule II prescription is issued on May 5 with instructions not to fill until June 5, it must be filled by June 26. The day after June 5 (i.e., June 6) is considered as day one.

H. Quantity/Refill Limits and Treatment of Pain
1. Although insurance companies and some pharmacies instituted their own limits on the quantities of certain controlled substance prescriptions, until 2019 neither the FCSA nor the TCSA had any specific quantity limits for a single Schedule II (or any other schedule) controlled substance prescription. The exceptions to this are that advanced practice registered nurses and physician assistants in Texas are limited to only prescribing up to a 90-day supply (including refills) of a Schedule III–V controlled substance. (*See Chapter C. in this book.*) Additionally, there is a 90-day supply limit when a practitioner issues multiple Schedule II prescriptions to be filled at a later date.
2. Effective September 1, 2019, the following limitations apply to prescriptions for opioid drugs:
    Note: The limitations are for opioid drugs. Not all opioid drugs are Schedule II controlled substances and not all Schedule II controlled substances are opioids.
    a. For the treatment of acute pain, a practitioner may not:
        (1) Issue a prescription for an opioid in an amount that exceeds a 10-day supply or
        (2) Provide for a refill of an opioid.
    Note: The Texas Medical Board interprets this section to mean a practitioner may write an opioid prescription for up to 10 days without a refill. However, the patient may see the practitioner in a follow-up appointment and receive

another opioid prescription for up to 10 days. The law does not limit how many times this may occur. See guidance issued by the Texas Medical Board on August 30, 2019.
- b. "Acute pain" means the normal, predicted, physiological response to a stimulus such as trauma, disease, and operative procedures. Acute pain is time limited. The term does not include:
  - (1) Chronic pain;
  - (2) Pain being treated as part of cancer care;
  - (3) Pain being treated as part of hospice or other end-of-life care; or
  - (4) Pain being treated as part of palliative care.
3. The quantity and refill limits above do not apply to a prescription for an opioid approved by the FDA for the treatment of substance addiction that is issued by a practitioner for the treatment of substance addiction.
4. Because it may be difficult for a pharmacist to know if a prescription for greater than a 10-day supply or with refills is for acute pain, the law provides that a dispenser is not subject to criminal, civil, or administrative penalties for dispensing or refusing to dispense a controlled substance under a prescription that exceeds the limits provided above.
5. It is a pharmacist's responsibility to determine that a controlled substance prescription is legitimate, and it is also a pharmacist's responsibility to ensure that patients obtain appropriate pain medication for their condition. Just because a prescription for a narcotic medication contains a large quantity or exceeds recommended doses, it does not necessarily mean the prescription is not legitimate.
6. TSBP Position Statement on Treatment of Pain can be found at *http://www.tsbp.state.tx.us/files_pdf/Pain_Policy.PDF*.
7. DEA Policy Statement on Dispensing Controlled Substances for the Treatment of Pain can be found at *http://www.deadiversion.usdoj.gov/fed_regs/notices/2006/fr09062.htm*.
8. Pain Management Clinics in Texas must be certified by the Texas Medical Board.
   - a. The names of certified Pain Management Clinics are posted on the Texas Medical Board's website. The website also lists Pain Management Clinics whose certificates have been revoked.
   - b. Individual physicians do not need to be certified to prescribe controlled substances. Just because a prescription is written by a practitioner employed by a certified Pain Management Clinic does not ensure that the prescription is authentic and is valid. The pharmacist must use his or her professional judgment to determine if the prescription was issued in the usual course of professional practice and for a legitimate medical purpose.

I. TCSA Required Notification on Safe Disposal of Schedule II Controlled Substances
   1. Unless exempted by 2. or 3. below, a pharmacy that dispenses a Schedule II controlled substance prescription must provide the patient a notification on the safe disposal of controlled substances. The notice must provide information on locations where Schedule II controlled substances are accepted for safe disposal or provide an Internet address specified by the Board that provides a searchable database of such locations. *See Board Rule 315.3(a)(5) for details.*
   2. A pharmacy that is registered with DEA as an "authorized collector" of controlled substances and regularly accepts controlled substances for safe disposal does not have to provide the notice in 1. above.
   3. A pharmacy that provides to the patient at the time of dispensing and at no cost to the patient either a mail-in pouch for surrendering unused controlled substances or chemicals to render any unused controlled substances unusable or non-retrievable does not have to provide the notification in 1. above.

J. Texas Official Prescription Form
1. Unless a specific exemption applies, all written Schedule II controlled substance prescriptions in Texas must be written on an official prescription form.
   a. The original "official" prescription form was a triplicate prescription issued by the Texas Department of Public Safety (DPS).
   b. In 2000, the official prescription forms became single copies with security features to prevent fraud.
   c. On September 1, 2016, the official prescription program and the prescription monitoring program were transferred from DPS to TSBP. The forms are still single forms but are now issued by TSBP.
   d. On September 1, 2018, TSBP issued new official prescription forms with additional security features. Effective June 1, 2019, all versions of the official prescription form issued prior to September 1, 2018 are invalid.
2. Accountability (TSBP Rule 315.13)
   a. A practitioner who obtains from the Board an official prescription form is accountable for each numbered form.
   b. A practitioner may not:
      (1) Allow another practitioner to use the individual practitioner's official prescription form;
      (2) Pre-sign an official prescription blank;
      (3) Postdate an official prescription; or
      (4) Leave an official prescription blank in a location where the practitioner should reasonably believe another could steal or misuse a prescription.
   c. While an official prescription blank is not in immediate use, a practitioner may not maintain or store the book at a location so the book is easily accessible for theft or other misuse.
   d. A practitioner must account for each voided official prescription form by sending the voided form to the Board.
3. Official Prescription Format
   a. Each official prescription form has a unique control number which is tied to the prescriber's name and DEA number.
   b. The forms come preprinted with the full name, address, and phone number of the prescriber and the prescriber's DEA number.
4. Security Features—Schedule II official prescription forms issued by the Texas State Board of Pharmacy are blue and contain the State of Texas seal. The prescription forms contain the following safety features:
   a. Control number—This number is located in the uppermost portion of the form just above the line for the patient's name and is unique for each prescription form. This number must be reported in the record transmitted when a Schedule II prescription is filled.
   b. Pantograph—This is a security feature that produces the word "VOID" multiple times on the face of the prescription form when someone attempts to copy or scan the prescription. If this feature is missing, the prescription form is not a valid official prescription.
   c. Thermochromic ink—This feature is found on the front of the prescription form as the symbol Rx. Applying heat or vigorously rubbing the area between the thumb and forefinger will cause the Rx symbol to disappear briefly and then reappear. If any other results are obtained when rubbing the thermochromic ink area, the prescription form should be considered suspect.
   d. Watermark—The seal for the State of Texas appears as a watermark on the face of the prescription and is visible from either side in regular light. Without this feature, the prescription form is not considered valid.

5. Prescriber's Information to Complete Official Prescription Form
   a. Date prescription is issued and earliest fill date if applicable.
      Note: The earlier versions of the form issued by DPS had a preprinted space for the earliest fill date, but the new forms issued by TSBP do not have this feature. This change means a prescriber who wishes to indicate an earlier fill date must write that information manually on the prescription.
   b. Name of patient (or animal owner).
   c. Address of patient (or animal owner).
   d. Species if an animal.
   e. Age of patient.
   f. Drug prescribed.
   g. Quantity—Numerically and written as a word (not required to be written as a word if an electronic prescription).
   h. Drug dosage.
   i. Instructions for use.
   j. Intended use of the drug unless the practitioner determines the information is not in the best interest of the patient.
   k. Signature of the prescriber.
6. Pharmacist's Responsibilities (TSBP Rule 315.5)
   a. Upon receiving a properly completed prescription form, a dispensing pharmacist must:
      (1) Ensure the date the prescription is presented is no later than 21 days after the date of issuance;
      (2) If multiple prescriptions are issued by the prescribing practitioner allowing up to a 90-day supply of Schedule II controlled substances, ensure each prescription is neither dispensed prior to the earliest date intended by the practitioner nor dispensed beyond 21 days from the earliest date the prescription may be dispensed;
      (3) Enter the date dispensed and the pharmacy prescription number and sign the prescription where indicated;
      (4) Indicate whether the pharmacy dispensed to the patient a quantity less than the quantity prescribed; and
      (5) Enter the following information if different from the prescribing practitioner's information:
         (a) The brand name or, if none, the generic name of the controlled substance dispensed or
         (b) The strength, quantity, and dosage form of the Schedule II controlled substance used to prepare the mixture or compound.
   b. The prescription presented for dispensing is void, and a new prescription is required if the prescription is presented more than 21 days after issuance or more than 21 days after any earliest dispense date.
7. Only One Prescription Per Form
   a. Official Prescription Forms are valid for prescriptions for all controlled substances. However, they are only required for Schedule II controlled substances.
      Note: TSBP does not recommend prescribers use the official form for Schedule III–V controlled substance prescriptions because pharmacies are not required to transmit the control number of those prescriptions. This practice would result in the control number remaining "open" or "not used." TSBP has confirmed that a non-Schedule II controlled substance prescription written on an official form is valid and may be filled. (See TSBP FAQs issued October 2018 on TSBP website.)
   b. If a physician has written a prescription for a Schedule II drug and another lower schedule (Schedule III, IV, or V) drug or a dangerous

drug, the pharmacist can cross out the non-Schedule II and transfer it to a pharmacy prescription pad as follows:
   (1) Dispense and file the Schedule II prescription and make sure the non-Schedule II drug is marked out.
   (2) Fill the non-Schedule II prescription as a verbal prescription, transfer it to a pharmacy prescription pad, and file it with Schedule III–V prescriptions.
8. Electronically Transmitting Controlled Substance Prescription Information From the Pharmacy to TSBP
   Schedule II prescription information must be transmitted to TSBP by the next business day after the prescription is completely filled. (*See Section XVIII.C. below.*)
9. Exceptions to the Use of an Official Prescription Form (When an official prescription form is NOT required)
   a. Hospital inpatient medication orders for patients admitted to a hospital, hospital clinic, hospital emergency room, licensed ambulatory surgical center, surgical suite in a dental office, or veterinary medical school.
   b. Hospital inpatients requiring an emergency quantity of a Schedule II drug upon release from the hospital.
      (1) Limited to a seven-day supply or minimum amount needed until patient can obtain access to a pharmacy, whichever is less.
      (2) Must be in an appropriately labeled container.
      (3) Must be dispensed by the hospital pharmacy while the patient is still admitted.
   c. Persons receiving treatment with a Schedule II drug from a member of a life flight helicopter medical team, emergency medical ambulance crew, or a paramedic/emergency medical technician.
   d. Persons receiving treatment with a Schedule II drug while an inmate in a correctional facility operated by the Texas Department of Criminal Justice.
   e. Animals admitted to an animal hospital including animals that are residents of zoos, wildlife parks, exotic game ranches, wildlife management programs, or state or federal research facilities.
   f. Administration of a Schedule II drug from a long term care facility's emergency kit.
   g. Therapeutic optometrists administering topical ocular cocaine as permitted under the Texas Optometry Act. (*See Chapter C in this book.*)
   h. Prescriptions from out-of-state practitioners but only if the pharmacy has submitted a plan which has been approved by TSBP.
   i. Electronic Schedule II prescriptions.

XVII. Schedule III, IV, and V Prescriptions

Note: Several of the requirements below will no longer be applicable once the Texas requirements for mandatory electronic prescriptions go into effect which is scheduled to occur January 1, 2021. In the interim or if that date gets postponed, pharmacists need to know the requirements for written, faxed, and verbal Schedule III–V prescriptions.

A. Schedule III, IV, and V Prescriptions
   1. Written Prescriptions
      a. All Schedule III and Schedule IV drugs require a prescription with the same federal requirements as for Schedule II prescriptions.
      b. Some Schedule V drugs may be available without a prescription. However, because Texas laws are stricter than federal law, there are no commercially available Schedule V products that can be sold without a prescription in Texas. (*See B. below.*)
   2. Verbal (telephonic) Prescriptions and Fax Prescriptions (either from a fax machine or computer generated by a practitioner or his or her agent)

a. Handled just like verbal or fax prescriptions for dangerous drugs.
b. May not be dispensed after six months from date of issuance.
c. Faxed prescriptions may serve as the original prescription for Schedule III, IV, and V products as long as the faxed prescription is manually signed by the practitioner. If the fax has a computer-generated signature, it is not valid and must be treated as an electronic prescription and meet those requirements.
3. Electronic Prescriptions (computer to computer)
   a. Schedule III, IV, and V prescriptions may be transmitted electronically so long as DEA requirements outlined in Section XV.D. of this chapter are met.
   b. A comprehensive opioid bill passed by Congress in 2018 will require electronic prescriptions for all controlled substances for Medicare and Medicaid patients by 2021. There are several exceptions in the law where an electronic prescription will not be required.
4. Refills
   a. Both federal and state law limit refills of Schedule III and Schedule IV prescriptions to five full refills within six months from the date of initial issuance if authorized by the practitioner.
   b. Federal law does not apply this restriction to Schedule V products. However, Texas law does apply the five refills in a six-month limitation to Schedule V products in addition to Schedule III and Schedule IV products.
   c. After five authorized refills of the full quantity prescribed are dispensed or after expiration of six months from date of issuance (whichever comes first), the prescription is not refillable. A new prescription is required for additional quantities.
   d. If fewer than five refills were authorized on the original prescription, additional refills may be authorized on the original prescription if the total of all refills does not exceed the five-refill limit or extend beyond the six-month period.
   e. Each refill is recorded on the back of the prescription with the pharmacist's initials and the date filled if the pharmacy is maintaining manual records or the refill must be recorded in the pharmacy's computer system.
   f. If a patient wants the original quantity increased, the pharmacist must obtain the prescriber's permission to generate a new prescription.
   g. DEA does not allow pharmacists to prepopulate a prescription for controlled substances with all required information and then fax or electronically send the prescription to a practitioner to be signed. (*See Section XV.C.4. in this chapter.*)
   h. Texas laws and rules permit emergency refills of controlled substances in Schedules III–V under specific circumstances. (*See Chapter G in this book.*)
   i. Automatic refills—TSBP rules permit pharmacies to implement automatic refill programs for controlled substance prescriptions in Schedules IV and V but not those in Schedule III.
   j. Emergency refills—TCSA and TSBP permit emergency refills of Schedule III–V prescriptions in certain situations. (*See Chapter G in this book.*)
5. Partial Filling
   a. Each partial filling must be recorded manually on the back of the prescription with the date, pharmacist's initials, and quantity or electronically in the pharmacy's computer system.
   b. The prescription order and dispensing of all refills must be within the six-month limit, and the total quantity dispensed cannot exceed the total quantity authorized on the prescription.

6. Transfers Between Pharmacies of Prescription Information for Schedule III–V Controlled Substances for Refill Purposes
   a. Under federal and Texas law, prescription information for Schedule III–V controlled substances may be transferred between pharmacies only one time. Once a Schedule III–V prescription has been transferred, all remaining refills must be obtained from the new pharmacy.
   b. There is an exception for pharmacies sharing a real-time, online database. Both federal and Texas law allow pharmacies that electronically share a real-time, online database to transfer a Schedule III–V prescription more than one time up to the maximum number of refills permitted by law (five times/six months) and the number of refills authorized by the prescriber.
   c. The transfer of controlled substance prescription information between pharmacies is for "refill purposes" only. (*See 21 CFR 1306.25.*) Therefore, a pharmacy may not transfer a controlled substance prescription that it has received but has not yet filled.
   Note: By policy, DEA has made an exception to this rule for controlled substance prescriptions that have been received by a pharmacy electronically. In the preamble to Notice of Proposed Rulemaking (73 FR 36750 (June 27, 2008)) and again in the Interim Final Rule on Electronic Prescriptions for Controlled Substances (75 FR 16268 (March 31, 2010)), DEA stated that it is acceptable for a pharmacy to transfer (or forward) an original unfilled electronic prescription for a controlled substance to another pharmacy. In later correspondence to the National Association of Boards of Pharmacy in 2017, DEA reiterated this policy and stated that this exception also applies to all electronic controlled substance prescriptions including Schedule II drugs. Since this procedure is allowed only by DEA policy, some pharmacies may choose not to allow this practice. Pharmacists should follow the policy of the pharmacy where they work regarding this procedure.

B. OTC Sale of Schedule V Products Under FCSA and TCSA
Note: By policy, TSBP is not enforcing this part of the law since all commercially available Schedule V products in Texas require a prescription. (See 4. below.) For example, TSBP will not inspect pharmacy records pertaining to Schedule V OTC Requirements listed below.
   1. Both federal and Texas laws allow certain Schedule V drugs to be provided under the direction of a pharmacist. After the pharmacist has completed his or her responsibilities, the actual cash transfer and delivery of the drug may be done by a non-pharmacist employee.
   2. Quantity and Dosage Unit Restrictions
      a. Cannot sell more than 8 oz. (240 cc) or 48 dosage units of any controlled substance containing opium.
      b. Cannot sell more than 4 oz. (120 cc) or 24 dosage units of any other controlled substance (i.e., codeine).
      Note: In Texas, a prescription is required for any codeine-containing product.
      c. Cannot sell more than 48 dosage units of any controlled substance containing opium.
      d. Cannot sell more than 24 dosage units of any other controlled substance.
   3. Other Requirements
      a. Sale to the same person is limited to once within 48 hours. A pharmacy cannot sell to the same patient within 48 hours.
      b. Purchaser has to be at least 18 years of age.
      c. Identification is necessary for proof of age.

d. Transaction must be recorded in a bound record book including:
      (1) Name and address of purchaser.
      (2) Name and quantity of controlled substance.
      (3) Date of purchase.
      (4) Name or initials of pharmacist (pharmacist must enter).
   e. Records must be kept by pharmacy for two years.
4. Texas Restrictions
   a. All codeine-containing products require a prescription in Texas. Even if they are Schedule V, they cannot be sold using the procedure in B. above.
   b. Most of the opium-containing Schedule V anti-diarrheal products have been removed from the market. Also, because the maximum opium concentration for a Schedule V product under Texas law is stricter than the federal limit, any such products would likely be a Schedule III product in Texas.
5. Conclusion—There are no commercially Schedule V products available that can be sold in Texas using the procedures outlined in B.1.-4. above.

XVIII. Texas Prescription Program for Controlled Substances (Texas Prescription Monitoring Program)

A. Overview and History
   1. As part of Ross Perot's "Texans' War on Drugs" legislative package, the Texas Prescription Program was created by the Texas Legislature in 1982 to monitor Schedule II controlled substance prescriptions. It included:
      a. A required triplicate prescription form for all Schedule II prescriptions and
      b. Reporting of all Schedule II prescriptions dispensed by pharmacies.
   2. The intent of the original legislation was to reduce drug diversion of Schedule II controlled substances from four sources:
      a. Patients "shopping" different prescribers;
      b. Prescribers with non-therapeutic prescribing patterns;
      c. Pharmacies with non-therapeutic dispensing patterns; and
      d. Forged prescriptions.
   3. In 2008, the program was expanded to include monitoring of Schedule III–V controlled substances. Although no special prescription forms are required for Schedule III–V drugs, pharmacies are required to electronically report dispensing of all controlled substance prescriptions including refills.
   4. In 2016, responsibility for the Official Prescription Form Program and Prescription Monitoring Program was transferred from the Department of Public Safety to the Texas State Board of Pharmacy.
B. Texas Prescription Monitoring Program (PMP)
   1. The Texas PMP collects prescription dispensing data on all Schedule II, III, IV, and V controlled substances dispensed by a pharmacy in Texas or to a Texas resident from an out-of-state pharmacy.
   2. Wholesale distributors also must report to the PMP the distribution of all Schedule II, III, IV, and V controlled substances to persons in Texas.
   3. The PMP is designed to assist pharmacists and physicians in identifying patients who may be getting prescriptions for controlled substances from multiple physicians or having prescriptions filled by multiple pharmacies.
   4. All approved PMP users have access to an advanced analytics and patient support tool called NarxCare. In addition to the existing PMP functionality, NarxCare aggregates and analyzes prescription information from providers and pharmacies and presents visual, interactive information, as well as advanced analytic insights, machine learning risk scores, and more to help physicians, pharmacists, and care teams provide better patient safety and

outcomes. NarxCare also provides tools and resources that support patients' needs and connects them to treatment when appropriate.

5. Effective March 1, 2020, practitioners (other than veterinarians) and pharmacists must check the PMP to review the patient's controlled substance history before prescribing or dispensing opioids, benzodiazepines, barbiturates, or carisoprodol. The dispensing pharmacist of a prescription shall be responsible for the review of the PMP database prior to dispensing the prescription, unless the pharmacy has designated another pharmacist whose identity has been recorded in the pharmacy's data processing system as responsible for PMP review.
    a. This check is not required if it is clearly indicated on the prescription record that the patient has been diagnosed with cancer, sickle cell disease, or is receiving hospice care.
    b. This check is also not required if the practitioner or pharmacist is unable to access the PMP after making and documenting a good faith effort to do so.
6. If a pharmacist uses a pharmacy management system that integrates data from the PMP, a review of the pharmacy management system with the integrated data shall be deemed compliant with the review of the PMP database requirement.
7. The Texas State Board of Pharmacy's contracted vendor for the PMP program is Appriss, Inc. and access is through the PMP AWARxE portal which can be found at the TSBP website.
8. Access to the PMP is restricted. *See TCSA Section 481.076 for details.*
    a. Pharmacists and pharmacist interns, pharmacy technicians, or pharmacy technician trainees acting at the direction of a pharmacist who are inquiring about a recent Schedule II, III, IV, or V prescription history of a particular patient may access the PMP to inquire about their own patients or own dispensing history.
    b. State regulatory boards also have access for purposes of investigating license holders or monitoring potentially harmful prescribing or dispensing patterns.
    c. A person who is authorized to access the PMP may only do so using that person's assigned identifier (i.e., login and password) and may not use the assigned identifier of another person.
    d. Unauthorized access or use of PMP information is a criminal misdemeanor and a violation of the TCSA, the Texas Pharmacy Act, and Board rules.
    e. A patient or a patient's parent or legal guardian, if the patient is a minor, may request a copy of his or her prescription record in the PMP, including a list of persons who have accessed that record, if a completed patient data request form and any supporting documentation required by the Board is submitted to the Board.
9. Notifications and Red Flags
    a. The PMP system identifies prescribing practices that may be potentially harmful and patient prescription patterns that may suggest drug diversion or drug abuse. The system sends electronic notifications to prescribers or dispensers indicating a potential harmful prescribing pattern or practices that may indicate drug diversion or abuse may be occurring.
    b. TSBP has also developed a list of "red flags" including behavior that suggests drug diversion or drug abuse may be occurring. Pharmacists who observe such behavior should access the PMP for such patients. These red flags can be found under Professional Responsibility of Pharmacists, TSBP Rule 291.29(f). (*See Chapter E in this book.*)

10. The Board shall establish a PMP Advisory Committee to make recommendations regarding information submitted to the Board and access to that information including recommendations for:
    a. Operational improvements to the electronic system that stores the information including implementing best practices and improvements that address system weaknesses and workflow challenges;
    b. Resolutions to identified data concerns;
    c. Methods to improve date accuracy, integrity, and security and to reduce technical difficulties; and
    d. The addition of any new data set or service to the information submitted to the Board or the access to that information.
11. The Texas PMP program is also part of the National Association of Boards of Pharmacy's PMP Interconnect® program which facilitates the transfer of PMP data across state lines. With over 40 states participating, this program provides the means for physicians and pharmacists to more easily identify patients with prescription drug abuse and misuse problems, especially if those patients are crossing state lines to obtain drugs.
12. The Texas PMP vendor provides an integration option to pharmacies and prescribers called PMP Gateway. This option allows a streamlined clinical workflow for pharmacies and prescribers. The integration eliminates the need for pharmacies and providers to log in separately to the PMP. Instead, the prescriber's electronic health record (EHR) system or the pharmacy's management system automatically initiates a patient query and returns the patient's controlled substance prescription record directly within the provider's EHR or pharmacy management system. However, not all systems can be integrated.

C. Electronically Transmitting Controlled Substance Prescription Information From the Pharmacy to TSBP
    1. Dispensing information must be transmitted to TSBP through the PMP Clearinghouse. Detailed information on how this is done through the AWARxE PMP Clearinghouse can be found at TSBP's PMP website *https://www.pharmacy.texas.gov/PMP/*.
    2. Pharmacies may transmit more frequently. However, they are required to transmit controlled substance dispensing information to TSBP no later than the next business day after the date the prescription is dispensed.
    Note: The reporting requirement applies after the controlled substance prescription is completely filled in cases where a partial fill is made.
    3. Although it is normally done automatically by a pharmacy's software program, it is still the pharmacist's responsibility to make sure that the following prescription information is transmitted to TSBP for all controlled substance prescriptions dispensed:
        a. The official prescription control number;
        b. The prescriber's DEA registration number;
        c. The patient's (or the animal owner's) name, age (or date of birth), and address (including city, state, and zip code);
        d. The date the prescription was issued and filled;
        e. The NDC number of the controlled substance dispensed;
        f. The quantity of the controlled substance dispensed;
        g. The pharmacy's prescription number; and
        h. The pharmacy's DEA registration number.
    4. If a pharmacy does not dispense any controlled substance prescriptions during a period of seven consecutive days, the pharmacy must send a report to the Board indicating that the pharmacy did not dispense any controlled substance prescriptions during that period, unless the pharmacy has obtained a waiver or permission to delay reporting to the Board.

5. A pharmacy must electronically correct dispensing data submitted to the Board within seven business days of identifying an omission, error, or inaccuracy in previously submitted dispensing data.

XIX. Methadone and Treatment of Narcotic Dependence
A. Generally, a physician may prescribe methadone or any other narcotic for a patient for analgesic purposes only. A narcotic-dependent patient who is to be or is being maintained or detoxified cannot receive a narcotic prescription order for this purpose. Narcotic prescriptions are only valid for treating pain.
B. Narcotic Treatment Programs
1. The administering and dispensing (but not prescribing) of narcotic drugs listed in any schedule to a narcotic-dependent person for detoxification or maintenance treatment are only permissible by a narcotic treatment program registered with DEA and FDA and licensed in Texas by the Texas Commission on Alcohol and Drug Abuse. These programs must also possess a permit issued by the Texas Department of Health. However, the Drug Addiction Treatment Act of 2000 (DATA) does allow office-based physicians to apply for a waiver to prescribe certain Schedule III–V drugs for opioid dependence. (*See C. below.*)
2. Maintenance treatment means the dispensing for a period in excess of 21 days of a narcotic drug in the treatment of an individual for dependence upon heroin or other morphine-like drugs.
3. Short-term detoxification treatment means the dispensing for a period not in excess of 30 days of a narcotic drug in decreasing doses to an individual to alleviate adverse physiological or psychological effects. These effects occur due to withdrawal from the continuous or sustained use of a narcotic drug. The goal of short-term detoxification treatment is to bring the individual to a narcotic drug-free state within 30 days.
4. Long-term detoxification treatment means the dispensing for a period in excess of 30 days but not in excess of 180 days of a narcotic drug in decreasing doses to an individual to alleviate adverse physiological or psychological effects. These effects occur due to withdrawal from the continuous or sustained use of a narcotic drug. The goal of long-term detoxification treatment is to bring the individual to a narcotic drug-free state within 180 days.
5. Only four individuals employed by the narcotic treatment program can dispense or administer narcotics to the patients: (1) the licensed physician, (2) a registered nurse under the direction of the licensed physician, (3) a licensed practical nurse under the direction of the licensed physician, or (4) a pharmacist under the direction of the licensed physician.
6. A physician who is not part of a narcotic treatment program may administer (not prescribe) narcotic drugs to an addicted individual on a daily basis for no more than a three (3)-day period to relieve that individual's acute withdrawal symptoms while the physician makes arrangements to enroll the individual in a narcotic treatment program. This treatment cannot last more than three (3) days and may not be renewed or extended.
7. A hospital that has no narcotic treatment program on the premises or a physician who is not part of a treatment program may administer narcotics to a drug-dependent individual for either detoxification or maintenance purposes if the individual is being treated in the hospital for a condition other than the addiction (i.e., surgery). It is assumed that the physician or hospital staff will not take advantage of this situation and detoxify or maintain a drug-dependent person who has sustained a very minor injury or illness which would not prevent the person from going to a registered narcotic treatment program.
C. Office-Based Treatment of Opiate Dependence
1. The Drug Addiction Treatment Act of 2000 allows for the treatment of opiate dependence from a physician's office with less restrictive controls than for

Schedule II drugs. The law allows specially trained physicians to prescribe certain narcotic Schedule III–V drugs to treat opiate dependence through a risk management program which includes close monitoring of drug distribution channels.
2. A practitioner authorized to issue prescriptions to treat opiate dependence under the Act is given a Drug Addiction Treatment Act of 2000 (DATA 2000) waiver identification code or "X" number. The "X" number of the practitioner must be on the prescription in addition to the practitioner's DEA registration number. Pharmacists can confirm a practitioner's waiver status on the Substance Abuse and Mental Health Services Administration (SAMHSA) website.
3. Authorized practitioners (sometimes called DATA 2000-waived practitioners) may treat 30, 100, or 275 patients at any one time, dependent on individual authorization from SAMHSA. Physicians who submitted the notification for initial authorization at least one year prior may submit a second notification of the need and intent to increase the patient limit from 30 patients up to 100 patients. Upon authorization by SAMHSA, DEA will issue a new DEA certificate of registration with a business activity code to identify whether the physician is authorized to treat 30 or 100 patients. To increase access to treatment, physicians who have had authorization to treat 100 patients for at least one year may apply for authorization to treat 275 patients if specific eligibility criteria are met.
4. Drugs approved under the act are Subutex® (buprenorphine) and Suboxone® (buprenorphine/naloxone combination). Subutex® is used for treatment while Suboxone® is used for maintenance therapy. These drugs, both Schedule III controlled substances, are available in sublingual form and may be dispensed by a pharmacy upon a prescription from a qualified practitioner.
5. The Comprehensive Addiction and Recovery Act of 2016 (CARA) expanded prescribing privileges for these products to treat opioid use disorder to Advanced Practice Registered Nurses (APRNs) and Physician Assistants (PAs) until October 1, 2021. APRNs and PAs must complete 24 hours of training to obtain a DATA 2000 waiver and can initially treat up to 30 patients. SAMHSA has indicated it intends to initiate rulemaking to allow APRNs and PAs who have prescribed at the 30-patient limit to apply for a waiver to prescribe for up to 100 patients.

Note: The Texas Board of Nursing and the Texas Medical Board have agreed that the supervising physician for any APRN or PA that prescribes these buprenorphine-containing products must also be a DATA 2000-waived practitioner.

XX. State and Federal Methamphetamine Controls
A. The Comprehensive Methamphetamine Control Act of 1996 and the Methamphetamine Anti-Proliferation Act of 2000 were passed by Congress in response to concerns over the illegal manufacturing of methamphetamines. The laws increased penalties for trafficking and manufacturing methamphetamines and attempted to control the distribution of certain over-the-counter precursor chemicals used to manufacture methamphetamines. The laws and regulations set forth registration requirements, recordkeeping, and reporting requirements for sales involving significant quantities of these precursor chemicals called List 1 chemicals. The law creates "threshold" amounts for single retail transactions involving list chemicals that trigger these requirements. Included as List 1 chemicals are ephedrine, pseudoephedrine, and phenylpropanolamine.

Note: A number of states have enacted even stricter laws and regulations on precursor chemicals. As usual, the stricter law must be followed.

B. Current Federal and Texas Law on Scheduled Listed Chemicals

The Combat Methamphetamine Epidemic Act of 2005 law was passed by Congress in 2006 to further control the sale of OTC products containing precursor chemicals used in the illicit manufacturing of methamphetamine. The law classifies all products (including multiple ingredient products) containing ephedrine, pseudoephedrine, and phenylpropanolamine as "scheduled listed chemical products." Products containing a "scheduled listed chemical" are subject to the following requirements:

1. Display Restrictions—Although the products may be sold by any retailer, covered products must be placed behind a counter (not necessarily a pharmacy counter) or in a locked cabinet if located on the selling floor,

   Note: Texas law specifies a locked cabinet must be within 30 feet of and in a direct line of sight from a pharmacy counter (if in a pharmacy) or a sales counter staffed by an employee of the establishment (if in a retail establishment that is not a pharmacy).

2. A retail establishment that is not a licensed pharmacy must obtain a Certificate of Authority from the State Department of Health Services to sell ephedrine, pseudoephedrine, and norpseudoephedrine products.

3. Retail Sales Limits
   a. Both Texas and federal law limit sales of covered products to an individual to 3.6 grams of base product per day and 9 grams of base product per 30 days.
   b. The amount of base product varies depending on the salt form of the drug involved (i.e., pseudoephedrine HCL vs. pseudoephedrine sulfate).
   c. For pseudoephedrine HCL, the retail daily sales limit of 3.6 grams is as follows:
      (1) 146 of the 30 mg tablets
      (2) 73 of the 60 mg tablets
      (3) 36 of the 120 mg tablets
   d. For pseudoephedrine HCL, the 30-day retail sales limit of 9 grams is as follows:
      (1) 366 of the 30 mg tablets
      (2) 183 of the 60 mg tablets
      (3) 91 of the 120 mg tablets

4. Product Packaging—Covered products (other than liquids including gel caps) must either be in blister or unit-dose packaging.

5. Logbook Requirements
   a. A retailer must maintain an electronic or written logbook that identifies the products by name, quantity sold, names and addresses of purchasers, and dates and times of sales.
   b. There is an exception for the logbook requirement for individual sales of a single "convenience" package of less than 60 mg of pseudoephedrine.
   c. A purchaser must present a photo identification issued by a state or federal government, sign the logbook, and enter his or her name, address, and date and time of sale.
   d. A retailer must verify that the name entered in the logbook corresponds to the customer identification.
   e. There are privacy protections for information in the logbooks which will be further detailed in regulations.
   f. If information from the logbook is provided to law enforcement in good faith, then the retailer is immune from civil liability claims.
   g. The Methamphetamine Production Prevention Act of 2008 made it easier for pharmacies to comply with these requirements by allowing for electronic signature capture and electronic logbooks.

6. Real-Time Electronic Logging System
    a. Prior to completing the sale of a product containing ephedrine, pseudoephedrine, or norpseudoephedrine, business establishments (including pharmacies) in Texas must submit a record of the sale to a real-time electronic logging system, including the name and date of birth of the person making the purchase, the address of the purchaser, the date and time of the purchase, the type of identification displayed by the person, the identification number, and the item and number of grams purchased.
    b. A real-time electronic logging system communicates with systems in other states to ensure that the purchase does not violate state or federal law regarding the purchase of those substances.
    c. An employee of a business establishment may override such a system to permit a prohibited sale only if the employee has a reasonable fear of imminent bodily harm or death from the person attempting to make the purchase.
7. Employee Training and Self-Certification
    a. Employers must self-certify that they:
        (1) Train employees who deal directly with customers to ensure they understand the requirements of the law;
        (2) Maintain training records;
        (3) Enforce sales limits;
        (4) Keep scheduled products behind the counter or in a locked cabinet; and
        (5) Maintain a written or electronic logbook.
    b. All distributors of listed chemicals may only sell listed chemicals to entities that are registered with the DEA or that are included on the self-certification list on the DEA's website.
8. Mail Service Limitations
    a. Mail service companies must confirm the identity of purchasers.
    b. Sales are limited to 7.5 grams per 30-day period.
9. Mobile Retail Vendors ('flea markets")
    a. Product must be placed in a locked cabinet.
    b. Sales are limited to no more than 7.5 grams of base product per customer per 30 days.
10. There is no age restriction under the federal act, but Texas law requires purchasers to be 16 years or older.

XXI. Online Resources
A. DEA Forms
The Drug Enforcement Administration (DEA) has available selected reports and applications required by the Federal Controlled Substances Act on the DEA website at *www.deadiversion.usdoj.gov*. The following forms are currently available:

DEA Form	Description
41	Registrants' Inventory of Drugs Surrendered
106	Report of Theft or Loss of Controlled Substance
161	Application for Permit to Export Controlled Substances
189	Application for Individual Manufacturing Quota
224	A Renewal Application for Registration—Retail
225	New Application for Registration—Wholesale
225	A Renewal Application for Registration—Wholesale
236	Controlled Substances Import/Export Declaration
250	Application for Procurement Quote for Controlled Substances
357	Application for Permit to Import Controlled Substances

363 New Application for Registration—Narcotic Treatment Program
363 A Renewal Application for Registration—Narcotic Treatment Program
486 Import/Export Declaration—Chemical
510 New Application for Registration—Chemical
510 A Renewal Application for Registration—Chemical

The forms are available in PDF format, so it will be necessary to have Adobe Acrobat or Adobe Acrobat Reader installed on the pharmacy's computer. Two versions of each form are available:
1. An interactive version, which will allow the user to complete the form online and print it on his or her printer for signature and mailing and
2. A blank form, which can be printed and completed manually.

The DEA recommends completing forms online to reduce errors.

B. *DEA Pharmacist's Manual*

The DEA Office of Diversion Control publishes a guidebook outlining the major provisions of the Federal Controlled Substances Act and regulations impacting the practice of pharmacy.

The Manual can be downloaded at *http://www.deadiversion.usdoj.gov/pubs/manuals/index.html*.

C. Questions and Answers

The DEA Office of Diversion Control website contains several question and answer documents that can assist pharmacists. It may be accessed at *http://www.deadiversion.usdoj.gov/faq/index.html*.

Summary of Major Differences Between Federal Controlled Substances Act (FCSA) and Texas Controlled Substances Act (TCSA) and Texas Pharmacy Act and Rules

I. **Codeine and Opium Products**
   A. Codeine-Containing Products
      1. FCSA—Allows OTC "exempt" sales of Schedule V products containing codeine.
      2. TCSA—Does not allow OTC "exempt" sales of Schedule V products containing codeine.
   B. Opium-Containing Products
      1. FCSA—Maximum amount for Schedule V = 100 mg/100 ml.
      2. TCSA—Maximum amount for Schedule V = 50 mg/100 ml.
      3. Any product containing more than 50 mg/100 ml of opium in Texas would be Schedule III or Schedule II (depending on the amount).

II. **Schedule V Controlled Substance Prescriptions**
   A. FCSA—Refills not limited to 5 refills/6 months
   B. TCSA—Refills limited to 5 refills/6 months

III. **Schedule II Controlled Substances**
   A. Special official prescription form required in Texas
   B. Time limit for filling Schedule II prescriptions
      1. FCSA—No time limit.
      2. TCSA—21 days after the date issued or the first date authorized to be filled if multiple prescriptions are issued on the same day with the instruction not to fill until a later date.

IV. **Automatic Refills**
   A. FCSA—Not addressed
   B. TSCA—Not addressed
   C. TSBP—Allows pharmacies to implement automatic refill programs for controlled substances in Schedules IV and V but not Schedule III

V. **Inventories**
   A. FCSA—Required biennially (every 2 years)
   B. TCSA—Required biennially (every 2 years)
   C. TSBP—Required annually (every year) and includes a requirement that most inventories be signed by the pharmacist-in-charge and notarized within three days of the day the inventory is taken, excluding Saturdays, Sundays, and federal holidays
   D. Perpetual Inventory Requirements
      1. Required for Schedule II controlled substances in Class C (institutional) pharmacies.
      2. Required for all controlled substances in remote pharmacies (*see Rule 291.20*).
      3. Required for all controlled substances in Class C Ambulatory Surgical Centers (ASCs). (*See Chapter I in this book.*)
      4. Required for all controlled substances in Class F-FEMCF (Freestanding Emergency Medical Care Facility) pharmacies. (*See Chapter J in this book.*)

VI. **Security**
   A. FCSA—Controlled substances may be stored in a secure cabinet that is locked or by dispersal throughout the noncontrolled drug stock to deter theft.
   B. TCSA—Same requirements but TSBP rules specifically require Class C (institutional), Class C-S (institutional preparing sterile products), Class C-ASC

(Ambulatory Surgical Center), and Class F-FEMCF (Freestanding Emergency Medical Care Facility) pharmacies to have locked storage for Schedule II controlled substances.

VII. Records
   A. Prescription Records
      1. Federal—Three options allowed:
         a. Two files—One with all controlled substances; one with all noncontrolled substances.
         b. Two files—One with Schedule II controlled substances; one with all other prescriptions (Schedule III–V and noncontrolled substances).
         c. Three files as required by TSBP (*see below*).
      2. Texas—TSBP requires three separate files for storage of controlled substance prescriptions; no other options are allowed.
         a. File 1—Schedule II prescriptions.
         b. File 2—Schedule III–V prescriptions.
         c. File 3—Dangerous drugs and other noncontrolled prescriptions (OTC).
   B. Invoices—Texas
      Invoices of controlled substances received by a pharmacy in Texas must have the initials of the pharmacist and the actual date of receipt recorded on the invoice.
      Note: In Class C-ASC (Ambulatory Surgical Center) pharmacies and Class F-FEMCF (Freestanding Emergency Medical Care Facility) pharmacies, invoices of dangerous drugs and controlled substances must be initialed by the person actually receiving the drugs since a pharmacist may not be present to initial the invoice.

VIII. Prescription Requirements
   A. Quantity and Refill Limits for Controlled Substances
      1. FCSA—No quantity limit on single prescription.
      2. TCSA—No refills and 10-day supply limit for opioid prescriptions for acute pain.
   B. Mandatory Electronic Prescriptions for Controlled Substances
      1. FCSA—Not required.
      2. TCSA—Required effective March 1, 2021 (with exceptions).
   C. Prescription quantity must be written out in Texas (e.g., #20 (twenty)) for written prescriptions.
   D. Delivered prescriptions must record either the name of the authorized delivery person, the person known to the pharmacist, the intern, the delivery person, or the address if mailed.
   E. Intended use is required on a prescription in Texas (required on all prescriptions); however, prescriber can opt out.
   F. Name and quantity of drug are required on all prescriptions in Texas.

IX. Methamphetamine Controls (e.g., pseudoephedrine)
   A. Display Restrictions
      1. Federal law requires a locked cabinet.
      2. Texas law specifies a locked cabinet within 30 feet of and in a direct line of sight from a pharmacy counter staffed by an employee of the establishment.
   B. Age
      1. Federal law—No age requirement.
      2. Texas law—Requires purchaser to be 16 years or older.
   C. Texas law requires nonpharmacy retailers to obtain a Certificate of Authority from the Texas Department of State Health Services.
   D. Texas law requires confirming legality of sale through a real-time electronic logging system.

CHAPTER B HIGHLIGHTS
Federal Controlled Substances Act (FCSA)
and
Texas Controlled Substances Act (TCSA)

1. The FCSA is administered by the Drug Enforcement Administration (DEA), and the TCSA is administered by the Texas Department of Public Safety (DPS) and the Texas State Board of Pharmacy (TSBP).
2. Federal Versus State Law—The more stringent law or regulation must be followed in all cases unless the two cannot consistently stand together. In that case, the state law must yield to the federal law.
3. Controlled substances are classified according to their abuse potential from Schedule I products (have the highest abuse potential and no accepted medical use) to Schedule V products (the lowest level of abuse potential).
4. Scheduled Listed Chemicals include products that contain ephedrine, pseudoephedrine, or phenylpropanolamine that may be marketed or distributed lawfully in the United States under the Food, Drug, and Cosmetic Act as nonprescription drugs. These products are subject to certain sales limitations and other restrictions.
5. Every person or firm who manufactures, distributes, dispenses, or performs various other functions with controlled substances must register with DEA.
6. A separate DEA registration is required for each general physical location where controlled substances are manufactured, distributed, imported, exported, or dispensed.
7. Compounding Controlled Substances
    a. DEA generally allows pharmacists to compound narcotic-controlled substances in Schedules II–V without being registered as a manufacturer if the concentration of the final solution, compound, or mixture is not greater than 20%.
    b. A prescription calling for compounding using a narcotic-containing product may be classified as Schedule II, III, or V depending on the concentration. The narcotic substance must be compounded in combination with one or more nonnarcotic therapeutic ingredients in recognized therapeutic amounts. (*See chart in this chapter for concentration limits for each schedule and for various narcotics.*)
8. Ordering Schedule II Controlled Substances
    a. Schedule II controlled substances must be ordered using a DEA Form 222 or electronically using an approved Controlled Substance Ordering System (CSOS).
    b. Only the registrant (individual, partner, or officer) may sign DEA Forms 222 unless that person has designated someone else to sign using a Power of Attorney.
9. Ordering With a Triplicate DEA Form 222
    a. Copy 1—Retained by a supplier (which may be a wholesaler selling to a pharmacy or a pharmacy selling to a practitioner or to another pharmacy).
    b. Copy 2—Sent by supplier to divisional DEA administrator.
    c. Copy 3—Retained by pharmacy (in separate file or attached to Schedule II invoices).
10. Ordering With a Single DEA Form 222
    a. Pharmacy makes a copy of the original DEA Form 222 before sending the original to the suppler.
    b. When the product arrives, the pharmacy records on its retained copy of DEA Form 222 the number of containers received and the date received for each item.
11. The 5% Rule—A pharmacy does not have to register with DEA as a distributor as long as the total quantities of controlled substances distributed during a 12-month period in which the pharmacy is registered do not exceed 5% of the total quantity of all controlled substances dispensed and distributed during that same 12-month period.
12. Storage of Controlled Substances in a Pharmacy—A pharmacy may store controlled substances in a secure cabinet that is locked or by dispersing the controlled substances throughout the noncontrolled drug stock to deter theft. However, Class C (institutional), Class C-S (institutional preparing sterile products), Class C-ASC

(Ambulatory Surgical Center), and Class F-FEMCF (Freestanding Emergency Medical Care Facility) pharmacies must have separate locked storage for Schedule II controlled substances.
13. A theft or significant loss of controlled substances must be reported to DEA and TSBP. DEA also recommends reporting the theft or loss to local police. DEA requires initial notification to be within one business day, but the Report of Theft or Loss (DEA Form 106) may be sent later after a determination of the extent of the theft or loss. These notifications should also be sent to TSBP.
14. Controlled Substance Disposal by a Pharmacy—Transfer to a reverse distributor is the preferred method of disposal and is simply a transfer from one DEA registrant (the pharmacy) to another DEA registrant (the reverse distributor).
15. Pharmacies and hospitals may amend their DEA registration to serve an "Authorized Collector" for unwanted controlled substances from patients. Special rules apply to authorized collectors.
16. TSBP rules require an annual inventory of all controlled substances, and the inventory must be signed by the pharmacist-in-charge and notarized within three days of the day the inventory is completed. This rule is stricter than the DEA requirement of a biennial (every 2 years) inventory.
17. TSBP rules require a perpetual inventory for Schedule II controlled substances in Class C (institutional) and Class C-S (institutional preparing sterile products) pharmacies and all controlled substances stored in Class C-ASC (Ambulatory Surgical Center) pharmacies, Class F-FEMCF (Freestanding Emergency Medical Care Facility) pharmacies, and at remote locations under the Remote Pharmacy Rules. (*See Chapter D in this book.*)
18. In Texas pharmacies, the original written prescriptions must be stored in three separate files:
    a. File #1—Schedule II.
    b. File #2—Schedule III, IV, and V.
    c. File #3—Dangerous drugs and OTC drugs.
19. Texas law allows advanced practice registered nurses and physician assistants in Texas to prescribe up to a 90-day supply of controlled substances in Schedules III–V (and in certain practice settings Schedule II controlled substances) with some restrictions. (*See Chapter C in this book.*)
20. Limitations on Opioid Prescriptions for Acute Pain
    a. For the treatment of acute pain, a practitioner may not issue a prescription for an opioid in an amount that exceeds a 10-day supply or provide for a refill.
    b. A pharmacist cannot be liable for dispensing or refusing to dispense a controlled substance under a prescription that exceeds the limits provided above.
21. Mandatory Electronic Prescriptions for Controlled Substances
    a. Prescriptions for controlled substances must be issued electronically starting January 1, 2021.
    b. There are many exceptions to this requirement.
22. A pharmacist may not change the following items on a Schedule II controlled substance prescription:
    a. Name of the patient.
    b. Name of the drug.
    c. Name of the prescribing physician.
    d. Date of the prescription.
23. Corresponding Responsibility—For a controlled substance prescription to be valid, it must be issued for a legitimate medical purpose by an individual practitioner acting in the usual course of professional practice. The responsibility for the proper prescribing and dispensing of controlled substances is upon the prescribing practitioner but a corresponding responsibility rests with the pharmacist who fills the prescription. Pharmacists should be aware of "red flags" that may indicate a prescription is not valid.
24. Schedule II Prescriptions
    Note: Some of these rules will change when mandatory electronic prescription requirements become effective on January 1, 2021.
    a. Must be written on a Texas Official Prescription Form or sent electronically and may not be taken verbally unless it is an emergency.

b. May not be refilled. However, DEA and Texas rules allow multiple prescriptions for Schedule II drugs to be issued the same day with instructions that they be filled at a later date under certain conditions including that the total quantity is not more than a 90-day supply.
c. A fax of the Texas Official Prescription Form may serve as the original Schedule II prescription only for
   (1) Narcotic-controlled substances to be administered by parenteral, intravenous, intramuscular, subcutaneous, or intraspinal infusion;
   (2) Any Schedule II controlled substance for residents of a long term care facility; or
   (3) Narcotic-controlled substances for a patient enrolled in a hospice care program.
d. Must be filled within 21 days after the date issued or the first date authorized to be filled.
e. May be sent electronically if both the prescriber's and pharmacy's computers systems meet all DEA security requirements.
f. If a pharmacy is unable to supply the full quantity ordered on a Schedule II prescription, a partial filling may be given as long as the remaining quantity is dispensed within 72 hours. On request of the patient or prescriber a partial fill may be provided for up to 30 days. If a prescription is for a long term care facility patient or terminally ill hospice patient, partial fills may be provided for up to 60 days.

25. Schedule III–V Prescriptions
    a. May be written, verbal, fax, or electronic (until January 1, 2021).
    b. May be refilled up to five times in six months.
    c. May be transferred to another pharmacy one time only unless the pharmacies share a common database.
    d. Prescriptions from out-of-state advanced practice nurses or physician assistants are not valid in Texas even if these nurses and physician assistants are registered with DEA and have prescriptive authority in their state. As a result, these prescriptions cannot be filled by Texas pharmacies. (*See this chapter and Chapter C.*)
26. Records of electronic controlled substance prescriptions must be maintained electronically.
27. Although federal law allows some Schedule V products to be sold without a prescription, all codeine products require a prescription under Texas law. There are no other commercially available Schedule V products that can be sold without a prescription in Texas.
28. The Texas Prescription Monitoring Program (PMP) is administered by the Texas State Board of Pharmacy (TSBP) and requires data regarding dispensing of controlled substances to be transmitted to TSBP no later than the next business day after a prescription is dispensed. Corrections to PMP reporting must be made electronically within seven business days of discovering an omission, error, or inaccuracy previously submitted. Checking the PMP will become mandatory for prescribers (other than veterinarians) and pharmacists when a prescription for an opioid, benzodiazepine, barbiturate, or carisoprodol is prescribed or dispensed starting March 1, 2020. There is an exception for cancer patients and patients in hospice care. Pharmacists are also required to check the PMP when specific patient/practitioner behavior is observed as required by TSBP rules.
29. A prescription written for methadone or any other controlled substance to treat addiction is not a valid prescription. The only exceptions are prescriptions written for Subutex® (buprenorphine) and Suboxone® (buprenorphine/naloxone combination) by specially trained practitioners under the Drug Addiction Treatment Act of 2000 and CARA 2016.
30. Nonprescription products containing certain List Chemicals such as pseudoephedrine must be placed behind a counter or in a locked cabinet, and they are subject to retail sales limits. Additionally, in Texas the purchaser must be at least 16 years of age.

CHAPTER C

CHAPTER 483 TEXAS HEALTH and SAFETY CODE

Texas Dangerous Drug Act (TDDA)

(Administered and Enforced by TSBP)

and Related Texas Laws and Rules

CHAPTER C

CHAPTER 483 TEXAS HEALTH and SAFETY CODE
Texas Dangerous Drug Act (TDDA)
(Administered and Enforced by TSBP)
and Related Texas Laws and Rules

Section 483.001 Definitions and Practice Issues
A. Dangerous Drug
   Any drug or device that is unsafe for self-medication and is not included in Schedules I through V or Penalty Groups I through IV of Chapter 481 (Texas Controlled Substances Act). The term includes a device or a drug that bears or is required to bear the legend:
   1. "Caution: Federal law prohibits dispensing without prescription" or "Rx only" or another legend that complies with federal law.
   2. "Caution: Federal law restricts this drug to use by or on the order of a licensed veterinarian."
B. Designated Agent
   1. A licensed nurse, physician assistant, pharmacist, or other individual designated by a practitioner to communicate prescription drug orders to a pharmacist;
   2. A licensed nurse, physician assistant, or pharmacist employed in a healthcare facility to whom the practitioner communicates a prescription drug order;
   3. A registered nurse or physician assistant authorized by a practitioner to carry out (or sign) a prescription drug order for dangerous drugs under the Medical Practice Act; or
   4. A person who is a licensed vocational nurse or has an education equivalent to or greater than that required for a licensed vocational nurse who is designated by the practitioner to communicate prescriptions for an advanced practice registered nurse or physician assistant authorized by the practitioner to sign prescription drug orders under Chapter 157 of the Medical Practice Act (Subtitle B, Occupations Code).
   Note: B.4. is included here for clarity although it is actually found in Section 483.022(f).
C. Pharmacy
   A facility at which prescription drug or medication orders are received, processed, or dispensed under this chapter, Chapter 481, and the Texas Pharmacy Act. The term does not include a narcotic drug treatment program that is regulated by Chapter 466, Health and Safety Code.
D. Practice of Pharmacy
   1. Provision of those acts or services necessary to provide pharmaceutical care.
   2. Interpretation and evaluation of prescription drug orders or medication orders.
   3. Participation in drug and device selection as authorized by law, drug administration, drug regimen review, or drug or drug-related research.
   4. Provision of patient counseling.
   5. Responsibility for:
      a. Dispensing of prescription drug orders or distribution of medication orders in the patient's best interest;
      b. Compounding and labeling of drugs and devices, except labeling by a manufacturer, repackager, or distributor of nonprescription drugs and commercially packaged prescription drugs and devices;

c. Proper and safe storage of drugs and devices; or
d. Maintenance of proper records for drugs and devices.
6. Performance of a specific act of drug therapy management for a patient delegated to a pharmacist by a written protocol from a physician licensed under the Texas Medical Practice Act.

E. Practitioner
A person licensed:
1. By the Texas Medical Board, State Board of Dental Examiners, State Board of Podiatry Examiners, Texas Optometry Board, or State Board of Veterinary Medical Examiners to prescribe and administer dangerous drugs;
2. By another state in a health field in which, under the laws of this state, a licensee may legally prescribe dangerous drugs;
3. In Canada or Mexico in a health field in which, under the laws of this state, a licensee may legally prescribe dangerous drugs; and
Note: Prescriptions from Canadian and Mexican practitioners can be legally filled only if the pharmacist has the original written prescription.
4. An advanced practice registered nurse or physician assistant to whom a physician has delegated the authority to prescribe or order a drug or device.

F. Prescription
An order from a practitioner or an agent of the practitioner designated in writing as authorized to communicate prescriptions or an order from an advanced practice registered nurse or physician's assistant to a pharmacist for a dangerous drug to be dispensed that states:
1. The date of the order's issue;
2. The name and address of the patient;
3. If the drug is prescribed for an animal, the species of such animal;
4. The name and quantity of the drug prescribed;
5. The directions for use of the drug;
6. The intended use of the drug unless the practitioner determines the furnishing of this information is not in the best interest of the patient;
7. The name, address, and telephone number of the practitioner at the practitioner's usual place of business, legibly printed or stamped; and
8. The name, address, and telephone number of the advanced practice registered nurse or physician assistant, legibly printed or stamped, if signed by an advanced practice registered nurse or physician assistant.

G. Scope of Practice of a Practitioner
A physician (D.O. or M.D.) may legally prescribe a drug to treat any disease or illness. Although a pharmacist should exercise caution, it is legal to fill a prescription written outside of a physician's specialty such as a hypertension medication written by an orthopedic surgeon or an oncologist. However, dentists, podiatrists, and veterinarians may only prescribe drugs used within their scope of practice. For example, a veterinarian cannot prescribe drugs for humans, and a prescription from a dentist for birth control pills would not likely be a valid prescription. Prescriptive authority for optometrists is restricted to specific drug classes. (*See Limited Independent Prescriptive Authority of Therapeutic Optometrists and Optometric Glaucoma Specialists in this chapter.*)

H. Self-Prescribing
Texas law does not specifically prohibit a physician from prescribing a dangerous drug or a controlled substance for himself or herself or for family members. However, the Texas Medical Board provides the following guidance to physicians:
1. It may be appropriate to undertake self-treatment or treatment of immediate family members in emergency situations. In addition, while physicians should not serve as primary or regular care providers for immediate family

members, there are situations in which routine care is acceptable for short-term, minor problems. There are significant risks for physicians who write prescriptions for controlled substances for themselves or immediate family members. Physicians should always document any treatment provided to avoid legal sanctions by the Texas Medical Board (TMB).
2. Texas Medical Board Rule 190.8(1)(M) states that inappropriate prescribing of dangerous drugs or controlled substances to oneself, family members, or others in which there is a close personal relationship is a violation of the Medical Practice Act. The rule states that (1) prescribing or administering dangerous drugs or controlled substances without taking an adequate history, performing a proper physical examination, and creating and maintaining adequate records and (2) prescribing controlled substances in the absence of immediate need (no more than 72 hours) constitute inappropriate prescribing.
I. Prescriptions may only be issued to a patient. Prescriptions may not be written "For Office Use." If a practitioner wishes to obtain drugs for office use, he or she may order the drugs from a wholesaler, a manufacturer, or a pharmacy and must use appropriate forms for ordering controlled substances (an invoice or DEA Form 222).
J. What happens to existing refills on a prescription if the prescriber dies? While there are no specific rules on this topic, it has been discussed by the Texas Medical Board and the Texas State Board of Pharmacy. Both have agreed that it is acceptable for the pharmacist to provide a 30-day supply to the patient and inform him or her to find a new doctor. However, DEA has not given an opinion on this, so pharmacists should use professional judgment if it is for a controlled substance. If there are no refills remaining on the prescription, it may be best to use the existing emergency refills rules. Documentation of these procedures by the pharmacist is crucial.

Section 483.002 Rules

The Texas State Board of Pharmacy may adopt rules to administer and enforce this chapter.

Section 483.003 Department of State Health Services Hearings Regarding Certain Drugs

A. The Texas Department of State Health Services may hold public hearings to determine if a dangerous drug is being abused.
B. Upon the Texas Department of State Health Services finding that a drug is being abused, dispensing of such drug may be limited to prescriptions issued by practitioners licensed in Texas or another U.S. state or territory (i.e., prescriptions from Canadian or Mexican practitioners cannot be dispensed).

Section 483.004 Commissioner of State Health Services

Emergency Authority Relating to Dangerous Drugs. If the Commissioner of State Health Services determines an immediate danger to public health exists as a result of dangerous drug prescriptions issued by practitioners in Canada or Mexico, emergency authority may be used to limit prescriptions to practitioners in Texas or other states of the United States.

Section 483.021 Determination by Pharmacist on Request to Dispense Certain Drugs

A. A pharmacist who is requested to dispense a dangerous drug under a prescription issued by a practitioner shall determine in the exercise of the pharmacist's professional judgment that the prescription is a valid prescription. A pharmacist may not dispense a dangerous drug if the pharmacist knows or should have known that the prescription was issued without a valid patient-physician relationship.

Note: This is similar to the corresponding responsibility for pharmacists for controlled substances.
   B. Therapeutic Optometrist
   A pharmacist who is requested to dispense a dangerous drug prescription issued by a therapeutic optometrist shall determine in the exercise of the pharmacist's professional judgment whether the prescription is for a dangerous drug that a therapeutic optometrist is authorized to prescribe under the Texas Optometry Act.

Section 483.022 Practitioner's Designation of Agent; Practitioner's Responsibilities
   A. A practitioner shall provide in writing the name of each designated agent.
   B. The practitioner shall maintain at the practitioner's usual place of business a list of the designated agents.
   C. The practitioner shall provide a pharmacist with a copy of the practitioner's written authorization for a designated agent on the pharmacist's request.
   D. A practitioner remains personally responsible for the actions of a designated agent who communicates a prescription to a pharmacist.
   E. This section does not relieve a practitioner from complying with the requirements of Subchapter A, Chapter 562, Occupations Code (relating to generic substitution).
   F. A practitioner may designate a person licensed as a licensed vocational nurse or has an education equivalent to or greater than a licensed vocational nurse to communicate prescriptions of an advanced practice registered nurse or physician's assistant.

Section 483.023 Retention of Prescriptions
Pharmacies must retain prescriptions for two years from the initial dispensing or the last date of refilling.

Section 483.024 Records of a Drug Acquisition or Disposal
The following persons shall maintain a record of each acquisition and each disposal of a dangerous drug for two years after the date of the acquisition or disposal:
   A. Pharmacies
   B. Practitioners
   C. Persons obtaining drugs for lawful research, teaching, or testing but not for resale
   D. Hospitals
   E. Manufacturers and wholesalers

Section 483.025 Inspections and Inventories
A person required to keep records of dangerous drugs shall:
   A. Provide records for inspection and copying.
   B. Allow the inventorying of drugs.

Section 483.041 Possession of Dangerous Drugs
   A. A person commits an offense if the person possesses a dangerous drug unless the person obtains the drug from a pharmacist acting in the manner described by Section 483.042A.1. below or from a practitioner as described by Section 483.042A.2. below.
   Note: This means the dangerous drug must be delivered by a pharmacist pursuant to a valid prescription and be appropriately labeled or, in limited situations, delivered by a practitioner. Delivery by a practitioner should only meet a patient's immediate needs (72-hour supply) or in rural areas where under specific circumstances physicians can dispense dangerous drugs.
   B. Except as provided by this chapter, a person commits an offense if the person possesses a dangerous drug for the purpose of selling the drug.

C. The following or their agents or employees may possess drugs if acting in the usual course of business or practice or in the performance of official duties:
  1. A pharmacy licensed by the Board (not pharmacist unless acting as an agent of the pharmacy).
  2. A practitioner: M.D., D.O., D.D.S., Podiatrist, Veterinarian, or Optometrist.
  3. A person who obtains a dangerous drug for lawful research, teaching, or testing but not for resale.
  4. A hospital that obtains a dangerous drug for lawful administration by a practitioner.
  5. An officer or employee of federal, state, or local government.
  6. A manufacturer or wholesaler licensed by the Commissioner of Health under Chapter 431 (Texas Food, Drug, and Cosmetic Act).
  7. A carrier or warehouseman.
  8. A Home and Community Support Services Agency (HCSSA) licensed under Chapter 142.
  9. A midwife who obtains oxygen or a dangerous drug for administration to a mother or newborn.
  10. A salvage broker or operator.
D. Offense: Illegal possession of dangerous drugs is a Class A misdemeanor.

Section 483.042 Delivery (Sale) or Offer to Deliver a Drug
A. It is unlawful for anyone to deliver a dangerous drug unless:
  1. Delivered by a pharmacist pursuant to:
     a. A prescription issued by a practitioner;
     b. A prescription issued by an advanced practice registered nurse (APRN) or physician assistant (PA) in compliance with the Medical Practice Act; or
     c. An original written prescription issued by a practitioner described in Section 483.001(12)(C) (i.e., a practitioner in Mexico or Canada).
  2. Delivered by:
     a. A practitioner in the course of practice or
     b. An advanced practice registered nurse (APRN) or physician assistant (PA) in the course of practice and pursuant to the Medical Practice Act.
B. Labeling of Container
  1. A pharmacist must attach a label to the immediate container. The label must contain the following information:
     a. Name and address of the pharmacy;
     b. Date dispensed;
     c. Prescription number;
     d. Name of the practitioner who prescribed the drug;
     e. Name of the patient and, if for an animal, the species of the animal; and
     f. Directions for the use of the drug.
  2. A practitioner, advanced practice registered nurse, or physician assistant must attach a label to the immediate container. The label must contain the following information:
     a. Name and address of the practitioner who prescribed the drug;
     b. Date dispensed;
     c. Name of the patient and, if for an animal, the species of the animal;
     d. Name of the practitioner who prescribed the drug; and
     e. Name, strength, and directions for the use of the drug.
C. Subsection A. above does not apply to the delivery or offer to deliver a dangerous drug to a person listed in Section 483.041(C) for use in the usual course of business or practice or the performance of official duties by the person (e.g., pharmacy, practitioner, TSBP, etc.).

D. The labeling provisions of B. do not apply to a dangerous drug prescribed or dispensed for administration to a patient who is institutionalized.
E. The offense of an illegal delivery (sale) is a state jail felony.

Section 483.043 Manufacture of a Dangerous Drug
A. It is unlawful to manufacture a dangerous drug unless so authorized.
B. An offense is a state jail felony.

Section 483.045 Forging or Altering Prescriptions
A. It is unlawful to:
   1. Forge a prescription or increase the prescribed quantity of a prescription (without a physician's authorization).
      Note: A pharmacist may increase the quantity of most dangerous drug prescriptions as permitted under the Texas Pharmacy Act Section 562.0545. (See Chapter D in this book.)
   2. Issue a prescription with a forged signature.
   3. Possess or obtain or attempt to obtain dangerous drugs:
      a. By a forged, fictitious, or altered prescription or
      b. By a fictitious or fraudulent telephone call.
B. The offense is a:
   1. Class B misdemeanor or
   2. Class A misdemeanor if the defendant has been previously convicted for a dangerous drug offense.

Section 483.046 Failure to Retain a Prescription
A. A pharmacist commits an offense if the pharmacist delivers a dangerous drug under a prescription and fails to retain the prescription.
B. The offense is a Class B misdemeanor or a Class A misdemeanor if previously convicted.

Section 483.047 Refilling a Prescription Without Authorization (Emergency Refills)
See Chapter G for detailed rules on emergency refills.

Section 483.048 Unauthorized Communication of Prescription
A. It is unlawful for a practitioner's agent to telephonically communicate a prescription unless the agent is designated as such in writing.
B. The offense is a:
   1. Class B misdemeanor or
   2. Class A misdemeanor if previously convicted.

Section 483.049 Failure to Maintain Records
A. A person commits an offense if the person is required to maintain a record under Section 483.023 (Retention of Prescription Records) or Section 483.024 (Records of Drug Acquisition or Disposal) and the person fails to maintain the record in the manner required by those sections.
B. The offense is a:
   1. Class B misdemeanor or
   2. Class A misdemeanor if previously convicted.

Section 483.050 Refusal to Permit Inspection
A. A person commits an offense if the person is required to permit an inspection under Section 483.025 and fails to permit the inspection.
B. The offense is a:
   1. Class B misdemeanor or
   2. Class A misdemeanor if previously convicted.

Section 483.073 Search Warrant
A peace officer may obtain a warrant to search for illegally possessed dangerous drugs.

Section 483.074 Seizure and Destruction
Dangerous drugs that are illegally manufactured, sold, or possessed may be seized and destroyed.

Note: Sections 483.101–483.107 below permit a physician to prescribe and a pharmacist to dispense an opioid antagonist pursuant to a prescription or a standing order to a person at risk of experiencing an opioid-related drug overdose or to a family member, friend, or other person in a position to assist a person at risk of an opioid-related drug overdose. It also provides protection from civil and criminal liability and disciplinary action to prescribers or pharmacists who choose to prescribe/dispense or not to prescribe/dispense such drugs.

Section 483.101 Definitions (Subchapter E—Opioid Antagonists)
A. "Emergency services personnel" includes firefighters, emergency medical services personnel as defined by Section 773.003, emergency room personnel, and other individuals who in the course and scope of employment or as a volunteer provide services for the benefit of the general public during emergency situations.
B. "Opioid antagonist" means any drug that binds to opioid receptors and blocks or otherwise inhibits the effects of opioids acting on those receptors.
C. "Opioid-related drug overdose" means a condition evidenced by symptoms such as extreme physical illness, decreased level of consciousness, constriction of the pupils, respiratory depression, or coma that a layperson would reasonably believe to be the result of the consumption or use of an opioid.
D. "Prescriber" means a person authorized by law to prescribe an opioid antagonist.

Section 483.102 Prescription for an Opioid Antagonist; Standing Order From a Prescriber
A. A prescriber may directly or by standing order prescribe an opioid antagonist to:
   1. A person at risk of experiencing an opioid-related drug overdose or
   2. A family member, friend, or other person in a position to assist a person described by A. 1. above.
B. A prescription issued under this section is considered as issued for a legitimate medical purpose in the usual course of professional practice.
C. A prescriber who acting in good faith with reasonable care prescribes or does not prescribe an opioid antagonist is not subject to any criminal or civil liability or any professional disciplinary action for:
   1. Prescribing or failing to prescribe the opioid antagonist or
   2. If the prescriber chooses to prescribe an opioid antagonist, any outcome resulting from the eventual administration of the opioid antagonist.

Note: A pharmacy must have a standing order with a physician to dispense an opioid antagonist such as naloxone without an individual prescription. Many chain pharmacies have standing orders that cover all their pharmacies in the state. The Texas Pharmacy Association also has a standing order that members can access after completing training. A prescription for an opioid antagonist issued by a pharmacist under a standing order is considered a valid prescription.

Section 483.103 Dispensing of an Opioid Antagonist by a Pharmacist
A. A pharmacist may dispense an opioid antagonist under a valid prescription to:
   1. A person at risk of experiencing an opioid-related drug overdose or
   2. A family member, friend, or other person in a position to assist a person described by A.1. above.
B. A prescription filled under this section is considered as filled for a legitimate medical purpose in the usual course of professional practice.
C. A pharmacist who acting in good faith and with reasonable care dispenses or does not dispense an opioid antagonist under a valid prescription is not subject to any criminal or civil liability or any professional disciplinary action for:
   1. Dispensing or failing to dispense the opioid antagonist or

2. If the pharmacist chooses to dispense an opioid antagonist, any outcome resulting from the eventual administration of the opioid antagonist.

> **Board of Pharmacy Rule 295.14**
> **Dispensing of Opioid Antagonist by a Pharmacist**

(a) Purpose. The purpose of this section is to provide standards for pharmacists engaged in the dispensing of opioid antagonists as authorized in Chapter 483, Health and Safety Code.
(b) Definitions.
  (1) **Opioid antagonist**—Any drug that binds to opioid receptors and blocks or otherwise inhibits the effects of opioids acting on those receptors.
  (2) **Opioid-related drug overdose**—A condition evidenced by symptoms such as extreme physical illness, decreased level of consciousness, constriction of the pupils, respiratory depression, or coma that a layperson would reasonably believe to be the result of the consumption or use of an opioid.
  (3) **Prescriber**—A person authorized by law to prescribe an opioid antagonist.
(c) Dispensing.
  (1) A pharmacist may dispense an opioid antagonist under a valid prescription including a prescription issued by a standing order to:
    (A) A person at risk of experiencing an opioid-related drug overdose or
    (B) A family member, friend, or other person in a position to assist a person described by (A) above.
  (2) A prescription dispensed under this section is considered as dispensed for a legitimate medical purpose in the usual course of professional practice.
  (3) A pharmacist who acting in good faith and with reasonable care dispenses or does not dispense an opioid antagonist under a valid prescription is not subject to any criminal or civil liability or any professional disciplinary action for:
    (A) Dispensing or failing to dispense the opioid antagonist or
    (B) If the pharmacist chooses to dispense an opioid antagonist, any outcome resulting from the eventual administration of the opioid antagonist.

Section 483.104 Distribution of Opioid Antagonist; Standing Order

A person or organization acting under a standing order issued by a prescriber may store an opioid antagonist and may distribute an opioid antagonist provided the person or organization does not request or receive compensation for storage or distribution.

Section 483.105 Possession of Opioid Antagonist

Any person may possess an opioid antagonist regardless of whether the person holds a prescription for the opioid antagonist.

Section 483.106 Administration of Opioid Antagonist

A. A person who acting in good faith and with reasonable care administers or does not administer an opioid antagonist to another person whom the person believes is suffering an opioid-related drug overdose is not subject to criminal prosecution, sanction under any professional licensing statute, or civil liability for an act or omission resulting from the administration of or failure to administer the opioid antagonist.
B. Emergency services personnel are authorized to administer an opioid antagonist to a person who appears to be suffering an opioid-related drug overdose as clinically indicated.

Prescriptive Authority for Advanced Practice Registered Nurses and Physician Assistants

I. General
   A. Texas law allows Advanced Practice Registered Nurses (APRNs) and Physician Assistants (PAs) to prescribe under what is essentially "dependent" prescriptive authority. Although they are recognized as practitioners, they must be working under the supervision of a physician under rules developed by the Board of Nursing and the Texas Medical Board.
   B. The term Advanced Practice Registered Nurse includes a nurse practitioner, a nurse-midwife, a nurse anesthetist, and a clinical nurse specialist. The term is synonymous with "advanced nurse practitioner."
   C. Prescribing by APRNs and PAs includes prescribing or ordering nonprescription drugs, dangerous drugs or devices, and controlled substances subject to the limitations described below including the issuing of a prescription drug order or a medication order.
   D. Prescriptive Authority Agreement or Facility Protocol
      1. A physician may delegate to an APRN or PA acting under adequate physician supervision the act of prescribing or ordering a drug or device as authorized in a prescriptive authority agreement between the physician and the APRN or PA. A prescriptive authority agreement must identify the practice locations and types or categories of drugs or devices that may be prescribed or the types or categories of drugs or devices that may not be prescribed. For detailed requirements on prescriptive authority agreements, see Texas Occupations Code Sections 157.0512, 157.0513, and 157.0514 and Texas Medical Board rules.
      2. The Texas Medical Board shall maintain and make available to the public a searchable online list of physicians, APRNs, and PAs with whom each physician, APRN, or PA has entered into a prescriptive authority agreement.
      3. In a hospital or long term care facility, prescriptive authority may be delegated to APRNs and PAs through a protocol rather than a prescriptive authority agreement. However, free standing clinics or other medical practices that are owned or operated by or associated with a hospital or long term care facility that are not physically located within the hospital or long term care facility are not considered facility-based practices. Prescriptive authority agreements are required in these settings.
   E. Controlled Substances
   An APRN or PA may prescribe controlled substances under the following conditions:
   1. The APRN or PA must be registered with the DEA.
   2. Schedule III, IV, and V Prescriptions
      a. Section 157.0511(b) of the Texas Medical Practices Act states that for Schedule III, IV, and V controlled substances prescribed by an APRN or PA, the prescription including a refill of the prescription may not exceed a 90-day supply.
      b. Although it states "a refill," both the Texas State Board of Pharmacy and the Texas Medical Board have agreed that a prescription for a Schedule III–V controlled substance from an APRN or PA can have more than one refill, but the prescription and any refills are only valid for 90 days. A controlled substance prescription from an APRN or PA is limited to a 90-day supply and expires after 90 days. After that, a new prescription would be required.

Notes

      c. Refills of Schedule III, IV, or V prescriptions may be authorized after consultation with the delegating physician, and the consultation is noted in the patient's chart.
      d. For controlled substance prescriptions for a child fewer than two years of age, the APRN or PA must consult with the delegating physician, and the consultation must be noted in the patient's chart.
      e. A physician may also delegate to a PA who provides board-certified obstetrical services or a certified nurse midwife (CNM) the administering or providing of controlled substances to a patient during intrapartum and immediate postpartum care.
   3. Schedule II Prescriptions
      a. Most APRNs and PAs cannot prescribe Schedule II controlled substances.
      b. One exception to this rule is a physician may delegate to an APRN or PA the authority to prescribe or order a Schedule II controlled substance in a hospital-based practice (not a nursing home or clinic that is not part of the hospital) in accordance with policies approved by the hospital's medical staff to a patient who has been admitted to the hospital for an intended length of stay of 24 hours or greater. Other exceptions are to a patient receiving services in the emergency department of the hospital or as part of a plan of care for the treatment of a person who has executed a written certification of a terminal illness, has elected to receive hospice care, and is receiving hospice treatment from a qualified hospice provider.

II. Mandated Information to be Provided on Each Prescription Issued by an APRN or PA
   A. Patient's name and address;
   B. Date issued;
   C. Name, strength, and quantity of drug prescribed;
   D. Directions for use;
   E. Intended use of the drug if appropriate;
   F. Number of refills permitted; and
   G. Name, address, and telephone number of the APRN or PA signing the prescription as well as the name, address, and telephone number of the delegating physician.
   Note: The signature of the physician is not required.
   H. If the prescription is for a controlled substance, the DEA number of the APRN or PA and the DEA number of the delegating physician must be on the prescription.

III. Supervision
   A. Except as provided in B. below, the combined number of APRNs and PAs with whom a physician may enter into a prescriptive authority agreement may not exceed seven APRNs and PAs or their full-time equivalents.
   B. The limitation in A. above does not apply to a prescriptive authority agreement if it is exercised in:
      1. A practice serving a medically underserved population or
      2. A facility-based practice in a hospital or long term care facility. (This does not apply to a freestanding clinic, center, or practice of the facility.)
   C. A physician must provide continuous supervision of the prescribing or ordering of a drug or device, but the constant physical presence of the physician is not required.

IV. Out-of-State APRNs and PAs
   A. Dangerous Drugs—Prescriptions for dangerous drugs from out-of-state APRNs or PAs can be filled in Texas. However, the APRN or PA must have prescriptive authority for these drugs in his or her own state.

B. Controlled Substances—Prescriptions for controlled substances from out-of-state APRNs or PAs are not valid prescriptions and cannot be filled in Texas.

Limited Independent Prescriptive Authority of Therapeutic Optometrists and Optometric Glaucoma Specialists

I. **Introduction**
   A. There are three separate types of licenses for Texas optometrists, each with different prescribing authority. The three types are: (1) Optometrists, (2) Therapeutic Optometrists, and (3) Optometric Glaucoma Specialists.
   B. Optometrists do not have any prescriptive authority and can be identified by their license number because it does not contain the letter "T" or "G."

II. **Therapeutic Optometrists**
   A. Therapeutic Optometrists may administer or prescribe drugs to treat the eye and adnexa (tissue surrounding the eye) but may not prescribe drugs to treat glaucoma nor controlled substances.
   B. Therapeutic Optometrists may only prescribe and administer:
      1. OTC oral medications;
      2. Ophthalmic devices; and
      3. Certain topical ocular pharmaceutical agents (*see chart below*).
   C. Therapeutic Optometrists can be identified by the letter "T" in their license. Most licensed optometrists are therapeutic optometrists.

III. **Optometric Glaucoma Specialists**
   A. Optometric Glaucoma Specialists are Therapeutic Optometrists who may treat glaucoma and other diseases of the eye. They have all of the privileges of a Therapeutic Optometrist but have an expanded formulary of drugs including certain oral prescription drugs and controlled substances from which they may prescribe.
   B. Optometric Glaucoma Specialists can be identified by the letter "G" in their license.
   C. Optometric Glaucoma Specialists may prescribe and administer:
      1. All medications included in the formulary for a Therapeutic Optometrist (see chart below);
      2. Antiglaucoma drugs; and
      3. The following oral drugs:
         a. One 10-day supply of oral antibiotics;
         b. One 72-hour supply of oral antihistamines;
         c. One 7-day supply of oral nonsteroidal anti-inflammatories; and
         d. One 3-day supply of any analgesic in Schedule III, IV, and V.
   D. Glaucoma Restrictions
      1. The law to allow Optometric Glaucoma Specialists to prescribe medication to treat glaucoma contains a number of restrictions and requirements. Optometric Glaucoma Specialists must consult with an ophthalmologist within 30 days after diagnosing glaucoma in a patient.
      2. Before prescribing a beta blocker, an Optometric Glaucoma Specialist must take a complete case history and determine whether the patient has received a physical examination within the past 180 days. If the patient has not had a physical examination or if the patient has a history of congestive heart failure, bradycardia, heart block, asthma, or chronic obstructive pulmonary disease, the Optometric Glaucoma Specialist must refer the patient to a physician for a physical examination before initiating beta blocker therapy.
   E. Optometric Glaucoma Specialists must be registered with DEA to prescribe and administer controlled substances.

Notes

Copyright © 2020 Fred S. Brinkley, Jr., and Gary G. Cacciatore

IV. Out-of-State Prescriptions From Optometrists

If a Texas pharmacy receives a prescription from an out-of-state optometrist, the prescription can be filled if the drug is one that may be prescribed by a Texas licensed Therapeutic Optometrist. Although some states may allow a broader formulary of drugs to be prescribed by optometrists, a Texas pharmacy may only dispense a drug that is allowed to be prescribed by an optometrist licensed in Texas. As with any out-of-state prescription, the pharmacist must first determine if the optometrist is authorized to prescribe the drug in his or her home state.

V. Cocaine Eye Drops for Diagnostic Purposes

A. Therapeutic Optometrists and Optometric Glaucoma Specialists can administer (but not prescribe or dispense) cocaine eye drops not greater than a 10% solution in prepackaged liquid form for diagnostic purposes.

B. Therapeutic Optometrists and Optometric Glaucoma Specialists must have a controlled substance registration certificate from DEA to possess and administer cocaine eye drops.

C. Pharmacist's Information
1. A pharmacist may only distribute cocaine to Therapeutic Optometrists or Optometric Glaucoma Specialists pursuant to a DEA Form 222.
2. A pharmacist may not distribute a controlled substance (other than a 10% solution of cocaine in prepackaged liquid form) to a Therapeutic Optometrist.
3. The 10% cocaine solution may not be compounded.

DRUGS THAT MAY BE PRESCRIBED BY OPTOMETRISTS

The type of drugs that may be prescribed depends on whether the licensee is an Optometrist, a Therapeutic Optometrist, or an Optometric Glaucoma Specialist.

OPTOMETRISTS (identified by a license number without letters): May not prescribe any prescription drugs.

THERAPEUTIC OPTOMETRISTS (identified by a license number ending in the letter T): May prescribe the appropriate **topical medication** for the purpose of diagnosing and treating visual defects, abnormal conditions, and diseases of the human vision system, including the eye and adnexa (associated anatomic parts). The following is a partial list of topical medications that Therapeutic Optometrists may prescribe.

Therapeutic Class	Type or Mechanism of Action	Generic Name (Partial List)
Anti-Allergy	Antihistamine	Levocabastine HCL, Olopatadine HCL, Pyrilamine Maleate, Lodoxamide Tromethamine, Pheniramine Maleate
	Membrane Stabilizer	Cromolyn Sodium
Anti-Fungal	Imidazoles	
	Polyenes	Natamycin
Anti-Infective	Agents Affecting Intermediary Metabolism	Sodium Sulfacetamide, Sulfisoxazole, Trimethoprim
	Aminoglycoside	Gentamicin, Tobramycin, Neomycin
	Anti-ACHase	
	Anti-Cell Membrane	Gramicidin, Polymyxin B Sulfacte
	Anti-Cell Wall Synthesis	Bacitracin
	Anti-DNA Synthesis	Ciprofloxacin
	Anti-Protein Synthesis (excluding chloramphenicol)	Erythromycin, Oxytetracycline HCL, Mupirocin
	Anti-Viral	Idoxuridine, Tribluridine, Vidarabine
	Cephalosporin	Cefazolin
Anti-Inflammatory	Nonsteroidal Anti-Inflammatory (NSAID)	Diclofenac Sodium, Flurbiprofen Sodium, Ketorolac Tromethamine, Suprofen
	Steroid	Dexamethasone, Hydrocortisone, Prednisolone Acetate, Remixolone, Fluorometholone, Medrysone, Prednisolone Sodium
Antiseptic		Zinc Sulfate
Chelating Agent		Deferoxamine, EDTA (Edetate Disocium)
Chemical Cautery		Silver Nitrate
Cycloplegic	Parasympatholytic	Atropine Sulfate, Homatropine HBr, Cyclopentolate HCL, Scopolamine HBr
Hyperosmotic		Glucose, Soium Chloride, Glycerin
Miotic	Anti-ACHase	
	Parasympathomimetic	Pilocarpine HCL (0.25–0.5% only)
Mucolytic		
Mydriatic	Sympathomimetic Alpha 1 Agonists only	Hydroxyamphetamine HBr, Phenylephrine
Vasoconstrictor	Sympathomimetic Alpha 1 Agonists only	Naphazoline HCL, Tetrahydroxoline HCL, Oxymetazoline HCL

If properly registered with DEA, Therapeutic Optometrists may **possess for administration** no more than 2 vials of prepackaged cocaine 10% eye drops.

OPTOMETRIC GLAUCOMA SPECIALISTS (identified by a license number ending in the letters TG) may prescribe everything a Therapeutic Optometrist may prescribe **and the following drugs:**
1. Appropriate **oral pharmaceutical agents** used for diagnosing and treating visual defects, abnormal conditions, and diseases of the human vision system, including the eye and adnexa, which are included in the following classification or are combinations of agents in the classifications:
    A. One 10-day supply of oral antibiotics;
    B. One 72-hour supply of oral antihistamines;
    C. One 7-day supply of oral nonsteroidal anti-inflammatories;
    D. One 3-day supply of any analgesic in controlled substance Schedules III, IV, and V (if properly registered with DEA); and
2. Antiglaucoma drugs.

Texas Health and Safety Code Chapter 488
Over-the-Counter Sales of Dextromethorphan

Note: This law prohibits over-the-counter sales of products containing dextromethorphan to customers under 18 years of age.

Section 488.001. Definitions
A. In this chapter:
   1. "Dextromethorphan" means any compound, mixture, or preparation containing any detectable amount of that substance, including its salts, optical isomers, and salts of optical isomers.
   2. "Sale" includes a conveyance, exchange, barter, or trade.
B. A term that is used in this chapter but is not defined by A. above has the meaning assigned by Section 481.002 if the term is defined in that section.

Section 488.002 Nonapplicability
A. This chapter does not apply to the sale of any product dispensed or delivered by a pharmacist according to a prescription issued by a practitioner for a valid medical purpose within the scope of the practitioner's practice as authorized by the practitioner's license issued under Title 3, Occupations Code.
B. This chapter does not require a business establishment to:
   1. Keep specific records of transactions covered by this chapter or
   2. Store dextromethorphan in a specific location in a business establishment or otherwise restrict the availability of dextromethorphan to customers.

Section 488.003 Distribution to Minors Prohibited; Prerequisite to Sale
A. A business establishment may not dispense, distribute, or sell dextromethorphan to a customer under 18 years of age.
B. Before dispensing, distributing, or selling dextromethorphan over the counter, a business establishment must require the customer obtaining the drug to display a driver's license or other form of identification containing the customer's photograph and indicating that the customer is 18 years of age or older, unless from the customer's outward appearance the person making the sale may reasonably presume the customer to be 27 years of age or older.

Section 488.004 Violation; Civil Penalty
A. A county or district attorney shall issue a warning to a business establishment for a first violation of this chapter.
B. After receiving a warning for the first violation under A. above, a business establishment is liable to the state for a civil penalty of:
   1. $150 for the second violation and
   2. $250 for each subsequent violation.
C. It is a defense in an action brought under this section that the person to whom the dextromethorphan was dispensed, distributed, or sold presented to the business establishment apparently valid proof of identification.
D. A proof of identification satisfies the requirements of C. above if it contains a physical description and photograph consistent with the person's appearance, purports to establish that the person is 18 years of age or older, and was issued by a governmental agency. The proof of identification may include a driver's license issued by this state or another state, a passport, or an identification card issued by a state or the federal government.
E. It is a defense in an action brought under this section that the business establishment made a good faith effort to comply with this section.

Section 488.005 Prohibited Local Regulation
- A. A political subdivision of this state may not adopt or enforce an ordinance, order, rule, regulation, or policy that governs the sale, distribution, or possession of dextromethorphan.
- B. An ordinance, order, rule, regulation, or policy described by A. above is void and unenforceable.

Possession and Administration of Certain Dangerous Drugs by Home and Community Support Services Agencies

- A. The Health and Safety Code authorizes Home and Community Support Services Agencies (HCSSA) and its employees who are registered nurses or licensed vocational nurses under physician's standing orders to purchase, store, or transport for the purpose of administering to:
  1. Their home health or hospice patients:
     a. Sterile water for injection and irrigation and
     b. Sterile saline for injection and irrigation.
  2. The agency's employees, home health or hospice patients, or patient's family members:
     a. Hepatitis B vaccine;
     b. Influenza vaccine; and
     c. Tuberculin purified protein derivative for tuberculosis testing.
- B. Possession
  An HCSSA and its employees who are registered nurses or licensed vocational nurses may purchase, store, or transport for the purpose of administering:
  1. The following items in a sealed portable container of a size determined by the dispensing pharmacist:
     a. 1,000 ml of 0.9% sodium chloride intravenous infusion;
     b. 1,000 ml of 5% dextrose in water for injection; or
     c. Sterile saline.
  2. Not more than 5 dosage units of:
     a. Heparin sodium lock flush—10 units/ml or 100 units/ml;
     b. Epinephrine HCl solution 1:1,000;
     c. Diphenhydramine HCl 50mg/ml;
     d. Methylprednisolone 125mg/2ml;
     e. Naloxone 1mg/ml in a 2ml vial;
     f. Promethazine 25mg/ml;
     g. Glucagon injection 1mg/ml;
     h. Furosemide 10mg/ml;
     i. Lidocaine 2.5% and prilocaine 2.5% in a 5 gram tube; or
     j. Lidocaine HCl solution 1% in a 2ml vial.
- C. Sealed Container
  An HCSSA and its authorized employees may purchase, store, or transport the drugs in a sealed container only if the agency has established policies to ensure that:
  1. The container is handled properly with respect to storage, transportation, and temperature stability;
  2. A drug is removed from the container only on a physician's order;
  3. Administration of any drug in the container is performed in accordance with a specific treatment protocol; and
  4. The agency maintains a written record of the dates/times the container is in the possession of a RN or LVN.

D. Administering in a Patient's Home
An HCSSA or its authorized employees who administer drugs listed under A. above may administer the drugs only in the patient's residence under a physician's orders with the provision of emergency treatment or the adjustment of:
1. Parenteral drug therapy;
2. Vaccine or tuberculin administration; and
3. If the drug is administered pursuant to a physician's order, the physician shall promptly send a signed copy of the order to the agency, and the agency shall:
    a. No later than 24 hours after receipt of the order reduce the order to written form and send a copy to the dispensing pharmacy and
    b. No later than 20 days after receipt of the order send a copy of the order as signed by and received from the physician to the dispensing pharmacy.
E. A pharmacist that dispenses a sealed portable container under this section shall ensure that the container:
1. Is designed to allow access to the contents of the container only if a tamper-proof seal is broken;
2. Bears a label that lists the drugs in the container and provides notice of the container's expiration date, which is the earlier of:
    a. The date that is six months after the date on which the container is dispensed or
    b. The earliest expiration date of any drug in the container; and
3. Remains in the pharmacy or under the control of a pharmacist, RN, or LVN.
F. If an HCSSA or an authorized employee purchases, stores, or transports a sealed container, the agency shall deliver the container to the dispensing pharmacy for verification of drug quality, quantity, integrity, and the expiration dates no later than the earlier of:
1. The 7th day after the date on which the seal on the container is broken or
2. The date for which notice is provided on the container label.
G. A pharmacy that dispenses a sealed portable container shall take reasonable precautionary measures to ensure that the HCSSA receiving the container complies with F. above. On receipt of a container under F., the pharmacy shall perform an inventory of the drugs used from the container and shall restock and reseal the container before delivering the container to the agency for reuse.

Texas Food, Drug, and Cosmetic Act
(Chapter 431, Health and Safety Code, Title 6, Subtitle A)
Subchapter M Drug Donation Program
(Administered by the Texas Department of State Health Services)

The Texas Food, Drug, and Cosmetic Act allows a charitable drug donor to donate unused prescription drugs to a charitable medical clinic, and the clinic can accept, dispense, or administer the donated drugs. A summary of the law follows.
A. Definitions
1. **Charitable drug donor** means:
    a. A licensed convalescent or nursing home;
    b. A licensed hospice;
    c. A hospital;
    d. A physician;
    e. A pharmacy; or
    f. A pharmaceutical seller or manufacturer.

Note: A seller or manufacturer may not donate drugs except pursuant to a qualified patient assistance program that donates drugs to a charitable medical clinic.

    2. **Charitable medical clinic** means a clinic that:
       a. Provides medical care without charge or for a substantially reduced charge;
       b. Complies with the insurance requirements of Chapter 84, Civil Practice and Remedies Code;
       c. Is exempt from federal income tax; and
       d. Is operated exclusively for the promotion of social welfare by being primarily engaged in promoting the common good and general welfare of the people in a community.

B. A charitable drug donor must use appropriate safeguards established by the Texas Department of State Health Services (TDSHS) to ensure that the drugs are not compromised or illegally diverted while being stored or transported to the charitable medical clinic.

C. A charitable medical clinic may not accept the drugs unless:
    1. It certifies that the drugs have been properly stored while in possession of the donor;
    2. The donor provides the clinic with a verifiable address and telephone number; and
    3. The person transferring possession of the drugs presents photographic identification.

D. The donated drugs must be:
    1. Prescription drugs but may not be controlled substances;
    2. Approved by FDA and individually packaged or packaged in unit-dose packaging;
    3. Oral or parenteral medication in sealed single-dose containers approved by FDA;
    4. Topical or inhalant drugs in sealed unit-of-use containers approved by FDA; or
    5. Parenteral medication in a sealed multiple-dose container approved by FDA from which no doses have been withdrawn.

E. The donated drugs may not be the subject of a mandatory or voluntary recall.

F. The charitable medical clinic may dispense or administer the donated drugs only:
    1. Before the expiration date of the drug and
    2. After a licensed pharmacist has determined that the drugs are of an acceptable integrity.

G. The law also establishes a limitation on liability for charitable drug donors, charitable medical clinics, and their employees if they comply with the terms of the law and rules.

H. TDSHS adopted the following Rule 229.22 to implement these provisions.

TDSHS RULE 229.22
Donation of Drugs to Charitable Medical Clinics

A charitable medical clinic may receive a drug donated by a charitable drug donor for dispensing to a patient of the charitable medical clinic provided that the following requirements are met.

    (1) The charitable drug donor must be licensed with TDSHS as a wholesale drug distributor. Manufacturers who participate in a patient assistance program and physicians who donate samples will not be required to be licensed with the department.

(2) The donated drugs must be dangerous drugs as defined in Health and Safety Code Chapter 483 entitled "Texas Dangerous Drug Act."
(3) Donated drugs may not be controlled substances as defined in Health and Safety Code Chapter 481 entitled "Texas Controlled Substances Act."
(4) All donated drugs must be approved by the Food and Drug Administration (FDA) and intended for human use.
(5) Donation of drug samples must comply with Title 21, Code of Federal Regulations (CFR), 203.39.
(6) Previously dispensed drugs shall not be donated.
(7) The charitable drug donor must verify that the requesting charity is legitimate.
   (A) Verification shall include copies of documents proving the charitable medical clinic's status as exempt from federal income tax and the address, telephone number, and name of the contact person at the charitable medical clinic.
   (B) Documentation of verification must be retained by the charitable drug donor for three years.
(8) A drug donated by a charitable drug donor shall be received by a charitable medical clinic in the manufacturer's unopened original tamper-evident packaging with its labeling intact.
(9) Delivery of a donated drug to a recipient charitable medical clinic shall be completed by an authorized agent or employee of the recipient charitable medical clinic or by the charitable drug donor. All deliveries shall be made in person. The authorized agent or employee shall present his or her official state identification to the recipient upon delivery.
(10) The recipient charitable medical clinic shall prepare at the time of collection or delivery of drugs a complete and accurate donation record. A copy of this record shall be retained by the recipient charitable medical clinic for at least three years and contain the following information:
   (A) A signed written statement from the charitable drug donor that the drugs have been properly stored in accordance with the manufacturer's instructions;
   (B) A verifiable name, address, and telephone number of the charitable drug donor;
   (C) The manufacturer, brand name, quantity, and lot or control number of the drugs donated;
   (D) The date of the donation; and
   (E) A copy of the official state identification of the authorized agent or employee of the charitable drug donor.
(11) A donated drug shall not be dispensed to a patient until it has been examined by a registered pharmacist at the recipient charitable medical clinic to confirm that the donation record accurately describes the drug delivered and to confirm in his or her professional judgment that no drug is adulterated or misbranded for any reason including, but not limited to, the following:
   (A) The drug is out of date;
   (B) The labeling has become mutilated, obscured, or detached from the drug packaging;
   (C) The drug shows evidence of having been stored or shipped under conditions that might adversely affect its stability, integrity, or effectiveness;
   (D) The drug has been recalled or is no longer marketed; or
   (E) The drug is otherwise possibly contaminated, deteriorated, or adulterated.
(12) Documentation of the examination of the drug and the drug donation record by the registered pharmacist shall be retained by the charitable medical clinic for three years after the date of examination.

(13) The recipient charitable medical clinic shall dispose of any drug found to be adulterated/misbranded by destroying it. The charitable medical clinic shall retain complete records of the disposition of all destroyed drugs for three years from the date of destruction.

(14) Each recipient charitable medical clinic shall conduct at least annually an inventory of drug stocks and shall prepare a report reconciling the results of each inventory with the most recent prior inventory. Drug inventory discrepancies and reconciliation problems shall be investigated by the charitable medical clinic and outcomes documented. All reports of reconciliation, investigation, and outcome shall be retained by the charitable medical clinic for three years.

(15) All charitable drug donors shall comply with the existing statutory standards contained in the Texas Health and Safety Code Chapter 431 and the requirements of 229.253 of this title (relating to Minimum Standards for Licensing) for "Licensing of Wholesale Distributors of Drugs," which includes "Good Manufacturing Practices."

(16) A charitable medical clinic shall immediately notify the Drugs and Medical Devices Division using the toll-free telephone number 888-839-6676 when it becomes aware of a significant loss or theft of drugs. A copy of the inventory reconciliation, investigation, and outcome report shall be forwarded to the Drugs and Medical Devices Division, 1100 West 49th Street, Austin, Texas 78756 within five days of the telephone notification.

(17) A charitable drug donor shall promptly notify in writing a charitable medical clinic to which donations have been made if the donor becomes aware of a recall or other situation pertaining to the safety and efficacy of the previously donated drugs. Documentation of this notice shall be retained for three years after the date of notification.

Texas Food, Drug, and Cosmetic Act
(Chapter 442, Health and Safety Code, Title 6, Subtitle A)
Donation of Prescription Drugs

A. This new chapter passed by the Texas Legislature requires the Executive Commissioner of the Texas Department of State Health Services to adopt standards and procedures for:
   1. Accepting, storing, labeling, and dispensing donated prescription drugs and
   2. Inspecting donated prescription drugs to determine whether the drugs are safe and suitable for redistribution (Section 442.052).
B. Donors may donate unused prescription drugs to participating providers who may be healthcare facilities, pharmacies, or pharmacists who are employees of a facility or pharmacy that elects to participate in the collection and redistribution of donated prescription drugs (Section 442.001 and Section 442.051).
C. Participating providers may dispense donated prescription drugs to a recipient in accordance with rules to be developed. A recipient is a person who voluntarily receives donated prescription drugs under the chapter (Section 442.001 and Section 442.051).
D. Donated prescription drugs may be accepted or dispensed only if the drug is in its original, unopened, sealed, and tamper-evident unit-dose packaging. A donated prescription drug may not be accepted or dispensed under the Act if the drug is a controlled substance, is adulterated or misbranded, is not stored in compliance with the product's labeling, or the FDA requires the drug to have a risk evaluation and mitigation strategy (REMS) (Section 442.053).

E. Before being dispensed to a recipient, a prescription drug donated under the chapter must be inspected by the participating provider to determine if the drug is adulterated or misbranded and whether the drug has been stored in compliance with the requirements of the drug's label (Section 442.054).
F. The Act provides a limitation of liability from criminal, administrative, and civil liability for donors, participating providers, and drug manufacturers (Section 442.057).

Note: See TDSHS website for additional information.

Medical Gases (Oxygen)

Any pharmacy involved in the manufacturing or filling of medical gases for patient use is required to be licensed with the Texas Department of State Health Services (TDSHS) and the FDA as a drug manufacturer and must comply with CGMPs. However, a hospital pharmacy that fills and provides oxygen for inpatient use would not have to be licensed as a manufacturer.

QUICK REFERENCE GUIDE
PRESCRIPTIONS WHICH MAY BE DISPENSED IN TEXAS

Prescriber Type / Rx Format	Written Rx (Paper Prescription)	Verbal/Telephonic (Oral/Spoken) Rx	Facsimile (Faxed) Rx*	Electronic (Electronic Data File) Rx	May be refilled if authorized verbally	Refills may be transferred between Texas pharmacies	Refills may be transferred from an out-of-state pharmacy to a Texas pharmacy
DANGEROUS DRUG RX ISSUED BY:							
Texas Physician, Dentist, Veterinarian, or Podiatrist	YES • Manual signature; or • Electronic replica of manual signature printed on secured paper, required.	YES	YES	YES	YES	YES for authorized refills.	YES for authorized refills.
Authorized Texas Advanced Practice Registered Nurse (APRN) or Physician Assistant (PA)	YES • Manual signature; or • Electronic replica of manual signature printed on secured paper, required; and • Delegating Physician information.	YES Delegating Physician information required.	YES Delegating Physician information required.	YES Delegating Physician information required.	YES	YES for authorized refills.	YES for authorized refills.
Texas Pharmacist Performing Drug Therapy Management (DTM) Under Written Protocol of a Physician	YES • Manual signature; • Written Protocol; • Issued at Hospital, Hospital-based clinic, or Academic health-care Institution	NO	NO	YES • Manual signature; • Written Protocol; • Issued at Hospital, Hospital-based clinic, or Academic health-care Institution	NO	YES	NO
Out-of-State[1] Physician, Dentist, Veterinarian, or Podiatrist	YES • Manual signature; or • Electronic replica of manual signature printed on secured paper, required.	YES	YES	YES	YES	YES for authorized refills.	YES for authorized refills.
Out-of-State[1] Advanced Practice Registered Nurse or Physician Assistant	YES • Manual signature; or • Electronic replica of manual signature printed on secured paper, required; and • Delegating Physician information.	YES Delegating Physician information required.	YES Delegating Physician information required.	YES Delegating Physician information required.	YES	YES for authorized refills.	YES for authorized refills.
Canadian or Mexican Practitioner	YES • Manual signature; or • Electronic replica of manual signature printed on secured paper, required.	NO	NO	NO	NO only refills authorized on original written Rx may be dispensed.	YES for authorized refills.	NO
CIII-V CONTROLLED SUBSTANCE RX ISSUED BY:							
Texas Physician, Dentist, Veterinarian, or Podiatrist	YES Manual signature required.	YES	YES of a manually signed paper prescription.	YES via application in compliance with DEA rules for EPCS**	YES	YES on a one-time basis (Exception***).	YES on a one-time basis (Exception***).
Authorized Texas Advanced Practice Registered Nurse (APRN) or Physician Assistant (PA)	YES • Manual signature required; and • for a period not to exceed 90 days; and • Delegating Physician information, including DEA #.	YES • for a period not to exceed 90 days; and • Delegating Physician information, including DEA#.	YES • of a manually signed paper prescription; and • for a period not to exceed 90 days; and • Delegating Physician information, including DEA#.	YES • via application in compliance with DEA rules for EPCS**; and • for a period not to exceed 90 days; and • Delegating Physician information, including DEA#.	YES after onsulting with delegating physician & the consultation is noted in the patient's chart.	YES on a one-time basis (Exception***).	YES on a one-time basis (Exception***).
Out-of-State[1] Physician, Dentist, Veterinarian, or Podiatrist	YES Manual signature required.	YES	YES of a manually signed paper prescription.	YES via application in compliance with DEA rules for EPCS**.	YES	YES on a one-time basis (Exception***).	YES on a one-time basis (Exception***).
Out-of-State[1] APRN or PA	NO	NO	NO	NO	NO	NO	NO
Canadian or Mexican Practitioner	NO	NO	NO	NO	NO	NO	NO

SCHEDULE II CONTROLLED SUBSTANCE PRESCRIPTIONS (CII Rxs):
- CII Rxs may be dispensed only if written on an "official form" provided by the Texas State Board of Pharmacy (TSBP) or if transmitted electronically by a practitioner to a pharmacy in compliance with DEA regulations.**
- CII Rxs issued by Out-of-State Practitioners[1] may be filled only by Texas pharmacies that have submitted a plan to TSBP and approved.
- Authorized Texas APRNs/PAs may issue CII Rxs for:
  1) a terminally ill patient who is receiving hospice treatment from a qualified hospice provider; or
  2) a patient hospitalized for 24 hours or greater, provided that the CII Rx is filled at the in-hospital pharmacy; or
  3) a patient receiving emergency services in the hospital's emergency department, provided that the CII Rx is filled at the in-hospital pharmacy.

* **Faxed Rxs** – All must include a statement indicating that the Rx has been faxed (e.g., "Faxed to...") and the name of the designated agent, if faxed by a designated agent.

** **EPCS** – Electronic Prescriptions for Controlled Substances (Code of Federal Regulations, Part 1311).

*** **Exception** – Pharmacies electronically sharing a real-time, on-line database may transfer up to the maximum refills permitted by law and the prescriber's authorization.

(1) - Includes the United States other than TX & U.S.Territories (Puerto Rico, U.S. Virgin Islands, American Samoa, Guam, Northern Mariana Islands).

NOTE: For Therapeutic Optometrists (T) & Optometric Glaucoma Specialists (TG), visit: www.pharmacy.texas.gov/files_pdf/Optometrists.pdf

CHAPTER C HIGHLIGHTS
Texas Dangerous Drug Act (TDDA)

1. Dangerous drugs are drugs other than controlled substances that are required to be dispensed pursuant to a valid prescription and are labeled "Rx only."
2. The following practitioners have prescriptive authority in Texas:
   a. Physicians
   b. Dentists
   c. Podiatrists
   d. Veterinarians
   e. Optometrists
   f. Advanced Practice Registered Nurses and Physician Assistants (delegated authority)
3. Although not included in the definition of practitioner under the TDDA, pharmacists in certain practice settings can sign prescriptions for dangerous drugs under delegated authority. (*See Drug Therapy Management in Chapter E.*) Class A pharmacy rules define and include these pharmacists as practitioners, so prescriptions signed by those pharmacists can be filled.
4. Pharmacists can fill prescriptions from out-of-state practitioners for dangerous drugs and Schedule III–V controlled substances, except that controlled substance prescriptions from out-of-state advanced practice registered nurses (APRNs) and physician assistants (PAs) cannot be filled in Texas.
5. A pharmacy must obtain special permission from the Texas State Board of Pharmacy if it wishes to fill prescriptions for Schedule II controlled substances from out-of-state practitioners.
6. Prescriptions for dangerous drugs (not controlled substances) from practitioners in Canada and Mexico can be filled only pursuant to a written prescription. Verbal, faxed, or electronic prescriptions are not valid.
7. Designated agents can communicate prescriptions on behalf of a practitioner.
8. A pharmacist may dispense an opioid antagonist under a valid prescription including a prescription issued by a standing order to a person at risk of experiencing an opioid-related drug overdose or to a family member, friend, or other person in a position to assist such person.
9. Texas Advanced Practice Registered Nurse (APRN) and Physician Assistant (PA) prescriptive authority is as follows:
   a. APRNs and PAs can prescribe under prescriptive authority agreements or under facility protocols in hospitals and long term care facilities.
   b. APRNs and PAs can prescribe controlled substances in Schedule III–V but the total quantity (including any refills) may not exceed a 90-day supply.
   c. Controlled substance prescriptions from out-of-state APRNs and PAs are not valid in Texas.
   d. APRNs and PAs in a hospital-based practice may prescribe Schedule II controlled substances in accordance with policies approved by the hospital's medical staff to a patient who has been admitted to the hospital for an intended length of stay of 24 hours or greater or is receiving services in the emergency department of the hospital or as part of a plan of care for the treatment of terminally ill/hospice patients.
10. Therapeutic Optometrists can prescribe certain topical ocular pharmaceutical agents, over-the-counter drugs, and ocular devices. (*See chart in this chapter for a list of ocular agents.*) In addition to these drugs, Optometric Glaucoma Specialists can also prescribe a limited formulary of dangerous drugs and controlled substances and can possess and administer cocaine eye drops for diagnostic purposes.
11. Pharmacies (and other business establishments) may not sell over-the-counter products containing dextromethorphan to customers under 18 years of age.

CHAPTER D

Texas Pharmacy Act (TPA)
(and Selected Board of Pharmacy Rules)

CHAPTER D

Texas Pharmacy Act (TPA)
(and Selected Board of Pharmacy Rules)

Where possible, we have attempted to link various Texas State Board of Pharmacy (TSBP) rules to the sections of the Act to which they relate. For example, rules on generic substitution have been placed immediately following Sections 562.001–562.015 (Prescription and Substitution Requirements) of the Act. Where only a portion of a rule is applicable to a particular part of the Act, only that part of the rule is placed there rather than the entire rule. Language taken from TSBP rules can be identified by a "shaded" number and title.

Chapter 551 General Provisions

Section 551.001 Short Title—The "Texas Pharmacy Act" (Act)

Section 551.002 Legislative Declaration
- A. The Texas Pharmacy Act (TPA) shall be liberally construed to regulate in the public interest the practice of pharmacy in this state as a professional practice that affects the public health, safety, and welfare.
- B. It is a matter of public interest and concern that the practice of pharmacy merits and receives the confidence of the public and that only qualified persons be permitted to engage in the practice of pharmacy in this state.
- C. The purpose of the Texas Pharmacy Act is to promote, preserve, and protect the public health, safety, and welfare through:
  1. Effectively controlling and regulating the practice of pharmacy and
  2. Licensing pharmacies engaged in the sale, delivery, or distribution of prescription drugs and devices used in diagnosing and treating injury, illness, and disease.

Section 551.003 Definitions

When used in this chapter, the following words and terms shall have the following meanings unless the context clearly indicates otherwise.
1. **Administer**—To directly apply a prescription drug to the body of a patient by any means including injection, inhalation, or ingestion by a person authorized by law to administer the drug. These individuals include a practitioner or an authorized agent under a practitioner's supervision or the patient at the direction of a practitioner.
2. **Board**—The Texas State Board of Pharmacy.
3. **Class A pharmacy license**—A community pharmacy license.
4. **Class B pharmacy license**—A nuclear pharmacy license.
5. **Class C pharmacy license**—An institutional pharmacy license.
6. **Class D pharmacy license**—A clinic pharmacy license.
7. **Class E pharmacy license**—A nonresident pharmacy license.
8. **College of pharmacy**—A school, college, or university that satisfies ACPE requirements as adopted by the Board or meets accreditation standards set by the Board.
9. **Compounding**—The preparation, mixing, assembling, packaging, or labeling of a drug or device:
   a. As a result of a practitioner's prescription drug order based on the practitioner-patient-pharmacist relationship in the course of professional practice;
   b. For administration to a patient by a practitioner as the result of a practitioner's initiative based on the practitioner-patient-pharmacist relationship in the course of professional practice;

c. In anticipation of prescription drug orders based on routine, regularly observed prescribing patterns; or
d. For or as an incident to research, teaching, or chemical analysis and not for selling or dispensing, except as allowed under Section 562.154 or Chapter 563 of the Act.
10. **Confidential record**—A health-related record including a patient medication record, prescription drug order, or medication order that contains information identifying an individual and that is maintained by a pharmacy or pharmacist.
11. **Controlled substance**—A substance including a drug or immediate precursor listed in Schedules I–V of the Texas Controlled Substances Act or the Federal Controlled Substances Act.
12. **Dangerous drug**—A drug or device that is not included in penalty group I–IV of the Texas Controlled Substances Act and is unsafe for self-medication or is required to bear the legend: "Caution: federal law prohibits dispensing without prescription" or "Rx only" or "Caution: federal law restricts this drug to use by or on the order of a licensed veterinarian."
13. **Deliver or delivery**—The actual, constructive, or attempted transfer of a prescription drug or device or controlled substance from one person to another with or without consideration.
14. **Designated agent**—
    a. An individual including a licensed nurse, physician assistant, or pharmacist designated by a practitioner and authorized to communicate a prescription drug order to a pharmacist and for whom the practitioner assumes legal responsibility.
    b. A licensed nurse, physician assistant, or pharmacist employed in a healthcare facility to whom the practitioner communicates a prescription drug order.
    c. A registered nurse or physician assistant authorized by a practitioner to administer a prescription drug order for a dangerous drug under Chapter 157, Subchapter B (Texas Medical Practice Act).
    d. A person who is a licensed vocational nurse or has an education equivalent to or greater than that required for a vocational nurse may be designated by the practitioner to communicate prescriptions of an advanced practice registered nurse or physician assistant authorized by the practitioner to sign prescription drug orders.
15. **Device**—An instrument, apparatus, implement, machine, contrivance, implant, in vitro reagent, or other similar or related article, including a component part or accessory, that is required under federal or state law to be ordered or prescribed by a practitioner.
15a. **Direct supervision**—Supervision by a pharmacist who directs the activities of a pharmacist intern, pharmacy technician, or pharmacy technician trainee to a sufficient degree to ensure that activities are performed accurately, safely, and without risk of harm to patients as specified by Board rule.
16. **Dispense**—To prepare, package, compound, or label in the course of professional practice a prescription drug or device for delivery to an ultimate user or the user's agent under a practitioner's lawful order.
17. **Distribute**—To deliver a prescription drug or device other than by administering or dispensing.
18. **Drug**—A substance recognized as a drug in a drug compendium, including the current official United States Pharmacopeia, official National Formulary, or official Homeopathic Pharmacopeia, or in a supplement to a drug compendium; a substance intended for use in the diagnosis, cure, mitigation,

treatment, or prevention of disease in a human or other animal; a substance other than food intended to affect the structure or a function of the body of a human or another animal; or a substance intended for use as a component of a substance described above.

19. **Drug regimen review**—Includes evaluation of a prescription drug or a medication order and a patient medication record for:
    a. A known allergy;
    b. A rational therapy-contraindication;
    c. A reasonable dose and route of administration;
    d. Reasonable directions for use;
    e. Duplication of therapy;
    f. Drug-drug interactions;
    g. Drug-food interactions;
    h. Drug-disease interactions;
    i. Adverse drug reactions; and
    j. Proper use including overuse or underuse.
20. **Internship**—A practical experience program approved by the Board.
21. **Label**—Written, printed, or graphic matter on the immediate container of a drug or device.
22. **Labeling**—The process of affixing a label, including all information required by federal and state statute or regulation, to a drug or device container. The term does not include the labeling by a manufacturer, packer, or distributor of a nonprescription drug or commercially packaged prescription drug or device or unit-dose packaging.
23. **Manufacturing**—The production, preparation, propagation, conversion, or processing of a drug or device either directly or indirectly by extraction from a substance of natural origin or independently by chemical or biological synthesis. The term includes packaging or repackaging a substance or labeling or relabeling a container and promoting and marketing the drug or device and preparing and promoting a commercially available product from a bulk compound for resale by a person, including a pharmacy or practitioner. The term does not include compounding.
24. **Medication order**—An order from a practitioner or a practitioner's designated agent for administration of a drug or device.
25. **Nonprescription drug**—A nonnarcotic drug or device that may be sold without a prescription and that is labeled and packaged in compliance with applicable state or federal law.
26. **Patient counseling**—Communication by a pharmacist of information, as specified in Board rules, to a patient or caregiver to improve therapy by ensuring proper use of a drug or device.
27. **Pharmaceutical care**—Providing drug therapy and other pharmaceutical services defined by Board rules and intended to assist curing or preventing a disease, eliminating or reducing a patient's symptoms, or arresting or slowing a disease process.
28. **Pharmacist**—A person licensed by the Board to practice pharmacy.
29. **Pharmacist-in-charge (P.I.C.)**—The pharmacist designated on a pharmacy license as the pharmacist who has the authority or responsibility for the pharmacy's compliance with statutes and rules relating to the practice of pharmacy.
30. **Pharmacist intern**—An undergraduate student enrolled in the professional sequence of a college of pharmacy approved by the Board and who is participating in a Board-approved internship program. A pharmacist intern also can be a graduate of a college of pharmacy who is participating in a Board-approved internship.

31. **Pharmacy**—A facility at which a prescription drug or medication order is received, processed, or dispensed under this Act, the Dangerous Drug Act, or the Controlled Substances Act. The term does not include a narcotic drug treatment program that is regulated by Chapter 466, Health and Safety Code.
32. **Pharmacy technician**—An individual employed by a pharmacy whose responsibility is to provide technical services that do not require professional judgment for preparing and distributing drugs and who works under the direct supervision of and is responsible to a pharmacist.
32a. **Pharmacy technician trainee**—An individual who is registered with the Board as a pharmacy technician trainee and is authorized to participate in a pharmacy technician training program.
33. **Practice of pharmacy**—
    a. Providing an act or service necessary to provide pharmaceutical care;
    b. Interpreting or evaluating a prescription drug order or medication order;
    c. Participating in drug or device selection as authorized by law and participating in drug administration, drug regimen review, or drug or drug-related research;
    d. Providing patient counseling;
    e. Being responsible for:
        (1) Dispensing a prescription drug order or distributing a medication order;
        (2) Compounding or labeling a drug or device, other than labeling by a manufacturer, repackager, or distributor of a nonprescription drug or commercially packaged prescription drug or device;
        (3) Properly and safely storing a drug or device; and
        (4) Maintaining proper records for a drug or device;
    f. Performing for a patient a specific act of drug therapy management delegated to a pharmacist by a written protocol from a practitioner licensed in this state in compliance with Chapter 157, Subchapter B (The Texas Medical Practice Act); and
    g. Administering an immunization or vaccination under a physician's written protocol.
34. **Practitioner**—
    a. A person licensed or registered to prescribe, distribute, administer, or dispense a prescription drug or device in the course of professional practice in this state, including a physician, dentist, podiatrist, or veterinarian but excluding a person licensed under this Act (i.e., pharmacists); or other person licensed or registered to prescribe, distribute, administer, or dispense a prescription drug or device in the course of professional practice in this state;
    b. A person licensed by another state, Canada, or the United Mexican States in a health field in which, under the law of this state, a license holder in this state may legally prescribe a dangerous drug;
    c. A person practicing in another state and licensed by another state as a physician, dentist, veterinarian, or podiatrist who has a current federal Drug Enforcement Administration registration number and who may legally prescribe a Schedule II, III, IV, or V controlled substance in that other state; or
    d. An advanced practice registered nurse or physician assistant to whom a physician has delegated the authority to prescribe a drug or device.
35. **Preceptor**—A pharmacist licensed in this state to practice pharmacy who meets the preceptor requirements specified by rules and who is certified by the Board to supervise pharmacist interns.

36. **Prescription drug**—
    a. A substance for which federal or state law requires a prescription before it may be legally dispensed to the public;
    b. A drug or device that under federal law is required, before being dispensed or delivered, to be labeled with one of the following statements:
       (1) "Caution: federal law prohibits dispensing without prescription";
       (2) "Rx only" or another legend that complies with federal law; or
       (3) "Caution: federal law restricts this drug to use by or on order of a licensed veterinarian"; or
    c. A drug or device that is required by federal or state statute or regulation to be dispensed on a prescription or that is restricted to use by a practitioner only.
37. **Prescription drug order**—An order from a practitioner or practitioner's designated agent to a pharmacist for a drug or a device to be dispensed or an order under Chapter 157, Subchapter B (Orders from Physician Assistants and Advanced Practice Registered Nurses).
38. **Prospective drug use review**—The review of a patient's drug therapy and prescription drug order or medication order as defined by Board rules before dispensing or distributing a drug to the patient.
39. **Provide**—To supply one or more unit doses of a nonprescription drug or dangerous drug to a patient.
40. **Radioactive drug**—A drug that exhibits spontaneous disintegration of unstable nuclei with the emission of nuclear particles or photons, including a nonradioactive reagent kit or nuclide generator that is intended to be used in the preparation of the substance.
41. **Substitution**—The dispensing of a drug or a brand of drug other than the drug or brand of drug ordered or prescribed.
42. **Texas trade association**—A cooperative and voluntarily joined statewide association of business or professional competitors in this state designed to assist its members and its industry or profession in dealing with mutual business or professional problems and in promoting their common interest.
43. **Ultimate user**—A person who obtains or possesses a prescription drug or device for the person's own use or for the use of a member of the person's household or for administering to an animal owned by the person or by a member of the person's household.
44. **Unit-dose packaging**—The ordered amount of a drug in a dosage form ready for administration to a particular patient by the prescribed route at the prescribed time and properly labeled with the name, strength, and expiration date of the drug.
45. **Written protocol**—A physician's order, standing medical order, standing delegation order, or other order or protocol as defined by rule of the Texas Medical Board under Chapter 157, Subchapter B.

Section 551.004 Applicability of the Act (The Texas Pharmacy Act)
A. This Act does not apply to (who cannot be regulated by TSBP):
   1. A practitioner licensed by the appropriate state board who supplies a patient of the practitioner with a drug in a manner authorized by state or federal law and who does not operate a pharmacy for the retailing of prescription drugs;
   2. A member of the faculty of a college of pharmacy recognized by the Board who is a pharmacist and who performs the pharmacist's services only for the benefit of the college;
   3. A person who procures prescription drugs for lawful research, teaching, or testing and not for resale; or

4. A home and community support services agency that possesses a dangerous drug as authorized by Section 141.0061, 142.0062, or 142.0063, Health and Safety Code. (*See Chapter C.*)
B. This Act does not prevent a practitioner from administering a drug to a patient of the practitioner.
C. This Act does not prevent the sale by a person other than a pharmacist, firm, joint stock company, partnership, or corporation of:
1. A nonprescription drug that is harmless if used according to instructions on a printed label on the drug's container and that does not contain a narcotic;
2. An insecticide, a fungicide, or a chemical used in the arts if the insecticide, fungicide, or chemical is properly labeled; or
3. An insecticide or fungicide that is mixed or compounded only for an agricultural purpose.
D. A wholesaler or manufacturer may distribute a prescription drug as provided by state or federal law.

Section 551.005 Application of the Sunset Act
Unless continued in existence (as provided under the Texas Sunset Act), the Texas State Board of Pharmacy is abolished, and this Act expires September 1, 2029.

Section 551.006 Exclusive Authority
Notwithstanding any other law, a pharmacist has the exclusive authority to determine whether to dispense a drug.

Section 551.008 Prohibition on Rule Violating Sincerely Held Religious Belief
A. All rules, regulations, or policies adopted by the Board may not violate Chapter 110, Civil Practice and Remedies Code (The Texas Religious Freedom Act).
B. A person may assert a violation of A. above as an affirmative defense in an administrative hearing or as a claim or defense in a judicial proceeding under Chapter 37, Civil Practice and Remedies Code (Texas Declaratory Judgments Act).

Note: Sections 551.006 and 551.008 of this Act arguably create a pharmacist's right of conscientious objection which has most often surfaced in the context of pharmacists refusing to dispense certain drugs such as oral contraceptives or Plan B "morning after" drugs based on religious beliefs. While this provision prevents the Board from adopting a rule or policy that violates the Texas Religious Freedom Act, pharmacists should still check their employer's policy on refusal to fill a prescription based on moral or religious beliefs.

Chapter 552 State Board of Pharmacy

Section 552.001 Membership
A. The Texas State Board of Pharmacy consists of eleven members appointed by the governor with the advice and consent of the senate as follows:
1. Seven members who are pharmacists;
2. One member who is a pharmacy technician; and
3. Three members who represent the public.
B. Appointments to the Board shall be made without regard to the race, color, disability, sex, religion, age, or national origin of the appointee.

Section 552.002 Qualifications
A. The Board must include representation for pharmacists employed in Class A pharmacies and Class C pharmacies.
B. A pharmacist board member must at the time of appointment:
1. Be a resident of this state;
2. Been licensed for the five years preceding appointment;
3. Be in good standing to practice pharmacy in this state; and
4. Be practicing pharmacy in this state.

C. A pharmacy technician board member must at the time of appointment:
   1. Be a resident of this state;
   2. Been registered as a pharmacy technician for the five years preceding appointment;
   3. Be in good standing to act as a pharmacy technician in this state; and
   4. Be acting as a pharmacy technician in this state.
D. Each person appointed to the Board shall, no later than the 15th day after the date of appointment, qualify by taking the constitutional oath of office.

Section 552.003 Public Member Eligibility
A person is not eligible for appointment as a public member of the Board if the person or person's spouse:
   1. Is registered, certified, or licensed by an occupational regulatory agency in the field of health care (e.g., nurse or physician);
   2. Is employed by or participates in the management of a business entity or other organization regulated by or receiving funds from the Board;
   3. Owns or controls directly or indirectly more than a 10 percent interest in a business entity or other organization regulated by or receiving funds from the Board; or
   4. Uses or receives a substantial amount of tangible goods, services, or funds from the Board other than compensation or reimbursement authorized by law for board membership, attendance, or expenses.

Section 552.004 Membership Restrictions
A. A person may not be a member of the Board if the person is required to register as a lobbyist under Chapter 305, Government Code, and its subsequent amendments because of the person's activities for compensation on behalf of a profession related to the operation of the Board (i.e., a person acting as a lobbyist for the Texas Pharmacy Association, Texas Medical Association, etc.).
B. A person may not be a member of the Board if the person is an officer, employee, or paid consultant of a Texas trade association in the field of health care or the person's spouse is an officer, employee, or paid consultant of a Texas trade association in the field of health care.

Section 552.005 Terms; Vacancy
A. Members of the Board are appointed for staggered six-year terms. The terms of either three or four members' terms as applicable expire every other year at midnight on the last day of the state fiscal year in the last year of the member's term.
B. If a vacancy occurs during a member's term, the governor shall appoint a replacement to fill the unexpired term.
C. A Board member may not serve more than two consecutive full terms. The completion of the unexpired portion of a full term is not a full term for purposes of this section.
D. A person appointed by the governor to a full term before the expiration of the term of the member being succeeded becomes a member of the Board on the first day of the next state fiscal year following the appointment.
E. A person appointed to an unexpired portion of a full term becomes a member of the Board on the day after the date of appointment.

Section 552.006 Board Member Training
A. A person who is appointed to and qualifies for office as a member of the Board may not vote, deliberate, or be counted as a member in attendance at a meeting of the Board until the person completes a training program that complies with this section.
B. The training program must provide the person with information regarding:
   1. The law governing the Board's operation;
   2. The programs, functions, rules, and budget of the Board;

3. The scope of and limitations on the rulemaking authority of the Board;
4. The types of Board rules, interpretations, and enforcement actions that may implicate federal antitrust law by limiting competition or impacting prices charged by persons engaged in a profession or business the Board regulates, including rules, interpretations, and enforcement actions that:
   a. Regulate the scope of practice of a person in a profession or business the Board regulates;
   b. Restrict advertising by persons in a profession or business the Board regulates;
   c. Affect the price of goods or services provided by persons in a profession or business the Board regulates; and
   d. Restrict participation in a profession or business the Board regulates;
5. The results of the most recent formal audit of the Board;
6. The requirements of:
   a. Laws relating to open meetings, public information, administrative procedure, and disclosing conflicts of interest and
   b. Other laws applicable to members of the Board in performing their duties; and
7. Any applicable ethics policies adopted by the Board or the Texas Ethics Commission.
C. A person appointed to the Board is entitled to reimbursement, as provided by the General Appropriations Act, for the travel expenses incurred in attending the training program regardless of whether the attendance at the program occurs before or after the person qualifies for office.
D. The executive director shall create a training manual that includes the information required by B. above. The executive director shall distribute a copy of the training manual annually to each board member. On receipt of the training manual, each board member shall sign and submit to the executive director a statement acknowledging receipt of the training manual. The Board shall publish a copy of each signed statement on the Board's Internet website.

Section 552.007 Officers
A. The governor shall designate a member of the Board as the president of the Board to serve in that capacity at the pleasure of the governor. The Board shall elect from its members for one-year terms a vice president, treasurer, and other officers the Board considers appropriate and necessary to conduct Board business.
B. The Board's president shall preside at each Board meeting and is responsible for the performance of the Board's duties and functions.
C. An officer, other than the president, shall perform the duties normally associated with the officer's position and other duties assigned to the officer by the Board.
D. The term of an officer begins on the first day of the state fiscal year following the officer's election and ends on election of a successor.
E. A member elected as an officer may not serve more than two consecutive full terms in each office to which the member is elected.

Section 552.008 Grounds for Removal
A. It is a ground for removal from the Board that a member:
   1. Does not have at the time of appointment the qualifications required for appointment to the Board;
   2. Does not maintain during service on the Board the qualifications required for appointment to the Board;
   3. Violates a prohibition established by Section 552.004 (related to being a lobbyist or an officer, employee, or paid consultant of a trade association in a healthcare field);

4. Cannot, because of illness or disability, discharge the member's duties for a substantial part of the member's term; or
5. Is absent from more than half of the regularly scheduled Board meetings that the member is eligible to attend during a calendar year unless the absence is excused by a majority vote of the Board.

B. If the executive director has knowledge that a potential ground for removal exists, the executive director shall notify the president of the Board of the ground. The president shall then notify the governor that a potential ground for removal exists.

C. The validity of an action of the Board is not affected by the fact that it is taken when a ground for removal of a Board member exists.

Section 552.009 Per Diem; Reimbursement
A. Each member of the Board is entitled to a per diem set by the legislative appropriation for each day the member engages in Board business.
B. A member is entitled to reimbursement for travel expenses as prescribed by the General Appropriations Act.

Section 552.010 Meetings
A. The Board shall meet at least once every four months to transact Board business.
B. The Board may meet at other times at the call of the Board's president or two-thirds of the Board's members.

Section 552.011 Executive Session
A. The Board may, in accordance with Chapter 551, Government Code (Open Meetings Act), conduct a portion of a Board meeting in executive session (closed session—not open to the public).
B. The Board may conduct in executive session a deliberation relating to the discipline of a license holder. At the conclusion of the deliberation and in open session, the Board shall vote and announce the decision.
C. The Board may also conduct in executive session disciplinary hearings related to impaired pharmacists or pharmacy students.

Section 552.012 Quorum; Validity of Board Action
Except where a greater number is required by this Act or by rule, an action of the Board must be by a majority of a quorum.

Chapter 553 Executive Director and Other Board Personnel

Section 553.001 Executive Director
The Board shall employ an executive director.

Section 553.002 Qualifications of the Executive Director
The executive director must be a pharmacist.

Section 553.003 General Duties of the Executive Director
A. The executive director is an ex officio member of the Board without vote.
B. The executive director is a full-time employee of the Board and shall:
 1. Serve as secretary to the Board;
 2. Perform the regular administrative functions of the Board and any other duty the Board directs; and
 3. Under the direction of the Board, perform the duties required by this Act or designated by the Board.
C. The executive director may not perform a discretionary or decision making function for which the Board is solely responsible.
D. The executive director shall keep the seal of the Board. The executive director may affix the seal only in the manner prescribed by the Board.

Section 553.004 Personnel
The Board may employ persons in positions or capacities the Board considers necessary to properly conduct the Board's business and fulfill the Board's responsibilities under this Act.

Section 553.005 Employee Restrictions

Section 553.006 Possession By Employee of a Regulated Substance
A Board employee may possess a dangerous drug or controlled substance when acting in the employee's official capacity.

Section 553.007 Division of Responsibility

Section 553.008 Qualifications and Standards of Conduct

Section 553.009 Career Ladder Program; Performance Evaluations

Section 553.010 Equal Employment Opportunity Policy; Report

Chapter 554 Board Powers and Duties; Rulemaking Authority
SUBCHAPTER A. Powers and Duties

Note: Four state laws affect TSBP's activities including disciplinary procedures, rulemaking procedures, meeting procedures, and availability of records.

A. Administrative Procedures Act (APA) (Chapter 2001, Texas Government Code)
All disciplinary action and rulemaking must be conducted in compliance with the provisions of this law.
B. Texas Open Meetings Act (Chapter 551, Texas Government Code)
All meetings and hearings are open to the public except for:
1. Executive sessions authorized by the Open Meetings Act;
2. TSBP deliberations relative to licensee disciplinary actions (however, the Board must vote and announce its decision in open session); and
3. TSBP disciplinary hearings relating to impaired pharmacists or pharmacy students.
C. Texas Public Information Act (Chapter 552, Texas Government Code)
All records of hearings or meetings are open records except for records relating to executive sessions, impaired pharmacists, certain licensure information, Board investigative records or complaints, and identity of complainants.
D. Texas Pharmacy Act (Occupations Code, Subtitle J) and Rules
Identifies Board responsibilities, practice standards, pharmacy standards, and disciplinary grounds and procedures.

Section 554.001 General Powers and Duties of the Board
A. The Board shall:
1. Administer and enforce this Act and rules adopted under this Act and enforce other laws relating to the practice of pharmacy and other powers and duties granted under other law;
2. Cooperate with other state and federal agencies in the enforcement of any law relating to the practice of pharmacy or any drug or drug-related law;
3. Maintain an office in which permanent records are kept; and
4. Preserve a record of the Board's proceedings.
B. The Board may:
1. Join a professional organization or association to promote the improvement of standards of the practice of pharmacy for protecting the health and welfare of the public and
2. Appoint committees from the Board's membership, an advisory committee from the pharmacy profession, and any other group to assist in administering this Act.

C. The Board may:
1. Issue a duplicate copy of a license to practice pharmacy or a license renewal certificate on a request from the holder and on payment of a fee determined by the Board and
2. Inspect a facility licensed under this Act for compliance with this Act.
D. The Board may be represented by counsel, including the attorney general, district attorney, or county attorney, in a legal action taken under this Act.
E. The Board shall develop formal policies outlining the structure, role, and responsibilities of each committee established under B.2. above that contains Board members. The Board may adopt rules to implement B.2.

Section 554.0011 Use of Alternative Rulemaking and Dispute Resolution
A. The Board shall develop a policy to encourage the use of:
1. Negotiated rulemaking procedures under Chapter 2008, Government Code for the adoption of Board rules and
2. Appropriate alternative dispute resolution procedures under Chapter 2009, Government Code to assist in the resolution of internal and external disputes under the Board's jurisdiction.
B. The Board's procedures relating to alternative dispute resolution must conform to the extent possible to any model guidelines issued by the State Office of Administrative Hearings for the use of alternative dispute resolution by state agencies.
C. The Board shall:
1. Coordinate the implementation of the policy adopted by A. above;
2. Provide training as needed to implement the procedures for negotiated rulemaking or alternative dispute resolution; and
3. Collect data concerning the effectiveness of those procedures.

Section 554.002 Regulation of the Practice of Pharmacy
The Board shall regulate the practice of pharmacy in this state by:
1. Issuing a license after examination or by reciprocity to an applicant qualified to practice pharmacy and issuing a license to a pharmacy under this Act;
2. Renewing a license to practice pharmacy and a license to operate a pharmacy;
3. Determining and issuing standards for recognizing and approving degree requirements of colleges of pharmacy whose graduates are eligible for a license in this state;
4. Specifying and enforcing requirements for practical training including an internship;
5. Enforcing the provisions of this Act relating to:
   a. The conduct or competence of a pharmacist practicing in this state and the conduct of a pharmacy operating in this state and
   b. The suspension, revocation, retirement, or restriction of a license to practice pharmacy or to operate a pharmacy or the imposition of an administrative penalty or reprimand on a license holder;
6. Regulating the training, qualifications, and employment of a pharmacist intern, pharmacy technician, and pharmacy technician trainee; and
7. Determining and issuing standards for recognizing and approving a pharmacy residency program for purposes of Subchapter T, Chapter 61, Education Code;

Board of Pharmacy Rule 291.27
Pharmacy Residency Programs

For the purposes of Subchapter T, Chapter 61, Education Code, the standards for pharmacy residency programs shall be the standards required by the American Society of Health-System Pharmacists' Commission on Credentialing. The pharmacy residency

Notes

programs approved by the Board shall be published periodically in the minutes of the Board.

(Continued from Section 554.002)

8. Regulating the training, qualifications, and employment of a pharmacist intern; and
9. Regulating the training qualifications and employment of pharmacy technicians.

Section 554.003 Procedures

The Board by rule shall specify the licensing procedures and fees for filing an application for a pharmacy license.

Section 554.004 Administration of Medication (*See also Section 554.052 for Immunizations and Vaccinations and Section 562.057 for Epinephrine Auto Injectors.*)

A. The Board shall specify conditions under which a pharmacist may administer medications, including an immunization and a vaccination. The conditions must ensure that:
   1. A licensed healthcare provider authorized to administer the medication is not reasonably available to administer the medication;
   2. Failure to administer the medication, other than an immunization or a vaccination, might result in a significant delay or interruption of a critical phase of drug therapy;
   3. The pharmacist possesses the necessary skill and education to administer the medication;
   4. Within a reasonable time after administering the medication, the pharmacist notifies the licensed healthcare provider responsible for the patient's care that the medication was administered;
   5. The pharmacist may not administer medications to a patient at the patient's residence, except at a licensed nursing home or hospital;
   6. The pharmacist administers an immunization or a vaccination under a physician's written protocol and meets the standards established by the Board; and
   7. The authority of the pharmacist to administer medications may not be delegated.
B. This section does not prohibit a pharmacist from preparing or manipulating a biotechnological agent or device.
C. This section does not prohibit a pharmacist from performing an act delegated by a physician in accordance with Chapter 157 (Medical Practice Act). The pharmacist performing a delegated medical act under that chapter is considered to be performing a medical act and not to be engaging in the practice of pharmacy.

Section 554.005 Prescription Drugs and Devices

A. In regulating the practice of pharmacy and the use in this state of prescription drugs and devices in the diagnosis, mitigation, or treatment or prevention of injury, illness, or disease, the Board shall:
   1. Regulate the delivery or distribution of a prescription drug or device;
   2. Specify the minimum standards for the professional environment, technical equipment, and security in a prescription dispensing area;
   3. Specify minimum standards for:
      a. Drug storage;
      b. Maintenance of prescription drug records; and
      c. Procedures for the:
         (1) Delivering and dispensing in a suitable, appropriately labeled container;
         (2) Providing of prescription drugs or devices;

(3) Monitoring of drug therapy; and
(4) Counseling of patients on proper use of a prescription drug or device in the practice of pharmacy;
4. Adopt rules regulating a prescription drug order or medication order transmitted by electronic means; and
5. Register a balance used for compounding drugs in a pharmacy licensed in this state and periodically inspect the balance to verify accuracy.
B. In implementing A.1. above, the Board may, after notice and a hearing, seize any prescription drug or device that poses a hazard to the public health and welfare.
C. In implementing A.1. above, the Board may not regulate:
1. Any manufacturer's representative or employee acting in the normal course of business;
2. A person engaged in the wholesale drug business and licensed by the Commissioner of Public Health as provided by Chapter 431, Health and Safety Code; or
3. An employee of a person described in 2. above, if the employee is acting in the normal course of business.

Section 554.006 Fees

Section 554.007 Funds; State Pharmacy Account

Section 554.008 Surety Bonds

Section 554.009 Lease or Purchase of Vehicles

Section 554.010 Peace Officers (TSBP investigators who are commissioned peace officers may carry weapons and make arrests.)

Section 554.011 Pilot and Demonstration Research Projects
A. The Board may approve pilot and demonstration research projects for innovative applications in the practice of pharmacy.
B. The Board shall specify the procedures to be followed in applying for approval of a project.
C. The approval may include a provision granting an exception to any rule adopted under this Act. The Board may extend the time an exception to a rule is granted as necessary for the Board to adopt an amendment or modification of the rule. The Board may condition approval of a project in compliance with this section and rules adopted under this section.
D. A project may not include therapeutic substitution or substitution of a medical device used in patient care.
E. This section does not expand the definition of pharmacy under this Act.

Board of Pharmacy Rule 291.23
Pilot or Demonstration Research Projects
for Innovative Applications in the Practice of Pharmacy

A. Purpose.
The purpose of this section is to specify the procedures to be followed in applying for approval of a pilot or demonstration research project for innovative applications in the practice of pharmacy as authorized by Section 554.011 of the Texas Pharmacy Act. In reviewing projects, the Board will only consider projects that expand pharmaceutical care services which contribute to positive patient outcomes. The Board will not consider any project intended only to provide a competitive advantage.

Notes

B. Scope of Pilot or Demonstration Research Projects and the Board's Approval of Such Projects.
   1. Pilot or demonstration research projects may not:
      a. Expand the definition of the practice of pharmacy as provided in the Act or
      b. Include therapeutic substitution or substitution of medical devices used in patient care.
   2. The Board's approval of pilot or demonstration research projects may include the granting of an exception to the rules adopted under this Act but may not include an exception from any law relating to the practice of pharmacy. Such exception to the rules shall be for a specified period of time, and such period may not exceed 18 months.
   3. The Board may extend the time an exception to a rule is granted as necessary for the Board to adopt an amendment or modification of the rule.
C. Procedures for Applying for Approval of Pilot or Demonstration Research Projects. A person who wishes the Board to consider approval of a pilot or demonstration research project shall submit to the Board a petition for approval which contains at least the following information:
   1. Name, address, telephone number, and license number of the pharmacist responsible for overseeing the project;
   2. Specific location and, if a pharmacy, the pharmacy license number where the proposed pilot or demonstration project will be conducted; and
   3. A detailed summary of the proposed pilot or demonstration project which includes:
      a. The goals, hypothesis, and/or objectives of the proposed project;
      b. A full explanation of the project and how it will be conducted;
      c. The time frame for the project including the proposed start date and length of study (such time frame may not exceed 18 months);
      d. Background information and/or literature review to support the proposal;
      e. The rule(s) that will have to be waived to complete the project and a request to waive the rule(s); and
      f. Procedures to be used during the project to ensure that the public's health and safety are not compromised as a result of the rule waiver.
D. Review and Approval or Denial of the Proposed Projects.
   1. On receipt of a petition for approval of a pilot or demonstration research project, Board staff shall initially review the petition for completeness and appropriateness. If the petition is incomplete or inappropriate for Board consideration for any reason, staff shall return the petition with a letter of explanation. Such review shall be completed within 30 working days of the receipt of the petition.
   2. Once Board staff has determined that the petition is complete and appropriate, a task force composed of Board staff, at least one Board member, and, if deemed necessary, resource personnel appointed by the Board president shall review the petition and make a written recommendation to the Board regarding approval. Such recommendation shall be presented to the Board at the next regularly scheduled meeting of the Board that occurs at least three weeks after completion of the review and written recommendation.
   3. A copy of the recommendation shall be provided to the petitioner and Board at least two weeks prior to the Board meeting.
   4. Both the petitioner and a representative of the task force shall be given equal time for presentations to the Board.
   5. Upon hearing the presentations, the Board shall either approve or deny the petition. If the Board approves the petition, the approval:
      a. Shall be specific for that project and for a specific time period and

b. May include conditions or qualifications if deemed appropriate by the Board.
   6. The Board or its representatives shall be allowed to inspect and review the project documentation and site at any time during the review process and after the project is approved.
E. Presentation of Results to the Board.
   1. The pharmacist responsible for overseeing the project shall forward to the Board a summary of the results of the project and conclusions drawn from the results within three months after completion of the project.
   2. A task force composed of Board staff, at least one Board member, and, if deemed necessary, resource personnel appointed by the Board president shall review the results and make written recommendations to the Board regarding the results of the project.
   3. The Board will receive the report of the task force at the next regularly scheduled meeting of the Board that occurs at least three weeks after the task force has completed its review and issued written recommendations.
   4. A copy of the task force recommendation shall be provided to the petitioner and Board at least two weeks prior to the Board meeting.
   5. Both the petitioner and a representative of the task force shall be given equal time for presentations to the Board.

Section 554.012 Notification Relating to Therapeutic Optometrists

The Board shall inform each holder of a license to practice pharmacy and each holder of a license to operate a pharmacy of the authority of a therapeutic optometrist to prescribe a drug under Section 351.357 by annually mailing to each license holder a notice that:
   1. Describes the authority of a therapeutic optometrist to prescribe a drug and
   2. Lists each drug that a therapeutic optometrist may lawfully prescribe.

Section 554.018 Comprehensive Substance Use Disorder Approach

The Board shall encourage pharmacists to participate in a program that provides a comprehensive approach to the delivery of early intervention and treatment services for persons with substance use disorders and persons who are at risk of developing substance use disorders, such as a program promoted by the Substance Abuse and Mental Health Services Administration within the United States Department of Health and Human Services.

SUBCHAPTER B. Rulemaking

Section 554.051 Rulemaking; General Powers and Duties
A. The Board shall adopt rules consistent with this Act for the administration and enforcement of this Act.
B. If the Board determines it necessary to protect the health and welfare of the citizens of this state, the Board may make a rule concerning the operation of a licensed pharmacy located in this state applicable to a pharmacy licensed by the board that is located in another state.
C. The Board shall adopt rules regarding records to be maintained by a pharmacist performing a specific act under a written protocol.
D. The Board by rule shall specify the minimum standards for professional responsibility in the conduct of a pharmacy.

Section 554.052 Immunizations and Vaccinations; Physician Supervision
A. The Board by rule shall require a pharmacist to notify a physician who prescribes an immunization or a vaccination within 24 hours after the pharmacist administers the immunization or vaccination.

B. The Board shall establish minimum education and continuing education standards for a pharmacist who administers an immunization or a vaccination. The standards must include Centers for Disease Control and Prevention training, basic life support training, and hands-on training in techniques for administering immunizations and vaccinations.
C. Supervision by a physician is adequate if the delegating physician:
   1. Is responsible for formulating or approving an order or protocol, including the physician's order, standing medical order, or standing delegation order, and periodically reviews the order or protocol and the services provided to a patient under the order or protocol;
   2. Except as provided by D. below, has established a physician-patient relationship with each patient under 14 years of age and referred the patient to the pharmacist;
   3. Is geographically located to be easily accessible to the pharmacy where an immunization or a vaccination is administered;
   4. Receives, as appropriate, a periodic status report on the patient, including any problem or complication encountered; and
   5. Is available through direct telecommunication for consultation, assistance, and direction.
D. A pharmacist may administer an influenza vaccination to a patient over seven years of age without an established physician-patient relationship.
E. The Texas Medical Board by rule shall establish the minimum content of a written order or protocol. The order or protocol may not permit the delegation of a medical diagnosis.

Board of Pharmacy Rule 295.15
Administration of Immunizations or Vaccinations by a Pharmacist Under Written Protocol of a Physician

A. Basic Requirements.
   1. Pharmacists may only administer immunizations or vaccinations pursuant to a written protocol from an authorizing physician.
   2. Pharmacists may administer immunizations or vaccinations to patients under 14 years of age only if referred to the pharmacist from a physician who has an established physician-patient relationship with the child except that a pharmacist may administer an influenza vaccination to a patient over the age of seven without an established physician-patient relationship.
   3. Immunizations may be done within a pharmacy or other location identified in the protocol. Such other location may not include where the patient resides except for licensed nursing homes and hospitals.
   4. The authority to administer may not be delegated.
   5. Pharmacists may only administer when a licensed healthcare provider authorized to administer medication is not reasonably available to administer the medication (not immediately available).
   6. The administering pharmacist must keep specific records and provide specific notifications.
   7. Before preparing a vaccine and between each patient contact, the pharmacist shall cleanse his or her hands with an alcohol-based waterless antiseptic hand rub or shall wash his or her hands with soap and water. If gloves are worn, the pharmacist shall change gloves between patients.
B. Minimum Statements Required in a Written Protocol.
   1. Statement identifying the individual physician authorized to prescribe drugs and responsible for the delegation of administration of immunizations or vaccinations.

2. Statement identifying the individual pharmacist authorized to administer immunizations or vaccinations.
3. Statement identifying the location(s) at which the pharmacist may administer immunizations or vaccinations.
4. Statement identifying the immunizations or vaccinations that may be administered by the pharmacist.
5. Statement identifying the activities that a pharmacist shall follow in the course of administering immunizations or vaccinations including procedures to follow in case of reactions.
6. Statement that describes the content of and appropriate mechanisms for the pharmacist to report the administration of immunizations or vaccinations to the physician.

C. Pharmacist Certification Requirements.
   1. A pharmacist must be certified by completing an ACPE approved course which includes:
      a. Current certification in Basic Cardiac Life Support.
      b. An evidence-based course consisting of study material, hands-on training, and testing with a passing score.
      c. Meeting CDC training guidelines and providing for a minimum of 20 hours of instruction and experiential training in specified content areas.
   2. Must maintain documentation of:
      a. Completion of initial training.
      b. Three hours of continuing education every two years, which are designed to maintain competency in the disease states, drugs, and administration of immunizations and vaccinations.
      c. Current certification in Basic Cardiac Life Support.

D. Physician Supervision.
   Physician supervision is adequate if the delegating physician:
   1. Is responsible for formulation or the approval of a physician's order, standing medical order, standing delegation order, or other order or protocol;
   2. Has an established physician-patient relationship with each patient under 14 years of age that is referred to the pharmacist (however, a pharmacist may administer an influenza vaccination to a patient over seven years of age without an established physician-patient relationship);
   3. Is geographically located so as to be easily accessible to the pharmacist;
   4. Receives, as appropriate, a periodic status report on the patient, including any problem or complication encountered; and
   5. Is available through direct telecommunication for consultation, assistance, and direction.

E. Notifications.
   1. A pharmacist administering immunizations or vaccinations shall notify:
      a. The physician who issued the written protocol within 24 hours of administering the immunization or vaccination.
      b. The primary care physician of the patient within 14 days of administering the immunization or vaccination.
   2. The notification shall include:
      a. Name and address of the patient.
      b. Age of the patient if under 14 years of age.
      c. Name of the patient's primary care physician.
      d. Name, manufacturer, and lot number of the vaccine administered.
      e. Amount administered.
      f. Date administered.
      g. Site of administration.

h. Route of administration.
i. Name, address, and title of person administering.
F. Records and Confidentiality for Immunization Administration.
1. Pharmacists must maintain records of each administration, including notifications, for at least two years.
2. Pharmacists must provide adequate security to prevent indiscriminate or unauthorized access to confidential records including immunization and vaccination records. In addition to the confidentiality requirements specified in Board Rule 291.27 (Confidentiality), a pharmacist shall comply with:
    a. The privacy provisions of the federal Health Insurance Portability and Accountability Act of 1996 (Pub. L. No. 104-191) and any rules adopted pursuant to this act;
    b. The requirements of Medical Records Privacy contained in Chapter 181, Health and Safety Code;
    c. The Privacy of Health Information requirements contained in Chapter 28B of the Insurance Code; and
    d. Any other confidentiality provisions of federal or state laws.

Section 554.053 Rulemaking; Pharmacy Technician and Pharmacy Technician Trainee

A. The Board shall establish rules for the use and duties of a pharmacy technician and pharmacy technician trainee in a pharmacy licensed by the Board. A pharmacy technician and pharmacy technician trainee shall be responsible to and must be directly supervised by a pharmacist.
B. The Board may not adopt a rule establishing a ratio of pharmacists to pharmacy technicians and pharmacy technician trainees in a Class C pharmacy or limiting the number of pharmacy technicians or pharmacy technician trainees that may be used in a Class C pharmacy.
C. The Board may determine and issue standards for the recognition and approval of a training program for pharmacy technicians and maintain a list of training programs that meet those standards.

Section 554.054 Rules Restricting Advertising or Competitive Bidding

A. The Board may not adopt rules restricting advertising or competitive bidding by a person regulated by the Board except to prohibit false, misleading, or deceptive practices by that person.
B. The Board may not adopt a rule to prohibit false, misleading, or deceptive practices by a person regulated by the Board if the rule:
1. Restricts the use of any medium for advertising;
2. Restricts the person's personal appearance or use of the person's voice in an advertisement;
3. Relates to the size or duration of an advertisement used by the person; or
4. Restricts the use of a trade name in advertising by the person.

Section 554.055 Rulemaking: Electronic Media

The Board shall adopt rules regarding the sale and delivery of drugs by use of electronic media including the Internet.

Chapter 557 Pharmacist Interns

Section 557.001 Pharmacist Intern Registration

A person must register with the Board before beginning a Board-approved internship in this state.

Section 557.002 Application for Registration

An application for the registration as a pharmacist intern must be on a form prescribed by the Board.

Section 557.003 Duration of Registration

A person's registration as a pharmacist intern remains in effect as long as the person meets the qualifications for an internship specified by Board rule.

Section 557.004 Limitations on Registration

A. The Board may:
1. Refuse to issue a registration to an applicant or
2. Restrict, suspend, or revoke a pharmacist intern registration for a violation of this Act.

B. The Board may take disciplinary action against an applicant for a pharmacist intern registration or the holder of a current or expired pharmacist intern registration in the same manner as against an applicant for a license or a license holder by imposing a sanction authorized under Section 565.001 if the Board finds that the applicant or registration holder has engaged in conduct described by Section 565.001 of the Act.

Note: See Chapter F for disciplinary action.

Chapter 558 License to Practice Pharmacy
SUBCHAPTER A. License (Pharmacists)

Section 558.001 License Required

A. A person may not practice pharmacy unless the person holds a license to practice pharmacy under this Act.
B. A person may not:
1. Impersonate a pharmacist or
2. Use the title "Registered Pharmacist" or "R.Ph." or words of similar intent unless the person is licensed to practice pharmacy in this state.

C. A person may not dispense or distribute prescription drugs unless the person:
1. Is a pharmacist or
2. Is otherwise authorized by this Act to dispense or distribute prescription drugs.

Section 558.002 Unauthorized Acquisition of a License

A person may not:
1. Impersonate before the Board an applicant applying for a license under this Act or
2. Acquire, with the intent to fraudulently acquire the license, a license in a manner other than provided by this Act.

Board of Pharmacy Rule 281.12
Criminal History Evaluation Letter

A. A person, who is enrolled or planning to enroll in an educational program that prepares the person for a license as a pharmacist or a registration as a pharmacy technician or trainee, or planning to take an examination required for such a license or registration, and who has reason to believe that he or she may be ineligible due to a conviction or deferred adjudication for a felony or misdemeanor offense, may request a criminal history evaluation letter regarding his or her eligibility for a license or registration.

B. The person must submit an application for the criminal history evaluation letter on a form provided by the Board which includes:
1. A statement indicating the reasons and basis for potential ineligibility, including each criminal offense for which the person was arrested, charged, convicted, or received deferred adjudication;

2. All legal documents related to the reasons and basis for potential ineligibility including, but not limited to, police reports, indictments, orders of deferred adjudication, judgments, probation records, and evidence of completion of probation, if applicable;
3. All requirements necessary for the Board to access the criminal history record information including submitting fingerprint information and paying the required fees; and
4. A nonrefundable fee of $150 for processing the application.
C. The application is considered complete when all documents and other information supporting the potential reasons and basis for potential ineligibility have been received by the Board. If such documentation is not received within 120 days of the initial receipt of the application, the application is considered to be expired and must be refiled along with the appropriate fees.
D. The Board shall conduct an investigation of the application and the person's eligibility for a license or registration.
E. The person or the Board may amend the application to include additional grounds for potential ineligibility at any time before a final determination is made.
F. A determination of eligibility will be made by the Board or its designees. Notification of the determination will be provided to the person in writing.
1. If no grounds for ineligibility are identified, the notification shall address the determination regarding each ground of potential ineligibility.
2. If grounds for ineligibility exist, the notification shall set out each basis for potential ineligibility and the corresponding determination.
G. The Board shall mail the determination of eligibility no later than the 90th day after the complete application, as required by B. and C. above, has been received by the Board.
H. The determination of eligibility shall be made based on the law in effect on the date of the receipt of a complete application.
I. In the discretion of the Board, any information the person fails to disclose on the application or any information determined to be inaccurate or incomplete shall invalidate the determination of eligibility on the basis of the information.
J. The administrative rules regarding disciplinary guidelines and regarding considerations and sanctions for criminal conduct apply in determining eligibility.
K. If a person submits an application for a license or registration at the same time or within 90 days after the receipt of a complete application for a criminal history evaluation letter, the Board will process only the application for a license or registration and will not issue a separate determination of eligibility.

SUBCHAPTER B. Licensing by Examination (Pharmacists)

Section 558.051 Qualifications for a License by Examination

A. To qualify for a license to practice pharmacy, an applicant for licensing by examination must submit to the Board:
1. A license fee set by the Board and
2. A completed application on a form prescribed by the Board with satisfactory sworn evidence that the applicant:
    a. Is at least 18 years old;
    b. Has completed a minimum of a 1,000-hour internship or other program that has been approved by the Board or has demonstrated, to the Board's satisfaction, experience in the practice of pharmacy that meets or exceeds the Board's minimum internship requirements;
    Note: The Act (law) requires 1,000 hours minimum; however, 1,500 hours are required by rule of the Board.

  c. Has graduated and received a professional practice degree, as defined by Board rule, from an accredited pharmacy degree program approved by the Board;
  d. Has passed the examinations required by the Board (NAPLEX and Texas MPJE); and
  e. Has not had a pharmacist license granted by another state restricted, suspended, revoked, or surrendered for any reason.
B. Each applicant must obtain practical experience in the practice of pharmacy concurrent with college attendance or after college graduation or both under conditions the Board determines.

Section 558.052 Content, Preparation, and Validation of Examination
A. The Board shall determine the content and subject matter of a licensing examination.
B. The examination shall be prepared to measure the competence of the applicant to practice pharmacy.
C. The Board may employ and cooperate with an organization or consultant in preparing an appropriate examination.
D. A written examination prepared or offered by the Board, including a standardized national examination, must be validated by an independent testing professional.

Board of Pharmacy Rule 283.7
Examination Requirements

A. Prior to taking the required examinations, the applicant shall meet minimum educational and age requirements and may be required to meet all requirements necessary for the Board to access the criminal history record information, including submitting fingerprint information and being responsible for all associated costs.
B. Applicant must pass NAPLEX which includes the following subject areas:
 1. Chemistry;
 2. Mathematics;
 3. Pharmacy;
 4. Pharmacology; and
 5. Practice of pharmacy.
C. To pass NAPLEX, the applicant must score 75 on a scaled score. NABP uses a mathematically-based weighted scoring model to calculate an ability measure for each NAPLEX examinee. The ability measures are transformed to a reporting scaled score that ranges from 0 to 150. Scaled scores do not represent a percentage or the raw number of correct answers. If the applicant fails, he or she may retake the exam four additional times for a total of five exams. Prior to any subsequent retakes, the applicant must comply with Rule 283.11 (Exam Retake Requirements).
D. To pass the Texas MPJE, the applicant must score 75 on a scaled score. NABP uses a mathematically-based weighted scoring model to calculate an ability measure for each MPJE candidate. These ability measures are transformed to a reporting scale that ranges from 0 to 100. Scaled scores do not represent a percentage or the raw number of correct answers. If the applicant fails, he or she may retake the exam four additional times for a total of five exams. Prior to any subsequent retakes, the applicant must comply with Rule 283.11 (Exam Retake Requirements).
E. NAPLEX and Texas MPJE exams are scored separately and can be retaken independently. A passing grade on an examination may be used for the purpose of licensure for a period of two years from the date of passing the examination.

F. A person who has failed the NAPLEX or Texas MPJE five times must present documentation of additional training before he or she can retake the exam as required by Board Rule 283.11 (Examination Retake Requirements).
G. Score Transfer Program.
Note: The Score Transfer Program allows a person to take the NAPLEX one time and have the score count toward licensure by examination in more than one state. (See NABP NAPLEX Registration Bulletin.)
Each applicant for licensure by examination using NAPLEX scores transferred from another state to Texas shall meet the following requirements for licensure in addition to the requirements above.
  1. The applicant shall request NABP to transfer NAPLEX scores to TSBP. Such a request shall be in accordance with NABP policy.
  2. The applicant shall pay the fee set out in Board Rule 283.9 (Fee Requirements for Licensure by Examination and Reciprocity).
  3. The applicant must pass the Texas Pharmacy Jurisprudence Examination (MPJE).
H. The NAPLEX and Texas MPJE shall be administered in compliance with the Americans with Disability Act of 1990 and in accordance with NABP policy.
I. The Board, in accordance with NABP policy, shall provide reasonable accommodations for an applicant diagnosed as having dyslexia as defined in 51.970, Texas Education Code. The applicant shall provide:
  1. Written documentation from a licensed physician which indicates that the applicant has been diagnosed as having dyslexia and
  2. A written request outlining the reasonable accommodations requested.

Section 558.053 Grading of the Examination
A. The Board may employ and cooperate with an organization or consultant in grading the examination.
B. The Board shall determine whether an applicant has passed the examination. The Board has sole discretion and responsibility for that determination.

Section 558.054 Frequency of Offering Examinations
The Board shall give the examination at least two times during each state fiscal year.

Section 558.055 Failure to Pass; Reexamination
A. An applicant who on the applicant's first attempt fails the examination may take the examination four additional times.
B. Before an applicant who has failed the examination five times is allowed to retake the examination, the applicant must provide documentation from a college of pharmacy that the applicant has successfully completed additional college course work in each examination area that the applicant failed.
C. If requested in writing by a person who fails the examination, the Board shall furnish the person with an analysis of the person's performance on the examination.

Board of Pharmacy Rule 283.11
Examination Retake Requirements

A. Licensing by Examination.
If an applicant fails to make a passing grade (75) on the NAPLEX and/or the Texas MPJE, the applicant may retake the exam(s) four additional times for a total of five exam administrations. Prior to any subsequent retakes for the exam(s), the applicant must:
  1. Complete course work in the subject areas recommended by the Board;
  2. Submit documentation to the Board which specifies that the applicant has successfully completed the course work specified; and
  3. Comply with the requirements of Board Rule 283.7 (Examination Requirements).

B. Licensing by Reciprocity.
If an applicant fails to make a passing grade (75) on the Texas MPJE, the applicant may retake the exam four additional times for a total of five exam administrations. Prior to any subsequent retakes for the exam, the applicant must:
1. Complete course work in the subject areas recommended by the Board;
2. Submit documentation to the Board which specifies that the applicant has successfully completed the course work specified; and
3. Comply with the requirements of Board Rule 283.8 (Reciprocity Requirements).
C. Course Work.
Course work consists of:
1. One or more standard courses or self-paced work offered in a college of pharmacy's academic program;
2. One or more courses presented by a Board-approved provider of continuing education as specified in Board Rule 295.8 (Continuing Education Requirements); or
3. Any course specified by the Board.

Section 558.056 Notification
The Board must notify each person taking an examination of the results of the examination no later than 30 days after the date the Board receives the results.

Section 558.057 Internship or Other Program to Qualify for Examination
A. In this section, "preceptor" means a pharmacist licensed in this state to practice pharmacy or another healthcare professional who meets the preceptor requirements specified by rule and who is recognized by the Board to supervise and be responsible for the activities and functions of a pharmacist intern in an internship program.
B. The Board shall:
1. Establish standards for an internship or other program necessary to qualify an applicant for the licensing examination and
2. Determine the qualifications necessary for a preceptor used in the program.

Board of Pharmacy Rule 283.2
Internship—Definitions

Note: There are four types of pharmacist interns—intern trainees, student interns, resident interns, and extended interns.

The following words and terms shall have the following meanings unless the context clearly indicates otherwise.
1. **ACPE**—Accreditation Council for Pharmacy Education.
2. **Applicant**—An individual having applied for licensure to act as a pharmacist in Texas.
3. **Approved Continuing Education**—Continuing education (C.E.) which meets the requirements of Board Rule 295.8 (Continuing Education Requirements).
4. **Board**—The Texas State Board of Pharmacy; all members, divisions, departments, sections, and employees thereof.
5. **College/School of pharmacy**—A college/school of pharmacy that has a professional degree program approved by the Board and accredited by:
   a. ACPE or
   b. The Canadian Council for Accreditation of Pharmacy Programs for 1993–2004 graduates.
6. **Competency**—A demonstrated state of preparedness for the realities of professional pharmacy practice.

7. **Direct supervision**—A pharmacist preceptor or healthcare professional preceptor who is physically present and on-site at the licensed location of the pharmacy where the pharmacist intern is performing pharmacist intern duties.
8. **Didactic**—Systematic classroom instruction.
9. **Extended intern**—An intern registered with the Board who has:
   a. Applied to the Board for licensure by examination and has successfully passed the NAPLEX and Texas MPJE but lacks the required number of hours of internship for licensure; or
   b. Applied to the Board to take the NAPLEX and Texas MPJE within six calendar months after graduation and has:
      (1) Graduated and received a professional degree from a college/school of pharmacy and
      (2) Completed all of the requirements for graduation and for receipt of a professional degree from a college/school of pharmacy, the professional degree program of which has been accredited by ACPE and approved by the Board; or
   c. Applied to take the NAPLEX and Texas MPJE within six calendar months after obtaining full certification from the Foreign Pharmacy Graduate Equivalency Commission; or
   d. Applied to the Board for reissuance of a pharmacist license which has been expired for more than two years but less than ten years and has successfully passed the Texas MPJE but lacks the required number of hours of internship or continuing education required for licensure; or
   e. Been ordered by the Board to complete an internship.
10. **Foreign pharmacy graduate**—An individual whose pharmacy degree was conferred by a pharmacy school whose professional degree program has not been accredited by ACPE and approved by the Board. An individual whose pharmacy degree was conferred by a pharmacy school that was accredited by the Canadian Council for Accreditation of Pharmacy Programs between 1993 and 2004 is not considered a foreign pharmacy graduate.
11. **FPGEC**—The Foreign Pharmacy Graduate Equivalency Commission.
12. **Healthcare professional**—An individual licensed as a physician, dentist, podiatrist, veterinarian, advanced practice registered nurse, or physician assistant in Texas or another state or a pharmacist in a state other than Texas but not licensed in Texas.
13. **Healthcare professional preceptor**—A healthcare professional serving as an instructor for a Texas college/school-based internship program which is recognized by a Texas college/school of pharmacy to supervise and be responsible for the activities and functions of a student intern or intern trainee in the internship program.
14. **Intern trainee**—An individual registered with the Board who is enrolled in the first year of the professional sequence of a Texas college/school of pharmacy and who may only work in a site assigned by a Texas college/school of pharmacy.
15. **Internship**—A practical experience program approved by the Board.
16. **MPJE**—Multistate Pharmacy Jurisprudence Examination.
17. **NABP**—The National Association of Boards of Pharmacy.
18. **NAPLEX**—The North American Pharmacy Licensing Examination or its predecessor, National Association of Boards of Pharmacy Licensing Examination.
19. **Pharmaceutical care**—The provision of drug therapy and other pharmaceutical services defined in the rules of the Board and intended to assist in the care, prevention of a disease, elimination or reduction of a patient's symptoms, or arresting or slowing of a disease process.
20. **Pharmacist intern**—An intern trainee, a student intern, a resident intern, or an extended intern who is participating in a Board-approved internship program.

21. **Pharmacist preceptor**—A pharmacist licensed in Texas to practice pharmacy who meets requirements under Board rules and is recognized by the Board to supervise and be responsible for the activities and functions of a pharmacist intern in an internship program.
22. **Preceptor**—A pharmacist preceptor or a healthcare professional preceptor.
23. **Professional degree**—A bachelor of science degree in pharmacy (B.S.) or a doctorate of pharmacy (Pharm.D.).
24. **Resident intern**—An individual who is registered with the Board and:
    a. Has graduated from a college/school of pharmacy and
    b. Is completing a residency program accredited by the American Society of Health-System Pharmacists in the state of Texas.
25. **State**—One of the 50 states in the United States of America, the District of Columbia, Puerto Rico, American Samoa, Guam, Northern Mariana Islands, and U.S. Virgin Islands.
26. **Student intern**—An individual registered with the Board who is enrolled in the professional sequence of a college/school of pharmacy, has completed the first professional year and obtained a minimum of 30 credit hours of work toward a professional degree in pharmacy, and is participating in a Board-approved internship program.
27. **Texas Pharmacy Jurisprudence Examination**—A licensing exam developed or approved by the Board which evaluates an applicant's knowledge of the drug and pharmacy requirements to practice pharmacy legally in the state of Texas.

Board of Pharmacy Rule 283.3
Educational and Age Requirements

An applicant for licensure as a pharmacist must be at least 18 years of age and meet one of the following:
1. Have graduated and received a professional degree (B.S. or Pharm.D.) from a college of pharmacy or
2. Have graduated from a foreign college of pharmacy and obtained full certification from the FPGEC.

Board of Pharmacy Rule 283.4
Internship Requirements

A. Goals and Objectives of Internship.
   1. The goal of internship is for the pharmacist intern to attain the knowledge, skills, and abilities to safely, efficiently, and effectively provide pharmacist-delivered patient care to a diverse patient population and practice pharmacy under the laws and rules of the state of Texas.
   2. The following competency objectives are necessary to accomplish the goal of internship in A.1. above:
      a. Provides drug products.
         The pharmacist intern shall demonstrate competence in determining the appropriateness of prescription drug orders and medication orders; evaluating and selecting products; and assuring the accuracy of the product/prescription dispensing process.
      b. Communicates with patients and/or patients' agents about prescription drugs.
         The pharmacist intern shall demonstrate the competence in interviewing and counseling patients and/or the patients' agents on drug usage, dosage, packaging, routes of administration, intended drug use, and storage; discussing drug cautions, adverse effects, and patient conditions;

explaining policies on fees and services; relating to patients in a professional manner; and interacting to confirm patient understanding.

c. Communicates with patients and/or patients' agents about nonprescription products, devices, dietary supplements, diet, nutrition, traditional nondrug therapies, complementary and alternative therapies, and diagnostic aids.

The pharmacist intern shall demonstrate competence in interviewing and counseling patients and/or patients' agents on conditions, intended drug use, and adverse effects; assisting in and recommending drug selection; triaging and assessing the need for treatment referral, including referral for a patient seeking pharmacist-guided self-care; providing information on medical/surgical devices and home diagnostic products; and providing poison control treatment information and referral.

d. Communicates with healthcare professionals and patients and/or patients' agents.

The pharmacist intern shall demonstrate competence in obtaining and providing accurate and concise information in a professional manner and using appropriate oral, written, and nonverbal language.

e. Practices as a member of the patient's interdisciplinary healthcare team.

The pharmacist intern shall demonstrate competence in collaborating with physicians, other healthcare professionals, and patients and/or patients' agents to formulate a therapeutic plan; demonstrate competence in establishing and interpreting databases; identify drug-related problems and recommend appropriate pharmacotherapy specific to patient needs; monitor and evaluate patient outcomes; and devise follow-up plans.

f. Maintains professional ethical standards.

The pharmacist intern is required to comply with laws and rules pertaining to pharmacy practice; to apply professional judgment; to exhibit reliability and credibility in dealing with others; to deal professionally and ethically with colleagues and patients; to demonstrate sensitivity and empathy for patients/caregivers; and to maintain confidentiality.

g. Compounding.

The pharmacist intern shall demonstrate competence in using acceptable professional procedures; selecting appropriate equipment and containers; appropriately preparing compound nonsterile and sterile preparations; and documenting calculations and procedures. Pharmacist interns engaged in compounding nonsterile preparations shall meet the training requirements for pharmacists specified in Board Rule 291.131 (Pharmacies Compounding Nonsterile Preparations). Pharmacist interns engaged in compounding sterile preparations shall meet the training requirements for pharmacists specified in Board Rule 291.133 (Pharmacies Compounding Sterile Preparations).

h. Retrieves and evaluates drug information.

The pharmacist intern shall demonstrate competence in retrieving, evaluating, managing, and using the best available clinical and scientific publications for answering a drug-related request in a timely fashion and assessing, evaluating, and applying evidence-based information to promote optimal health care. The pharmacist intern shall perform investigations on relevant topics to promote inquiry and problem solving with dissemination of findings to the healthcare community and/or the public.

i. Manages general pharmacy operations.

The pharmacist intern shall develop a general understanding of planning, personnel and fiscal management, leadership skills, and policy

development. The pharmacist intern shall have an understanding of drug security, drug storage, control procedures, the regulatory requirements associated with these procedures, and maintaining quality assurance and performance improvement. The pharmacist intern shall observe and document discrepancies and irregularities, keep accurate records, and document actions. The pharmacist intern shall attend meetings requiring pharmacy representation.
   j. Participates in public health, community service, or professional activities.
   The pharmacist intern shall develop basic knowledge and skills needed to become an effective healthcare educator and a responsible participant in civic and professional organizations.
   k. Demonstrates scientific inquiry.
   The pharmacist intern shall develop skills to expand and/or refine knowledge in the areas of pharmaceutical and medical sciences or pharmaceutical services. These skills and knowledge may include data analysis of scientific, clinical, sociological, and/or economic impacts of pharmaceuticals (including investigational drugs), pharmaceutical care, and patient behaviors, with dissemination of findings to the scientific community and/or the public.
B. Hours Requirement.
   1. The Board requires 1,500 hours of internship for licensure which may be obtained through the following methods:
      a. In a Board-approved student internship as specified in C. below; or
      b. In a Board-approved, extended internship program as specified in D. below; and/or
      c. Graduation from a college/school of pharmacy after July 1, 2007. Persons graduating from such programs shall be credited 1,500 hours or the number of hours actually obtained and reported by the college; and/or
      d. Through internship hours approved and certified to the Board by another state board of pharmacy.
   2. Pharmacist interns participating in an internship may be credited no more than 50 hours per week of internship experience.
   3. Internship hours may be used for the purpose of licensure for no longer than two years from the date the internship is completed.
C. College/School-Based Internship Programs.
   1. Internship Experience Acquired by Student Interns.
      a. An individual may be designated a student intern provided he or she meets all of the following requirements:
         (1) Submits an application to the Board with required information;
         (2) Is enrolled in the professional sequence of a college/school of pharmacy that has a professional degree program accredited by ACPE and approved by the Board;
         (3) Has successfully completed the first professional year and obtained a minimum of 30 credit hours of work towards a professional degree in pharmacy; and
         (4) Has met all requirements necessary for the Board to access the criminal history record information, including submitting fingerprint information and being responsible for all associated costs.
      b. The terms of the student internship shall be as follows:
         (1) The student internship shall be gained concurrent with college attendance which may include:
            (a) Partial semester breaks such as spring breaks;
            (b) Between semester breaks; and

(c) Whole semester breaks provided the student intern attended the college/school in the immediate preceding semester and is scheduled with the college/school to attend in the immediate subsequent semester.
            (2) The student internship shall be obtained in pharmacies licensed by the Board, federal government pharmacies, or in a Board-approved program.
            (3) The student internship shall be in the presence of and under the supervision of a healthcare professional preceptor or a pharmacist preceptor.
        c. None of the internship hours acquired outside of a school-based program may be substituted for any of the hours required in a Texas college/school of pharmacy internship program.
    2. Expiration Date for Student Intern Designation.
        a. The student internship expires:
            (1) If the student intern voluntarily or involuntarily ceases enrollment, including suspension, in a college/school of pharmacy;
            (2) The student intern fails either the NAPLEX or Texas MPJE specified in this rule; or
            (3) The student intern fails to take either the NAPLEX or Texas MPJE or both within six calendar months after graduation.
        b. The executive director of the Board, in his or her discretion, may extend the term of the student internship if the administration of the NAPLEX or Texas MPJE is suspended or delayed.
    3. Texas Colleges of Pharmacy Internship Programs.
        a. Intern trainees and student interns completing a Board-approved Texas college/school-based structured internship shall be credited the actual number of hours obtained and reported by the college. No credit shall be awarded for didactic experience.
        b. No more than 600 hours of the required 1,500 hours may be obtained under a healthcare professional preceptor except when a pharmacist intern is working in a federal government pharmacy.
        c. Individuals enrolled in the professional sequence of a Texas college/school of pharmacy may be designated as an intern trainee provided he or she meets all of the following requirements:
            (1) Submits an application to the Board with the required information;
            (2) Is enrolled in the professional sequence of a college/school of pharmacy; and
            (3) Has met all requirements necessary for the Board to access the criminal history record information, including submitting fingerprint information and being responsible for all associated costs. Such internship shall remain in effect during the time the intern trainee is enrolled in the first year of the professional sequence and shall expire upon completion of the first year of the professional sequence or upon separation from the professional sequence.
D. Extended Internship Program.
    1. A person may be designated an extended intern provided he or she has met one of the following requirements:
        a. Passed the NAPLEX and Texas MPJE but lacks the required number of internship hours for licensure;
        b. Applied to the Board to take the NAPLEX and Texas MPJE within six calendar months after graduation and has:
            (1) Graduated and received a professional degree from a college/school of pharmacy or

  (2) Completed all of the requirements for graduation and received a professional degree from a college/school of pharmacy;
 c. Applied to the Board to take the NAPLEX and Texas MPJE within six calendar months after obtaining full certification from the Foreign Pharmacy Graduate Equivalency Commission;
 d. Applied to the Board for reissuance of a pharmacist license which has expired for more than two years but less than ten years and has successfully passed the Texas MPJE but lacks the required number of hours of internship or continuing education required for licensure;
 e. Is a resident in a residency program accredited by the American Society of Health-System Pharmacists in the state of Texas; or
 f. Been ordered by the Board to complete an internship.
2. In addition to meeting one of the requirements in D.1. above, an applicant for an extended internship must:
 a. Submit an application to the Board with required information and
 b. Meet all requirements necessary for the Board to access the criminal history record information, including submitting fingerprint information and being responsible for all associated costs.
3. The terms of the extended internship are as follows:
 a. The extended internship shall be Board-approved and attained in a pharmacy licensed by the Board or a federal government pharmacy participating in a Board-approved internship program.
 b. The extended internship shall be in the presence of and under the direct supervision of a pharmacist preceptor.
4. The extended internship remains in effect for two years. However, the internship expires immediately upon:
 a. The failure of the extended intern to take the NAPLEX and Texas MPJE within six calendar months after graduation or Foreign Pharmacy Graduate Equivalency Commission (FPGEC) certification;
 b. The failure of the extended intern to pass the NAPLEX and Texas MPJE specified in this rule;
 c. Upon termination of the residency program; or
 d. Obtaining a Texas pharmacist license.
5. The executive director of the Board in his or her discretion may extend the term of the extended internship if administration of the NAPLEX and/or Texas MPJE is suspended or delayed.
6. An applicant for licensure who has completed fewer than 500 hours of internship at the time of application shall complete the remainder of the 1,500 hours of internship and have the preceptor certify that the applicant has met the objectives listed in A. above.

E. Pharmacist Intern Identification.
1. Pharmacist interns shall keep documentation of designation as a pharmacist intern with them when serving as an intern and make it available for inspection by Board agents.
2. Pharmacist interns shall wear an identification tag or badge which bears the person's name and identifies him or her as a pharmacist intern.

F. Change of Address and/or Name.
1. A pharmacist intern shall notify the Board electronically or in writing within 10 days of a change of address giving the old and new address.
2. A pharmacist intern shall notify the Board in writing within 10 days of a change of name by:
 a. Sending a copy of the official document reflecting the name change (e.g., marriage certificate, divorce decree, etc.);

b. Returning the current pharmacist intern certificate which reflects the previous name; and
c. Paying a fee as determined by the Board.

Board of Pharmacy Rule 283.5
Pharmacist Intern Duties

A pharmacist intern participating in a Board-approved internship program may perform any duty of a pharmacist provided the duties are delegated and under the supervision of a pharmacist preceptor or healthcare professional preceptor with the exception that he or she cannot sign a document required to be signed by a pharmacist.

A. A pharmacist preceptor serving as an instructor for a Texas college/school-based internship program may delegate any duty of a pharmacist to an intern trainee as long as the duties are performed in a site assigned by a Texas college/school of pharmacy and under the direct supervision of a pharmacist preceptor assigned by a Texas college/school of pharmacy.

Note: While there are no differences in the duties that may be delegated to an intern trainee versus a student intern, the intern trainee may only perform his or her duties at a site assigned by the school and under the direct supervision of a pharmacist preceptor.

B. When not under the supervision of a pharmacist preceptor, a pharmacist intern may function as a pharmacy technician and perform all of the duties of a pharmacy technician without registering as a pharmacy technician provided the pharmacist intern:
  1. Is registered with the Board as a pharmacist intern;
  2. Is under the direct supervision of a pharmacist;
  3. Has completed the pharmacy's onsite technician training program;
  4. Has completed the training required for pharmacists in Board Rule 291.133 (Pharmacies Compounding Sterile Preparations) if the pharmacist intern is compounding sterile preparations; and
  5. Is not counted as a pharmacy technician in the ratio of pharmacists to pharmacy technicians. The ratio of pharmacists to pharmacy interns shall be 1:1 when performing pharmacy technician duties.

C. A pharmacist intern may not:
  1. Present or identify himself or herself as a pharmacist;
  2. Sign or initial any document which is required to be signed or initialed by a pharmacist (e.g., dispensed official prescription) unless a preceptor cosigns the document; or
  3. Independently supervise pharmacy technicians.

Board of Pharmacy Rule 283.6
Preceptor Requirements and Ratio of Preceptors to Pharmacist Interns

A. Preceptor Requirements.
  1. Preceptors shall be:
     a. A pharmacist whose license to practice pharmacy in Texas is current and not on inactive status with the Board or
     b. A healthcare professional preceptor.
  2. To be recognized as a pharmacist preceptor, a pharmacist must:
     a. Have at least one year of experience or six months of residency training if the pharmacy resident is in a program accredited by the American Society of Health-System Pharmacists;
     b. For initial certification, have completed three hours of pharmacist preceptor training provided by an ACPE approved provider within the

previous two years. Such training shall be developed by a Texas college/school of pharmacy or be approved by a committee comprised of the Texas colleges/schools of pharmacy or the Board;
      c. To continue certification, have completed three hours of pharmacist preceptor training provided by an ACPE approved provider within the preceptor pharmacist's current license renewal period. Such training shall be developed by a Texas college/school of pharmacy or be approved by a committee comprised of the Texas colleges/schools of pharmacy or the Board; and
      d. Meet the requirements of C. below.
  B. Ratio of Preceptors to Pharmacist Interns.
    1. A preceptor may supervise only one pharmacist intern at any given time (1:1 ratio) except as provided in 2. below.
    2. The following is applicable to a Texas college/school of pharmacy internship program only.
      a. Supervision of a pharmacist intern shall be:
        (1) Direct supervision when the student intern or intern trainee is engaged in functions associated with the preparation and delivery of prescription or medication drug orders and
        (2) General supervision when the student intern or intern trainee is engaged in functions not associated with the preparation and delivery of prescription or medication drug orders.
      b. Exceptions to the 1:1 ratio. There is no ratio requirement for preceptors supervising pharmacist interns as a part of a Texas college/school of pharmacy program.
  C. No pharmacist may serve as a pharmacist preceptor if his or her pharmacist license has been the subject of an order of the Board imposing a penalty during the time he or she is serving as a pharmacist preceptor or within the three-year period immediately preceding application for approval as a pharmacist preceptor. However, a pharmacist may petition the Board in writing for approval to act as a pharmacist preceptor. The Board may consider the following items in approving a pharmacist's petition to act as a preceptor:
    1. The type and gravity of the offense for which the pharmacist's license was disciplined;
    2. The length of time since the action that caused the order;
    3. The length of time the pharmacist has previously served as a preceptor;
    4. The availability of other preceptors in the area;
    5. The reason(s) the pharmacist believes he or she should serve as a preceptor;
    6. A letter of recommendation from a Texas college/school of pharmacy if the pharmacist will be serving as a preceptor for a Texas college/school of pharmacy; and
    7. Any other factor presented by the pharmacist demonstrating good cause why the pharmacist should be allowed to act as a pharmacist preceptor.

Section 558.058 Accessibility of Examination
The Board by rule shall ensure that an examination under this Act is administered to applicants with disabilities in compliance with the Americans with Disabilities Act of 1990 (42 U.S.C. Section 12101 et seq.).

Section 558.059 Examination Fee Refund
  A. The Board may retain all or part of an examination fee paid by an applicant who is unable to take the examination.
  B. The Board shall adopt policies allowing the Board to refund the examination fee paid by an applicant who:

1. Provides advance notice of the applicant's inability to take the examination or
2. Is unable to take the examination because of an emergency.
C. The Board's policy must establish the required notification period and the emergencies that warrant a refund.
D. The Board shall make efforts to ensure that the policy does not conflict with the policy of a national testing body involved in administering the examination.

SUBCHAPTER C. Licensing by Reciprocity

Section 558.101 Qualifications for License by Reciprocity

A. To qualify for a license to practice pharmacy, an applicant for licensing by reciprocity must:
 1. Submit to the Board:
    a. A reciprocity fee set by the Board and
    b. A completed application in the form prescribed by the Board given under oath;
 2. Have graduated and received a professional practice degree as defined by Board rule from an accredited pharmacy degree program approved by the Board;
 3. Have presented to the Board:
    a. Proof of current or initial licensing by examination (This means an applicant can reciprocate a license to Texas from a state regardless if the applicant received that license by examination or reciprocity.) and
    b. Proof that the current license and any other license granted to the applicant by another state has not been restricted, suspended, revoked, or surrendered for any other reason; and
 4. Pass the Texas Pharmacy Jurisprudence Examination (MPJE).
B. An applicant is not eligible for licensing by reciprocity unless the state in which the applicant was originally licensed as a pharmacist grants reciprocal licensing to pharmacists licensed by examination in this state under like circumstances and conditions.

Board of Pharmacy Rule 283.8
Reciprocity Requirements

A. All applicants for licensure by reciprocity:
 1. Shall meet educational and age requirements set out in Board Rule 283.3.
 2. May be required to meet all requirements necessary for the Board to access the criminal history record information, including submitting fingerprint information and being responsible for all associated costs.
 3. Shall complete Texas and NABP reciprocity applications.
    (Fraudulent statements are grounds for denial or, if application is granted, grounds for suspension, revocation, and cancellation.)
 4. Shall provide proof of initial licensing by examination and proof that their current license and any other license or licenses have not been suspended, revoked, cancelled, surrendered, or otherwise restricted for any reason.
 5. Shall pass the Texas Pharmacy Jurisprudence Exam (MPJE) with a minimum score of 75. (The passing grade may be used for the purpose of licensure by reciprocity for a period of two years from the date of passing the examination.) If the applicant fails, he or she may retake the exam four additional times for a total of five exams. Prior to any subsequent retakes, the applicant must comply with Board Rule 283.11 (Exam Retake Requirements).

B. An applicant originally licensed in another state after 1978 and who has graduated and received a professional degree from a college of pharmacy shall show proof such applicant has passed the NAPLEX or an equivalent exam based on criteria no less stringent than the criteria in force in Texas.
C. A foreign pharmacy graduate shall submit written documentation that such applicant has obtained full certification from FPGEE and has passed NAPLEX or an equivalent examination based on criteria no less stringent than the criteria in force in Texas.
D. If a reciprocity applicant should fail the Texas MPJE, written notification of intent to retake the exam shall be received in the Board office no later than three weeks prior to the examination date.
E. An applicant is not eligible for licensing by reciprocity unless the state in which the applicant is currently or was initially licensed as a pharmacist also grants reciprocal licensing to pharmacists duly licensed by examination in this state under like circumstances and conditions.

Board of Pharmacy Rule 283.9
Fee Requirements for Licensure by Examination, Score Transfer, and Reciprocity

A. Fees for Licensure by Examination, Score Transfer, and Reciprocity. (*See details of Board Rule 283.9 on TSBP website.*)
B. Fees for Applicant Who Fails Exam and Retakes Exam. (*See details of Board Rule 283.9 on TSBP website.*)
C. Rescheduling an Examination. (*See details of Board Rule 283.9 on TSBP website.*)
D. A person who takes NAPLEX and/or the Texas MPJE will be notified of the results of the examination(s) within two weeks of receipt of the results of the examination(s) from the testing service. If both NAPLEX and the Texas MPJE are taken, the applicant will not be notified until the results of both examinations have been received. Such notification will be made within two weeks after receipt of the results of both examinations.
E. Once an applicant has successfully completed all requirements of licensure, the applicant will be notified of licensure as a pharmacist and of his or her pharmacist license number. The following is applicable:
   1. The notice letter shall serve as authorization for the person to practice pharmacy in Texas for a period of 30 days from the date of the notice letter.
   2. The applicant shall complete a pharmacist license application and pay one pharmacist license fee as specified in Board Rule 295.5 (Pharmacist License or Renewal Fees).
   3. The provisions of Board Rule 295.7 (Pharmacist License Renewal) apply to the timely receipt of an application and licensure fee.
   4. If the application and payment of the pharmacist license fee are not received by the Board within 30 days from the date of the notice letter, the person's license to practice pharmacy shall expire. A person may not practice pharmacy with an expired license.

Board of Pharmacy Rule 283.12
Licenses for Military Service Members, Military Veterans, and Military Spouses

This rule establishes an alternative licensing procedure, including additional time to renew a license, for military service members, military veterans, and military spouses who are applying for or renewing a pharmacist license. It also allows these same individuals to place their license on inactive status if they are not engaged in the practice of pharmacy in Texas without having to pay a fee. (*See details of Board Rule 283.12 on TSBP website.*)

SUBCHAPTER D. Provisional and Temporary Licensing

Section 558.151 Qualifications for Provisional License

Section 558.152 Duration of Provisional License

Section 558.153 Processing of License Application

Section 558.154 Issuance of License to Provisional License Holder and Section 558.155 Temporary Pharmacist License

These sections authorize and set forth the requirements for TSBP to grant a provisional license to individuals licensed in another state and applying for licensure in Texas or issue a temporary pharmacist license. TSBP has adopted the following rule for issuing an emergency temporary pharmacist license.

Board of Pharmacy Rule 295.6
Emergency Temporary Pharmacist License

A. Definitions.
The following words and terms shall have the following meanings unless the context clearly indicates otherwise.
 1. **Emergency situation**—An emergency caused by a natural or manmade disaster or any other exceptional situation that causes an extraordinary demand for pharmacist services.
 2. **State**—One of the 50 states in the United States of America, the District of Columbia, and Puerto Rico.
 Note: The word "state" also includes American Samoa, Guam, Northern Mariana Islands, and U.S. Virgin Islands although they are not included in this rule language.
B. Emergency Temporary Pharmacist License. In an emergency situation, the Board may grant a pharmacist who holds a license to practice pharmacy in another state an emergency temporary pharmacist license to practice in Texas. The following is applicable for the emergency temporary pharmacist license.
 1. An applicant for an emergency temporary pharmacist license under this rule must hold a current pharmacist license in another state and that license and other licenses held by the applicant in any other state may not be suspended, revoked, canceled, surrendered, or otherwise restricted for any reason.
 2. To qualify for an emergency temporary pharmacist license, the applicant must submit an application including the following information:
  a. Name, address, and phone number of the applicant and
  b. Any other information required by the Board.
 3. An emergency temporary pharmacist license shall be valid for a period as determined by the Board not to exceed six months. The executive director of the Board in his or her discretion may renew the license for an additional six months if the emergency situation still exists.
C. Exception. This rule is not applicable to pharmacists enrolled in a volunteer health registry maintained by the Texas Department of State Health Services.

SUBCHAPTER E. Certain Prohibited Acts

Section 558.201 Duplicating a License or Certificate

Except as expressly provided under this Act, a person may not in any manner duplicate a license to practice pharmacy or a license renewal certificate.

Note: It is permissible to copy the "pocket" license card that is provided with a pharmacist renewal certificate.

Section 558.202 False Affidavit

A person who falsely makes an affidavit prescribed by Section 558.051 (Qualifications for a License by Examination) or Section 558.101 (Qualifications for License by Reciprocity) of the Act is guilty of fraudulent and dishonorable conduct and malpractice.

Chapter 559 Renewal of License to Practice Pharmacy (Pharmacists)

SUBCHAPTER A. General Provisions

Section 559.001 Expiration of License

A. Except as provided by B. below, a license to practice pharmacy expires on December 31 of each year or every other year as determined by the Board.
B. The Board may adopt a system under which licenses to practice pharmacy expire on various dates during the year.
   Note: TSBP rules require that pharmacist licenses expire every two years on the last day of the month of the pharmacist's birthday month.
C. If the Board changes the expiration date of a license, the Board shall prorate the license renewal fee to cover the months for which the license is valid for the year in which the date is changed. The total license renewal fee is due on the new expiration date.

Section 559.002 Renewal Period

A license to practice pharmacy may be renewed for one or two years as determined by the Board.

Note: TSBP renews licenses every two years as stated in B. above.

Section 559.003 Requirements for Renewal

A. To renew a license to practice pharmacy, the license holder (before the expiration date of the license) must:
   1. Pay a renewal fee as determined by the Board;
   2. Comply with the continuing education requirements prescribed by the Board; and
   3. File with the Board a completed application for a license renewal certificate that is given under oath and is accompanied by a certified statement executed by the license holder that the license holder has satisfied the continuing education requirements during the preceding license period.
B. A person whose license has been expired for 90 days or less may renew the expired license by paying to the Board a renewal fee that is equal to one and one-half times the normally required renewal fee for the license.
   Note: The person must also report the required number of continuing education hours. (See Board Rule 283.10A. in this chapter.)
C. A person whose license has been expired for more than 90 days but less than one year may renew the expired license by paying to the Board a renewal fee that is equal to two times the normally required renewal fee for the license.
   Note: The person must also report the required number of continuing education hours. (See Board Rule 283.10B. in this chapter.)

D. A person whose license has been expired for one year or more may not renew the license. The person may obtain a new license by complying with the requirements and procedures for obtaining an original license including the examination requirement.
Note: See Section 559.005 and Board Rule 283.10 summarized below for alternatives to retaking the NAPLEX.
E. A person may not renew a license to practice pharmacy if the person holds a license to practice pharmacy in another state that has been suspended, revoked, cancelled, or subject to an action that prohibits the person from practicing pharmacy in that state.
F. The Board may refuse to renew a license to practice pharmacy for a license holder who is in violation of a Board Order.

Board of Pharmacy Rule 295.5
Pharmacist License or Renewal Fees

A. Biennial Registration. The Board requires all pharmacist licenses to be renewed every two years.
B. License fees are subject to change. (*See the Board's website for current fees.*)
C. Fees consist of:
   1. A processing and licensing fee;
   2. A surcharge to fund the pharmacist and pharmacy student impairment program (evaluation only, not treatment);
   3. A surcharge to fund Texas Online; and
   4. A surcharge to fund the Office of Patient Safety.
D. Exemption From the Fee. The license of a pharmacist who has been licensed by TSBP for at least 50 years or who is at least 72 years old shall be renewed without payment of the fee provided such pharmacist is not actively practicing pharmacy. The renewal certificate of such pharmacist shall reflect an inactive status. A person whose license is renewed under this section may not engage in the active practice of pharmacy without first paying the renewal fee.

Section 559.005 Issuance of a New License
A. The Board may issue a new license to practice pharmacy to a person who is prohibited under Section 559.003D. of the Act from renewing a license (because the license has been expired for one year or more) if the person has not had a license granted by any other state restricted, suspended, revoked, canceled, or surrendered for any reason and qualifies under this section.
B. A person qualifies under this section if the person:
   1. Was licensed as a pharmacist in this state, moved to another state, and is licensed and has been practicing in the other state for the two years preceding the date the application for a new license is submitted;
   2. Pays to the Board an amount equal to the examination fee for the license; and
   3. Passes the Texas MPJE.
C. A person qualifies for a license under this section if the person:
   1. Was licensed as a pharmacist in this state;
   2. Pays to the Board an amount equal to the examination fee for the license;
   3. Passes the Texas MPJE and any other examination required by the Board; and/or
   4. Instead of passing the examination required by the Board, participates in continuing pharmacy education and practices under conditions set by the Board.
D. A person qualifies for a license under this section if the person:
   1. Submits to reexamination and
   2. Completes the requirements and procedures for obtaining an original license.

Board of Pharmacy Rule 283.10
Requirements for Application for a Pharmacist License Which Has Expired

Note: Board Rule 283.10 has been summarized in several areas to provide clarity. Additionally, a pharmacist cannot practice with an expired license, but these provisions allow for an expired license to be reinstated under certain circumstances.

A. Expired fewer than 90 days: The person may renew the license by paying to the Board a renewal fee that is equal to one and one-half times the renewal fee for the license as specified in Board Rule 295.5 and by reporting the completion of required contact hours of approved continuing education.
B. Expired more than 90 days but less than one year: The person may renew the license by paying to the Board all unpaid renewal fees and a fee that is equal to the examination fee for a license and by reporting the completion of required contact hours of approved continuing education.
C. Expired for one year or more: The person may not renew the license and shall apply for a new license.

Board Rule 283.10 provides the requirements for pharmacists whose Texas license has been expired for one year or more to obtain a new license without having to retake the NAPLEX.

1. If a pharmacist moved to another state, has a license in good standing in another state, has been actively practicing pharmacy in that state for the immediate two years prior to applying for a new Texas license, and has completed the minimum of 30 contact hours of continuing education during the preceding two years, he or she may obtain a new Texas license by:
   a. Passing the Texas MPJE and
   b. Paying the examination fee.
2. If a pharmacist has not practiced pharmacy for the two years preceding application for a new Texas license, he or she may obtain a new Texas license if his or her license has not been expired for 10 years or more by:
   a. Passing the Texas MPJE;
   b. Paying the examination fee; and
   c. Meeting the required continuing education requirements and internship hours as set forth in the chart below.

Number of Years	Expired Number of CE Hours	Number of Internship Hours
>1–<2	15	N/A
>2–<3	30	N/A
>3–<4	45	N/A
>4–<5	45	500
>5–<6	45	700
>6–<7	45	900
>7–<8	45	1,100
>8–<9	45	1,300
>9–<10	45	1,500

3. If a pharmacist's license has been expired for 10 years or more, there is no alternative other than retaking the NAPLEX and Texas MPJE and meeting all internship requirements.

Notes

Section 559.006 License Expiration Notice

At least 30 days before the expiration of a person's license, the Board shall send a written notice of the impending license expiration to the person at the license holder's last known address according to the Board's records.

Section 559.007 Practicing Pharmacy Without a Renewal Certificate

A person who practices pharmacy without a current license renewal certificate as required by this Act is practicing pharmacy without a license and is subject to all penalties for practicing pharmacy without a license.

Subchapter B. Mandatory Continuing Education

Section 559.051 Satisfaction of Continuing Education Requirement

A. A holder of a license to practice pharmacy may meet the continuing education requirement by:
  1. Completing continuing education programs approved by the Board or
  2. Passing a standardized pharmacy examination approved by the Board.
B. A license holder who takes the examination under A.2. above must pay the examination fee assessed by the Board.

Section 559.052 Rules Relating to Continuing Education

A. The Board shall adopt rules relating to:
  1. The adoption or approval of mandatory continuing education programs;
  2. The approval of providers and the operation of continuing education programs; and
  3. The evaluation of the effectiveness of continuing education programs and a license holder's participation and performance in those programs.
B. In establishing the requirement for continuing education, the Board shall consider:
  1. Factors that lead to the competent performance of professional duties and
  2. The continuing education needs of license holders.
C. In adopting rules relating to the approval of continuing education programs or providers, the Board may consider:
  1. Programs approved by the Texas Pharmacy Foundation and
  2. Providers approved by the Accreditation Council for Pharmacy Education.
D. The Board shall approve home study courses, correspondence courses, or other similar programs.
E. The Board by rule may grant an extension for the completion of a continuing education requirement for good cause.
F. The Board by rule may exempt a person from all or part of the continuing education requirements.

Section 559.0525 Continuing Education Relating to Opioid Drugs

A. The Board shall develop a continuing education program regarding opioid drug abuse and the delivery, dispensing, and provision of tamper-resistant opioid drugs after considering input from interested persons.
B. The Board by rule may require a license holder to satisfy a number of the continuing education hours required by Section 559.003 of the Act through attendance of a program developed under this section.

Note: The Board developed this continuing education program and adopted a rule that required pharmacists to complete one hour of continuing education related to opioid abuse. That rule was repealed in late 2019 and has been replaced by some new required courses. See TSBP Rule 295.8 in this chapter.

Section 559.053 Program Hours Required

A license holder satisfies the continuing education requirement by presenting evidence satisfactory to the Board of the completion of at least 30 hours of continuing education during the preceding 24 months of the person's license period.

Section 559.054 Certificate of Completion

Each continuing education provider approved by the Board shall issue a certificate of completion to a license holder who satisfactorily completes the program.

Section 559.055 Records

Each license holder shall maintain records for three years showing the continuing education programs completed by the license holder.

Note: This record is one of the few records that must be kept for three years.

Section 559.056 Demonstration of Compliance

On an audit by the Board, a license holder is in compliance with the continuing education requirements if the license holder submits to the Board:
1. An affidavit stating that the license holder has complied with those requirements and
2. Records showing completion of the continuing education programs.

Note: All pharmacists should register with the CPE Monitor Service, a collaborative effort of the National Association of Boards of Pharmacy (NABP) and the Accreditation Council for Pharmacy Education (ACPE), that allows pharmacists to electronically keep track of continuing pharmacy education (CPE) credits from ACPE accredited providers. More information on CPE Monitor is available on the NABP website. A pharmacist must maintain his or her records for any non-ACPE accredited continuing education since those would not be tracked or identified by the CPE Monitor Service.

Board of Pharmacy Rule 295.8
Continuing Education Requirements

A. Authority and Purpose.
 1. Authority. In accordance with Section 559.053 of the Act, all pharmacists must complete and report 30 contact hours (3.0 CEUs) of approved continuing education during the previous license period to renew their license to practice pharmacy.
 2. Purpose. The Board recognizes that the fundamental purpose of continuing education is to maintain and enhance the professional competency of pharmacists licensed to practice in Texas for the protection of the health and welfare of the citizens of Texas.
B. Definitions.
 1. **ACPE**—Accreditation Council for Pharmacy Education.
 2. **Act**—The Texas Pharmacy Act, Chapters 551–569, Occupations Code.
 3. **Approved programs**—Live programs, home study, and other mediated instruction delivered by an approved provider or a program specified by the Board and listed as an approved program in E. below.
 4. **Approved provider**—An individual, institution, organization, association, corporation, or agency that is approved by the Board.
 5. **Board**—The Texas State Board of Pharmacy.
 6. **Certificate of completion**—A certificate or other official document presented to a participant upon the successful completion of an approved continuing education program.
 7. **Contact hour**—A unit of measure of educational credit which is equivalent to approximately 60 minutes of participation in an organized learning experience.
 8. **Continuing Education Unit (CEU)**—A unit of measure of education credit which is equivalent to 10 contact hours (i.e., one CEU = 10 contact hours).
 9. **CPE monitor**—A collaborative service from the National Association of Boards of Pharmacy and ACPE that provides an electronic system for pharmacists to track their completed CPE credits.

10. **Credit hour**—A unit of measurement for continuing education equal to 15 contact hours.
11. **Enduring materials (home study)**—Activities that are printed or recorded or computer-assisted instructional materials that do not provide for direct interaction between faculty and participants.
12. **Initial license period**—The time period between the date of issuance of a pharmacist's license and the next expiration date following the initial 30-day expiration date. This time period ranges from 18 to 30 months depending on the birth month of the licensee.
13. **License period**—The time period between consecutive expiration dates of a license.
14. **Live programs**—Activities that provide for direct interaction between faculty and participants and may include lectures, symposia, live teleconferences, workshops, etc.
15. **Standardized pharmacy examination**—The North American Pharmacy Licensing Examination (NAPLEX).

C. Methods for a Pharmacist to Obtain Continuing Education.
1. Successfully completing 30 contact hours (3.0 CEUs) of Board-approved programs during the preceding license period (*see approved programs listed in E. below*);
2. Successfully completing during the preceding license period one credit hour for each year of his or her license period, which is a part of the professional degree program in a college of pharmacy. The professional degree program must be accredited by ACPE (e.g., participants in a nontraditional Pharm.D. program); or
3. Taking and passing NAPLEX during the preceding license period as a Texas-licensed pharmacist, which is equivalent to 30 contact hours of continuing education.

D. Reporting Requirements.
1. To renew a license to practice pharmacy, a pharmacist must report the completion of at least 30 contact hours (3.0 CEUs) of continuing education on the renewal application. The following is applicable to the reporting of continuing education contact hours:
   a. At least one contact hour (0.1 CEUs) shall be related to Texas pharmacy laws or rules;
   b. For renewals received after January 1, 2020 and before August 31, 2023, at least one contact hour (0.1 CEUs) annually for a total of two contact hours (0.2 CEUs) during that timeframe. The two contact hours shall be related to best practices, alternative treatment options, and multi-modal approaches to pain management;
   c. At least two contact hours (0.2 CEUs) shall be related to approved procedures of prescribing and monitoring controlled substances, shall be obtained by September 1, 2021, and must be reported on the next license renewal after September 1, 2021;
   d. Any continuing education requirements which are imposed upon a pharmacist as part of a Board Order or Agreed Board Order shall be in addition to the required 30 hours; and
   e. For renewals received after August 31, 2020 and before September 1, 2022, a pharmacist must have completed the human trafficking prevention course required in Section 116.002 of the Texas Occupations Code.

   Note: The statute requires that such course is approved by the Texas Health and Human Services Commission and that a list of approved courses be posted on the commission's website.

2. Failure to Report Completion of Required Continuing Education.
   The following is applicable if a pharmacist fails to report the completion of the required continuing education.
   a. The license of a pharmacist who fails to report the completion of the required number of hours shall not be renewed, and the pharmacist shall not be issued a renewal certificate until such time as the pharmacist successfully completes the required continuing education.
   b. A pharmacist who practices pharmacy without a current renewal certificate is subject to all penalties of practicing pharmacy without a license including delinquent fees.
3. Extension of Time for Reporting.
   A pharmacist who has had a physical disability, an illness, or other extenuating circumstance prohibiting him or her from obtaining continuing education credit during the preceding license year may be granted an extension of time to complete the continuing education requirement. (*See Board Rule 295.8 for details on requesting such an extension.*)
4. Exemptions From Reporting Requirements.
   a. All pharmacists licensed in Texas shall be exempt from the continuing education requirements during their initial license period.
   b. Pharmacists who are not actively practicing pharmacy shall be granted an exemption to the reporting requirements for continuing education provided the pharmacists submit a completed renewal application for each license period which states that they are not practicing pharmacy. Upon submission of the completed renewal application, the pharmacist shall be issued a renewal certificate which states that the pharmacist is inactive. Pharmacists who wish to return to the practice of pharmacy after being exempted from the continuing education requirements as specified in this subparagraph must:
      (1) Notify the Board of their intent to actively practice pharmacy;
      (2) Pay the fee as specified in Board Rule 295.9 (Inactive License); and
      (3) Provide copies of completion certificates from approved continuing education programs as specified in E. below for 30 contact hours (3.0 CEUs). For applications to reactivate received before September 1, 2023, at least one contact hour (0.1 CEU) shall be related to best practices, alternative treatment options, and multi-modal approaches to pain management as specified in Chapter 481.0764 of the Texas Health and Safety Code. Approved continuing education earned within two years prior to the licensee applying for the return to active status may be applied toward the continuing education requirement for reactivation of the license but may not be counted toward subsequent renewal of the license.

E. Approved Programs.
   1. Any program presented by an ACPE approved provider shall be an approved program subject to the following conditions.
      a. Pharmacists may receive credit for the completion of the same ACPE course only once during a license period.
      b. Pharmacists who present approved CE programs may receive credit for the time expended during the actual presentation of the program. Pharmacists may receive credit for the same presentation only once during a license period.
      c. Proof of completion of an ACPE course shall contain the following:
         (1) Name of the participant;
         (2) Title and completion date of the program;

Notes

Copyright © 2020 Fred S. Brinkley, Jr., and Gary G. Cacciatore

(3) Name of the approved provider sponsoring or cosponsoring the program;
(4) Number of contact hours and/or CEUs awarded;
(5) Assigned ACPE universal program number and a "P" designation indicating that the CE is targeted to pharmacists; and
(6) Either a dated certifying signature of the approved provider and the official ACPE logo or the CPE Monitor logo.

2. Courses which are part of a professional degree program or an advanced pharmacy degree program offered by a college of pharmacy that has a professional degree program accredited by ACPE.
    a. Pharmacists may receive credit for the completion of the same course only once during a licensure period. A course is equivalent to one credit hour for each year of the renewal period.
    b. Pharmacists who teach these courses may receive credit toward their continuing education, but such credit may be received only once for teaching the same course during a licensure period.
3. Basic cardiopulmonary resuscitation (CPR) courses which lead to CPR certification by the American Red Cross or the American Heart Association or its equivalent are approved programs. Pharmacists may receive credit for one contact hour (0.1 CEU) toward their CE requirement for completion of a CPR course and may receive credit for a CPR course only once during a licensure period. Proof of completion of a CPR course shall be the certificate issued by the American Red Cross or the American Heart Association.
4. Advanced cardiovascular life support (ACLS) courses or pediatric advanced life support (PALS) courses which lead to initial ACLS or PALS certification by the American Heart Association or its equivalent shall be recognized as approved programs. Pharmacists may receive credit for 12 contact hours (1.2 CEUs) toward their continuing education requirement for completion of an ACLS or PALS course only once during a licensure period. Proof of completion of an ACLS or PALS course shall be the certificate issued by the American Heart Association.
5. Advanced cardiovascular life support (ACLS) courses or pediatric advanced life support (PALS) courses which lead to ACLS or PALS recertification by the American Heart Association or its equivalent shall be recognized as approved programs. Pharmacists may receive credit for 4 contact hours (0.4 CEUs) toward their continuing education requirement for completion of an ACLS or PALS recertification course only once during a licensure period. Proof of completion of an ACLS or PALS recertification course shall be the certificate issued by the American Heart Association.
6. Attendance at TSBP meetings shall be recognized for continuing education credit as follows:
    a. Pharmacists shall receive credit for three contact hours (0.3 CEUs) toward their continuing education requirements for attending a full public Board meeting in its entirety.
    b. A maximum of six contact hours (0.6 CEUs) are allowed for attendance at a Board meeting during a license period.
    c. Proof of attendance for a complete Board meeting shall be a certificate issued by TSBP.
7. Participation in a TSBP appointed Task Force shall be recognized for continuing education credit as follows:
    a. Pharmacists shall receive credit for three contact hours (0.3 CEUs) toward their continuing education requirements for participating in a TSBP appointed Task Force.
    b. Proof of participation in a Task Force shall be a certificate issued by TSBP.

8. Attendance at programs presented by TSBP or courses offered by TSBP as follows:
   a. Pharmacists shall receive credit for the number of hours for the program or course as stated by TSBP.
   b. Proof of attendance at a program presented by TSBP or completion of a course offered by TSBP shall be a certificate issued by TSBP.
9. Pharmacists shall receive credit toward their continuing education requirements for programs or courses approved by other state boards of pharmacy as follows:
   a. Pharmacists shall receive credit for the number of hours for the program or course as specified by the other state board of pharmacy.
   b. Proof of attendance at a program or course approved by another state board of pharmacy shall be a certificate or other documentation that indicates:
      (1) Name of the participant;
      (2) Title and completion date of the program;
      (3) Name of the approved provider sponsoring or cosponsoring the program;
      (4) Number of contact hours and/or CEUs awarded;
      (5) Dated certifying signature of the provider; and
      (6) Documentation that the program is approved by the other state board of pharmacy.
10. Completion of an Institute for Safe Medication Practices (ISMP) Medication Safety Self-Assessment for hospital pharmacies or for community/ambulatory pharmacies shall be recognized for continuing education credit as follows:
    a. Pharmacists shall receive credit for three contact hours toward their continuing education requirement for completion of an ISMP Medication Safety Self-Assessment.
    b. Proof of completion of an ISMP Medication Safety Self-Assessment shall be a continuing education certificate provided by an ACPE approved provider for completion of an assessment or a document from ISMP showing completion of an assessment.
11. Pharmacists shall receive credit for three contact hours (0.3 CEUs) toward their continuing education requirements for taking and successfully passing an initial Board of Pharmaceutical Specialties certification examination administered by the Board of Pharmaceutical Specialties. Proof of successfully passing the examination shall be a certificate issued by the Board of Pharmaceutical Specialties.
12. Programs approved by the American Medical Association (AMA) as Category 1 Continuing Medical Education (CME) and accredited by the Accreditation Council for Continuing Medical Education subject to the following conditions.
    a. Pharmacists may receive credit for the completion of the same CME course only once during a licensure period.
    b. Pharmacists who present approved CME programs may receive credit for the time expended during the actual presentation of the program. Pharmacists may receive credit for the same presentation only once during a licensure period.
    c. Proof of the completion of a CME course shall contain the following information:
       (1) Name of the participant;
       (2) Title and completion date of the program;
       (3) Name of the approved provider sponsoring or cosponsoring the program;
       (4) Number of contact hours and/or CEUs awarded; and
       (5) Dated certifying signature of the approved provider.

F. Retention of Continuing Education Records and Audit of Records by the Board.
  1. Retention of Records.
     Pharmacists shall maintain certificates of completion of approved CE for three years from the date of reporting the contact hours on a license renewal application. Such records may be retained in hard copy or electronic format. *Note: All CE provided by ACPE approved providers is tracked by NABP through NABP's CPE Monitor allowing pharmacists to electronically track all ACPE approved CE completed. All pharmacists should obtain an NABP CPE Monitor number and provide that number when registering for an ACPE approved CE program.*
  2. Audit of Records by the Board.
     The Board shall audit the records of pharmacists for the verification of reported continuing education credit. The following is applicable for such audits.
     a. Upon a written request, a pharmacist shall provide to the Board documentation of proof for all continuing education contact hours reported during a specified license year(s). Failure to provide all requested records during the specified time period constitutes prima facie evidence of failure to keep and maintain records and shall subject the pharmacist to disciplinary action by the Board.
     b. Credit for continuing education contact hours shall only be allowed for approved programs for which the pharmacist submits documentation of proof reflecting that the hours were completed during the specified license year(s). Any other reported hours shall be disallowed. A pharmacist who has received credit for continuing education contact hours disallowed during an audit shall be subject to disciplinary action.
     c. A pharmacist who submits false or fraudulent records to the Board shall be subject to disciplinary action by the Board.
  3. Dates.
     If pharmacists attend a live CE program, the completion date and the credit date for the course is the day that the pharmacist attended the program. Regarding correspondence courses, these courses are not considered complete until a certificate of completion is received from the provider with a dated certifying signature. Credit for the correspondence course is awarded on the date specified on the certificate, not the date the CE was completed. This can be important when reporting hours to the Board for a specified renewal period.

SUBCHAPTER C. Inactive Status (Inactive Pharmacist License)

Section 559.101 Eligibility for Inactive Status

The Board by rule shall adopt a system for placing on inactive status a license held by a person who:
1. Is licensed by the Board to practice pharmacy;
2. Is not eligible to renew the license because of failure to comply with the continuing education requirements; and
3. Is not practicing pharmacy in this state.

Section 559.102 Restriction on Length of Inactive Status

The Board may restrict the length of time a license may remain on inactive status.

Section 559.103 Application for Inactive Status

A license holder may place the holder's license on inactive status by:
1. Applying for inactive status on a form prescribed by the Board before the expiration date of the license and

2. Complying with all other requirements for the renewal of a license other than the continuing education requirements.

Section 559.104 Return to Active Status
A holder of a license that is on inactive status may return to active status by:
1. Applying for active status on a form prescribed by the Board and
2. Providing evidence satisfactory to the Board that the license holder has completed the number of hours of continuing education (up to 36 hours) that would otherwise have been required for renewal of the license.

Section 559.105 Practicing Pharmacy During Inactive Status
A. A holder of a license that is on inactive status may not practice pharmacy in this state.
B. A license holder who practices pharmacy while the holder's license is on inactive status is practicing pharmacy without a license.

Board of Pharmacy Rule 295.9
Inactive Status (License)

A. Placing a License on Inactive Status. A person who is licensed by the Board but who is not eligible to renew the pharmacist license for failure to comply with the continuing education requirements of Section 559.053 of the Act and who is not engaged in the practice of pharmacy in this state may place the license on inactive status at the time of the license renewal or during a license year.
   1. To place a license on inactive status at the time of renewal, the licensee shall:
      a. Complete and submit before the expiration date a pharmacist license renewal application;
      b. State on the renewal application that the license is to be placed on inactive status and that the licensee shall not practice pharmacy in Texas while the license is inactive; and
      c. Pay the fee issuing an amended license as specified in Board Rule 295.5E. *Note: Special rules apply to military service members, military veterans, and military spouses who may place their license on inactive status without having to pay the fee.*
   2. To place a license on inactive status at a time other than the time of the license renewal, the licensee shall:
      a. Return the current renewal certificate to the Board;
      b. Submit a signed statement stating that the licensee shall not practice pharmacy in Texas while the license is inactive and the date the license is to be placed on inactive status; and
      c. Pay the fee for issuance of an amended license.
B. A pharmacist who is on inactive status shall not practice pharmacy in this state. The practice of pharmacy by a pharmacist whose license is on inactive status constitutes the practice of pharmacy without a license.
C. Reactivating a License. A pharmacist whose license is on inactive status may return the license to active status by:
   1. Applying for active status on a form prescribed by the Board;
   2. Providing copies of completion certificates from approved continuing education programs as specified in Board Rule 295.8E. (Continuing Education Requirements) for 30 hours. For applications to reactivate received before September 1, 2023, at least one contact hour (0.1 CEU) shall be related to best practices, alternative treatment options, and multi-modal approaches to pain management as specified in Chapter 481.0764 of the Texas Health and Safety Code. Approved continuing education earned within two years prior to the licensee applying for the return to active status may be applied toward

the continuing education requirement for reactivation of the license but may not be counted toward the subsequent renewal of the license; and
   3. Paying the pharmacist license renewal fee.
D. In an emergency caused by a natural or manmade disaster or any other exceptional situation that causes an extraordinary demand for pharmacist services, the executive director of the Board in his or her discretion may allow a pharmacist whose license has been inactive for no more than two years to reactivate his or her license prior to obtaining the required continuing education specified in C.2. above, provided the pharmacist completes the continuing education requirement within six months of the reactivation of the license. If the required continuing education is not provided within six months, the license shall return to an inactive status.
E. A person who is exempt from the renewal fee under Board Rule 295.5 (licensed for 50 years or 72 years of age and not practicing) is also considered inactive.

Chapter 560 Licensing of Pharmacies
SUBCHAPTER A. License Required

Section 560.001 License Required
A. A person may not operate a pharmacy in this state unless the pharmacy is licensed by the Board.
B. A pharmacy located in another state may not ship, mail, or deliver to this state a prescription drug or device dispensed under a prescription drug order or dispensed or delivered as authorized by Chapter 562 of the Act (compounded and prepackaged drugs including compounded products for office use) unless the pharmacy is licensed by the Board or is exempt under Section 560.004 of the Act.

Section 560.002 Use of "Pharmacy"; Providing Pharmacy Services Without a License
A. A person may not display in or on a place of business the word "pharmacy" or "apothecary" in any language, any word or combination of words of the same or similar meaning, or a graphic representation that would lead the public to believe that the business is a pharmacy unless the facility is a pharmacy licensed under this Act.
B. A person may not advertise a place of business as a pharmacy or provide pharmacy services unless the facility is a pharmacy licensed under this Act.

Section 560.003 Prohibited Advertising of Pharmacy
A. A pharmacy that is not licensed under this Act may not advertise the pharmacy's services in this state.
B. A person who is a resident of this state may not advertise the pharmacy services of a pharmacy that is not licensed by the Board if the pharmacy or person makes the advertisement with the knowledge that the advertisement will or is likely to induce a resident of this state to use the pharmacy to dispense a prescription drug order.

Section 560.004 Exemption
The Board may grant an exemption from the licensing requirements of this Act on the application of a pharmacy located in another state that restricts to isolated transactions the pharmacy's dispensing of a prescription drug or device to a resident of this state.

SUBCHAPTER B. Pharmacy Classifications and Licensure

Section 560.051 License Classifications
A. Each applicant for a pharmacy license shall apply for a license in one or more of the following classifications:

1. Class A;
2. Class B;
3. Class C;
4. Class D;
5. Class E; or
6. Another classification established by Board rule under Section 560.053 of the Act. The Board has established the following additional classes of pharmacy by Board rule:
    a. Class F;
    b. Class G; and
    c. Class H.
B. A Class A pharmacy license or community pharmacy license authorizes a pharmacy to dispense a drug or device to the public under a prescription drug order.
C. A Class B pharmacy license or nuclear pharmacy license authorizes a pharmacy to dispense a radioactive drug or device for administration to the ultimate user.
D. A Class C pharmacy license or institutional pharmacy license may be issued to:
    1. A pharmacy located in an inpatient facility, including a hospital licensed under Chapter 241 or 577, Health and Safety Code, or a hospital maintained by the state.
    2. A hospice inpatient facility licensed under Chapter 142, Health and Safety Code.
    3. An ambulatory surgical center licensed under Chapter 243, Health and Safety Code.
E. A Class D pharmacy license or clinic pharmacy license authorizes a pharmacy to dispense a limited type of drug or device under a prescription drug order.
F. A Class E pharmacy license or nonresident pharmacy license may be issued to a pharmacy located in another state whose primary business is to:
    1. Dispense a prescription drug or device under a prescription drug order and deliver the drug or device to a patient, including a patient in this state, by United States mail, common carrier, or delivery service;
    2. Process a prescription drug order for a patient, including a patient in this state; or
    3. Perform another pharmaceutical service as defined by Board rule.
G. A Class F pharmacy (Freestanding Emergency Medical Center Pharmacy) license may be issued to a pharmacy as stated in Board Rule 291.151.
H. A Class G pharmacy (Central Prescription Drug Order or Medication Order Processing Pharmacy) license may be issued to a pharmacy as stated in Board Rule 291.153.
I. A Class H pharmacy (Limited Prescription Delivery Pharmacy) license may be issued to a pharmacy as stated in Board Rule 291.155.
J. The Board may determine the classification under which a pharmacy may be licensed.

Section 560.052 Qualifications
A. The Board by rule shall establish the standards that each pharmacy and the pharmacy's employees involved in the practice of pharmacy must meet to qualify for licensing as a pharmacy in each classification.
B. To qualify for a pharmacy license, an applicant must submit to the Board:
    1. A license fee set by the Board, except as provided by D. below and
    2. A completed application that:
        a. Is on a form prescribed by the Board;
        b. Includes notice that a surety bond may be required under Section 565.0551;
        c. Is given under oath;

d. Includes proof that:
   (1) A pharmacy license held by the applicant in this state or another state, if applicable, has not been restricted, suspended, revoked, or surrendered for any reason and
   (2) No owner of the pharmacy for which the application is made has held a pharmacist license in this state or another state, if applicable, that has been restricted, suspended, revoked, or surrendered for any reason; and
e. Includes a statement of:
   (1) The ownership;
   (2) The location of the pharmacy;
   (3) The license number of each pharmacist who is employed by the pharmacy, if the pharmacy is located in this state, or who is licensed to practice pharmacy in this state, if the pharmacy is located in another state;
   (4) The pharmacist license number of the pharmacist-in-charge; and
   Note: Since "pharmacist" is defined as a person licensed by TSBP, Class E (nonresident) pharmacies are required to have a Texas-licensed PIC.
   (5) Any other information the Board determines necessary; and
3. A disclosure statement required under Section 560.0521 unless:
   a. The pharmacy for which the application is made is operated by a publicly traded company;
   b. The pharmacy for which the application is made is wholly owned by a retail grocery store chain; or
   c. The applicant is applying for a Class B or Class C pharmacy license.
C. A pharmacy located in another state that applies for a license, in addition to satisfying the requirements of this chapter, must provide to the Board:
   1. Evidence that the applicant holds a pharmacy license, registration, or permit in good standing issued by the state in which the pharmacy is located;
   2. The name of the owner and pharmacist-in-charge of the pharmacy for service of process;
   3. Evidence of the applicant's ability to provide the Board a record of a prescription drug order dispensed or delivered as authorized by Chapter 562 of the Act (compounded and prepackaged drugs including compounded products for office use) by the applicant to a resident of or practitioner in this state no later than 72 hours after the time the Board requests the record;
   4. An affidavit by the pharmacist-in-charge that states that the pharmacist has read and understands the laws and rules relating to the applicable license;
   5. Proof of creditworthiness; and
   6. An inspection report issued:
      a. Not more than two years before the date the license application is received and
      b. By the pharmacy licensing board in the state of the pharmacy's physical location, except as provided by F. below.
D. A pharmacy operated by the state or a local government that qualifies for a Class D pharmacy license is not required to pay a fee to obtain a license.
E. With respect to a Class C pharmacy license, the Board may issue a license to a pharmacy on certification by the appropriate agency that the facility in which the pharmacy is located has substantially completed the requirements for licensing.
F. A Class E pharmacy may submit an inspection report issued by an entity other than the pharmacy licensing board of the state in which the pharmacy is physically located if:

  a. The state's licensing board does not conduct inspections;
  b. The inspection is substantively equivalent to an inspection conducted by the Board as determined by Board rule; and
  c. The inspecting entity meets specifications adopted by the Board for inspecting entities.
G. A license may not be issued to a pharmacy that compounds sterile preparations unless the pharmacy has been inspected by the Board to ensure that the pharmacy meets the safety standards and other requirements of the Act and rules.
H. The Board may accept, as satisfying the inspection requirement in G. above for a pharmacy located in another state, an inspection report issued by the pharmacy licensing board in the state in which the pharmacy is located if:
 1. The Board determines that the other state has comparable standards and regulations applicable to pharmacies, including standards and regulations related to health and safety and
 2. The pharmacy provides to the Board any requested documentation related to the inspection.

Section 560.0521 Sworn Disclosure Statement

A. A disclosure statement included with an application under Section 560.052B.2. must include:
 1. The name of the pharmacy;
 2. The name of each person who has a direct financial investment in the pharmacy;
 3. The name of each person who:
  a. Is not an individual;
  b. Has any financial investment in the pharmacy; and
  c. Is not otherwise disclosed under 2. above;
 4. The total amount or percentage of the financial investment made by each person described by 2. above; and
 5. The name of each of the following persons, if applicable, connected to the pharmacy if the person is not otherwise disclosed under 2. or 3. above:
  a. A partner;
  b. An officer;
  c. A director;
  d. A managing employee;
  e. An owner or person who controls the owner; and
  f. A person who acts as a controlling person of the pharmacy through the exercise of direct or indirect influence or control over the management of the pharmacy, the expenditure of money by the pharmacy, or a policy of the pharmacy, including:
   (1) A management company, landlord, marketing company, or similar person who operates or contracts for the operation of a pharmacy and, if the pharmacy is a publicly traded corporation or is controlled by a publicly traded corporation, an officer or director of the corporation but not a shareholder or lender of the corporation;
   (2) An individual who has a personal, familial, or other relationship with an owner, manager, landlord, tenant, or provider of a pharmacy that allows the individual to exercise actual control of the pharmacy; and
   (3) Any other person the Board by rule requires to be included based on the person's exercise of direct or indirect influence or control.
B. An applicant shall notify the Board no later than the 60th day after the date any administrative sanction or criminal penalty is imposed against a person described by A. above.

C. The Board may adopt rules regarding the disclosure of the source of a financial investment under A. above.
D. A disclosure statement under this section shall be given under oath as prescribed by Board rule.
E. Information contained in a disclosure statement under this section is confidential and not subject to disclosure under Chapter 552, Government Code (Texas Public Information Act).

Board of Pharmacy Rule 291.1
Pharmacy License Application

A. To qualify for a pharmacy license, the applicant must submit an application which includes any information requested on the application.
Note: See Pharmacy License Application on the TSBP website for requirements.
B. The applicant may be required to meet all requirements necessary for the Board to access the criminal history record information, including submitting fingerprint information and being responsible for all associated costs. The criminal history information may be required for each individual owner or, if the pharmacy is owned by a partnership or closely held corporation, for each managing officer.
C. A fee as specified under Board Rule 291.6 for issuing initial, renewal, and duplicate or amended pharmacy licenses will be charged.
D. For the purpose of this rule, managing officers are the top four executive officers, including the corporate officer in charge of pharmacy operations, who are designated by the partnership or corporation to be jointly responsible for the legal operation of the pharmacy.
E. Prior to the issuance of a license for a pharmacy located in Texas, the Board shall conduct an onsite inspection of the pharmacy in the presence of the pharmacist-in-charge and owner or representative of the owner to ensure that the pharmacist-in-charge and owner can meet the requirements of the Texas Pharmacy Act and rules.
F. If the applicant holds an active pharmacy license in Texas on the date of application for a new pharmacy license or for another good cause shown as specified by the Board, the Board may waive the pre-inspection as set forth in E. above.

Board of Pharmacy Rule 291.6
Pharmacy License Fees

A. License fees are subject to change. Contact TSBP or check the Board's website for current fees.
B. Biennial Registration. The Board requires all pharmacy licenses to be renewed every two years.
C. Fees consist of:
   1. A processing and licensing fee;
   2. A surcharge to fund the pharmacist and pharmacy student impairment program (evaluation only, not treatment);
   3. A surcharge to fund Texas Online; and
   4. A surcharge to fund the Office of Patient Safety.
D. Duplicate or amended licenses or renewal certificates can be obtained from TSBP by contacting TSBP or checking the Board's website.

Section 560.053 Establishment of Additional Pharmacy Classifications

The Board by rule may establish classifications of pharmacy licenses in addition to the classifications under Section 560.051 of the Act if the Board determines that:

1. The practice setting will provide pharmaceutical care services to the public;
2. The existing classifications of pharmacy licenses are not appropriate for that practice setting; and
3. Establishment of a new classification of pharmacy license is necessary to protect the public health, safety, and welfare.

Note: The Board has established Class F, G, and H pharmacies by rule. See Chapter J in this book.

Board of Pharmacy Rule 291.22
Petition to Establish an Additional Class of Pharmacy

A. Purpose. The purpose of this section is to specify the procedures to be followed in petitioning the Board to establish an additional class of pharmacy as authorized by 560.053 of the Texas Pharmacy Act (Chapters 551–566 and 568–569, Texas Occupations Code). In reviewing petitions, the Board will only consider petitions that provide pharmaceutical care services which contribute to positive patient outcomes. The Board will not consider any petition intended only to provide a competitive advantage.

B. Procedures for Petitioning the Board to Establish an Additional Class of Pharmacy. A person who wishes the Board to consider establishing an additional class of pharmacy shall submit to the Board a petition for which contains at least the following information:
  1. Name, address, telephone number, and pharmacist's license number of the pharmacist responsible for submitting the petition;
  2. A detailed summary of the additional class of pharmacy which includes:
     a. A description of the type of pharmacy and the pharmaceutical care services provided to the public;
     b. If a pharmacy of this type currently exists, the name, address, and license number of the pharmacy; and
     c. A full explanation of the reasons:
        (1) The existing classifications of pharmacy licenses are not appropriate for this practice setting and
        (2) The establishment of a new classification of pharmacy license is necessary to protect the public health, safety, and welfare.

C. Review and Approval or Denial of the Petition.
  1. On receipt of a petition to establish an additional class of pharmacy, the Board staff shall initially review the petition for completeness and appropriateness. If the petition is incomplete or inappropriate for Board consideration for any reason, the Board staff shall return the petition with a letter of explanation. Such review shall be completed within 30 working days of receipt of the petition.
  2. Once the Board staff has determined that the petition is complete and appropriate, a task force composed of Board staff, at least one Board member, and, if deemed necessary, resource personnel appointed by the Board president shall review the petition and make a written recommendation to the Board regarding approval. Such recommendation shall be presented to the Board at the next regularly scheduled meeting of the Board that occurs at least three weeks after completion of the review and written recommendation.
  3. A copy of the recommendation shall be provided to the petitioner and the Board at least two weeks prior to the Board meeting.
  4. Both the petitioner and a representative of the task force shall be given equal time for presentations to the Board.
  5. Upon hearing the presentations, the Board shall approve or deny the petition. If the Board approves the petition, the Board shall direct staff to

develop rules for the new class of pharmacy or appoint a task force to work with the staff to assist in developing rules for the new class of pharmacy. The Board shall approve or deny any petition to establish an additional class of pharmacy no later than the Board meeting following the meeting at which the petition is heard.

SUBCHAPTER C. Restrictions on a Pharmacy License

Section 560.101 License Not Transferable

A pharmacy license issued under this chapter is not transferable or assignable.

Note: Although a pharmacy license is not transferable, the Board does have rules requiring notification to the Board of a change in location or name. See Board Rule 291.3A. in Chapter E in this book.

Section 560.102 Separate License for Each Location

A. A separate pharmacy license is required for each principal place of business of a pharmacy.
B. Only one pharmacy license may be issued for a specific location.

Board of Pharmacy Rule 291.127
Emergency Remote Pharmacy License

A. Definitions.
The following words and terms shall have the following meanings unless the context clearly indicates otherwise.
1. **Emergency remote pharmacy**—A pharmacy not located at the same Texas location as a home pharmacy at which pharmacy services are provided during an emergency situation.
2. **Emergency situation**—An emergency caused by a natural or manmade disaster or any other exceptional situation that causes an extraordinary demand for pharmacy services.
3. **Home pharmacy**—A currently licensed Class A (community), Class C (institutional), or Class D (clinic) pharmacy that is providing emergency pharmacy services through an emergency remote pharmacy.
B. Emergency Remote Pharmacy License. In an emergency situation, the Board may grant a holder of a Class A (community), Class C (institutional), or Class D (clinic) pharmacy license the authority to operate a pharmacy and provide pharmacy services at an alternate location. The following is applicable for the emergency remote pharmacy.
1. The emergency remote pharmacy will not be issued a separate pharmacy license but shall operate under the license of the home pharmacy. To qualify for an emergency remote pharmacy license, the applicant must submit an application including the following information:
   a. License number, name, address, and phone number of the home pharmacy;
   b. Name, address, and phone number of the emergency remote pharmacy;
   c. Name and Texas pharmacist license number of the pharmacist-in-charge of the home pharmacy and of the pharmacist-in-charge of the emergency remote pharmacy; and
   d. Any other information required by the Board.
2. The Board will notify the home pharmacy of the approval of an emergency remote pharmacy license.
3. The emergency remote pharmacy license shall be valid for a period as determined by the Board not to exceed six months. The executive director of the Board in his or her discretion may renew the remote license for an

additional six months if the emergency situation still exists and the holder of the license shows good cause for the emergency remote pharmacy to continue operation.
4. The emergency remote pharmacy shall have a written contract or agreement with the home pharmacy which outlines the services to be provided and the responsibilities and accountabilities of the remote and home pharmacy in fulfilling the terms of the contract or agreement in compliance with federal and state laws and regulations.
5. The home pharmacy shall designate a pharmacist to serve as the pharmacist-in-charge of the emergency remote pharmacy.
6. The emergency remote pharmacy shall comply with the rules for the class of pharmacy under which the pharmacy is licensed as follows:
   a. Class A (Community Pharmacy)—*See Chapter G in this book.*
   b. Class C (Institutional Pharmacy)—*See Chapter I in this book.*
   c. Class D (Clinic Pharmacy)—*See Chapter J in this book.*
7. The records of services provided at the emergency remote pharmacy shall be maintained at the home pharmacy for a period of two years from the date of provision of the service. Such records shall be produced by the pharmacy within 48 hours if requested by an authorized agent of TSBP or DEA.

Section 560.103 False Affidavit
A person who falsely makes the affidavit prescribed by Section 560.052 of the Act is guilty of fraudulent and dishonorable conduct and malpractice.

Chapter 561 Renewal of a Pharmacy License

Section 561.001 Expiration of a License
A. A pharmacy license expires on May 31 of each year.
B. The Board may adopt a system under which the pharmacy licenses expire on various dates during the year (or every other year as appropriate).
C. If the Board changes the expiration date of a license, the Board shall prorate the license renewal fee to cover the number of months for which the license is valid for the year in which the date is changed. The total license renewal fee is due on the new expiration date.

Section 561.002 Annual Renewal
A pharmacy license must be renewed annually or biannually as determined by the Board.
Note: TSBP by rule requires pharmacy licenses to be renewed every two years.

Section 561.003 Requirements for Renewal
A. The Board by rule shall establish:
   1. Procedures to be followed for the renewal of a pharmacy license;
   2. The fees to be paid for the renewal of a pharmacy license; and
   3. The standards in each classification that each pharmacy and the pharmacy's employees involved in the practice of pharmacy must meet to qualify for relicensing as a pharmacy.
B. A pharmacy license may be renewed by:
   1. Payment of a renewal fee set by Board Rule 291.6 and
   2. Filing with the Board a completed application for a license renewal certificate given under oath before the expiration date of the license or license renewal certificate.
C. A pharmacy whose license has been expired for 90 days or fewer may renew the expired license by paying to the Board a renewal fee that is equal to one and one-half times the normally required renewal fee for the license.

Notes

D. Not in effect; repealed by legislative action.
E. If a pharmacy's license has been expired for one year or more, the pharmacy may not renew the license. The pharmacy may obtain a new license by complying with the requirements and procedures for obtaining an original license.

Board of Pharmacy Rule 291.14
Pharmacy License Renewal

A. Renewal Requirements.
   1. A license to operate a pharmacy expires on the last day of the assigned expiration month.
   2. The provisions of Section 561.005 (Suspension of License) of the Act shall apply if the completed application and a renewal fee are not received on or before the last day of the assigned expiration month.
   3. An expired license may be renewed according to the following schedule:
      a. If the license has been expired for 90 days or fewer, the license may be renewed by paying to the Board a renewal fee that is equal to one and one-half times the required renewal fee as specified in Board Rule 291.6 (Pharmacy License Fees).
      b. If the license has been expired for 91 days or more, the license may not be renewed. The pharmacy may apply for a new license as specified in Board Rule 291.1 (Pharmacy License Application).
B. If the Board determines on inspection at the pharmacy's address on or after the expiration date of the license that no pharmacy is located or exists at the pharmacy's address (e.g., the building is vacated or for sale or lease or another business is operating at the location), the Board shall not renew the license.
C. Additional Renewal Requirements for Class E Pharmacies.
   See Chapter J in this book.

Section 561.0031 Additional Renewal Requirement for a Class E Pharmacy
See Chapter J on Class E Pharmacies.

Section 561.0032 Additional Renewal Requirements for a Compounding Pharmacy
A. In addition to the renewal requirements under Section 561.003 of the Act, a pharmacy that compounds sterile preparations may not renew a pharmacy license unless the pharmacy:
   1. Has been inspected as provided by Board rule and
   2. Has reimbursed the Board for all expenses including travel incurred by the Board in inspecting the pharmacy (if located in another state) during the term of the expiring license.
B. The Board may accept, as satisfying the inspection requirement in A. above for a pharmacy located in another state, an inspection report issued by the pharmacy licensing board in the state in which the pharmacy is located if:
   1. The Board determines that the other state has comparable standards and regulations applicable to pharmacies including standards and regulations related to health and safety and
   2. The pharmacy provides to the Board any requested documentation related to the inspection.

Section 561.004 Issuance of a License Renewal Certificate
On timely receipt of a completed application and renewal fee, the Board shall issue a license renewal certificate that contains:
   1. The pharmacy license number;
   2. The period for which the license is renewed; and
   3. Other information the Board determines necessary.

Section 561.005 Suspension of a Pharmacy License for Nonrenewal
   A. The Board shall suspend the license and remove from the register of licensed pharmacies the name of a pharmacy that does not file a completed application and pay the renewal fee on or before the date the license expires.
   B. After review by the Board, the Board may determine that A. above does not apply if the license is the subject of a pending investigation or a disciplinary action.

Chapter 562 Practice by a License Holder (Pharmacist)
SUBCHAPTER A. Prescription and Substitution Requirements

Section 562.001 Definitions
   1. **Biological product** has the same meaning assigned by Section 351, Public Health Act (42 U.S.C. Section 262).
   1a. **Generically equivalent** means a drug that is pharmaceutically equivalent and therapeutically equivalent to the drug prescribed.
   1b. **Interchangeable** in reference to a biological product has the meaning assigned by Section 351, Public Health Service Act (42 U.S.C. Section 262) or means a biological product that is designated as therapeutically equivalent to another product by the United States Food and Drug Administration in the most recent edition or supplement of the United States Food and Drug Administration's *Approved Drug Products with Therapeutic Equivalence Evaluations* (also known as the FDA Orange Book).
   Note: Although the Act references the FDA Orange Book as designating equivalency, the official FDA reference for biological products is the List of Licensed Biological Products with Reference Product Exclusivity and Biosimilarity or Interchangeability Evaluations (also known as the FDA Purple Book).
   2. **Pharmaceutically equivalent** means drug products that have identical amounts of the same active chemical ingredients in the same dosage form and that meet the identical compendia or other applicable standards of strength, quality, and purity according to the United States Pharmacopeia or other nationally recognized compendium.
   3. **Therapeutically equivalent** means pharmaceutically equivalent drug products that, if administered in the same amounts, will provide the same therapeutic effect, identical in duration and intensity.

Section 562.002 Legislative Intent
It is the intent of the legislature to save consumers money by allowing the substitution of lower-priced generically equivalent drug products for certain brand name drug products and the substitution of interchangeable biological products for certain biological products and for pharmacies and pharmacists to pass on the net benefit of the lower costs of the generically equivalent drug product or interchangeable biological product to the purchaser.

Section 562.003 Disclosure of Price; Patient's Option
If the price of a drug or a biological product to a patient is lower than the patient's copayment under the patient's prescription drug insurance plan, the pharmacist shall offer the patient the option of paying for the drug or biological product at the lower price instead of paying the amount of the copayment.

Section 562.004 Prescription Transmitted Orally by a Practitioner
A pharmacist to whom a prescription is transmitted orally shall:
   1. Note on the file copy of the prescription the dispensing instructions of the practitioner or the practitioner's agent and
   2. Retain the prescription for the period specified by law.

Section 562.005 Record of a Dispensed Drug or Biological Product

A pharmacist shall record on the prescription form the name, strength, and manufacturer or distributor of a drug dispensed as authorized by this Act.

Section 562.0051 Communication Regarding Certain Dispensed Biological Products

A. No less than the third business day after the date of dispensing a biological product, the dispensing pharmacist or the pharmacist's designee shall communicate to the prescribing practitioner the specific product provided to the patient, including the name of the product and the manufacturer or national drug code number.

Note: A. above has been interpreted by TSBP as only requiring this notification if the biological product dispensed has been substituted for the biological product prescribed. This is further described in B. below.

B. The communication must be conveyed by making an entry into an interoperable electronic medical records system or through electronic prescribing technology or a pharmacy benefit management system or a pharmacy record, which may include information submitted for payment of claims, that a pharmacist reasonably concludes is electronically accessible by the prescribing practitioner. Otherwise, the pharmacist or the pharmacist's designee shall communicate the biological product dispensed to the prescribing practitioner using facsimile, telephone, electronic transmission, or other prevailing means provided the communication is not required if:
   1. There is no interchangeable biological product approved by the FDA for the product prescribed or
   2. A refill prescription is not changed from the product dispensed on the prior filling of the prescription.

Section 562.006 Label

A. Unless otherwise directed by the practitioner, the label on the dispensing container must state the actual drug dispensed, indicated by either:
   1. The brand name or
   2. If there is not a brand name, the drug's generic name or the name of the biological product, the strength of the drug or biological product, and the manufacturer or distributor of the drug or biological product.
B. In addition to the information required by A. above, the label on the dispensing container of a drug or biological product dispensed by a Class A or Class E pharmacy must indicate:
   1. The name, address, and telephone number of the pharmacy;
   2. The date the prescription is dispensed;
   3. The name of the prescribing practitioner;
   4. The name of the patient or, if the drug or biological product was prescribed for an animal, the species of the animal and the name of the owner;
   5. Instructions for use;
   6. The quantity dispensed;
   7. If the drug or biological product is dispensed in a container other than the manufacturer's original container, the date after which the prescription should not be used, determined according to criteria established by Board rule based on standards in the United States Pharmacopeia/National Formulary; and
   8. Any other information required by Board rule.
C. The information required by B.7. above may be recorded on any label affixed to the dispensing container.
D. B. above does not apply to a prescription dispensed to a person at the time of his or her release from prison or jail if the prescription is for no more than a 10-day supply of medication.

E. If a drug or biological product has been selected other than the one prescribed, the pharmacist shall place on the container the words "Substituted for brand prescribed" or "Substituted for 'brand name'" where 'brand name' is the name of the brand name drug or biological product prescribed.
F. The Board shall adopt rules requiring the label on a dispensing container to be in plain language and printed in an easily readable font size for the consumer. (*See labeling requirements of Board Rule 291.33E. in Chapter G of this book.*)

Section 562.0061 Other Prescription Information
The Board shall adopt rules specifying the information a pharmacist must provide to a consumer when dispensing a prescription to the consumer for self-administration. The information must be:
1. Written in plain language;
2. Relevant to the prescription; and
3. Printed in an easily readable font size.

Section 562.0062 Required Statement Regarding Medication Disposal
The Board by rule shall require pharmacists when dispensing certain drugs to include on the dispensing container label or in the information required by Section 562.0061 of this Act the statement "Do not flush unused medications or pour down a sink or drain."

Section 562.007 Refills
A properly authorized prescription refill shall follow the original dispensing instruction unless otherwise indicated by the practitioner or the practitioner's agent.

Section 562.008 Generic Equivalent or Interchangeable Biological Product Authorized
A. If a practitioner certifies on the prescription form that a specific prescribed brand is medically necessary, the pharmacist shall dispense the drug or interchangeable biological product as written by the practitioner. The certification must be made as required by the dispensing directive adopted under Section 562.015 of this Act. The Act does not permit a pharmacist to substitute a generically equivalent drug or interchangeable biological product unless the substitution is made as provided by this Act.
B. Except as otherwise provided by this Act, a pharmacist who receives a prescription for a drug or biological product for which there is one or more generic equivalents or one or more interchangeable biological products may dispense any of the generic equivalents or interchangeable biological products.

Section 562.009 Requirements Concerning Selection of Generically Equivalent Drug or Interchangeable Biological Product
A. Before delivery of a prescription for a generically equivalent drug or interchangeable biological product, a pharmacist must personally or through the pharmacist's agent or employee:
1. Inform the patient or the patient's agent that a less expensive generically equivalent drug or interchangeable biological product is available for the brand prescribed and
2. Ask the patient or the patient's agent to choose between the generically equivalent drug or interchangeable biological product and the brand prescribed.
B. A pharmacy is not required to comply with the provisions of A. above:
1. In the case of the refill of a prescription for which the pharmacy previously complied with A. above with respect to the same patient or patient's agent or
2. If the patient's physician or physician's agent advises the pharmacy that:
   a. The physician has informed the patient or the patient's agent that a less expensive generically equivalent drug or interchangeable biological product is available for the brand prescribed and

b. The patient or the patient's agent has chosen either the brand prescribed or the less expensive generically equivalent drug or interchangeable biological product.
C. A pharmacy that supplies a prescription by mail is considered to have complied with the provisions of A. above if the pharmacy includes on the prescription order form completed by the patient or the patient's agent language that clearly and conspicuously:
   1. States that if a less expensive generically equivalent drug or interchangeable biological product is available for the brand prescribed, the patient or the patient's agent may choose between the generically equivalent drug and the brand prescribed and
   2. Allows the patient or the patient's agent to indicate the choice between the generically equivalent drug or interchangeable biological product and the brand prescribed.
D. If the patient or the patient's agent fails to indicate otherwise to a pharmacy on the prescription order form under C. above, the pharmacy may dispense a generically equivalent drug or interchangeable biological product.
E. If the prescription is for an immunosuppressant drug as defined by Section 562.0141(a)(1), the pharmacist must comply with the provisions of Section 562.0141. This provision expires if Section 562.0141 expires under the requirements of Section 562.0142.
Note: E. above is not currently in effect.

Section 562.010 Responsibility Concerning Generically Equivalent Drug or Interchangeable Biological Product; Liability

A. A pharmacist who selects a generically equivalent drug or interchangeable biological product to be dispensed under this Act assumes the same responsibility for selecting the generically equivalent drug or interchangeable biological product as the pharmacist does in filling a prescription for a drug or biological product prescribed by a generic name.
B. The prescribing practitioner is not liable for a pharmacist's act or omission in selecting, preparing, or dispensing a drug under this Act.

Section 562.011 Restriction on Selection of and Charging for Generically Equivalent Drug or Interchangeable Biological Product

A. A pharmacist may not select a generically equivalent drug or interchangeable biological product unless the generically equivalent drug or interchangeable biological product selected costs less than the prescribed drug or biological product.
B. A pharmacist may not charge for dispensing a generically equivalent drug or interchangeable biological product a professional fee higher than the pharmacist customarily charges for dispensing the brand name drug or biological product prescribed.

Section 562.012 Substitution of a Dosage Form Permitted

With the patient's consent, a pharmacist may dispense a dosage form of a drug different from that prescribed, such as a tablet instead of a capsule or a liquid instead of a tablet, if the dosage form dispensed:
1. Contains the identical amount of active ingredients as the dosage prescribed for the patient;
2. Is not an enteric-coated or timed-release product; and
3. Does not alter clinical outcomes.

Board of Pharmacy Rule 291.33(c)(4)(A)(B)
Substitution of a Dosage Form Permitted

(1) As specified in Section 562.012 of the Act, a pharmacist may dispense a dosage form of a drug product different from that prescribed such as tablets instead of capsules or liquid instead of tablets provided:
(A) The patient consents to the dosage form substitution and
(B) The dosage form so dispensed:
  (i) Contains the identical amount of the active ingredients as the dosage prescribed for the patient;
  (ii) Is not an enteric-coated or timed-release product; and
  (iii) Does not alter desired clinical outcomes.
(2) Substitution of a dosage form may not include the substitution of a product that has been compounded by the pharmacist unless the pharmacist contacts the practitioner prior to dispensing and obtains permission to dispense the compounded product.

Section 562.013 Applicability of Subchapter
Unless a drug is determined to be generically equivalent to or a biological product is determined to be interchangeable with the brand prescribed, drug selection as authorized by this Act does not apply to:
1. An enteric-coated tablet;
2. A controlled-release product;
3. An injectable suspension, other than an antibiotic;
4. A suppository containing active ingredients for which systemic absorption is necessary for therapeutic activity; or
5. A different delivery system for aerosol or nebulizer drugs.

Section 562.014 Narrow Therapeutic Index Drugs
Note: This section of the Act and Board Rule 309.3(e)(2) implementing this section are not currently in effect.

Section 562.0141 Transplant Immunosuppressant Drug Product Selection Prohibited
Note: This section of the Act is currently not in effect.

Section 562.0142 Adoption of Rules
Note: This section of the Act is currently not in effect.

Section 562.015 Dispensing Directive; Compliance with Federal Law
A. The Board shall adopt rules to provide a dispensing directive to instruct pharmacists on the manner in which to dispense a drug or biological product according to the contents of a prescription. The rules adopted under this section must:
  1. Require the use of the phrase "brand necessary" or "brand medically necessary" on a prescription form to prohibit the substitution of a generically equivalent drug or interchangeable biological product for a brand name drug or biological product;
  2. Be in a format that protects confidentiality as required by the Health Insurance Portability and Accountability Act of 1996 (Pub. L. No. 104-191) and its subsequent amendments;
  3. Comply with federal and state law, including rules, with regard to formatting and security requirements;
  4. Be developed to coordinate with 42 C.F.R. Section 447.512; and
  5. Include an exemption for electronic prescriptions as provided by B. below.
B. The Board shall provide an exemption from the directive adopted under this section for prescriptions transmitted electronically. The Board may regulate the use of electronic prescriptions in the manner provided by federal law including rules.

Section 562.016 List of Approved Interchangeable Biological Products

The Board shall maintain on the Board's website a link to the United States Food and Drug Administration's list of approved interchangeable biological products.

Chapter 309 Board of Pharmacy Generic Substitution Rules

Board of Pharmacy Rule 309.1
Objective

The following governs the substitution of lower-priced generically equivalent drug products for certain brand name drug products and the substitution of interchangeable biological products for certain biological products.

Board of Pharmacy Rule 309.2
Definitions

The following words and terms shall have the following meanings unless the context clearly indicates otherwise. Any term not defined in this rule shall have the definition set out in the Act, Chapter 551.003 and Chapter 562.001.

1. **Act**—The Texas Pharmacy Act, Occupations Code, Subtitle J, as amended.
2. **Biological product**—A virus, therapeutic serum, toxin, antitoxin, vaccine, blood, blood component or derivative, allergenic product, protein (except any chemically synthesized polypeptide), or analogous product, or arsphenamine or derivative of arsphenamine (or any other trivalent organic arsenic compound), applicable to the prevention, treatment, or cure of a disease or condition of human beings.
3. **Biosimilar**—A biological product that is highly similar to the reference product notwithstanding minor differences in clinically inactive components and there are no clinically meaningful differences between the biological product and the reference product in terms of the safety, purity, and potency of the product.
4. **Data communication device**—An electronic device that receives electronic information from one source and transmits or routes it to another (e.g., bridge, router, switch, or gateway).
5. **Electronic prescription drug order**—A prescription drug order which is transmitted by an electronic device to the receiver (pharmacy).
6. **Generically equivalent**—A drug that is pharmaceutically equivalent and therapeutically equivalent to the drug prescribed.
7. **Interchangeable**—Referencing a biological product that is:
    a. Biosimilar to the reference product and can be expected to produce the same clinical result as the reference product in any given patient; and if the biological product is administered more than once to an individual, the risk in terms of safety or diminished efficacy of alternating or switching between use of the biological product and the reference product is not greater than the risk of using the reference product without such alternation or switch may be substituted for the reference product without the intervention of the healthcare provider who prescribed the reference product or
    b. Designated as therapeutically equivalent to another product by the United States Food and Drug Administration in the most recent edition or supplement of the United States Food and Drug Administration's *Approved Drug Products with Therapeutic Equivalence Evaluations* (also known as the FDA Orange Book).

Note: Although the Act and Board rules reference the FDA Orange Book as designating equivalency, the official FDA reference for biological products is the List of Licensed Biological Products with Reference Product Exclusivity and Biosimilarity or Interchangeability Evaluations (also known as the FDA Purple Book).

8. **Pharmaceutically equivalent**—Drug products that have identical amounts of the same active chemical ingredients in the same dosage form and that meet the identical compendia or other applicable standards of strength, quality, and purity according to the United States Pharmacopeia or another nationally recognized compendium.
9. **Reference product**—A single biological product against which a biological product is evaluated and is found to be biosimilar.
10. **Therapeutically equivalent**—Pharmaceutically equivalent drug products that, if administered in the same amounts, will provide the same therapeutic effect, identical in duration and intensity.
11. **Original prescription**—The:
    a. Original written prescription drug order or
    b. Original verbal or electronic prescription drug order reduced to writing either manually or electronically by the pharmacist.

Board of Pharmacy Rule 309.3
Generic Substitution Requirements

A. General Requirements. In accordance with Chapter 562 of the Act, a pharmacist may dispense a generically equivalent drug product or interchangeable biological if:
   1. The generic drug or interchangeable biological product costs the patient less than the prescribed drug product;
   2. The patient does not refuse the substitution; and
   3. The practitioner does not certify on the prescription form that a specific prescribed brand is medically necessary as specified in the dispensing directive described in C. below.
B. Prescription Format for Written Prescription Drug Orders.
   1. A written prescription drug order issued in Texas may:
      a. Be on a form containing a single signature line for the practitioner and
      b. Contain the following reminder statement on the face of the prescription: "A generically equivalent drug product may be dispensed unless the practitioner handwrites the words 'Brand Necessary' or 'Brand Medically Necessary' on the face of the prescription."
   2. A pharmacist may dispense a prescription that is not issued on the form specified in B.1. above. However, the pharmacist may dispense a generically equivalent drug or interchangeable biological product unless the practitioner has prohibited substitution through a dispensing directive in compliance with C.1. below.
   3. The prescription format specified in B.1. above does not apply to the following types of prescription drug orders:
      a. Prescription drug orders issued by a practitioner in a state other than Texas;
      b. Prescriptions for dangerous drugs issued by a practitioner in the United Mexican States or the Dominion of Canada; or
      c. Prescription drug orders issued by practitioners practicing in a federal facility provided they are acting in the scope of their employment.
   4. In the event of multiple prescription orders appearing on one prescription form, the practitioner shall clearly identify which prescription(s) the

dispensing directive(s) apply. If the practitioner does not clearly indicate to which prescription(s) the dispensing directive(s) apply, the pharmacist may substitute all drugs listed on the prescription form.

C. Dispensing Directive.
1. General Requirements. The following is applicable to dispensing directives outlined in this rule.
   a. When a prescription is issued for a brand name product that has no generic equivalent product, the pharmacist must dispense the brand name product. If a generic equivalent or interchangeable biological product becomes available, a pharmacist may substitute the generically equivalent or interchangeable biological product unless the practitioner has specified on the initial prescription that the brand name product is medically necessary.
   b. If the practitioner has prohibited substitution through a dispensing directive, a pharmacist shall not substitute a generically equivalent drug or interchangeable biological product unless the pharmacist obtains verbal or written authorization from the practitioner, notes such authorization on the original prescription drug order, and notifies the patient in accordance with Board Rule 309.4 (Patient Notification).
2. Written Prescriptions.
   a. A practitioner may prohibit the substitution of a generically equivalent drug or interchangeable biological product for a brand name drug product by writing across the face of the written prescription in the practitioner's own handwriting the phrase "Brand Necessary" or "Brand Medically Necessary."
   b. The dispensing directive shall:
      (1) Be in a format that protects confidentiality as required by the Health Insurance Portability and Accountability Act of 1996 (29 U.S.C. Section 1181 et seq.) and its subsequent amendments and
      (2) Comply with federal and state law including rules with regard to formatting and security requirements.
   c. The dispensing directive specified in this paragraph may not be pre-printed, rubber stamped, or otherwise reproduced on the prescription form.
   d. A practitioner may only prohibit substitution on a written prescription by following the dispensing directive specified in this rule. Two-line prescription forms, check boxes, or other notations on an original prescription drug order which indicate "substitution instructions" are not valid methods to prohibit substitution, and a pharmacist may substitute on these types of written prescriptions.
3. Verbal Prescriptions.
   a. If a prescription drug order is transmitted to a pharmacist verbally, the practitioner or practitioner's agent shall prohibit substitution by specifying "Brand Necessary" or "Brand Medically Necessary." The pharmacist shall note any substitution instructions by the practitioner or practitioner's agent on the file copy of the prescription drug order. Such file copy may follow the one-line format indicated in B.1. above or any other format that clearly indicates the substitution instructions.
   b. If the practitioner or practitioner's agent does not clearly indicate that the brand name is medically necessary, the pharmacist may substitute a generically equivalent drug or interchangeable biological product.
   c. To prohibit substitution on a verbal prescription reimbursed through the medical assistance program specified in 42 C.F.R., Section 447.331 (Medicaid):

- (1) The practitioner or the practitioner's agent shall verbally indicate that the brand is medically necessary and
- (2) The practitioner shall mail or fax a written prescription to the pharmacy which complies with the dispensing directive for written prescriptions specified in C. above within 30 days.
  4. Electronic Prescription Drug Orders.
     a. To prohibit substitution, the practitioner or practitioner's agent shall clearly indicate substitution instructions in the electronic prescription drug order.
     b. If the practitioner or practitioner's agent does not indicate or does not clearly indicate in the electronic prescription drug order that the brand is necessary, the pharmacist may substitute a generically equivalent drug or interchangeable biological product.
     c. To prohibit substitution on an electronic prescription drug order reimbursed through the medical assistance program specified in 42 C.F.R., Section 447.331 (Medicaid), the practitioner shall comply with state and federal laws.
  5. Prescriptions Issued by Out-of-State, Mexican, Canadian, or Federal Facility Practitioners.
     a. The dispensing directive specified in C. above does not apply to the following types of prescription drug orders:
        (1) Prescription drug orders issued by a practitioner in a state other than Texas;
        (2) Prescriptions for dangerous drugs issued by a practitioner in the United Mexican States or the Dominion of Canada; or
        (3) Prescription drug orders issued by practitioners practicing in a federal facility provided they are acting in the scope of their employment.
     b. A pharmacist may not substitute on prescription drug orders identified in a. above unless the practitioner has authorized substitution on the prescription drug order. If the practitioner has not authorized substitution on the written prescription drug order, a pharmacist shall not substitute a generically equivalent drug product unless:
        (1) The pharmacist obtains verbal or written authorization from the practitioner (such authorization shall be noted on the original prescription drug order) or
        (2) The pharmacist obtains written documentation regarding substitution requirements from the state board of pharmacy in the state, other than Texas, in which the prescription drug order was issued. The following is applicable concerning this documentation.
            (a) The documentation shall state that a pharmacist may substitute on a prescription drug order issued in such other state unless the practitioner prohibits substitution on the original prescription drug order.
            (b) The pharmacist shall note on the original prescription drug order the fact that documentation from such other state board of pharmacy is on file.
            (c) Such documentation shall be updated yearly.
D. Refills.
  1. Original Substitution Instructions. All refills shall follow the original substitution instructions unless otherwise indicated by the practitioner or practitioner's agent.
  2. Narrow Therapeutic Index Drugs. This rule is not in effect.

Board of Pharmacy Rule 309.4
Patient Notification

A. Substitution Notification. Before delivery of a prescription for a generically equivalent drug or interchangeable biological product as authorized by Chapter 562, Subchapter A of the Act, a pharmacist must:
   1. Personally or through his or her agent or employee inform the patient or the patient's agent that a less expensive generically equivalent drug or interchangeable biological product is available for the brand prescribed, and ask the patient or the patient's agent to choose between the generically equivalent drug or interchangeable biological product and the brand prescribed.
   2. Offer the patient or the patient's agent the option of paying for a prescription drug at a lower price instead of paying the amount of the copayment under the patient's prescription drug insurance plan if the price of the prescribed drug is lower than the amount of the patient's copayment.
B. Exceptions. A pharmacy is not required to comply with the provisions of A. above:
   1. In the case of the refill of a prescription for which the pharmacy previously complied with A. above with regard to the same patient or patient's agent or
   2. If the patient's physician or physician's agent advises the pharmacy that:
      a. The physician has informed the patient or the patient's agent that a less expensive generically equivalent drug or interchangeable biological is available for the brand prescribed and
      b. The patient or the patient's agent has chosen either the brand prescribed or the less expensive generically equivalent drug or interchangeable biological.
C. Notification by Pharmacies Delivering Prescriptions by Mail.
   1. A pharmacy that supplies a prescription by mail is considered to have complied with the provision of A. above if the pharmacy includes on the prescription order form completed by the patient or the patient's agent language that clearly and conspicuously:
      a. States that if a less expensive generically equivalent drug or interchangeable biological is available for the brand prescribed, the patient or the patient's agent may choose between the generically equivalent drug or interchangeable biological and the brand prescribed and
      b. Allows the patient or the patient's agent to indicate the choice of the generically equivalent drug or interchangeable biological and the brand prescribed.
   2. If the patient or patient's agent fails to indicate otherwise to a pharmacy on the prescription order form under C.1. above, the pharmacy may dispense a generically equivalent drug or interchangeable biological.
D. Inpatient Notification Exemption. Class C (institutional) pharmacies shall be exempt from the labeling provisions and patient notification requirements of Sections 562.006 and 562.009 of the Act with respect to drugs distributed pursuant to medication orders.

Board of Pharmacy Rule 309.6
Records

A. When the pharmacist dispenses a generically equivalent drug or interchangeable biological product pursuant to Subchapter A, Chapter 562 of the Act, the following information shall be noted on the original written or hard copy of the oral prescription drug order:

Note: TSBP rules also allow these records to be maintained in the pharmacy's computer system.
  1. Any substitution instructions communicated orally to the pharmacist by the practitioner or practitioner's agent or a notation that no substitution instructions were given and
  2. The name and strength of the actual drug product dispensed noted on the original or hardcopy prescription drug order. The name shall be either:
     a. The brand name and strength or
     b. The generic name or name of the interchangeable biological, strength, and name of the manufacturer or distributor of such generic drug or interchangeable biological product. (The name of the manufacturer or distributor may be reduced to an abbreviation or initials provided the abbreviation or initials are sufficient to identify the manufacturer or distributor. For combination drug products having no brand name, the principal active ingredients shall be indicated on the prescription.)
B. If a pharmacist refills a prescription drug order with a generically equivalent product or interchangeable biological product from a different manufacturer or distributor than previously dispensed, the pharmacist shall record on the prescription drug order the information required in A. above for the product dispensed on the refill.
C. If a pharmacy uses patient medication records for recording prescription information, the information required in A. and B. above shall be recorded on the patient medication records.
D. The National Drug Code (NDC) of a drug or any other code may be indicated on the prescription drug order at the discretion of the pharmacist, but such code shall not be used in place of the requirements of A. and B above.

Board of Pharmacy Rule 309.7
Dispensing Responsibilities

A. The determination of the drug product to be substituted as authorized by Subchapter A, Chapter 562 of the Act is the professional responsibility of the pharmacist, and the pharmacist may not dispense any product that does not meet the requirements of Subchapter A, Chapter 562 of the Act.
B. Pharmacists shall use 1.-3. below as a basis for the determination of generic equivalency as defined in Subchapter A, Chapter 562 of the Act.
  1. For drugs listed in the publication, pharmacists shall use *Approved Drug Products with Therapeutic Equivalence Evaluations* and current supplements published by the federal Food and Drug Administration (the Orange Book) within the limitations stipulated in that publication to determine generic equivalency. Pharmacists may only substitute products that are rated therapeutically equivalent in the Orange Book and have an "A" rating. "A" rated drug products include but are not limited to those designated AA, AB, AN, AO, AP, or AT in the Orange Book.
  2. For drugs not listed in the Orange Book, pharmacists shall use their professional judgment to determine generic equivalency.
     Note: 2. above allows pharmacists to substitute pre-1938 drugs that are not listed in the Orange Book such as atropine sulfate, chloral hydrate, codeine, colchicine, digoxin, levothyroxine, morphine sulfate, nitroglycerin, phenobarbital, thyroid, and quinine.
  3. Although not currently referenced in the Act or rules, the official FDA reference for determining interchangeability of biological products is the FDA Purple Book.

> **Board of Pharmacy Rule 309.8**
> *Advertising of Generic Drugs by Pharmacies*

Prescription drug advertising comparing generic drugs or biological products and brand name drugs or biological products is subject to Section 554.054 of the Act and in compliance with federal law.

SUBCHAPTER B. Other Practice by Pharmacist

Section 562.052 Release of Confidential Records

A confidential record is privileged, and a pharmacist may release a confidential record only to:
1. The patient or the patient's agent;
2. A practitioner or another pharmacist if, in the pharmacist's professional judgment, the release is necessary to protect the patient's health and well-being;
3. The Board or to a person or to another state or federal agency authorized by law to receive the confidential record;
4. A law enforcement agency engaged in the investigation of a suspected violation of Chapter 481 or 483, Health and Safety Code, or the Comprehensive Drug Abuse Prevention and Control Act of 1970;
5. A person employed by a state agency that licenses a practitioner, if the person is performing the person's official duties; or
6. An insurance carrier or other third-party payor authorized by the patient to receive the information.

Section 562.053 Reports to the Board

A pharmacist shall report in writing to the Board no later than the 10th day after the date of a change of address or place of employment.

> **Board of Pharmacy Rule 295.1**
> *Change of Address and/or Name*

A. Notify the Board in writing within 10 days of a change of address, giving the old and new addresses and the license number.
B. Notify the Board in writing within 10 days of a change of name by:
  1. Sending a copy of the official document reflecting the name change (e.g., marriage certificate, divorce decree, etc.) and
  2. Paying a fee.
  3. Pharmacists who change their name may retain the original license to practice pharmacy (wall certificate). However, if the pharmacist wants an amended license (wall certificate) issued which reflects the pharmacist's name change, the pharmacist must:
     a. Return the original certificate and
     b. Pay a fee.
  4. An amended electronic renewal certificate reflecting the new name will be issued by the Board without a fee.

> **Board of Pharmacy Rule 295.2**
> *Change of Employment*

A. A pharmacist must notify the Board in writing within 10 days of a change of employment. The pharmacist is also responsible for ensuring that his or her name is removed from the previous pharmacy license and added to the license at

the new pharmacy of employment. The pharmacist-in-charge is also responsible for removing the name of the departing pharmacist from the pharmacy license.
B. For the purposes of this rule, the term "employment" means the pharmacy at which the pharmacist engages in work on a regular and routine basis, whether remunerative or not, including the practice of pharmacy, administrative or managerial duties, supervisory tasks, or direct or indirect contractual services for pay. The term does not include an isolated case of practicing pharmacy on a temporary basis in order to relieve another pharmacist, unless such isolated cases become regular and routine.

Section 562.054 Emergency Refills (also found in TCSA and TDDA)
See TSBP Rule on Emergency Refills in Chapter G.

Section 562.0545 90-Day Supply and Accelerated Refills
See TSBP Rule on Accelerated Refills in Chapter G.

Section 562.055 Report to the Texas Department of Health (now Texas Department of State Health Services (TDSHS))
A pharmacist shall report to the Texas Department of Health (now TDSHS) any unusual or increased prescription rates, unusual types of prescriptions, or unusual trends in pharmacy visits that may be caused by bioterrorism, epidemic or pandemic disease, or novel and highly fatal infectious agents or biological toxins that might pose a substantial risk of a significant number of human fatalities or incidents of permanent or long-term disability. Prescription-related events that require a report include:
A. An unusual increase in the number of:
  1. Prescriptions to treat respiratory or gastrointestinal complaints or fever;
  2. Prescriptions for antibiotics; and
  3. Requests for information on over-the-counter pharmaceuticals to treat respiratory or gastrointestinal complaints or fever.
B. Any prescription that treats a disease that is relatively uncommon and has bioterrorism potential.

Section 562.056 Practitioner-Patient Relationship Required
A. Before dispensing a prescription, a pharmacist shall determine in the exercise of sound professional judgment that the prescription is a valid prescription. A pharmacist may not dispense a prescription drug if the pharmacist knows or should know that the prescription was issued without a valid practitioner-patient relationship.
A1. To be a valid prescription, a prescription must be issued for a legitimate medical purpose by a practitioner acting in the usual course of the practitioner's professional practice. The responsibility for the proper prescribing and dispensing of prescription drugs is on the prescribing practitioner, but a corresponding responsibility rests with the pharmacist who dispenses the prescription.
B. This section does not prohibit a pharmacist from dispensing a prescription when a valid practitioner-patient relationship is not present in the case of an emergency.

Section 562.057 Administration of Epinephrine
A. A pharmacist may administer epinephrine through an auto-injector device in accordance with this section.
B. The Board shall adopt rules designed to protect the public health and safety to implement this section. The rules must provide that a pharmacist may administer epinephrine through an auto-injector device to a patient in an emergency situation.
C. A pharmacist may maintain, administer, and dispose of epinephrine auto-injector devices only in accordance with rules adopted by the Board under this section.

D. A pharmacist who administers epinephrine through an auto-injector device to a patient shall report the use to the patient's primary care physician, as identified by the patient, if the patient has a primary care physician.
E. A pharmacist who in good faith administers epinephrine through an auto-injector device in accordance with the requirements of this section is not liable for civil damages for an act performed in the administration unless the act is willfully or wantonly negligent. A pharmacist may not receive remuneration for the administration of epinephrine through an auto-injector device but may seek reimbursement for the cost of the epinephrine auto-injector device.
F. The administration of epinephrine through an auto-injector device to a patient in accordance with the requirements of this section does not constitute the unlawful practice of any healthcare profession.

Board of Pharmacy Rule 295.16
Administration of Epinephrine by a Pharmacist

A. Purpose. The purpose of this rule is to allow pharmacists to administer epinephrine through an auto-injector device to a patient in an emergency situation as authorized in Chapter 562 of the Act.
B. Definitions. The following words and terms shall have the following meanings unless the context clearly indicates otherwise.
   1. **Act**—The Texas Pharmacy Act, Chapter 551–569, Occupations Code, as amended.
   2. **Administer**—The direct application of a prescription drug to the body of an individual by any means including injection by a pharmacist.
   3. **Anaphylaxis**—A sudden, severe, and potentially life-threatening allergic reaction that occurs when a person is exposed to an allergen. Symptoms may include shortness of breath, wheezing, difficulty breathing, difficulty talking or swallowing, hives, itching, swelling, shock, or asthma. Causes may include, but are not limited to, an insect sting, food allergy, drug reaction, and exercise.
   4. **Epinephrine auto-injector**—A disposable drug delivery system that contains a premeasured single dose of epinephrine that is used to treat anaphylaxis in an emergency situation.
C. Administration Requirements.
   1. Pharmacists may administer epinephrine through an auto-injector to a patient in an emergency situation.
   2. The authority of a pharmacist to administer epinephrine through an auto-injector may not be delegated.
   3. Epinephrine administered by a pharmacist under the provisions of this rule shall be in the legal possession of a pharmacist or legal possession of a pharmacy, which shall be the pharmacy responsible for drug accountability, including the maintenance of records of administration of the epinephrine.
D. Limitation on Liability.
   1. A pharmacist who in good faith administers epinephrine through an auto-injector in accordance with this rule and Chapter 562 of the Act is not liable for civil damages for an act performed in the administration unless the act is willfully or wantonly negligent.
   2. A pharmacist may not receive remuneration for the administration of epinephrine through an auto-injector but may seek reimbursement for the cost of the epinephrine auto-injector.
   3. The administration of epinephrine through an auto-injector to a patient in accordance with the requirements of this rule and Chapter 562 of the Act does not constitute the unlawful practice of any healthcare profession.

E. Notifications.
1. A pharmacist who administers epinephrine through an auto-injector to a patient shall report the use to the patient's primary care physician, as identified by the patient, as soon as practical but in no event more than 72 hours from the time of administering the epinephrine.
2. Immediately after administering the epinephrine auto-injector, the pharmacist shall ensure that 911 is called and the patient is evaluated by emergency personnel for possible transfer to the nearest emergency department for additional evaluation, monitoring, and treatment.
3. The notifications required in 1. above shall include the:
   a. Name of the patient;
   b. Age of the patient if under 8 years of age;
   c. Name and manufacturer of the epinephrine auto-injector;
   d. Date the epinephrine was administered;
   e. Name and title of the person administering the epinephrine; and
   f. Name, address, and telephone number of the pharmacy.
F. Records.
1. The notification required to be made under this rule shall be kept by the pharmacy, and these records shall be available for at least two years from the date of each record for inspecting and copying by the Board or its representative and to other authorized local, state, or federal law enforcement or regulatory agencies.
2. The notification may be maintained in an alternative data retention system such as a data processing system or direct imaging system provided:
   a. The records maintained in the alternative system contain all of the information required on the manual record and
   b. The data processing system is capable of producing a hard copy of the record upon request of the Board, its representative, or other authorized local, state, or federal law enforcement or regulatory agencies.
G. Prescriptions for Epinephrine Auto-Injector and Asthma Medication for Various Entities.
1. Several laws also now allow pharmacists to dispense epinephrine auto-injectors (and in some cases asthma medication) to various entities based on prescriptions without requiring the name of or any other identifying information relating to the user.
2. An order from a physician or person who has been delegated prescriptive authority (APRN or PA) may issue an order for an epinephrine auto-injector to be stored at specific types of entities. Such order must contain:
   a. The name and signature of the prescribing physician or other person;
   b. The name of the entity to which the order is issued;
   c. The quantity of epinephrine auto-injectors to be obtained and maintained under the order; and
   d. The date the order was issued.
3. Prescriptions for epinephrine auto-injectors may be dispensed by a pharmacy pursuant to a valid prescription without requiring the name or any other identifying information of the user for:
   a. Law enforcement agencies;
   b. Day care centers;
   c. Child-care facilities;
   d. Day camps or youth camps;
   e. Private or independent institutions of higher education;
   f. Amusement parks;
   g. Restaurants;
   h. Sports venues;

i. Youth centers; and
   j. Any other entity designated by rule of the Texas Health and Human Services Commission.
   (*See HB 1849, HB 4260, and SB 1827 from 86th Texas Legislature of 2019.*)
4. Prescriptions for epinephrine auto-injectors and asthma medication may be dispensed by a pharmacy pursuant to a valid prescription without requiring the name or any other identifying information of the user for:
   a. A school district;
   b. An open-enrollment charter school; and
   c. A private school.
   (*See HB 2243 from 86th Texas Legislature of 2019.*)

SUBCHAPTER C. Practice by Pharmacy (Pharmacies)

Section 562.101 Supervision of Pharmacy
A. A pharmacy is required to be under the supervision of a pharmacist as provided by this section.
B. A Class A or Class B pharmacy is required to be under the continuous onsite supervision of a pharmacist during the time the pharmacy is open for pharmacy services.
C. A Class C pharmacy that is in an institution with more than 100 beds is required to be under the continuous onsite supervision of a pharmacist during the time the pharmacy is open for pharmacy services.
D. A Class C pharmacy that is in an institution with 100 beds or fewer is required to have the services of a pharmacist on a part-time or consulting basis according to the needs of the institution.
E. A Class D pharmacy is required to be under the continuous supervision of a pharmacist whose services are required according to the needs of the pharmacy. *Note: Onsite supervision is not required.*
F. A Class E pharmacy is required to be under the continuous onsite supervision of a pharmacist and shall designate one pharmacist licensed to practice pharmacy by the regulatory or licensing agency of the state in which the Class E pharmacy is located to serve as the pharmacist-in-charge of the Class E pharmacy.
Note: Section 560.052 of the Act also requires that the pharmacist-in-charge be a Texas licensed pharmacist. See Chapter J.
G. For a pharmacy license classification established under Section 560.053 of the Act, the Board shall adopt rules that provide for the supervision of the pharmacy by a pharmacist. Supervision under the Board rules must require at least continuous supervision by a pharmacist according to the needs of the pharmacy. (*See Board Rule 291.22 in this chapter.*)

Section 562.1011 Operation of a Class C Pharmacy in Certain Rural Hospitals
See Chapter I in this book.

Section 562.102 Confidential Record
A pharmacy shall comply with Section 562.052 of the Act concerning the release of a confidential record.

Section 562.103 Display of Licenses by a Pharmacy
A. A pharmacy shall display in the pharmacy in full public view the license under which the pharmacy operates.
B. A Class A or C pharmacy that serves the public shall:
   1. Display the word "pharmacy" or a similar word or symbol as determined by the Board in a prominent place on the front of the pharmacy and
   2. Display in public view the license of the pharmacist-in-charge of the pharmacy.

C. A pharmacy shall maintain and make available to the public on request proof that each pharmacist, pharmacist intern, pharmacy technician, and pharmacist technician trainee working in the pharmacy holds the appropriate license or registration.

Section 562.104 Toll-Free Telephone Number Required

A pharmacy whose primary business is to dispense a prescription drug or device under a prescription drug order to a patient located outside the area covered by the pharmacy's telephone area code shall provide a toll-free telephone line. That line must be answered during normal business hours to enable communication between a patient or the patient's physician and a pharmacist at the pharmacy who has access to the patient's records.

Section 562.1045 Linking Internet Sites

A. This section applies only to a pharmacy that:
  1. Maintains a generally accessible Internet site and
  2. Sells or distributes drugs through the Internet.
B. A pharmacy subject to this section shall link its site to the Internet site maintained by the Board. The link must be:
  1. On the pharmacy's initial home page and
  2. If the pharmacy sells drugs through its site, on the page where the sale occurs.
C. A pharmacy subject to this section shall post:
  1. On its initial home page, general information on how to file a complaint about the pharmacy with the Board and
  2. Specific information on how to file a complaint with the Board not more than two links away from its initial home page.
D. Information under C. above must include the Board's telephone number, mailing address, and Internet website address.

Section 562.105 Maintenance of Records

A pharmacy shall maintain a permanent record of:
  1. Any civil litigation initiated against the pharmacy by a resident of this state or
  2. A complaint that arises out of a prescription for a resident of this state that was lost during delivery.

Note: This section was originally written to apply to out-of-state (Class E) pharmacies, but it now applies to all pharmacies.

Section 562.106 Notification

A. A pharmacy shall report in writing to the Board no later than the 10th day after the date of:
  1. A permanent closing of the pharmacy;
  2. A change of ownership of the pharmacy;
  3. A change of the person designated as the pharmacist-in-charge of the pharmacy;
  4. A sale or transfer of any controlled substance or dangerous drug as a result of the permanent closing or change of ownership of the pharmacy;
  5. Any matter or occurrence that the Board requires by rule to be reported;
  6. As determined by the Board, an out-of-state purchase of any controlled substance (not currently required by the Board);
  7. A final order against the pharmacy license holder by the regulatory or licensing agency of the state in which the pharmacy is located if the pharmacy is located in another state; or
  8. A final order against a pharmacist who is designated as the pharmacist-in-charge of the pharmacy by the regulatory or licensing agency of the state in which the pharmacy is located in another state.

A1. A pharmacy shall report in writing to the Board no later than the 30th day before the date of a change of location of the pharmacy.
B. A pharmacy shall report in writing to the Board a theft or significant loss of any controlled substance immediately on discovery of the theft or loss. The pharmacy shall include with the report a list of all controlled substances stolen or lost.
Note: TSBP rules also require immediate notification to the Board of a significant loss or theft of dangerous drugs as well as a report of loss of data from a pharmacy computer system (data processing system) within 10 days.
C. A pharmacy shall report in writing to the Board a disaster, accident, or emergency that may affect the strength, purity, or labeling of a drug, medication, device, or other material used in the diagnosis or treatment of illness, injury, or disease immediately on the occurrence of the disaster, accident, or emergency. (Board rule allows up to 10 days.)
D. The reporting pharmacy shall maintain a copy of any notification required by the Act for two years and make the copy available for inspection.

Section 562.107 Written Consumer Information Required
A. Each pharmacy shall make available to the consumer written information designed for the consumer that provides at a minimum:
 1. The therapeutic use of a drug and
 2. The names of generically equivalent drugs.
B. The information must be in a conspicuous location that is easily accessible to pharmacy customers. The information shall be periodically updated as necessary to reflect a change in the information.
C. On request by a consumer, the pharmacy shall make available to the consumer the cost index ratio of the prescribed drug and any generic equivalents of the prescribed drug.

Introduction to Remote Pharmacy Services Laws and Rules

The Texas Pharmacy Act recognizes three types of remote pharmacy practice in which drugs may be stored and/or dispensed from locations where a pharmacist is not present. TSBP has also adopted a rule recognizing a fourth type of remote service. **These four types of remote pharmacy services include Emergency Medication Kits at nursing homes, Automated Pharmacy Systems for routine dispensing of drugs at certain healthcare facilities including nursing homes, Telepharmacy Systems at certain healthcare facilities and remote dispensing sites, and Automated Storage and Delivery Systems for delivery of dispensed prescriptions.** The Remote Pharmacy Services rules are not the rules for remote order entry. The rules for remote order entry can be found in Board Rule 291.123 (Centralized Prescription Drug and Medication Order Processing) in Chapter E of this book. The main provisions of the Act for these types of remote pharmacy services and a summary of the rules for all four types are provided below.

Section 562.108 Emergency Medication Kits (nursing homes)
A. A Class A or Class C pharmacy or a Class E pharmacy located no more than 20 miles from any institution in this state that is licensed under Chapter 242 (primarily nursing homes) or Chapter 252 (intermediate care facilities for mentally retarded), Health and Safety Code, may maintain controlled substances and dangerous drugs in an emergency medication kit used at an institution licensed under those chapters. A U.S. Department of Veterans Affairs pharmacy or another federally operated pharmacy may maintain controlled substances and dangerous drugs in an emergency medication kit used at an institution licensed under Chapter 242, Health and Safety Code, that is a veterans home, as defined

by Section 164.002, Natural Resources Code. The controlled substances and dangerous drugs may be used only for the emergency medication needs of a resident at the institution. A Class E pharmacy may not maintain drugs in an emergency medication kit for an institution that is located more than 20 miles from a pharmacy.
B. The Board shall adopt rules relating to emergency medication kits including:
1. The amount and type of dangerous drugs and controlled substances that may be maintained in an emergency medication kit;
2. Procedures regarding the use of drugs from an emergency medication kit;
3. Recordkeeping requirements; and
4. Security requirements.

Summary of Board of Pharmacy Rule 291.121(b)
Remote Pharmacy Services Using an Emergency Medication Kit

Note: The following is a summary of this rule. See the complete official language in Board Rule 291.121(b).

1. This rule allows a Class A or C pharmacy or a Class E pharmacy located within 20 miles of a facility to provide pharmacy services to facilities licensed under Chapter 242 (Convalescent Homes, Nursing Homes, and Related Institutions), Health and Safety Code, or Chapter 252 (Intermediate Care Facilities for the Mentally Retarded), Health and Safety Code, using an Emergency Medication Kit as outlined in Section 562.108 of the Texas Pharmacy Act. It also allows a U.S. Department of Veterans Affairs pharmacy or other federally operated pharmacy to provide pharmacy services using an Emergency Medical Kit at an institution licensed under Chapter 242 that is a Texas State Veterans Home.
2. An application to TSBP is required before providing these services.
3. According to Appendix H of the *DEA Pharmacist's Manual*, a DEA registration is not required for a nonautomated emergency kit such as a "tackle box" at a long term care facility. However, DEA does require a pharmacy using an automated dispensing system as an emergency kit with controlled substances contained in it to obtain a separate DEA registration at the address of the facility. (*See 21 CFR 1301.27(b)*.)
4. Access to the emergency medication kit is limited to pharmacists and healthcare personnel employed by the facility.
5. Contents of the emergency medication kit shall be determined by the consultant pharmacist, pharmacist-in-charge of the provider pharmacy, medical director, and director of nursing and shall be limited to those drugs necessary to meet the resident's emergency medication needs. This rule means a situation in which a drug cannot be supplied by a pharmacy within a reasonable time.
6. Stocking of drugs in an automated pharmacy system must be done by a pharmacist, pharmacy technician, or pharmacy technician trainee unless the system uses barcoding, microchip, or other technologies to ensure that the containers or unit-dose drugs are accurately loaded and other specific requirements of Board Rule 291.121(b)(4)(F)(ii) are met.
7. A record must be maintained of all drugs sent to and returned from the remote location and should be kept separate from the records of the provider pharmacy and from other remote site records.
8. A perpetual inventory of all controlled substances must be maintained for each remote location. Each remote location's controlled substances must be inventoried on the same day as the provider pharmacy's inventory.

Section 562.109 Automated Pharmacy Systems (primarily used in nursing homes)

A. In this section, "automated pharmacy system" means a mechanical system that:
   1. Dispenses prescription drugs and
   2. Maintains related transaction information.
B. A Class A or Class C pharmacy may provide pharmacy services through an automated pharmacy system in a facility that is not at the same location as the Class A or Class C pharmacy. The pharmacist-in-charge of the Class A or Class C pharmacy is responsible for filling and loading the storage containers for medication stored in bulk at the facility.
C. An automated pharmacy system is required to be under the continuous supervision of a pharmacist as determined by Board rule. To qualify as continuous supervision for an automated pharmacy system, the pharmacist is not required to be physically present at the site of the automated pharmacy system and may supervise the system electronically.
D. An automated pharmacy system may be located only at a healthcare facility regulated by the state.
E. The Board shall adopt rules regarding the use of an automated pharmacy system under this section including:
   1. The types of healthcare facilities at which an automated pharmacy system may be located, which shall include a facility regulated under Chapter 142 (home health and hospice), Chapter 242 (primarily nursing homes), or Chapter 252 (intermediate care facilities for mentally retarded), Health and Safety Code;
   2. Recordkeeping requirements; and
   3. Security requirements.

Summary of Board of Pharmacy Rule 291.121(a) Remote Pharmacy Services Using Automated Pharmacy Systems (primarily used in nursing homes)

Note: The following is a summary of this rule. See the complete official language in Board Rule 291.121(a).

1. This rule allows a Class A or C pharmacy to provide pharmacy services to facilities licensed under Health and Safety Code Chapters 142 (Home and Community Support Service Agencies including hospices), 242 (Convalescent Homes, Nursing Homes, and Related Institutions), 247 (Assisted Living Facilities), and 252 (Intermediate Care Facilities for the Mentally Retarded) as well as jails or prisons operated by the State of Texas or local government.
2. Drugs may only be maintained in an automated pharmacy system.
3. If controlled substances are to be stored at the remote location using an automated pharmacy system, a DEA registration must be obtained for the remote location in the name of the pharmacy providing the remote pharmacy services.
4. An application to TSBP is required prior to providing these services.
5. A pharmacist may supervise the operation of the system electronically, and a pharmacist shall control all operations of the automated pharmacy system and approve the release of the initial dose after receiving a valid prescription drug order.
6. Drugs dispensed using the automated pharmacy system must meet the labeling requirements or alternative labeling requirements found in Board Rule 291.33(c)7.
7. Drugs used in the automated pharmacy system must be in the original manufacturer's container or be prepackaged in the provider pharmacy.

8. Stocking of drugs in an automated pharmacy system must be done by a pharmacist, pharmacy technician, or pharmacy technician trainee unless the system uses removable cartridges or containers and other specific requirements of Board Rule 291.20(a)(4)(F)(ii) are met.
9. A record must be maintained of all drugs sent to and returned from the remote location and should be kept separate from the records of the provider pharmacy and from other remote site records.
10. A perpetual inventory of all controlled substances must be maintained for each remote location. Each remote location's controlled substances must be inventoried on the same day as the provider pharmacy's inventory.

Section 562.110 Telepharmacy Systems

A. The statutory definitions for "Provider Pharmacy," "Remote Dispensing Site," and "Telepharmacy System" are as follows.
  1. A "Provider Pharmacy" means a Class A pharmacy that provides pharmacy services through a telepharmacy system at a remote dispensing site.
  Note: By Board rule, a provider pharmacy includes either a Class A or Class C pharmacy that provides pharmacy services through a telepharmacy system at a remote healthcare site or a Class A pharmacy that provides pharmacy services through a telepharmacy system at a remote dispensing site.
  2. A "Remote Dispensing Site" means a location licensed as a telepharmacy that is authorized by a provider pharmacy through a telepharmacy system to store and dispense prescription drugs and devices, including dangerous drugs and controlled substances.
  3. A "Telepharmacy System" means a system that monitors the dispensing of prescription drugs and provides for related drug use review and patient counseling services by an electronic method, including the use of the following types of technology:
     a. Audio and video;
     b. Still image capture; and
     c. Store and forward.
B. A Class A or Class C pharmacy located in this state may provide pharmacy services, including the dispensing of drugs, through a telepharmacy system in locations separate from the Class A or Class C pharmacy.
C. A telepharmacy system is required to be under the continuous supervision of a pharmacist as determined by Board rule. To qualify as continuous supervision for a telepharmacy system, the pharmacist is not required to be physically present at the site of the telepharmacy system. The pharmacist shall supervise the system electronically by audio and video communication.
D. A telepharmacy system may be located only at a healthcare facility in this state that is regulated by this state or the federal government or at a remote dispensing site.
E. The Board shall adopt rules regarding the use of a telepharmacy system under this section, including:
  1. The types of healthcare facilities at which a telepharmacy system may be located, which must include the following facilities:
     a. A clinic designated as a rural health clinic regulated under 42 U.S.C. Section 1395x(aa);
     b. A health center as defined by 42 U.S.C. Section 254b; and
     c. A federally qualified health center as defined by 42 U.S.C. Section 1396d(l)(2)(B);
  2. The areas that qualify under F. below;
  3. Recordkeeping requirements; and
  4. Security requirements.

Notes

F. Except as provided in F.1. below, a telepharmacy system in a healthcare facility may not be located in a community in which a Class A or Class C pharmacy is located as determined by Board rule. If a Class A or Class C pharmacy is established in a community after a telepharmacy system has been located under this section, the telepharmacy system may continue to operate in that community.

F.1. A telepharmacy system located at a federally qualified health center as defined by 42 U.S.C. Section 1396d(l)(2)(B) may be located in a community in which a Class A or Class C pharmacy is located as determined by Board rule.

G. A telepharmacy system in a remote dispensing site may not be located within 22 miles by road of a Class A pharmacy.

Summary of TPA Section 562.110 and Board of Pharmacy Rule 291.121(c) Remote Pharmacy Services Using Telepharmacy Systems

Note: The following is a summary of this section of the Act and Board rule. See complete official language in TPA Section 562.110 and Board of Pharmacy Rule 291.121(c).

1. These provisions allow certain provider pharmacies to provide telepharmacy services at two types of remote sites—remote healthcare sites and remote dispensing sites.
2. A Class A or C pharmacy may provide pharmacy services through a telepharmacy system, including the dispensing of drugs at remote healthcare sites which include:
   a. Rural health clinics regulated under 42 U.S.C. Section 1395x(aa);
   b. Health centers as defined by 42 U.S.C. Section 254b (serving medically underserved populations);
   c. Federally qualified health centers as defined by 42 U.S.C. Section 1396d(l)(2)(B);
   d. Healthcare facilities located in a medically underserved area as determined by the United States Department of Health and Human Services; and
   e. Healthcare facilities located in a health professional shortage area as determined by the United States Department of Health and Human Services.
3. A Class A pharmacy (but not a Class C pharmacy) may provide pharmacy services through a telepharmacy system, including the dispensing of drugs, at remote dispensing sites.
4. A telepharmacy system is a system that monitors the dispensing of prescription drugs and provides for related drug use regimen and patient counseling services by an electronic method which includes the use of audio and video, still image capture, and store and forward.
5. If controlled substances are to be stored at the remote location, a DEA registration must be obtained for the remote location.
6. Drugs dispensed at the remote location through a telepharmacy system shall only be delivered to the patient or patient's agent at the remote location.
7. A provider pharmacy may not supervise more than two remote sites.
8. An application to TSBP is required before providing these services.
9. A perpetual inventory of all controlled substances must be maintained for each remote location. Each remote location's controlled substances must be inventoried on the same day as the provider pharmacy's inventory.
10. Original prescription records shall be kept at the remote site, and the provider pharmacy shall have electronic access to those records.
11. A pharmacy that provides remote pharmacy services through a telepharmacy system at a remote location shall operate according to a written program for quality assurance of the telepharmacy system.

Copyright © 2020 Fred S. Brinkley, Jr., and Gary G. Cacciatore

12. Remote Healthcare Sites.
    a. Except in federally qualified health centers, a pharmacy may not provide remote pharmacy services at a remote healthcare site if a Class A or Class C pharmacy that dispenses prescription drug orders to outpatients is located in the same community (as defined in the rule).
    Note: Community is defined by Board rule as within 10 miles if not in a metropolitan statistical area.
    b. Unlike a remote dispensing site, a remote healthcare site may have Schedule II controlled substances.
13. Remote Dispensing Sites.
    a. A remote dispensing site is a location licensed as a telepharmacy that is authorized by a provider pharmacy through a telepharmacy system to store and dispense drugs and devices, including dangerous drugs and controlled substances.
    b. A remote dispensing site must be staffed by an onsite pharmacy technician who is under the continuous supervision of a pharmacist employed by the provider pharmacy.
    c. Pharmacy technicians at a remote dispensing site must have worked at least one year at a retail pharmacy during the past three years and must complete a Board-approved training program on the proper use of a telepharmacy system.
    d. Pharmacy technicians at a remote dispensing site are included in the pharmacist-pharmacy technician ratio of the provider pharmacy. They may not perform extemporaneous sterile or nonsterile compounding but may prepare commercially available medications for dispensing, including reconstitution of orally administered powder antibiotics.
    e. Only a Class A pharmacy may serve as a provider pharmacy for a remote dispensing site.
    f. A remote dispensing site may not be located within 22 road miles of a Class A pharmacy. If a Class A pharmacy opens within that mileage restriction after a remote dispensing site is operating, the remote dispensing site may continue to operate.
    g. A remote dispensing site may not dispense Schedule II controlled substances.
    h. If a remote dispensing site dispenses an average of more than 125 prescriptions each day the site is open (calculated annually), it must apply for a Class A license.
    i. A pharmacist employed by a provider pharmacy must make at least monthly onsite visits to a remote dispensing site and must reconcile the perpetual inventory of controlled substances to the on-hand count at the remote dispensing site.
14. The chart below provides a summary and comparison of the two types of "remote sites" where telepharmacy is allowed.

Remote Healthcare Sites	Remote Dispensing Sites
Provider pharmacy may be a Class A or Class C pharmacy.	Provider pharmacy must be a Class A pharmacy.
Provider pharmacy may not supervise more than two remote sites.	Provider pharmacy may not supervise more than two remote sites.
No restriction on drug classes.	May not dispense Schedule II controlled substances.
Does not require a pharmacy technician.	Must be staffed by a pharmacy technician.

(continued)

Notes

Remote Healthcare Sites	Remote Dispensing Sites
Except in federally qualified health centers, may not be located if a Class A or Class C pharmacy dispensing to outpatients is within 10 miles (if not located in a metropolitan statistical area).	May not be located if a Class A pharmacy is within 22 road miles.
A DEA registration is required for controlled substances.	A DEA registration is required for controlled substances.
Perpetual inventory of controlled substances is required.	Perpetual inventory of controlled substances is required.
No special training for pharmacy technicians (if used).	Pharmacy technicians must have one year of retail experience and training on a telepharmacy system.
No requirement for pharmacist visits or reconciliation of controlled substances.	Pharmacist employed by a provider pharmacy must make at least monthly onsite visits to a remote dispensing site and must reconcile the perpetual inventory of controlled substances to the on-hand count.
No limit on prescriptions dispensed.	If a remote dispensing site dispenses an average of more than 125 prescriptions each day the site is open (calculated annually), it must apply for a Class A license.

Summary of Board of Pharmacy Rule 291.121(d) Remote Pharmacy Services Using Automated Storage and Delivery Systems

Note: The following is a summary of this section of the Board rule. See complete official language in Board Rule 291.121(d).

1. This rule allows a Class A or Class C pharmacy to provide pharmacy services using an automated storage and delivery system at a remote delivery site. These systems are for delivery of previously verified prescriptions that have been dispensed by the Class A or Class C provider pharmacy.
2. An automated storage and delivery system is a mechanical system that delivers dispensed prescription drugs to patients at a remote delivery site and maintains related transaction information. They are sometimes referred to as kiosks.
3. A provider pharmacy may only provide remote pharmacy services using an automated storage and delivery system at Board-approved remote delivery sites. An application for approval to provide such services must be submitted to the Board and be renewed every two years with the provider pharmacy's pharmacy license.
4. Only dispensed drugs may be stored in an automated storage and delivery system at a remote delivery site.
5. A provider pharmacy shall comply with appropriate controlled substance registrations for each remote delivery site if dispensed controlled substances are maintained within an automated storage and delivery system.
   Note: It is unclear if DEA considers the controlled substances in these remote automated storage and delivery systems to be already dispensed and therefore no DEA registration would be required or if a separate registration is required for each site. If a separate DEA registration is required, it is unclear how the transfer of controlled substances from the provider pharmacy to the remote location would be accounted for since, per Board rule, the drugs are already dispensed by the provider pharmacy. Pharmacists should be cautious about

providing controlled substance prescriptions using an automated storage and delivery system at a location that is not registered with DEA or should seek confirmation from DEA that this is allowed.

6. Patients obtaining their prescriptions from an automated storage and delivery system shall receive counseling via direct link to audio or video communication by a Texas-licensed pharmacist who has access to the complete patient medication records (patient profile) maintained by the provider pharmacy prior to release of any new prescription.
Note: Counseling is not required for refill prescriptions.
7. A pharmacist must be accessible at all times to respond to patients' or other healthcare professionals' questions and needs pertaining to drugs delivered through the use of the system.
8. An automated storage and delivery system must be locked by key, combination, or other mechanical or electronic means to prohibit access by unauthorized personnel. There must also be a security system including security camera(s) that records a digital image of the individual accessing the system to pick up a prescription.
9. Access to an automated storage and delivery system is limited to pharmacists and pharmacy technicians or pharmacy technician trainees under the direct supervision of a pharmacist. Stocking of dispensed prescriptions must be completed under the supervision of a pharmacist.
10. A pharmacy providing services through an automated storage and delivery system at a remote delivery site shall operate according to a written program of quality assurance and written policies and procedures.

Section 562.112 Practitioner-Patient Relationship Required

A. A pharmacy shall ensure that its agents and employees before dispensing a prescription determine in the exercise of sound professional judgment that the prescription is a valid prescription. A pharmacy may not dispense a prescription drug if an agent or employee of the pharmacy knows or should know that the prescription was issued on the basis of an Internet-based or telephone consultation without a valid practitioner-patient relationship.
Note: While this section still remains in the Texas Pharmacy Act, the practice of telemedicine/telehealth is a "legal" practice in the state of Texas. The Texas Medical Practice Act allows for the use of an Internet-based or telephone consultation between the prescriber and a patient. Prescriptions issued in these circumstances may be valid; however, pharmacists must still ensure that there is a valid practitioner-patient relationship. Texas Medical Board rules specify two prohibitions on telemedicine:
  1. *A practitioner-patient relationship is not present if a practitioner prescribes an abortifacient or any other drug or device that terminates a pregnancy and*
  2. *Treatment for chronic pain with scheduled drugs using telemedicine is not allowed. TSBP has a Telemedicine Frequently Asked Questions document on its website which provides more information about telemedicine for pharmacists.*
B. A. above does not prohibit a pharmacy from dispensing a prescription in an emergency when a valid practitioner-patient relationship is not present. (*See Board Rule 291.29 (Professional Responsibility of Pharmacists) in Chapter E of this book.*)

SUBCHAPTER D. Compounded and Prepackaged Drugs

Section 562.151 Definitions (*See Chapter H in this book.*)

Section 562.152 Compounding for Office Use (*See Chapter H in this book.*)

Section 562.153 Requirements for Office Compounding (*See Chapter H in this book.*)

Section 562.154 Distribution of Compounded and Prepackaged Products to Certain Pharmacies (*See Chapter H in this book.*)

Section 562.155 Compounding Service and Compounded Products (*See Chapter H in this book.*)

Section 562.156 Compounded Sterile Preparation; Notice to Board (*See Chapter H in this book.*)

Chapter 563 Prescription Requirements; Delegation of Administration and Provision of Dangerous Drugs
SUBCHAPTER B. Delegation of Administration and Provision of Dangerous Drugs by Physicians

Section 563.051 General Delegation of Administration and Provision of Dangerous Drugs

A. A physician may delegate to any qualified and properly trained person acting under the physician's supervision the act of administering or providing dangerous drugs in the physician's office, as ordered by the physician, that are used or required to meet the immediate therapeutic needs of the physician's patients. Texas Medical Board rules define "immediate need" as a 72-hour supply of a dangerous drug. (*See Texas Medical Board Rule 169.2(6).*) The administration or provision of the dangerous drugs must be performed in compliance with laws relating to the practice of medicine and state and federal laws relating to those dangerous drugs.

B. A physician may also delegate to any qualified and properly trained person acting under the physician's supervision the act of administering or providing dangerous drugs through a facility licensed by the Board (a Class D pharmacy), as ordered by the physician, that are used or required to meet the immediate therapeutic needs of the physician's patients. The administration of those dangerous drugs must be in compliance with laws relating to the practice of medicine, professional nursing, and pharmacy as well as state and federal drug laws. The provision of those dangerous drugs must be in compliance with:
   1. Laws relating to the practice of medicine, professional nursing, and pharmacy;
   2. State and federal drug laws; and
   3. Rules adopted by the Board.

C. The administration or provision of the drugs may be delegated through a physician's order, a standing medical order, a standing delegation order, or another order defined by the Texas Medical Board.

D. This section does not authorize a physician or a person acting under the supervision of a physician to keep a pharmacy, advertised or otherwise, for the retail sale of dangerous drugs, other than as authorized under Section 563.053 (exception for rural physicians) of the Act, without complying with the applicable laws relating to the dangerous drugs.

E. A practitioner may designate a licensed vocational nurse or a person having education equivalent to or greater than that required for a licensed vocational nurse to communicate the prescriptions of an advanced practice registered nurse or physician assistant authorized by the practitioner to sign prescription drug orders.

Section 563.052 Suitable Container Required

A drug or medicine provided under this Act must be supplied in a suitable container labeled in compliance with applicable drug laws. A qualified and trained person, acting under the supervision of a physician, may specify at the time of the provision of the drug the inclusion on the container of the date of the provision, the patient's name, and the address.

Section 563.053 Dispensing of Dangerous Drugs in Certain Rural Areas
A. In this section, "reimbursement for cost" means an additional charge, separate from that imposed for the physician's professional services, that includes the cost of the drug product and all other actual costs to the physician incidental to providing the dispensing service. The term does not include a separate fee imposed for the act of dispensing the drug itself.
B. This section applies to an area located in a county with a population of 5,000 or fewer or in a municipality or an unincorporated town with a population of fewer than 2,500. The area must be within a 15-mile radius of the physician's office and in which a pharmacy is not located. This section does not apply to a municipality or unincorporated town that is adjacent to a municipality with a population of 2,500 or more.
C. A physician who practices medicine in an area described in B. above may:
    1. Maintain a supply of dangerous drugs in the physician's office to be dispensed in the course of treating the physician's patients and
    2. Be reimbursed for the cost of supplying those drugs without obtaining a pharmacy license under Chapter 558 of this Act.
D. A physician who dispenses dangerous drugs under C. above shall:
    1. Comply with each labeling provision under this Act applicable to that class of drugs and
    2. Oversee compliance with packaging and recordkeeping provisions applicable to that class of drugs.
E. A physician who desires to dispense dangerous drugs under this section shall notify both TSBP and the Texas Medical Board that the physician practices in an area described by B. above. The physician may continue to dispense dangerous drugs in the area until the Board determines after notice and hearing that the physician no longer practices in an area described by B. above.

Section 563.054 Administration of Dangerous Drugs (Veterinarians)
A. A veterinarian may:
    1. Administer or provide dangerous drugs to a patient in the veterinarian's office or on the patient's premises if the drugs are used or required to meet the needs of the veterinarian's patients;
    2. Delegate the administration or provision of dangerous drugs to a person who:
        a. Is qualified and properly trained and
        b. Acts under the veterinarian's supervision; and
    3. Itemize and receive compensation for the administration or provision of the dangerous drugs under A.1. above.
B. This section does not permit a veterinarian to maintain a pharmacy for the retailing of drugs without complying with applicable laws.
Note: B. above means a veterinarian may dispense dangerous drugs to his or her own patients but may not dispense dangerous drugs prescribed by other veterinarians unless he or she obtains a Class A pharmacy license.
C. The administration or provision of dangerous drugs must comply with:
    1. Laws relating to the practice of veterinary medicine and
    2. State and federal laws relating to dangerous drugs.

Chapter 564 Program to Aid Impaired Pharmacists and Pharmacy Students: Pharmacy Peer Review
SUBCHAPTER A. Reporting and Confidentiality

Section 564.001 Reports
   A. An individual or entity, including a pharmaceutical peer review committee, who has knowledge relating to an action or omission of a pharmacist in this state or a pharmacy student who is enrolled in the professional sequence of an accredited pharmacy degree program approved by the Board that might provide grounds for disciplinary action under Section 565.001(a)(4) or (7) of the Act may report relevant facts to the Board.
   B. A committee of a professional society composed primarily of pharmacists, the staff of the committee, or a district or local intervener participating in a program established to aid pharmacists or pharmacy students impaired by chemical abuse or mental or physical illness may report in writing to the Board the name of an impaired pharmacist or pharmacy student and the relevant information relating to the impairment.
   C. The Board may report to a committee of the professional society or the society's designated staff information that the Board receives relating to a pharmacist or pharmacy student who may be impaired by chemical abuse or mental or physical illness.

Section 564.002 Confidentiality
   A. All records and proceedings of the Board, an authorized agent of the Board, or a pharmaceutical organization committee relating to the administration of this chapter are confidential and are not considered public information for purposes of Chapter 552, Government Code (Texas Public Information Act). Records considered confidential under this section include:
      1. Information relating to a report made under Section 564.001 above, including the identity of the individual or entity making the report;
      2. The identity of an impaired pharmacist or pharmacy student participating in a program administered under this Act except as provided by Section 564.003 below;
      3. A report, interview, statement, memorandum, evaluation, communication, or other information possessed by the Board, an authorized agent of the Board, or a pharmaceutical organization committee related to a potentially impaired pharmacist or pharmacy student;
      4. A policy or procedure of an entity that contracts with the Board relating to personnel selection; and
      5. A record relating to the operation of the Board, an authorized agent of the Board, or a pharmaceutical organization committee as the record relates to a potentially impaired pharmacist or pharmacy student.
   B. A record or proceeding described by this section is not subject to disclosure, subpoena, or discovery except to a member of the Board or an authorized agent of the Board involved in the discipline of an applicant or license holder.

Section 564.003 Disclosure of Certain Information
   A. The Board may disclose information that is confidential under Section 564.002 above only:
      1. During a proceeding conducted by the State Office of Administrative Hearings, the Board, or a panel of the Board or in a subsequent trial or appeal of a Board action or order;
      2. To a pharmacist licensing agency or disciplinary authority of another jurisdiction;
      3. Under a court order;

4. To a person providing a service to the Board, including an expert witness, investigator, or employee of an entity that contracts with the Board related to a disciplinary proceeding against an applicant or license holder, if the information is necessary for preparation for or presentation in the proceeding; or
5. As provided by B. below.

A1. Information that is disclosed under A. above remains confidential and is not subject to discovery or subpoena in a civil suit and may not be introduced as evidence in any action other than appeal of a Board action.

A2. Information that is confidential under Section 564.002 above and that is admitted under seal in a proceeding conducted by the State Office of Administrative Hearings is confidential information for the purpose of a subsequent trial or appeal.

B. The Board may disclose that the license of a pharmacist who is the subject of an order of the Board that is confidential under Section 564.002 above is suspended, revoked, canceled, restricted, or retired or that the pharmacist is in any other manner limited in the practice of pharmacy. The Board may not disclose the nature of the impairment or other information that resulted in the Board's action.

Section 564.004 Immunity

A. Any person, including a Board employee or member, peer review committee member, pharmaceutical organization committee member, or pharmaceutical organization district or local intervener, who provides information, reports, or records under Section 564.001A. or B. above to aid an impaired pharmacist or pharmacy student is immune from civil liability if the person provides the information in good faith.

B. A. above shall be liberally construed to accomplish the purposes of this section, and the immunity provided under A. above is in addition to any other immunity provided by law.

C. A person who provides information or assistance to the Board under this Act is presumed to have acted in good faith. A person who alleges a lack of good faith has the burden of proof on that issue.

Section 564.005 Record of Report

On a determination by the Board that a report submitted by a peer review committee or pharmaceutical organization committee under Section 564.001A. or B. above is without merit, the Board shall expunge the report from the pharmacist's or pharmacy student's individual record in the Board's office.

Section 564.006 Examination of Report

A pharmacist, a pharmacy student, or an authorized representative of the pharmacist or pharmacy student is entitled on request to examine the peer review or the pharmaceutical organization committee report submitted to the Board and to place into the record a statement of reasonable length of the pharmacist's or pharmacy student's view concerning information in the report.

SUBCHAPTER B. Program Administration

Section 564.051 Program Authorization; Funding

The funding for the impaired pharmacists and pharmacy students program is provided through a surcharge on pharmacists and pharmacy licenses and renewals. These fees cover evaluation but not treatment.

SUBCHAPTER C. Pharmacy Peer Review

The Act permits pharmacy societies or associations and pharmacy owners to establish pharmacy peer review committees. The purpose of these committees is to evaluate the quality of pharmacy services and to suggest improvements in pharmacy systems to enhance patient care. Importantly, the statute provides for proceedings and records of pharmacy peer review committees to remain confidential unless the committee agrees to release or the Board subpoenas the information. Because establishment of these pharmacy peer review committees is voluntary rather than mandatory, the Board has not issued any rules to implement the legislation. Instead, the Board has adopted guidelines for pharmacy organizations or owners to use in developing peer review guidelines. These guidelines are available on the Board's website (*www.pharmacy.texas.gov*) or by contacting the Board's office. (*See Section 564.101–106 of the Texas Pharmacy Act for detailed language of this law.*)

Chapter 568 Pharmacy Technicians and Pharmacy Technician Trainees

Section 568.001 Qualifications

A. In establishing rules under Section 568.001 of the Act, the Board shall require that:
1. A pharmacy technician:
    a. Have a high school diploma or a high school equivalency certificate or be working to achieve an equivalent diploma or certificate and
    b. Have passed a Board-approved pharmacy technician certification examination.
2. A pharmacy technician trainee have a high school diploma or a high school equivalency certificate or be working to achieve an equivalent diploma or certificate.
B. The Board shall adopt rules that permit a pharmacy technician and pharmacy technician trainee to perform only nonjudgmental technical duties under the direct supervision of a pharmacist.

Section 568.002 Registration Required

A. A person must register with the Board before beginning work in a pharmacy in this state as a pharmacy technician or a pharmacy technician trainee.
B. The Board may allow a pharmacy technician to petition the Board for a special exemption from the technician certification requirement if the pharmacy technician is in a county with a population of fewer than 50,000.
   Note: For details about this exemption from certification, see Board Rule 297.7 in this chapter.
C. An applicant for registration as a pharmacy technician or pharmacy technician trainee must:
1. Be of good moral character and
2. Submit an application on a form prescribed by the Board.
D. A person's registration as a pharmacy technician or pharmacy technician trainee remains in effect as long as the person meets the qualifications established by Board rule.

Section 568.003 Grounds for Disciplinary Action (*See Chapter F in this book.*)

Section 568.0035 Discipline Authorized, Effect on Pharmacy Technician Trainee (*See Chapter F in this book.*)

Section 568.0036 Submission to a Mental or Physical Examination (*See Chapter F in this book.*)

Section 568.0037 Temporary Suspension or Restriction of Registration (*See Chapter F in this book.*)

Section 568.004 Renewal of Registration
The Board may adopt a system in which the registrations of pharmacy technicians and pharmacy technician trainees expire on various dates during the year.

Section 568.005 Fees
The Board may adopt fees as necessary for the registration of pharmacy technicians and pharmacy technician trainees.

Section 568.006 Ratio of Pharmacists to Pharmacy Technicians and Pharmacy Technician Trainees
The ratio of onsite pharmacists to pharmacy technicians and pharmacy technician trainees in a Class A pharmacy must be at least one pharmacist for every five pharmacy technicians or pharmacy technician trainees if the Class A pharmacy dispenses no more than 20 different prescription drugs and does not produce intravenous or intramuscular drugs onsite.

Note: This law is a special and very limited law (and rule below) that only applies in specific circumstances for this unique type of Class A pharmacy. It doesn't apply to 99% of Class A pharmacies in Texas. See Class A rules (Chapter G in this book) for general rules relating to ratios of pharmacists to pharmacy technicians.

Board of Pharmacy Rule 291.32(d)(3)(B)
Ratio of Onsite Pharmacists to Pharmacy Technicians and Pharmacy Technician Trainees

A Class A pharmacy may have a ratio of onsite pharmacists to pharmacy technicians of 1:5 provided the pharmacy dispenses no more than 20 different prescription drugs, does not produce sterile pharmaceuticals including intravenous or intramuscular drugs onsite, and the following conditions are met:
1. At least four of the pharmacy technicians are registered pharmacy technicians and
2. The pharmacy has written policies and procedures regarding the supervision of pharmacy technicians, including requirements that the registered pharmacy technicians included in a 1:5 ratio may be involved only in one process at a time. For example, a technician who is compounding nonsterile pharmaceuticals or who is involved in the preparation of prescription drug orders may not also call physicians for the authorization of refills.

Section 568.007 Registration of a Pharmacy Technician Trainee
A. A person must register with the Board before beginning work in a pharmacy in this state as a pharmacy technician trainee.
B. An application for registration as a pharmacy technician trainee must be on a form prescribed by the Board.
C. A person's registration as a pharmacy technician trainee remains in effect as long as the person meets the qualifications specified by Board rule.
D. The Board may, on a determination that a ground for discipline exists under Section 568.003 of the Act, take disciplinary action against a pharmacy technician trainee under Section 568.0035 of the Act.

Section 568.008 Pharmacy Technicians in Hospitals with a Clinical Pharmacy Program
A. In this section, "clinical pharmacy program" means a program that provides pharmaceutical care services as specified by Board rule.
B. A Class C pharmacy that has an ongoing clinical pharmacy program may allow a pharmacy technician to verify the accuracy of work performed by another pharmacy technician relating to the filling of floor stock and unit-dose distribution systems for a patient admitted to the hospital if the patient's orders have previously been reviewed and approved by a pharmacist.

Notes

C. The pharmacist-in-charge of the clinical pharmacy program shall adopt policies and procedures for the verification process authorized by this section.
D. A hospital must notify the Board before implementing the verification process authorized by this section.
E. The Board shall adopt rules to implement this section including rules specifying:
  1. The duties that may be verified by another pharmacy technician;
  2. The records that must be maintained for the verification process; and
  3. The training requirements for pharmacy technicians who verify the accuracy of the work of other pharmacy technicians.

Note: See Board Rule 291.74 in Chapter I of this book.

Section 568.009 Change of Address or Employment

No later than the 10th day after the date of a change of address or employment, a pharmacy technician or a pharmacy technician trainee shall notify the Board in writing of the change.

Board of Pharmacy Rules—Chapter 297
Pharmacy Technicians and Pharmacy Technician Trainees

297.1 Purpose

The purpose of this rule is to provide a comprehensive and coherent regulatory scheme for the registration and training of pharmacy technicians and pharmacy technician trainees in Texas.

297.2 Definitions

1. **Act**—The Texas Pharmacy Act.
2. **Board**—Texas State Board of Pharmacy.
3. **Pharmacy technician**—An individual who is registered with the Board and whose responsibility in a pharmacy is to provide technical services that do not require professional judgment regarding preparing and distributing drugs and who works under the direct supervision of and is responsible to a pharmacist. Pharmacy technician includes registered pharmacy technicians and pharmacy technician trainees.
4. **Pharmacy technician trainee**—An individual who is registered with the Board as a pharmacy technician trainee and is authorized to participate in a pharmacy's technician training program.
5. **Registered pharmacy technician**—A pharmacy technician who is registered with the Board.

297.3 Registration Requirements

A. General.
  1. Individuals who are not registered with the Board may not be employed as or perform the duties of a pharmacy technician or a pharmacy technician trainee.
  2. Individuals who have previously applied and registered as a pharmacy technician, regardless of the pharmacy technician's current registration status, may not register as a pharmacy technician trainee.
  3. Individuals who apply and are qualified for both a pharmacy technician trainee registration and a pharmacy technician registration concurrently will not be considered for a pharmacy technician trainee registration.
B. Registration for Pharmacy Technician Trainees. An individual may register as a pharmacy technician trainee only once, and the registration may not be renewed.
  1. Each applicant for pharmacy technician trainee registration shall:
    a. Have a high school or equivalent diploma (e.g., GED) or be working to achieve a high school or equivalent diploma. For the purpose of this

clause, an applicant for registration may be working to achieve a high school or equivalent diploma for no more than two years and
   b. Complete the Texas application for registration that includes the following information:
      (1) Name;
      (2) Addresses, phone numbers, date of birth, and social security number; and
      (3) Any other information requested on the application; and
   c. Meet all requirements necessary for the Board to access the criminal history record information, including submitting fingerprint information and paying the required fees.
  2. Once an applicant has successfully completed all requirements of registration and the Board has determined there are no grounds to refuse registration, the applicant shall be notified of registration as a pharmacy technician trainee and of his or her pharmacy technician registration number.
  3. Pharmacy technician trainee registrations expire two years from the date of registration or upon notification of registration as a registered pharmacy technician, whichever is earlier. A pharmacy technician trainee registration is not renewable.
C. Initial Registration for Pharmacy Technicians.
  1. Each applicant for pharmacy technician registration shall:
     a. Have a high school or equivalent diploma (e.g., GED) or be working to achieve a high school or equivalent diploma. For the purpose of this clause, an applicant for registration may be working to achieve a high school or equivalent diploma for no more than two years;
     b. Either have:
        (1) Taken and passed a pharmacy technician certification examination approved by the Board and have a current certification certificate or
        (2) Been granted an exemption from certification by the Board as specified in Board Rule 297.7 below (Exemption from Pharmacy Technician Certification Requirements);
     c. Complete the Texas application for registration that includes the following information:
        (1) Name;
        (2) Addresses, phone numbers, date of birth, and social security number; and
        (3) Any other information requested on the application; and
     d. Pay the registration fee specified in Board Rule 297.4 (Fees).
  2. New pharmacy technician registrations shall be assigned an expiration date, and the fee shall be prorated based on the assigned expiration date.
  3. Once an applicant has successfully completed all requirements of registration and the Board has determined there are no grounds to refuse registration, the applicant shall be notified of registration as a pharmacy technician and of his or her pharmacy technician registration number. If the pharmacy technician applicant were registered as a pharmacy technician trainee at the time the pharmacy technician registration is granted, the pharmacy technician trainee registration expires.
D. Renewal.
   Note: Certification is not required for the renewal of a pharmacy technician registration.
  1. All applicants for the renewal of a pharmacy technician registration shall:
     a. Complete the Texas application for registration that includes the following information:
        (1) Name;
        (2) Addresses, phone numbers, date of birth, and social security number;

(3) Meet all requirements necessary for the Board to access the criminal history record information, including submitting fingerprint information and paying the required fees; and
(4) Any other information requested on the application;
   b. Pay the renewal fee specified in Board Rule 297.4; and
   c. Complete 20 contact hours of continuing education per renewal period as specified in Board Rule 297.8 (Continuing Education).
2. A pharmacy technician registration expires on the last day of the assigned expiration month.
3. If the completed application and renewal fee are not received in the Board's office on or before the last day of the assigned expiration month, the person's pharmacy technician registration shall expire. An expired registration shall be renewed according to the following schedule.
   a. If a pharmacy technician registration has expired for 90 days or fewer, the person may become registered by making application and paying to the Board a renewal fee that is equal to one and one-half times the renewal fee for the registration.
   b. If a pharmacy technician registration has been expired for more than 90 days but less than one year, the person may become registered by making application and paying to the Board a renewal fee that is equal to two times the renewal fee for the registration.
   c. If a pharmacy technician registration has expired for more than one year, the pharmacy technician may not renew the registration and must complete the requirements for an initial registration as specified in C. above.
4. After review, the Board may determine that 3.c. above does not apply if the registrant is the subject of a pending investigation or disciplinary action.
E. An individual may use the title "Registered Pharmacy Technician" or "Ph.T.R" if the individual is registered as a pharmacy technician in this state.

297.4 Fees
Fees are subject to change. (*See the Board's website for current fees.*)

297.5 Pharmacy Technician Trainees
A. A person designated as a pharmacy technician trainee shall be registered with the Board prior to beginning training in a Texas licensed pharmacy.
B. A person may be designated as a pharmacy technician trainee for no more than two years. The requirements for registration as a pharmacy technician must be completed within the two-year period.

297.6 Pharmacy Technician and Pharmacy Technician Trainee Training
A. Pharmacy technicians and pharmacy technician trainees shall complete initial training as outlined by the pharmacist-in-charge in a training manual. Such training:
   1. Shall meet the requirements of Board Rule 297.3D. above and
   2. May not be transferred to another pharmacy unless:
      a. The pharmacies are under common ownership and control and have a common training program and
      b. The pharmacist-in-charge of each pharmacy in which the pharmacy technician or pharmacy technician trainee works certifies that the pharmacy technician or pharmacy technician trainee is competent to perform the duties assigned in that pharmacy.
B. The pharmacist-in-charge shall assure the continuing competency of pharmacy technicians and pharmacy technician trainees through in-service education and training to supplement initial training.

C. The pharmacist-in-charge shall document the completion of the training program and certify the competency of pharmacy technicians and pharmacy technician trainees completing the training. A written record of initial and in-service training of pharmacy technicians and pharmacy technician trainees shall be maintained and contain the following information:
 1. Name of the person receiving the training;
 2. Date(s) of the training;
 3. General description of the topics covered;
 4. A statement that certifies that the pharmacy technician or pharmacy technician trainee is competent to perform the duties assigned;
 5. Name of the person supervising the training; and
 6. Signature of the pharmacy technician or pharmacy technician trainee and the pharmacist-in-charge or other pharmacist employed by the pharmacy and designated by the pharmacist-in-charge as responsible for the training of pharmacy technicians and pharmacy technician trainees.
D. A person who has previously completed the training program outlined in E. below, a licensed nurse, or a physician assistant is not required to complete the entire training program outlined in E. below if the person is able to show competency through a documented assessment of competency. Such competency assessment may be conducted by personnel designated by the pharmacist-in-charge, but the final acceptance of competency must be approved by the pharmacist-in-charge.
E. Pharmacy technician and pharmacy technician trainee training shall be outlined in a training manual. The training manual shall at a minimum contain the following:
 1. Written procedures and guidelines for the use and supervision of pharmacy technicians and pharmacy technician trainees. Such procedures and guidelines shall:
    a. Specify the manner in which the pharmacist responsible for the supervision of pharmacy technicians and pharmacy technician trainees will supervise such personnel and verify the accuracy and completeness of all acts, tasks, and functions performed by such personnel and
    b. Specify duties which may and may not be performed by pharmacy technicians and pharmacy technician trainees and
 2. Instruction in the following areas and any additional areas appropriate to the duties of pharmacy technicians and pharmacy technician trainees in the pharmacy:
    a. Orientation;
    b. Job descriptions;
    c. Communication techniques;
    d. Laws and rules;
    e. Security and safety;
    f. Prescription drugs:
       (1) Basic pharmaceutical nomenclature and
       (2) Dosage forms;
    g. Drug orders:
       (1) Prescribers;
       (2) Directions for use;
       (3) Commonly-used abbreviations and symbols;
       (4) Number of dosage units;
       (5) Strengths and systems of measurement;
       (6) Routes of administration;
       (7) Frequency of administration; and
       (8) Interpreting directions for use;

h. Drug order preparation:
    (1) Creating or updating patient medication records;
    (2) Entering drug order information into the computer or typing the label in a manual system;
    (3) Selecting the correct stock bottle;
    (4) Accurately counting or pouring the appropriate quantity of a drug product;
    (5) Selecting the proper container;
    (6) Affixing the prescription label;
    (7) Affixing auxiliary labels if indicated; and
    (8) Preparing the finished product for inspection and final check by pharmacists;
i. Other functions;
j. Drug product prepackaging;
k. Written policies and guidelines for the use of and supervision of pharmacy technicians and pharmacy technician trainees; and
l. Confidential patient medication records.

F. Pharmacy technicians and pharmacy technician trainees compounding non-sterile pharmaceuticals shall meet the training and education requirements specified in the rules for the class of pharmacy in which the pharmacy technician is working.

G. Pharmacy technicians and pharmacy technician trainees compounding sterile pharmaceuticals shall meet the training and education requirements specified in the rules for the class of pharmacy in which the pharmacy technician or pharmacy technician trainee is working.

297.7 Exemption from Pharmacy Technician Certification Requirements

Note: This is an exemption from certification, not TSBP registration.

A. Purpose. The Board encourages all pharmacy technician trainees to become certified by taking and passing a pharmacy technician certification exam approved by the Board. However, the Board will consider petitions for exemption on a case by case basis. This rule outlines procedures to petition the Board for an exemption to the certification requirements established by Section 568.002 of the Act (Pharmacy Technician Registration Required).

B. Long-term Exempt Pharmacy Technicians. Long-term exempt pharmacy technicians are technicians who on September 1, 2001 had been continuously employed as a pharmacy technician in this state for at least 10 years and who received an exemption from the Board.

C. Rural County Exempt Pharmacy Technicians. Rural county exempt pharmacy technicians are pharmacy technicians working in counties with a population of 50,000 or less. (*See complete official language in Board Rule 297.7(c) for details on eligibility, the petition process, and limitations of this exemption.*)

297.8 Continuing Education Requirements

A. Pharmacy Technician Trainees. Pharmacy technician trainees are not required to complete continuing education.

B. Pharmacy Technicians.
   1. All pharmacy technicians shall be exempt from the continuing education requirements during their initial registration period.
   2. All pharmacy technicians must complete and report 20 contact hours of approved continuing education obtained during the previous renewal period in pharmacy-related subjects to renew their registration as a pharmacy technician.
   3. A pharmacy technician may satisfy the continuing education requirements by

a. Successfully completing the number of continuing education hours necessary to renew a registration as specified in 2. above;
   b. Successfully completing during the preceding license period one credit hour for each year of the renewal period in a pharmacy-related college course(s); or
   c. Taking and passing a pharmacy technician certification exam during the preceding renewal period which shall be equivalent to the number of continuing education hours necessary to renew a registration as specified in 2. above.
4. To renew a registration, a pharmacy technician must report on the renewal application the completion of at least 20 contact hours of continuing education. The following is applicable to the reporting of continuing education contact hours.
   a. At least one contact hour of the 20 contact hours specified in 2. above shall be related to Texas pharmacy laws or rules.
   b. Any continuing education requirements which are imposed upon a pharmacy technician as part of a Board Order or Agreed Board Order shall be in addition to the requirements of this rule.
   c. For renewals received after August 31, 2020 and before September 1, 2022, a pharmacy technician must have completed the human trafficking prevention course required in Section 116.002 of the Texas Occupations Code.
   Note: The statute requires that this course be approved by the Texas Health and Human Services Commission and that a list of approved courses be posted on the commission's website.
5. Pharmacy technicians are required to maintain records of the completion of their continuing education for three years from the date of reporting the hours on a renewal application. The records must contain at least the following information:
   a. Name of participant;
   b. Title and date of program;
   c. Program sponsor or provider (the organization); and
   d. Dated signature of sponsor representative.
6. The Board shall audit the records of pharmacy technicians for verification of reported continuing education credit. The following is applicable for such audits.
   a. Upon a written request, a pharmacy technician shall provide to the Board copies of the record required to be maintained in 5. above or certificates of completion for all continuing education contact hours reported during a specified registration period. Failure to provide all requested records by the specified deadline constitutes prima facie evidence of a violation of this rule.
   b. Credit for continuing education contact hours shall only be allowed for programs for which the pharmacy technician submits copies of records reflecting that the hours were completed during the specified registration period(s). Any other reported hours shall be disallowed.
   c. A pharmacy technician who submits false or fraudulent records to the Board shall be subject to disciplinary action by the Board.
7. The following is applicable if a pharmacy technician fails to report the completion of the required continuing education.
   a. The registration of a pharmacy technician who fails to report the completion of the required number of continuing education contact hours shall not be renewed, and the pharmacy technician shall not be issued

a renewal certificate for the license period until such time as the pharmacy technician successfully completes the required continuing education and reports the completion to the Board.
    b. A person shall not practice as a pharmacy technician without a current renewal registration certificate.
8. A pharmacy technician who has had a physical disability, an illness, or other extenuating circumstances prohibiting the pharmacy technician from obtaining continuing education credit during the preceding license period may be granted an extension of time to complete the continued education requirement. The following is applicable for this extension.
    a. The pharmacy technician shall submit a petition to the Board with his or her registration renewal application which contains:
        (1) The name, address, and registration number of the pharmacy technician;
        (2) A statement of the reason for the request for extension;
        (3) If the reason for the request for extension is health related, a statement from the attending physician(s) treating the pharmacy technician which includes the nature of the physical disability or illness and the dates the pharmacy technician was incapacitated; and
        (4) If the reason for the request for the extension is for other extenuating circumstances, a detailed explanation of the extenuating circumstances and, if because of military deployment, documentation of the dates of the deployment.
    b. After review and approval of the petition, a pharmacy technician may be granted an extension of time to comply with the continuing education requirement which shall not exceed one license renewal period.
    c. An extension of time to complete continuing education credit does not relieve a pharmacy technician from the continuing education requirement during the current license period.
    d. If a petition for an extension to the reporting period for continuing education is denied, the pharmacy technician shall:
        (1) Have 60 days to complete and report completion of the required continuing education requirements and
        (2) Be subject to the requirements of 7. above relating to failure to report completion of the required continuing education if the required continuing education is not completed and reported within the required 60-day time period.
9. The following are considered approved programs for pharmacy technicians.
    a. Any program presented by an Accreditation Council for Pharmacy Education (ACPE) approved provider subject to the following conditions.
        (1) Pharmacy technicians may receive credit for the completion of the same ACPE course only once during a renewal period.
        (2) Pharmacy technicians who present approved ACPE continuing education programs may receive credit for the time expended during the actual presentation of the program. Pharmacy technicians may receive credit for the same presentation only once during a license period.
        (3) Proof of completion of an ACPE course shall contain the following information:
            (a) Name of the participant;
            (b) Title and completion date of the program;
            (c) Name of the approved provider sponsoring or cosponsoring the program;
            (d) Number of contact hours awarded;

- (e) Assigned ACPE universal program number and a "T" designation indicating that the CE is targeted to pharmacy technicians; and
- (f) Either a dated certifying signature of the approved provider and the official ACPE logo or the Continuing Pharmacy Education Monitor logo.

b. Pharmacy-related college courses which are part of a pharmacy technician training program or part of a professional degree program offered by a college of pharmacy.
   (1) Pharmacy technicians may receive credit for the completion of the same course only once during a license period. A course is equivalent to one credit hour for each year of the renewal period. One credit hour is equal to 15 contact hours.
   (2) Pharmacy technicians who teach these courses may receive credit toward their continuing education, but such credit may be received only once for teaching the same course during a license period.

c. Basic cardiopulmonary resuscitation (CPR) courses which lead to CPR certification by the American Red Cross or the American Heart Association or its equivalent shall be recognized as approved programs. Pharmacy technicians may receive credit for one contact hour toward their continuing education requirement for completion of a CPR course only once during a renewal period. Proof of the completion of a CPR course shall be the certificate issued by the American Red Cross or the American Heart Association or its equivalent.

d. Advanced cardiovascular life support (ACLS) courses or pediatric advanced life support (PALS) courses which lead to initial ACLS or PALS certification by the American Heart Association or its equivalent shall be recognized as approved programs. Pharmacy technicians may receive credit for twelve contact hours toward their continuing education requirement for completion of an ACLS or PALS course only once during a renewal period. Proof of the completion of an ACLS or PALS course shall be the certificate issued by the American Heart Association or its equivalent.

e. Advanced cardiovascular life support (ACLS) courses or pediatric advanced life support (PALS) courses which lead to ACLS or PALS recertification by the American Heart Association or its equivalent shall be recognized as approved programs. Pharmacy technicians may receive credit for four contact hours toward their continuing education requirement for completion of an ACLS or PALS recertification course only once during a renewal period. Proof of the completion of an ACLS or PALS recertification course shall be the certificate issued by the American Heart Association or its equivalent.

f. Attendance at TSBP Board Meetings shall be recognized for continuing education credit as follows:
   (1) Pharmacy technicians shall receive credit for three contact hours toward their continuing education requirement for attending a full, public Board business meeting in its entirety.
   (2) A maximum of six contact hours are allowed for attendance at a Board meeting during a renewal period.
   (3) Proof of attendance for a complete Board meeting shall be a certificate issued by TSBP.

g. Participation in a TSBP appointed Task Force shall be recognized for continuing education credit as follows:

(1) Pharmacy technicians shall receive credit for three contact hours toward their continuing education requirement for participating in a TSBP appointed Task Force.
(2) Proof of participation for a Task Force shall be a certificate issued by TSBP.

h. Attendance at programs presented by TSBP or courses offered by TSBP shall be recognized as follows:
(1) Pharmacy technicians shall receive credit for the number of hours for the program or course as stated by TSBP.
(2) Proof of attendance at a program presented by TSBP or completion of a course offered by TSBP shall be a certificate issued by TSBP.

i. Pharmacy technicians shall receive credit toward their continuing education requirements for programs or courses approved by other state boards of pharmacy as follows:
(1) Pharmacy technicians shall receive credit for the number of hours for the program or course as specified by the other state board of pharmacy.
(2) Proof of attendance at a program or course approved by another state board of pharmacy shall be a certificate or other documentation that indicates:
 (a) Name of the participant;
 (b) Title and completion date of the program;
 (c) Name of the approved provider sponsoring or cosponsoring the program;
 (d) Number of contact hours awarded;
 (e) Dated certifying signature of the provider; and
 (f) Documentation that the program is approved by the other state board of pharmacy.

j. Completion of an Institute for Safe Medication Practices (ISMP) Medication Safety Self-Assessment for hospital pharmacies or for community/ambulatory pharmacies shall be recognized for continuing education credit as follows:
(1) Pharmacy technicians shall receive credit for three contact hours toward their continuing education requirement for completion of an ISMP Medication Safety Self-Assessment.
(2) Proof of the completion of an ISMP Medication Safety Self-Assessment shall be:
 (a) A continuing education certificate provided by an ACPE approved provider for the completion of an assessment or
 (b) A document from ISMP showing the completion of an assessment.

k. Programs approved by the American Medical Association (AMA) as Category 1 Continuing Medical Education (CME) and accredited by the Accreditation Council for Continuing Medical Education shall be subject to the following conditions.
(1) Pharmacy technicians may receive credit for the completion of the same CME course only once during a license period.
(2) Pharmacy technicians who present approved CME programs may receive credit for the time expended during the actual presentation of the program. Pharmacy technicians may receive credit for the same presentation only once during a license period.
(3) Proof of the completion of a CME course shall contain the following information:
 (a) Name of the participant;
 (b) Title and completion date of the program;

(c) Name of the approved provider sponsoring or cosponsoring the program;
(d) Number of contact hours awarded; and
(e) Dated certifying signature of the approved provider.
l. In-service education provided under the direct supervision of a pharmacist shall be recognized as continuing education as follows:
(1) Pharmacy technicians shall receive credit for the number of hours provided by a pharmacist(s) at the pharmacy technician's place of employment.
(2) Proof of the completion of in-service education shall contain the following information:
(a) Name of the participant;
(b) Title or description of the program;
(c) Completion date of the program;
(d) Name of the pharmacist supervising the in-service education;
(e) Number of hours; and
(f) Dated signature of the pharmacist providing the in-service education.
10. Pharmacy technicians who are certified by a certification program approved by the Board and maintain this certification shall be considered as having met the continuing education requirements of this rule and shall not be subject to an audit by the Board provided one hour of continuing education is related to Texas pharmacy laws or rules.

297.9 Notifications

A. Change of Address and/or Name.
1. Change of Address. A pharmacy technician or pharmacy technician trainee shall notify the Board electronically or in writing within 10 days of a change of address, giving the old and new address and registration number.
2. Change of Name.
a. A pharmacy technician or pharmacy technician trainee shall notify the Board in writing within 10 days of a change of name by:
(1) Sending a copy of the official document reflecting the name change (e.g., marriage certificate, divorce decree, etc.) and
(2) Paying a fee.
b. An amended registration and/or certificate reflecting the new name of the pharmacy technician or pharmacy technician trainee will be issued by the Board.
B. Change of Employment. A pharmacy technician or pharmacy technician trainee shall report electronically or in writing to the Board within 10 days of a change of employment, giving the name and license number of the old and the new pharmacy and the registration number.

297.10 Registration for Military Service Members, Military Veterans, and Military Spouses

The same special accommodations for pharmacists' licensure, renewal, and continuing education requirements for military service members, military veterans and military spouses also apply to pharmacy technician registration and renewal. (*See complete official language of Board Rule 297.10 on the TSBP website.*)

297.11 Temporary Emergency Registration

A. Definitions.
The following words and terms shall have the following meanings unless the context clearly indicates otherwise.

1. **Emergency situation**—An emergency caused by a natural or manmade disaster or any other exceptional situation that causes an extraordinary demand for pharmacist services.
2. **State**—One of the 50 states in the United States of America, the District of Columbia, and Puerto Rico.

B. Emergency Temporary Pharmacy Technician Registration. In an emergency situation, the Board may grant a pharmacy technician who holds a current registration in another state an emergency temporary pharmacy technician registration to practice in Texas. The following is applicable for the emergency temporary pharmacy technician registration.
   1. An applicant for an emergency temporary pharmacy technician registration under this rule must hold a current pharmacy technician registration in another state and that registration and other registrations held by the applicant in any other state may not be suspended, revoked, canceled, surrendered, or otherwise restricted for any reason.
   2. To qualify for an emergency temporary pharmacy technician registration, the applicant must submit an application to TSBP including the following information:
      a. Name, address, and phone number of the applicant and
      b. Any other information required by the Board.
   3. An emergency temporary pharmacy technician registration shall be valid for a period as determined by the Board not to exceed six months. The executive director of the Board in his or her discretion may renew the registration for an additional six months if the emergency situation still exists.

C. Exception. This rule is not applicable to pharmacy technicians enrolled in a volunteer health registry maintained by the Texas Department of State Health Services.

Chapter 569 Reporting Requirements for Professional Liability Insurers

Section 569.001 Duty to Report
A. Every insurer or other entity providing pharmacist's professional liability insurance, pharmacy technician professional and supplemental liability insurance, or druggist's professional liability insurance covering a pharmacist, pharmacy technician, or pharmacy license holder in this state shall submit to the Board the information described in Section 569.002 of the Act at the time prescribed.
B. The information shall be provided with respect to a notice of claim letter or complaint filed against an insured in a court if the notice or complaint seeks damages relating to the insured's conduct in providing or failing to provide appropriate service within the scope of pharmaceutical care or services and with respect to settlement of a claim or lawsuit made on behalf of the insured.
C. If a pharmacist, a pharmacy technician, a pharmacy technician trainee, or a pharmacy licensed in this state does not carry or is not covered by pharmacist's professional liability insurance, pharmacy technician professional and supplemental liability insurance, or druggist's professional liability insurance and is insured by a non-admitted carrier or other entity providing pharmacy professional liability insurance that does not report under this Act, the duty to report information under Section 569.002 of the Act is the responsibility of the pharmacist, pharmacy technician, pharmacy technician trainee, or pharmacy license holder.

Section 569.002 Information to be Reported
A. The following information must be furnished to the Board no later than the 30th day after receipt by the insurer of the notice of claim letter or complaint from the insured:

1. The name of the insured and the insured's Texas pharmacy technician registration number, pharmacy technician trainee registration number, or pharmacist or pharmacy license number;
2. The policy number; and
3. A copy of the notice of claim letter or complaint.
B. The Board shall, in consultation with the Texas Department of Insurance, adopt rules for reporting additional information as the Board may require. Other claim reports required under state and federal law shall be considered in determining the information to be reported, the form of the report, and the frequency of reporting under the rules. Additional information that the Board may require may include:
    1. The date of any judgment, dismissal, or settlement and
    2. Whether an appeal has been taken and by which party.

Section 569.003 Immunity from Liability

An insurer reporting under this section, its agents or employees, the Board, or the Board's employees or representatives are not liable for damages in a suit brought by any person or entity for reporting as required by this section or for any other action taken under this section.

Section 569.004 Restriction on Use of Information Requested

A. Information submitted to the Board under this Act and the fact that the information has been submitted to the Board may not be:
    1. Offered in evidence or used in any manner in the trial of a suit described in this section or
    2. Used in any manner to determine the eligibility or credentialing of a pharmacy to participate in a health insurance plan defined by the Insurance Code.
B. Information submitted under this section is confidential and is not subject to disclosure under Chapter 552, Texas Public Information Act.
C. The Board shall adopt rules to ensure the confidentiality of information submitted under this section.

Section 569.005 Investigation of Report

A. Except as otherwise provided in this Act, a report received by the Board under this section is not a complaint for which a Board investigation is required.
B. The Board shall review the information relating to a pharmacist, a pharmacy technician, a pharmacy technician trainee, or a pharmacy license holder against whom at least three professional liability claims have been reported within a five-year period in the same manner as if a complaint against the pharmacist, pharmacy technician, pharmacy technician trainee, or pharmacy license holder had been made under Chapter 555 of this Act.

Section 569.006 Sanctions Imposed on Insurer

The Texas Department of Insurance may impose on any insurer subject to this Act sanctions authorized by Section 7, Article 1.10, Insurance Code, if the insurer fails to report information as required by this section.

Board of Pharmacy Rule 281.18
Reporting Professional Liability Claims

(a) Reporting Responsibilities.
    (1) Every insurer or other entity providing pharmacist's professional liability insurance, pharmacy technician professional and supplemental liability insurance, or druggist's professional liability insurance covering a pharmacist, pharmacy technician, or pharmacy license holder in this state shall submit to the Board the information described in (b) below at the time prescribed.

(2) The information shall be provided with respect to a notice of claim letter or complaint filed against an insured in a court if the notice or complaint seeks damages relating to the insured's conduct in providing or failing to provide appropriate service within the scope of pharmaceutical care or services and with respect to settlement of a claim or lawsuit made on behalf of the insured.

(3) If a pharmacist, a pharmacy technician, or a pharmacy licensed in this state does not carry or is not covered by pharmacist's professional liability insurance, pharmacy technician professional and supplemental liability insurance, or druggist's professional liability insurance or if a pharmacist, a pharmacy technician, or a pharmacy licensed in this state is insured by a non-admitted carrier or other entity providing pharmacy professional liability insurance that does not report under this Act, the duty to report information under (b) below is the responsibility of the particular pharmacist, pharmacy technician, or pharmacy license holder.

(4) For the purposes of this rule, a professional liability claim or complaint shall be defined as a cause of action against a pharmacist, pharmacy, or pharmacy technician for conduct in providing or failing to provide appropriate service within the scope of pharmaceutical care or services, which proximately results in injury to or death of the patient, whether the patient's claim or cause of action sounds in tort or contract, to include pharmacist's interns, pharmacy residents, supervising pharmacists, on-call pharmacists, and consulting pharmacists.

(b) Information to be Reported and Due Dates. The following reports are required for claims initiated or resolved on or after September 1, 1999.

(1) Initial Report. No later than the 30th day after receipt of the notice of claim letter or complaint by the insurer if the insurer has the duty to report or by the pharmacist, pharmacy technician, or a pharmacy if the license holder has the duty to report, the following information must be furnished to the Board on a form provided by the Board:
(A) Name and address of the insurer;
(B) Name and address of the insured and type of license or registration held (pharmacist, pharmacy, or pharmacy technician);
(C) Insured's Texas pharmacist or pharmacy license number or pharmacy technician registration number;
(D) Certification if applicable;
(E) Policy number;
(F) Name(s) of plaintiff(s);
(G) Date of injury;
(H) County of injury;
(I) Cause of injury (e.g., dispensing error);
(J) Nature of injury;
(K) Type of action (e.g., claim only or lawsuit);
(L) Name and phone number of the person filing the report; and
(M) A copy of the notice of claim letter or the lawsuit filed in court.

(2) Follow-up Report. Within 105 days after disposition of the claim, the following information must be provided to the Board on a form provided by the Board:
(A) Name and address of the insured and type of license or registration held (pharmacist, pharmacy, or pharmacy technician);
(B) Insured's Texas pharmacist or pharmacy license number or pharmacy technician registration number;
(C) Name(s) of plaintiff(s);
(D) Date of disposition;

- (E) Type of disposition (e.g., settlement, judgment);
- (F) Amount of disposition;
- (G) Whether an appeal has been taken and by which party; and
- (H) Name and phone number of the person filing the report.
  - (3) Definition. For the purpose of this rule, "disposition of a claim" shall include circumstances where a court order has been entered, a settlement agreement has been reached, or the complaint has been dropped or dismissed.
- (c) Report Format.
  - (1) Separate reports are required for each defendant licensee or registrant.
  - (2) The information shall be reported on a form provided by the Board.
  - (3) A court order or settlement agreement may be submitted as an attachment to the follow-up report.
- (d) Claims Not Required to be Reported. Examples of claims that are not required to be reported under this rule are the following:
  - (1) Product liability claims (i.e., where a licensee invented a medical device which may have injured a patient, but the licensee has no personal pharmacist-patient relationship with the specific patient claiming injury by the device);
  - (2) Antitrust allegations;
  - (3) Allegations involving improper peer review activities;
  - (4) Civil rights violations; or
  - (5) Allegations of liability for injuries occurring on a licensee's property but not involving a breach of duty (i.e., slip and fall accidents).
- (e) Liability.
  An insurer reporting under this rule, its agents or employees, the Board, or the Board's employees or representatives are not liable for damages in a suit brought by any person or entity for reporting as required by this rule or for any other action taken under this rule.
- (f) Limit on Use of Information Reported.
  - (1) Information submitted to the Board under this rule and the fact that the information has been submitted to the Board may not be:
    - (A) Offered in evidence or used in any manner in the trial of a suit described in this rule or
    - (B) Used in any manner to determine the eligibility or credentialing of a pharmacy to participate in a health insurance plan defined by the Insurance Code.
  - (2) A report received by the Board under this rule is not a complaint for which a Board investigation is required except that the Board shall review the information relating to a pharmacist, pharmacy technician, or pharmacy license holder against whom at least three professional liability claims have been reported within a five-year period in the same manner as if a complaint against the pharmacist, pharmacy technician, or pharmacy license holder had been made under Chapter 555 of the Act. The Board may initiate an investigation of the pharmacist, pharmacy technician, or pharmacy license holder based on the information received under this rule.
  - (3) The information received under this rule may be used in any Board proceedings as the Board deems necessary.
- (g) Confidentiality. Information submitted under this rule is confidential, except as provided in (f)(3) above, and is not subject to disclosure under Chapter 552, Texas Public Information Act.
- (h) Penalty. The Texas Department of Insurance may impose on any insurer subject to this Act sanctions authorized by Sections 82.051–82.055 (formerly Section 7, Article 1.10) of the Texas Insurance Code if the insurer fails to report information as required by this rule.

CHAPTER D HIGHLIGHTS
Texas Pharmacy Act (TPA)

1. The Texas State Board of Pharmacy (TSBP) is responsible for protecting the public health and safety by regulating the practice of pharmacy in Texas and administering and enforcing the Texas Pharmacy Act.
2. TSBP is composed of 11 members—seven pharmacists, one pharmacy technician, and three public members.
3. TSBP may approve pilot and demonstration research projects for innovations in pharmacy practice that may include a waiver or exemption from a Board rule, but the Board may not waive requirements of state or federal laws.
4. Texas pharmacists who meet certification and continuing education requirements may provide immunizations and vaccinations to patients under a written protocol with a physician.
    a. For influenza vaccines, patients must be over age seven.
    b. For all other immunizations, patients must be over age 14.
    c. Notifications must be sent to the physician providing the protocol and each patient's primary care physician.
5. Pharmacist Licensure by Examination
    a. Must have graduated from an accredited pharmacy degree program approved by the Board.
    b. Must be at least 18 years old.
    c. Must have completed 1500 hours of internship.
    d. Must pass the North American Pharmacist Licensure Exam (NAPLEX) and Multistate Pharmacy Jurisprudence Exam (MPJE) for Texas.
    e. Must not have had a pharmacist license in another state restricted, suspended, revoked or surrendered.

    Note: A pharmacist who takes and passes the NAPLEX and has that score transferred to Texas through NABP's Score Transfer Program is deemed to have obtained his or her license in Texas by examination once he or she passes the Texas MPJE.
6. Pharmacist Licensure by Reciprocity (from another state)
    a. Same requirements as above except instead of taking and passing NAPLEX the pharmacist must provide proof of current licensing in another state or of initial licensure by examination;
    b. Provide proof that current licenses in other states have not been restricted, suspended, revoked, or surrendered; and
    c. Pass the Texas MPJE.
7. Pharmacist Interns (includes intern trainees, student interns, extended interns, and resident interns)
    a. In the first professional year Texas college of pharmacy students must register as intern trainees. After completing the first professional year (30 semester hours), an intern trainee can register as a student intern.
    b. Pharmacist interns may perform any duty of a pharmacist provided the duties are delegated by and under the supervision of a pharmacist who is registered as a preceptor. The exception is they may not sign a document required to be signed by a pharmacist.
    c. When an intern is not working under the supervision of a preceptor, he or she functions as a pharmacy technician but does not count in any ratio of pharmacists to pharmacy technicians.
8. Pharmacist Continuing Education (CE) Requirements
    a. Pharmacists must obtain 30 contact hours (3.0 CEUs) of approved continuing education every two years to renew their license.
    b. One hour of the 30 contact hours must be related to Texas pharmacy laws and rules.
    c. For renewals received after January 1, 2020 and before August 31, 2023, at least one contact hour (0.1 CEUs) annually for a total of two contact hours (0.2 CEUs) during that timeframe must be obtained. The two contact hours shall be related to best practices, alternative treatment options, and multi-modal approaches to pain management;
    d. At least two contact hours (0.2 CEUs) shall be related to approved procedures of prescribing and monitoring controlled substances, shall be obtained by September 1, 2021, and must be reported on the next license renewal after September 1, 2021.

e. For renewals received after August 31, 2020 and before September 1, 2022, a pharmacist must have completed a human trafficking prevention course approved by the Texas Health and Human Services Commission.
   f. There are various approved ways to obtain CE (*see Board Rule 295.8C.*) but the most common is a program offered by an Accreditation Council for Pharmacy Education (ACPE) provider.
   g. Pharmacists shall maintain CE records for three years.
9. Pharmacy Licensure
   a. Class A and A-S*—community pharmacies
   b. Class B—nuclear pharmacies
   c. Class C and C-S*—institutional pharmacies (hospitals, ambulatory surgical centers, and inpatient hospices)
   d. Class D—clinic pharmacies
   e. Class E and E-S*—nonresident pharmacies that ship prescriptions to patients in Texas
   f. Class F—freestanding emergency medical facility (FEMC) pharmacies
   g. Class G—central prescription drug or medication order processing pharmacies
   h. Class H—limited prescription delivery pharmacies
   S*—indicates the pharmacy compounds sterile preparations
10. Substitution of Generic Drugs and Interchangeable (biosimilar) Biological Products
    a. Substitution is permissive (not mandatory) as long as the patient does not refuse and the prescriber has not prohibited the substitution through a "dispensing directive" in b. below.
    b. A practitioner may prohibit the substitution of a generically equivalent drug or interchangeable biological product for a brand name drug product by writing across the face of the written prescription in the practitioner's own handwriting the phrase "Brand Necessary" or "Brand Medically Necessary."
    c. No later than the third business day after the date of dispensing a biological product that has been substituted, the dispensing pharmacist or the pharmacist's designee shall communicate to the prescribing practitioner the specific product provided to the patient, including the name of the product and the manufacturer or national drug code number. This communication can be made electronically.
    d. Generic equivalency for drugs is determined by the FDA Orange Book. However, a pharmacist may dispense a generic for a product not found in the Orange Book using his or her professional judgment.
    e. Interchangeability of biological products is determined by the FDA Purple Book although the Act and TSBP rules reference the FDA Orange Book.
11. Substitution of Dosage Form
    Pharmacists may dispense a dosage form of a drug product different from that prescribed, such as tablets instead of capsules or liquid instead of tablets, provided the patient consents to the dosage form substitution, the dosage form dispensed contains the identical amount of the active ingredients as the dosage prescribed for the patient and is not an enteric-coated or a timed-release product, and does not alter desired clinical outcomes.
12. Remote Pharmacy Services Rules
    Texas recognizes four types of remote pharmacy services in which drugs can be stored and/or dispensed from locations that are not pharmacies and where a pharmacist is not present. They include the following;
    a. Emergency medication kits (primarily in nursing homes);
    b. Automated pharmacy systems (primarily in nursing homes);
    c. Telepharmacy systems (in remote healthcare facilities or remote dispensing sites); and
    d. Automated storage and delivery systems (for delivery of dispensed drugs at remote sites).
13. Physician Dispensing
    Unlike many states, physicians in Texas generally cannot dispense drugs. The only exceptions are as follows.
    a. Physicians may provide dangerous drugs to meet a patient's immediate therapeutic needs (defined as a 72-hour supply) and
    b. Physicians in rural areas where there is no pharmacy may dispense dangerous drugs and be reimbursed for costs.

14. Pharmacy Technicians and Pharmacy Technician Trainees
    a. Pharmacy technicians and pharmacy technician trainees must be registered with TSBP before working in a pharmacy.
    b. An individual may register as a pharmacy technician trainee for two years only and that registration cannot be renewed.
    c. To initially register as a pharmacy technician, an individual must take and pass a pharmacy technician certification exam and be certified by the Board-approved certification organization.
    d. A pharmacy technician does not need to maintain his or her certification to renew his or her Texas registration. However, the requirements to renew the registration with TSBP are similar to requirements for certification through a Board-approved certification organization.
    e. All pharmacy technicians and trainees must participate in documented training at each pharmacy where they work.
    f. The ratio of pharmacists to technicians allowed varies by the class of pharmacy. In Class A (community) pharmacies the ratio is 1 pharmacist to 4 technicians (1:4) as long as at least one of the technicians is registered (not all technicians can be trainees). If all the technicians are trainees, the ratio is 1:3. There is no ratio in Class C (institutional) pharmacies.
    g. Pharmacy Technician Continuing Education (CE) Requirements
        (1) A pharmacy technician must obtain 20 hours of approved continuing education per renewal period (every two years). One hour of the 20 hours must be related to Texas pharmacy laws and rules.
        (2) There are various approved ways to obtain CE, including most of the methods approved for pharmacists such as ACPE courses. However, pharmacy technicians can also receive credit for in-service programs provided they are under the direct supervision of a pharmacist.
15. The practice of telemedicine in Texas is a legal practice. However, pharmacists must still ensure that there is a valid practitioner-patient relationship for telemedicine prescriptions. Texas Medical Board rules specify two prohibitions on telemedicine:
    a. A practitioner-patient relationship is not present if a practitioner prescribes an abortifacient or any other drug or device that terminates a pregnancy and
    b. Treatment for chronic pain with scheduled drugs using telemedicine is not allowed.

CHAPTER E

Miscellaneous Texas Pharmacy and Drug Laws and Rules

General Rules for Pharmacists

Chapter 295

CHAPTER E

Miscellaneous Texas Pharmacy and Drug Laws and Rules
General Rules for Pharmacists
Chapter 295

Board of Pharmacy Rule 295.3
Responsibility of a Pharmacist

A. A pharmacist-in-charge shall ensure that the pharmacy is in compliance with all laws and rules governing the practice of pharmacy.
B. All pharmacists while on duty are responsible for complying with all laws/ rules governing the practice of pharmacy.

Board of Pharmacy Rule 295.4
Sharing Money Received for Prescriptions (Kickbacks)

No pharmacist may share or offer to share the money received from filling a prescription with the practitioner.

Board of Pharmacy Rule 295.12
Pharmacist Certification Programs

A. Purpose. The purpose of this section is to provide standards for the recognition and approval of pharmacist certification programs as authorized by Section 554.0021 of the Act.
B. Definitions.
   The following words and terms when used in this section shall have the following meanings, unless the context clearly indicates otherwise.
   1. **ACPE**—Accreditation Council for Pharmacy Education.
   2. **Approved provider of pharmacist certificate programs**—An individual, institution, organization, association, corporation, or agency that is approved by the Board and recognized by ACPE in accordance with its policy and procedures as having:
      a. Met criteria indicative of the ability to provide quality continuing education programs and
      b. Met the procedures outlined in the ACPE "Guidance Document for Practice Based Activities."
   3. **Board**—Texas State Board of Pharmacy.
C. Recognized Certification Programs.
   1. The Board shall recognize as certified any pharmacist who successfully completes:
      a. Any program offered by an approved provider of pharmacist certificate programs;
      b. Any program that meets the requirements of Board Rule 295.15 (Administration of Immunizations or Vaccinations by a Pharmacist Under Written Protocol of a Physician);
      c. Any certification offered by the:
         (1) Board of Pharmaceutical Specialties;
         (2) American Society of Consultant Pharmacists;
         (3) American Board of Clinical Pharmacology;

(4) American Board of Applied Toxicology;
(5) American Academy of Pain Management; or
d. Any additional certifications as published on the Board's website.
2. Texas pharmacists may not identify themselves as certified unless they have completed one of the programs specified in C.1. above.

> **Board of Pharmacy Rule 295.13**
> **Drug Therapy Management by a Pharmacist**
> **Under the Written Protocol of a Physician**

A. Purpose.
To provide standards for the maintenance of records of a pharmacist engaged in the provision of drug therapy management as authorized in the Texas Medical Practice Act and the Texas Pharmacy Act.

B. Definitions.
1. **Drug therapy management (DTM)**—The performance of specific acts by pharmacists as authorized by a physician through written protocol. Drug therapy management does not include the selection of drug products not prescribed by the physician, unless the drug product is named in the physician initiated protocol or the physician initiated record of deviation from a standing protocol. Drug therapy management may include the following:
   a. Collecting and reviewing patient drug use histories;
   b. Ordering or performing routine drug therapy related patient assessment procedures including temperature, pulse, and respiration;
   c. Ordering drug therapy related laboratory tests;
   d. Implementing or modifying drug therapy following diagnosis, initial patient assessment, and ordering of drug therapy by a physician as detailed in the protocol; or
   e. Implementing any other drug therapy related act delegated by a physician.
2. **Written protocol**—A physician's order, standing medical order, standing delegation order, or other order or protocol as defined by rule of the Texas Medical Board under the Texas Medical Practice Act.
   a. A written protocol must contain at a minimum the following:
      (1) A statement identifying the individual physician authorized to prescribe drugs and responsible for the delegation of drug therapy management;
      (2) A statement identifying the individual pharmacist authorized to dispense drugs and to engage in drug therapy management as delegated by the physician;
      (3) A statement identifying the types of drug therapy management decisions that the pharmacist is authorized to make which shall include:
         (a) A statement of the ailments or diseases involved, drugs, and types of drug therapy management authorized and
         (b) A specific statement of the procedures, decision criteria, or plan the pharmacist shall follow when exercising drug therapy management authority;
      (4) A statement of the activities the pharmacist shall follow in the course of exercising drug therapy management authority, including the method for documenting decisions made and a plan for communication or feedback to the authorizing physician concerning specific decisions made. Documentation shall be recorded within a reasonable time of each intervention and may be entered on the patient medication record, patient medical chart, or in a separate log book; and

(5) A statement that describes appropriate mechanisms and time schedule for the pharmacist to report to the physician monitoring the pharmacist's exercise of delegated drug therapy management and the results of the drug therapy management.
   b. A standard protocol may be used or the attending physician may develop a drug therapy management protocol for the individual patient. If a standard protocol is used, the physician shall record what deviations, if any, from the standard protocol are ordered for that patient.
C. Physician Delegation to a Pharmacist.
   1. As specified in Chapter 157 of the Texas Medical Practice Act, a physician may delegate to a properly qualified and trained pharmacist acting under adequate physician supervision the performance of specific acts of drug therapy management authorized by the physician through the physician's order, standing medical order, standing delegation order, or other order or protocol.
   2. A delegation under C.1. above may include the implementation or modification of a patient's drug therapy under a protocol if:
      a. The delegation follows a diagnosis, initial patient assessment, and drug therapy order by the physician and
      b. The pharmacist maintains a copy of the protocol for inspection until at least the seventh anniversary of the expiration date of the protocol.
   3. A pharmacist has the authority to sign a prescription for dangerous drugs for a patient if:
      a. The delegation follows a diagnosis, initial patient assessment, and drug therapy order by the physician;
      b. The pharmacist practices in a federally qualified health center, a hospital, a hospital-based clinic, or an academic healthcare institution; and
      c. The federally qualified health center, hospital, hospital-based clinic, or academic healthcare institution in which the pharmacist practices has bylaws and a medical staff policy that permit a physician to delegate the management of a patient's drug therapy to a pharmacist.

Note: A pharmacist in any practice setting may implement and modify drug therapy under 2. above, but only pharmacists in those practice settings specified in 3. above may sign a prescription drug order.

   4. A pharmacist who signs a prescription for a dangerous drug under authority granted under C.3. above shall:
      a. Notify the Board that a physician has delegated the authority to sign a prescription for dangerous drugs. Such notification shall:
         (1) Be made on an application provided by the Board;
         (2) Occur prior to signing any prescription for a dangerous drug;
         (3) Be updated annually; and
         (4) Include a copy of the written protocol.
      b. Include the pharmacist's name, address, and telephone number as well as the name, address, and telephone number of the delegating physician on each prescription for a dangerous drug signed by the pharmacist.
   5. The Board shall post the following information on its website:
      a. The name and license number of each pharmacist who has notified the Board that a physician has delegated authority to sign a prescription for a dangerous drug;
      b. The name and address of the physician who delegated the authority to the pharmacist; and
      c. The expiration date of the protocol granting the authority to sign a prescription.

Notes

D. Pharmacist Training Requirements.
   1. Initial Requirements. A pharmacist shall maintain records and provide to the Board within 24 hours of a request a statement attesting to the fact that the pharmacist has within the last year:
      a. Completed at least six hours of continuing education related to drug therapy offered by a provider approved by the Accreditation Council for Pharmacy Education (ACPE) or
      b. Engaged in drug therapy management as allowed under previous laws or rules. A statement from the physician supervising the acts shall be sufficient documentation.
   2. Continuing Requirements. A pharmacist engaged in drug therapy management shall annually complete six hours of continuing education related to drug therapy offered by a provider approved by ACPE.
      Note: These hours may be applied toward the CE hours required for renewal of a license to practice pharmacy.
E. Supervision.
   Physician supervision shall be as specified in the Medical Practice Act and shall be considered adequate if the delegating physician:
   1. Is responsible for the formulation or approval of the written protocol and any patient-specific deviations from the protocol. In addition, the delegating physician must review the written protocol and any patient-specific deviations from the protocol at least annually, outlining the services provided to a patient under the protocol on a schedule defined in the written protocol;
   2. Has established and maintains a physician-patient relationship with each patient provided drug therapy management by a delegated pharmacist and informs the patient that drug therapy will be managed by a pharmacist under written protocol;
   3. Is geographically located so as to be able to be physically present daily to provide medical care and supervision;
   4. Receives on a schedule defined in the written protocol a periodic status report on the patient including any problem or complication encountered;
   5. Is available through direct telecommunication for consultation, assistance, and direction; and
   6. Determines that the pharmacist to whom the physician is delegating drug therapy management establishes and maintains a pharmacist-patient relationship with the patient.
F. Records.
   1. Maintenance of Records.
      a. Every record required to be kept under this section shall be kept by the pharmacist and be available for at least two years from the date of such record for inspecting and copying by the Board or its representative and to other authorized local, state, or federal law enforcement or regulatory agencies.
      b. Records may be maintained in an alternative data retention system such as a data processing system or direct imaging system provided:
         (1) The records maintained in the alternative system contain all of the information required on the manual record and
         (2) The data processing system is capable of producing a hard copy of the record upon the request of the Board, its representative, or other authorized local, state, or federal law enforcement or regulatory agencies.
   2. Written Protocol.
      a. A copy of the written protocol and any patient-specific deviations from the protocol shall be maintained by the pharmacist.

  b. A pharmacist shall document all interventions undertaken under the written protocol within a reasonable time of each intervention. Documentation may be maintained in the patient medication record, patient medical chart, or a separate log.
  c. A standard protocol may be used for all patients or the attending physician may develop a drug therapy management protocol for the individual patient. If a standard protocol is used, the physician shall record what deviations if any from the standard protocol are ordered for that patient. A pharmacist shall maintain a copy of any deviations from the standard protocol ordered by the physician.
  d. Written protocols including standard protocols, any patient-specific deviations from a standard protocol, and any individual patient protocol shall be reviewed by the physician and pharmacist at least annually and revised if necessary. Such review shall be documented in the pharmacist's records. Documentation of all services provided to the patient by the pharmacist shall be reviewed by the physician on the schedule established in the protocol.
G. Confidentiality for Drug Therapy Management. (*See Board Rule 291.27 in this chapter for general confidentiality provisions.*)
 1. In addition to the confidentiality requirements specified in Board Rule 291.27 (Confidentiality), a pharmacist shall comply with:
  a. The privacy provisions of the federal Health Insurance Portability and Accountability Act (HIPAA) of 1996 (Pub. L. No. 104-191) and any rules adopted pursuant to this act;
  b. The requirements of Medical Records Privacy contained in Chapter 181, Texas Health and Safety Code;
  c. The Privacy of Health Information requirements contained in Chapter 28B of the Texas Insurance Code; and
  d. Any other confidentiality provisions of federal or state laws.
 2. This section shall not affect or alter the provisions relating to the confidentiality of the physician-patient communication as specified in the Medical Practice Act.
H. Construction and Interpretation.
 1. As specified in the Medical Practice Act, this section does not restrict the use of a pre-established healthcare program or restrict a physician from authorizing the provision of patient care by use of a pre-established healthcare program if the patient is institutionalized and the care is to be delivered in a licensed hospital with an organized medical staff that has authorized standing delegation orders, standing medical orders, or protocols.
 2. As specified in the Medical Practice Act, this section may not be construed to limit, expand, or change any provision of law concerning or relating to therapeutic drug substitution or administration of medication including the Pharmacy Act.

All Classes of Pharmacy
Chapter 291

Board of Pharmacy Rule 291.1
Pharmacy License Application

See Board Rule 291.1 (Pharmacy License Application) in Chapter D.

Board of Pharmacy Rule 291.3
Required Notifications

A. Change of Location.
   1. When a pharmacy changes location, the following is applicable.
      a. A new completed pharmacy application containing the information outlined in Board Rule 291.1 (Pharmacy License Application) must be filed with the Board no later than 30 days before the date of the change of location of the pharmacy.
      b. The previously issued license must be returned to the Board office.
      c. An amended license reflecting the new location of the pharmacy will be issued by the Board.
      d. A fee as specified in Board Rule 291.6 (Pharmacy License Fees) will be charged for issuance of the amended license.
   2. At least 14 days prior to the change of location of a pharmacy that dispenses prescription drug orders, the pharmacist-in-charge shall post a sign in a conspicuous place indicating that the pharmacy is changing locations. The sign shall be in the front of the prescription department and at all public entrance doors to the pharmacy and shall indicate the date the pharmacy is changing locations.
   3. Disasters, accidents, and emergencies which require the pharmacy to change location shall be immediately reported to the Board. If a pharmacy changes location suddenly due to disasters, accidents, or other emergency circumstances and the pharmacist-in-charge cannot provide notification 14 days prior to the change of location, the pharmacist-in-charge shall comply with the provisions of A.2. above as far in advance of the change of location as allowed by the circumstances.
   4. When a Class A-S, C-S, or E-S pharmacy changes location, the pharmacy's classification will revert to a Class A, Class C, or Class E unless or until the Board or its designee has inspected the new location to ensure the pharmacy meets the requirements as specified in 291.133 of this rule (relating to Pharmacies Compounding Sterile Preparations).
   5. When a Class B pharmacy changes location, the Board shall inspect the pharmacy at the new location to ensure the pharmacy meets the requirements as specified in this rule (relating to Nuclear Pharmacy (Class B)) prior to the pharmacy becoming operational.
B. Change of Name. When a pharmacy changes its name, the following is applicable.
   1. A new completed pharmacy application containing the information outlined in Board Rule 291.1 (Pharmacy License Application) must be filed with the Board within 10 days of the change of the name of the pharmacy.
   2. The previously issued license must be returned to the Board office.
   3. An amended license reflecting the new name of the pharmacy will be issued by the Board.
   4. A fee as specified in Board Rule 291.6 (Pharmacy License Fees) will be charged for issuance of the amended license.

C. Change of Managing Officers.
 1. The owner of a pharmacy shall notify the Board in writing within 10 days of a change of any managing officer of a partnership or corporation which owns a pharmacy. The written notification shall include the effective date of such change and the following information for all managing officers:
    a. Name and title;
    b. Home address and telephone number;
    c. Date of birth;
    d. Copy of social security card or other official document showing the social security number, as approved by the Board; and
    e. A copy of a current driver license, state-issued photo identification card, or passport.
 2. For purposes of C.1. above, managing officers are defined as the top four executive officers, including the corporate officer in charge of pharmacy operations, who are designated by the partnership or corporation to be jointly responsible for the legal operation of the pharmacy.
D. Change of Ownership.
 1. When a pharmacy changes ownership, a new pharmacy application must be filed with the Board following the procedures specified in Board Rule 291.1 (Pharmacy License Application). In addition, a copy of the purchase contract or mutual agreement between the buyer and seller must be submitted.
 2. The license issued to the previous owner must be returned to the Board.
 3. A fee as specified in Board Rule 291.6 will be charged for issuance of a new license.
E. Change of Pharmacist Employment.
 1. Change of Pharmacist Employed in a Pharmacy. When a change in pharmacist employment occurs, the pharmacist shall report such change in writing to the Board within 10 days.
 2. Change of Pharmacist-in-Charge of a Pharmacy. The incoming pharmacist-in-charge shall be responsible for notifying the Board within 10 days in writing on a form provided by the Board that a change of pharmacist-in-charge has occurred. The notification shall include the following:
    a. The name and license number of the departing pharmacist-in-charge;
    b. The name and license number of the incoming pharmacist-in-charge;
    c. The date the incoming pharmacist-in-charge became the pharmacist-in-charge; and
    d. A statement signed by the incoming pharmacist-in-charge attesting that:
       (1) An inventory has been conducted by the departing and incoming pharmacists-in-charge. If the inventory was not taken by both pharmacists, the statement shall provide an explanation and
       (2) The incoming pharmacist-in-charge has read and understands the laws and rules relating to this class of pharmacy.
F. Notification of Theft or Loss of a Controlled Substance or a Dangerous Drug.
 1. Controlled Substances. For the purposes of Section 562.106 of the Act, the theft or significant loss of any controlled substance by a pharmacy shall be reported in writing to the Board immediately on discovery of the theft or loss. A pharmacy shall be in compliance by submitting to the Board a copy of the Drug Enforcement Administration (DEA) report of theft or loss of controlled substances (DEA Form 106) or by submitting a list of all controlled substances stolen or lost.
    Note: Although the language in the Board rule states that the pharmacy can comply by sending a copy of DEA Form 106 to TSBP and DEA, this may not be feasible. The pharmacy must notify DEA and TSBP in writing immediately (within one business day) of the discovery of the theft or significant loss.

However, DEA Form 106 may be provided later to DEA and TSBP once the pharmacy has investigated and validated the extent of the theft or loss.
  2. Dangerous Drugs. A pharmacy shall report in writing to the Board immediately on the discovery of theft or significant loss of any dangerous drug by submitting a list of the name and quantity of all dangerous drugs stolen or lost.
 G. Fire or Other Disaster. If a pharmacy experiences a fire or other disaster, the following requirements are applicable.
  1. Responsibilities of the Pharmacist-in-Charge.
   a. The pharmacist-in-charge shall be responsible for reporting the date of a fire or other disaster which may affect the strength, purity, or labeling of drugs, medications, devices, or other materials used in the diagnosis or the treatment of an injury, illness, or disease. This notification shall be reported to the Board within 10 days from the date of the disaster.
   b. The pharmacist-in-charge or designated agent shall comply with the following procedures.
    (1) If controlled substances, dangerous drugs, or Drug Enforcement Administration (DEA) order forms are lost or destroyed in the disaster, the pharmacy shall:
     (a) Notify the DEA and the Board of the loss of the controlled substances or loss of DEA Forms 222 immediately upon discovery.
     (b) Notify the Board in writing of the loss of the dangerous drugs by submitting a list of the dangerous drugs lost.
    (2) If the extent of the loss of controlled substances or dangerous drugs is not able to be determined, the pharmacy shall:
     (a) Take a new, complete inventory of all remaining drugs specified in Board Rule 291.17(c) (Inventory Requirements);
     (b) Submit to DEA a statement attesting that the loss of controlled substances is indeterminable and that a new, complete inventory of all remaining controlled substances was conducted and state the date of such inventory; and
     (c) Submit to the Board a statement attesting that the loss of controlled substances and dangerous drugs is indeterminable and that a new, complete inventory of the drugs specified in Board Rule 291.17(c) was conducted and state the date of such inventory.
   c. If the pharmacy changes to a new, permanent location, the pharmacist-in-charge shall comply with A. above of this rule.
   d. If the pharmacy moves to a temporary location, the pharmacist shall comply with A. above of this rule. If the pharmacy returns to the original location, the pharmacist-in-charge shall again comply with A. above of this rule.
   e. If the pharmacy closes due to fire or other disaster, the pharmacy may not be closed for longer than 90 days as specified in Board Rule 291.11 (Operating a Pharmacy). (*See Chapter F.*)
   f. If the pharmacy discontinues business (ceases to operate as a pharmacy), the pharmacist-in-charge shall comply with Board Rule 291.5 (Closed Pharmacies). (*See Board Rule 291.5 below.*)
   g. The pharmacist-in-charge shall maintain copies of all inventories, reports, or notifications required by this section for a period of two years.
  2. Drug Stock.
   a. Any drug which has been exposed to excessive heat, smoke, or other conditions which may have caused deterioration shall not be dispensed.
   b. Any potentially adulterated or damaged drug shall only be sold, transferred, or otherwise distributed pursuant to the provisions of the Texas

Food, Drug, and Cosmetics Act (Chapter 431, Health and Safety Code) administered by the Bureau of Food and Drug Safety of the Texas Department of State Health Services.
H. Notification to Consumers (on how to file complaints). *See Chapter F.*
I. Notification of Licensees or Registrants Obtaining Controlled Substances or Dangerous Drugs by Forged Prescriptions.

If a licensee or registrant obtains controlled substances or dangerous drugs from a pharmacy by means of a forged prescription, the pharmacy shall report in writing to the Board immediately on discovery of such forgery. A pharmacy shall be in compliance with this subsection by submitting to the Board the following:
  1. Name of licensee or registrant obtaining controlled substances or dangerous drugs by a forged prescription;
  2. Date(s) of forged prescription(s);
  3. Name(s) and amount(s) of drug(s); and
  4. Copies of forged prescriptions.
J. Notification of Disciplinary Action Taken in Another State.

For the purpose of Section 562.106 of the Act, a pharmacy shall report in writing to the Board no later than the 10th day after the date of:
  1. A final order against the pharmacy license holder by the regulatory or licensing agency of the state in which the pharmacy is located if the pharmacy is located in another state or
  2. A final order against a pharmacist who is designated as the pharmacist-in-charge of the pharmacy by the regulatory or licensing agency of the state in which the pharmacy is located if the pharmacy is located in another state.

Summary Chart of Major Notifications Required by TSBP

Required Report	Who Reports	Time Frame	Source
Change of pharmacist name or address	Pharmacist	Within 10 days	Rule 295.1
Change of pharmacist employment	Pharmacist	Within 10 days	Rule 291.3(e)
Permanent closing of pharmacy	Pharmacy	Within 10 days after closing	TPA 562.106 and Rule 291.5
Change of pharmacy ownership	Pharmacy	Within 10 days and new license required	TPA 562.106 and Rule 291.3(d)
Change of pharmacy location	Pharmacy	New license filed 30 days prior to change	TPA 562.106 and Rule 291.3(a)
Change of pharmacy name	Pharmacy	New license filed 10 days prior to change	Rule 291.3(b)
Change of managing officers or partnership/corporation	Pharmacy	Within 10 days	Rule 291.3(c)
Change of pharmacist-in-charge (PIC)	Incoming PIC	Within 10 days	TPA 562.106 and Rule 291.3(e)(2)
Sale or transfer of drugs as a result of closing or change of ownership	Pharmacy	Within 10 days	TPA 562.106
Fire or other disaster, accident, or emergency that may affect the strength, purity, or labeling of a drug or medical device	Pharmacy/PIC	Within 10 days	TPA 562.106 and Rule 291.3(g)
Significant loss or theft of controlled substances or dangerous drugs	Pharmacy	Immediately upon discovery	Rule 291.3(f)
Significant loss of data from pharmacy computer system	Pharmacy	Within 10 days	Records requirements are in each class of pharmacy rules
A licensee or registrant obtaining dangerous drugs or controlled substances from a forged prescription	Pharmacy	Immediately upon discovery	Rule 291.3(i)
A final order against the pharmacy license holder or pharmacist-in-charge by the regulatory or licensing agency of the state in which the pharmacy is located if in another state.	Pharmacy	Within 10 days	TPA 561.106 and Rule 291.3(j)

Board of Pharmacy Rule 291.5
Closing a Pharmacy

Note: These rules apply when closing a pharmacy and no further pharmacy activities will take place at the location. If a pharmacy is being sold and pharmacy activities will continue at the location, the rules for change of ownership should be followed. Those rules include applying for a new pharmacy license and providing notification to TSBP at least 10 days in advance as required under Board Rule 291.3, as well as notification to DEA regarding the inventory and transfer of controlled substances. (See Termination of Registration and Transfer of Controlled Substances Upon Sale of a Pharmacy in Chapter B.)

A. Prior to Closing a Pharmacy.
   1. At least 14 days prior to the closing of a pharmacy that dispenses prescription drugs, the pharmacist-in charge shall post a closing notice sign in a conspicuous place in the front of the prescription department and at all public entrance doors to the pharmacy. Such closing notice sign shall contain the following information:
      a. The date of the closing and
      b. The name, address, and telephone number of the pharmacy acquiring the prescription drug orders including refill information and patient medication records of the pharmacy.
   2. The pharmacy shall notify DEA of any controlled substances being transferred to another registrant as specified in 21 CFR 1301.52(d).
B. Closing Day of a Pharmacy.
   On the date of closing, the pharmacist-in-charge shall comply with the following:
   1. Take an inventory as specified in Board Rule 291.17 (Inventory Requirements).
   2. Remove all prescription drugs from the pharmacy by one or a combination of the following methods:
      a. Return prescription drugs to manufacturer or supplier (for credit/disposal);
      b. Transfer (sell or give away) prescription drugs to a person who is legally entitled to possess drugs such as a hospital or another pharmacy; and
      c. Destroy the prescription drugs following procedures specified in Board Rule 303.2 (Disposal of Stock Prescription Drugs).
   3. If the pharmacy dispenses prescription drug orders:
      a. Transfer the prescription drug order files including refill information and patient medication records to a licensed pharmacy and
      b. Remove all signs or notify the landlord or owner of the property that it is unlawful to use the word "pharmacy" either in English or any other language or use any other word or combination of words of the same or similar meaning or use any graphic representation that would mislead or tend to mislead the public that a pharmacy is located at the address.
C. After Closing a Pharmacy.
   1. Within 10 days after the closing of the pharmacy, the pharmacist-in-charge shall forward to the Board a written notice of the closing which includes the following information:
      a. The actual date of closing;
      b. The license issued to the pharmacy;
      c. A statement attesting;
         (1) That an inventory as specified in Board Rule 291.17 (Inventory Requirements) has been conducted and
         (2) The manner by which the dangerous drugs and controlled substances possessed by the pharmacy were transferred or disposed; and
      d. If the pharmacy dispenses prescription drug orders, the name and address of the pharmacy to which the prescription drug orders including refill information and patient medication records were transferred.
   2. If the pharmacy is registered to possess controlled substances, a notification must be sent to a DEA divisional office explaining that the pharmacy has closed. In addition, the following items must be sent:
      a. DEA registration certificate and
      b. All unused DEA Forms 222 with the word "VOID" written on the face of each order form.

Notes

3. Once the pharmacy has notified the Board that the pharmacy is closed, the license may not be renewed. The pharmacy may apply for a new license as specified in Board Rule 291.1 (Pharmacy License Application).
D. Emergency Closing of a Pharmacy.
If a pharmacy is closed suddenly due to fire, destruction, natural disaster, death, property seizure, eviction, bankruptcy, or other emergency circumstances and the pharmacist-in-charge cannot provide notification 14 days prior to the closing, the pharmacist-in-charge shall comply with the provisions of A. above as far in advance of the closing as allowed by the circumstances.
E. Joint Responsibility.
If the pharmacist-in-charge is not available to comply with the requirements of this section, the owner shall be responsible for compliance with the provisions of this section.

Board of Pharmacy Rule 291.7
Prescription Drug Recalls

A. The pharmacist-in-charge shall develop and implement a written procedure for proper management of drug recalls which may include where appropriate contacting patients to whom the recalled drug products have been dispensed.
B. The written procedure shall include, but not be limited to, the following:
 1. The pharmacist-in-charge shall reasonably ensure that a recalled drug has been removed from inventory no more than 24 hours after receipt of the recall notice and quarantined until proper disposal or destruction of the drug and
 2. If the drug that is the subject to a recall is maintained by the pharmacy in a container without a lot number, the pharmacist-in-charge shall consider this drug included in the recall.

Board of Pharmacy Rule 291.8
Return of Prescription Drugs

Note: This section addresses drugs that have been dispensed. For rules on returning drugs to stock that were not dispensed, see Chapter G.
A. It is generally illegal for a pharmacist to accept a return of a prescription after it has been dispensed and left the control of the pharmacy for purposes of resale or redispensing. A pharmacist is permitted to accept a return of a dispensed dangerous drug in order to destroy the drug as allowed by Chapter 303, but the drugs cannot be resold. Controlled substances may only be returned for destruction if the pharmacy is designated as an "authorized collector" with DEA. (*See Chapter B in this book.*)
B. An exception to the general prohibition on accepting the return of dispensed drugs is the voluntary drug donation program under the Texas Food, Drug, and Cosmetic Act, Chapter 442. (*See Chapter C in this book.*)
C. Another exception to the general prohibition on accepting the return of dispensed drugs is for the return of certain unused drugs from healthcare facilities regulated under Chapter 242, Health and Safety Code (primarily nursing homes) or a penal institution to the dispensing pharmacy. The consultant pharmacist for the healthcare facility or a licensed healthcare professional for a penal institution may return to the pharmacy certain unused drugs, other than controlled substances, purchased from the pharmacy if the following conditions are met:
 1. The unused drugs must:
  a. Be approved by the federal Food and Drug Administration and be
   (1) Sealed in unopened tamper-evident packaging and either individually packaged or packaged in unit-dose packaging;

(2) Oral or parenteral medication in sealed unit-of-use containers approved by the federal Food and Drug Administration;
(3) Topical or inhalant drugs in sealed unit-of-use containers approved by the federal Food and Drug Administration; or
(4) Parenteral medications in sealed multiple-dose containers approved by the federal Food and Drug Administration from which doses have not been withdrawn;

b. Not be the subject of a mandatory recall by a state or federal agency or a voluntary recall by a drug seller or manufacturer; and
c. Have not been in the physical possession of the person for whom it was prescribed.

2. A healthcare facility or penal institution may not return any drug product that has been compounded, appears on inspection to be adulterated, requires refrigeration, or has fewer than 120 days until the expiration date or end of the shelf life.
3. The consultant pharmacist/licensed healthcare professional shall be responsible for assuring that an inventory of the drugs to be returned to a pharmacy is completed. The following information shall be included in the inventory:
   a. Name and address of the facility or institution;
   b. Name and pharmacist license number of the consultant pharmacist or name and license number of the licensed healthcare professional;
   c. Date of return;
   d. Date the prescription was dispensed;
   e. Prescription number;
   f. Name of dispensing pharmacy;
   g. Name, strength, and quantity of drug; and
   h. Signature of consultant pharmacist.
4. The healthcare facility/penal institution shall send a copy of the inventory to the pharmacy with the drugs returned and to the Health and Human Services Commission.
5. Dispensing/Receiving Pharmacy Responsibilities. If a pharmacy accepts the return of unused drugs from a healthcare facility/penal institution, the following is applicable:
   a. A pharmacist employed by the pharmacy shall examine the drugs to ensure the integrity of the drug product.
   b. The pharmacy shall reimburse or credit the entity that paid for the drug including the state Medicaid program for an unused drug returned to the pharmacy. The pharmacy shall maintain a record of the credit or reimbursement containing the following information:
      (1) Name and address of the facility or institution which returned the drugs;
      (2) Date and amount of the credit or reimbursement;
      (3) Name of the person or entity to whom the credit or reimbursement was issued;
      (4) Date the prescription was dispensed;
      (5) Prescription number;
      (6) Name, strength, and quantity of drug; and
      (7) Signature of the pharmacist responsible for issuing the credit.
   c. After the pharmacy has issued credit or reimbursement, the pharmacy may restock and redispense the unused drugs returned under this section.
6. Limitation on Liability.
   a. A pharmacy that returns unused drugs, a manufacturer that accepts unused drugs under these provisions, and the employees of the pharmacy or manufacturer are not liable for harm caused by the accepting,

Notes

dispensing, or administering of drugs returned in strict compliance with these provisions unless the harm is caused by:
(1) Willful or wanton acts of negligence;
(2) Conscious indifference or reckless disregard for the safety of others; or
(3) Intentional conduct.
b. This limitation on liability does not apply if harm results from the failure to fully and completely comply with these laws and rules relating to the return of prescriptions drugs.

Board of Pharmacy Rule 291.9
Prescription Pick Up Locations

A. Except as provided in Board Rule 291.155 (Limited Prescription Delivery Pharmacy—Class H), no person, firm, or business establishment may have, participate in, or permit an arrangement, branch, connection, or affiliation whereby prescriptions are solicited, collected, picked up, or advertised to be picked up from any location other than a pharmacy which is licensed and in good standing with the Board.
Note: Another exception to this rule is the use of an automated storage and delivery system or kiosk at a location outside of a pharmacy. (See Remote Pharmacy rules in Chapter D.)

B. A pharmacist or pharmacy by means of its employee or by use of a common carrier or the U.S. Mail at the request of the patient may:
1. Pick up prescription orders at the:
   a. Office or home of the prescriber;
   b. Residence or place of employment of the person for whom the prescription was issued; or
   c. Hospital or medical care facility in which the patient is receiving treatment; and
2. Deliver prescription drugs to the:
   a. Office of the prescriber if the prescription is for a dangerous drug or for a single dose of a controlled substance that is for administration to the patient in the prescriber's office;
   Note: Federal law is more restrictive and only allows a pharmacy to deliver a controlled substance prescription to a practitioner if it is to be administered by injection or implant for maintenance or detoxification treatment by a qualifying practitioner and the drug is administered within 14 days. The federal law allows DEA to reduce this requirement to fewer than 14 days but not fewer than 7 days for 2 years by regulation. Although this federal law became effective in late 2018, DEA has not yet passed such a regulation. TSBP may need to modify this rule to match the federal law.
   b. Residence of the person for whom the prescription was issued;
   c. Place of employment of the person for whom the prescription was issued if the person is present to accept delivery; or
   d. Hospital or medical care facility in which the patient is receiving treatment.

Board of Pharmacy Rule 291.10
Pharmacy Balance Registration/Inspection

A. Definitions.
Pharmacy balance—An instrument for weighing ingredients including balances and scales.

B. Registration.
   1. A pharmacy shall annually or biennially register each pharmacy balance.
   2. An annual registration fee is charged for each pharmacy balance. *See Board Rule 291.10 for specific fees.*
C. Inspection.
   1. The Board shall periodically inspect pharmacy balances to verify accuracy.
   2. If a pharmacy balance fails the accuracy inspection, the following is applicable.
      a. The pharmacy balance may not be used until it is repaired by an authorized repair person.
      b. A tag indicating that the pharmacy balance failed inspection and may not be used shall be placed on the pharmacy balance.

Board of Pharmacy Rule 291.15
Storage of Drugs

All drugs shall be stored at the proper temperature and conditions as defined by the following terms:
1. **Freezer**—A place in which the temperature is maintained thermostatically between minus 25 degrees Celsius and minus 10 degrees Celsius (minus 13 degrees Fahrenheit and 14 degrees Fahrenheit).
2. **Cold**—Any temperature not exceeding 8 degrees Celsius (46 degrees Fahrenheit). A refrigerator is a cold place in which the temperature is maintained thermostatically between 2 degrees Celsius and 8 degrees Celsius (36 degrees Fahrenheit and 46 degrees Fahrenheit).
3. **Cool**—Any temperature between 8 degrees Celsius and 15 degrees Celsius (46 degrees Fahrenheit and 59 degrees Fahrenheit). An article for which storage in a cool place is directed may alternatively be stored and distributed in a refrigerator unless otherwise specified by the individual monograph.
4. **Room temperature**—The temperature prevailing in a working area.
5. **Controlled room temperature**—A temperature maintained thermostatically between 15 degrees Celsius and 30 degrees Celsius (59 degrees Fahrenheit and 86 degrees Fahrenheit).
6. **Warm**—Any temperature between 30 degrees Celsius and 40 degrees Celsius (86 degrees Fahrenheit and 104 degrees Fahrenheit).
7. **Excessive heat**—Any temperature above 40 degrees Celsius (104 degrees Fahrenheit).
8. **Protection from freezing**—Where, in addition to the risk of breakage of the container, freezing subjects a product to loss of strength or potency or to destructive alteration of the dosage form and the container label bears an appropriate instruction to protect the product from freezing.
9. **Dry place**—A place that does not exceed 40% average relative humidity at controlled room temperature or the equivalent water vapor pressure at other temperatures.

Board of Pharmacy Rule 291.16
Samples

Unless otherwise specified, a pharmacy may not sell, purchase, trade, or possess prescription drug samples unless the pharmacy meets all of the following conditions:
A. The pharmacy is owned by a charitable organization described in the Internal Revenue Code of 1986 or by a city, state or county government;

B. The pharmacy is a part of a healthcare entity which provides health care primarily to indigent or low-income patients at no or reduced cost;
C. The samples are for dispensing or provision at no charge to patients of such a healthcare entity; and
D. The samples are possessed in compliance with the federal Prescription Drug Marketing Act of 1987.

Board of Pharmacy Rule 291.17
Inventory Requirements

A. General Requirements for a Pharmacist-in-Charge.
   1. Responsible for taking all required inventories. He or she may delegate this inventory responsibility to another person(s).
   2. Maintain the inventory in written, typewritten, or printed form. An inventory taken by oral recording device must be promptly transcribed.
   3. Keep the inventory in the pharmacy and have it available for inspection for two years.
   4. File the inventory separately from all other records.
   5. Include all stocks of all controlled substances on hand on the date of the inventory (including any which are out of date).
   6. Take the inventory either as of the opening of business or close of business on the inventory date.
   7. Indicate whether the inventory is taken as of the opening of business or at the close of business on the inventory date. If the pharmacy is open 24 hours a day, the inventory record shall indicate the time that the inventory was taken.
   8. Make an exact count or measure of all controlled substances listed in Schedule II.
   9. Make an estimated count or measure of controlled substances listed in Schedules III, IV and V. If a container holds more than 1,000 tablets or capsules, an exact count of the contents must be made (not necessary unless container has been opened).
   10. List Schedule II controlled substances separately from the inventory of Schedules III, IV, and V controlled substances.
   11. If the pharmacy maintains a perpetual inventory of controlled substances, reconcile this perpetual inventory on the date of the inventory.
B. Initial Inventory.
   1. A new Class A, A-S, C, C-S, or F pharmacy shall take an inventory on the opening day of business. The inventory shall include all stocks (including any out-of-date drugs) of all controlled substances.
   2. If a Class A, A-S, C, C-S, or F pharmacy commences business with no controlled substances, the pharmacy shall record this fact as the initial inventory.
   3. The initial inventory shall serve as the pharmacy's inventory until May 1 of the following year or until the pharmacy's regular general physical inventory date. At that time the Class A, A-S, C, C-S, or F pharmacy shall take an annual inventory as specified in C. below (Annual Inventory).
C. Annual Inventory.
   Note: TSBP annual inventory requirements are more stringent than DEA biennial inventory requirements. As a result, they must be followed in Texas.
   1. A Class A, A-S, C, C-S, or F pharmacy must take inventory of all controlled substances on hand on May 1 of each year or on the pharmacy's regular general physical inventory date. Such inventory may be taken within 4 days of

the specified inventory date and shall include all stocks of all controlled substances (including out-of-date drugs).
2. When renewing a Class A, A-S, C, C-S, or F pharmacy license, a statement must be included on the application that an annual inventory has been conducted, the date of the inventory, and the name of the person(s) taking the inventory.
3. The person(s) taking the annual inventory and the pharmacist-in-charge shall indicate the time the inventory was taken as specified in A.7. above and shall sign and date the inventory with the date the inventory was taken. The signature of the pharmacist-in-charge and the date of the inventory shall be notarized within three days of the day the inventory is completed, excluding Saturdays, Sundays, and federal holidays.

D. Change of Ownership of a Class A, A-S, C, C-S, or F Pharmacy.
1. A Class A, A-S, C, C-S, or F pharmacy that changes ownership shall take an inventory on the date of the change of ownership. Such inventory shall include all stocks of all controlled substances (including any out-of-date drugs).
2. The inventory constitutes the closing inventory for the seller and the initial inventory for the buyer.
3. All Schedule II controlled substances must be transferred from the seller to the buyer by use of a DEA Form 222.
4. The person(s) taking the change of ownership inventory and the pharmacist-in-charge shall indicate the time the inventory was taken as specified in A.7 above and shall sign and date the inventory with the date the inventory was taken. The signature of the pharmacist-in-charge and the date of the inventory shall be notarized within three days of the day the inventory is completed, excluding Saturdays, Sundays, and federal holidays.

E. Closed Pharmacies.
1. The pharmacist-in-charge of a closed Class A, A-S, C, C-S, or F pharmacy shall notify the Board within 10 days of the closing and shall forward to the Board a statement that an inventory of all controlled substances on hand has been taken, as well as the date of closing and the manner by which the dangerous drugs and controlled substances of the pharmacy were transferred or disposed.
2. The person(s) taking the closing inventory and the pharmacist-in-charge shall indicate the time the inventory was taken as specified in A.7. above and shall sign and date the inventory with the date the inventory was taken. The signature of the pharmacist-in-charge and the date of the inventory shall be notarized within three days of the day the inventory is completed, excluding Saturdays, Sundays, and federal holidays.

F. Additional Requirements for Class C and Class C-S Pharmacies.
1. Perpetual Inventory.
   a. A Class C and Class C-S pharmacy shall maintain a perpetual inventory of all Schedule II drugs.
   b. The perpetual inventory shall be reconciled on the date of the annual inventory.
   c. A Class C Ambulatory Surgical Center (ASC) pharmacy must maintain a perpetual inventory of all controlled substances that is reconciled at least once in every calendar week that the pharmacy is open.
2. Annual Inventory (Class C and Class C-S).
   The inventory shall be maintained in the pharmacy. The inventory shall include all controlled substances located in the pharmacy and, if applicable, all controlled substances located in other departments within the institution.

If an inventory is conducted in other departments within the institution, the inventory of the pharmacy shall be listed separately as follows:
   a. The inventory of drugs on hand in the pharmacy shall be listed separately from the inventory of drugs on hand in the other areas of the institution and
   b. The inventory of drugs on hand in all other departments shall be identified by department.

G. Inventory Required Upon the Change of a Pharmacist-in-Charge of a Class A, A-S, C, C-S, or F Pharmacy.
   1. On the date of the change of the pharmacist-in-charge of a Class A, A-S, C, C-S, or F pharmacy, an inventory shall be taken. Such inventory shall include all stocks of all controlled substances (including any out-of-date drugs).
   2. Inventory constitutes the closing inventory for the departing pharmacist-in-charge and the beginning inventory for the incoming pharmacist-in-charge.
   3. If the departing and the incoming pharmacists-in-charge are unable to conduct the inventory together, a closing inventory shall be conducted by the departing pharmacist-in-charge and a new and separate beginning inventory shall be conducted by the incoming pharmacist-in-charge.
   4. The incoming pharmacist-in-charge shall be responsible for notifying the Board within 10 days as specified in Board Rule 291.3 (Notifications) that a change of pharmacist-in-charge has occurred.

H. Inventory Requirements for Remote Pharmacies.
A provider pharmacy providing services at a different location under the remote pharmacy provisions found in Board Rule 291.121 shall:
   1. Keep a perpetual inventory of controlled substances and other drugs required to be inventoried under Board Rule 291.17 (Inventory Requirements for All Classes of Pharmacies) that are received and dispensed or distributed from each remote site.
   2. As specified in Board Rule 291.17, a provider pharmacy shall conduct an inventory at each remote site. The following is applicable to this inventory:
      a. The inventory of each remote site and the provider pharmacy shall be taken on the same day.
      b. The inventory of each remote site shall be included with, but listed separately from, the drugs of other remote sites and separately from the drugs of the provider pharmacy.

Note: Regarding TSBP inventories, the signature of the pharmacist-in-charge is required and must be notarized for the Annual, Change of Ownership, and Closing inventories but not for an Initial inventory or a Change in PIC inventory.

Board of Pharmacy Rule 291.24
Pharmacy Residency Programs

For the purposes of Subchapter T, Chapter 61, Education Code, the standards for pharmacy residency programs shall be the standards required by the American Society of Health-System Pharmacists' Commission on Credentialing. The pharmacy residency programs approved by the Board shall be published periodically in the minutes of the Board.

Board of Pharmacy Rule 291.27
Confidentiality

A. A pharmacist shall provide adequate security of prescription drug orders, medication orders, and patient medication records to prevent indiscriminate or unauthorized access to confidential health information. If prescription drug orders, requests for refill authorizations, or other confidential health information is not transmitted directly between a pharmacy and a physician but is transmitted through a data communication device, confidential health information may not be accessed or maintained by the operator of the data communication device unless specifically authorized to obtain the confidential information by this section.

B. Confidential records are privileged and may be released only to:
1. The patient or the patient's agent;
2. A practitioner or another pharmacist if in the pharmacist's professional judgment the release is necessary to protect the patient's health and well-being;
3. The Board or to a person or another state or federal agency authorized by law to receive the confidential record;
4. A law enforcement agency engaged in the investigation of a suspected violation of Chapter 481 or 483, Health and Safety Code, or the Comprehensive Drug Abuse Prevention and Control Act of 1970 (21 U.S.C. Section 801 et seq.);
5. A person employed by a state agency that licenses a practitioner if the person is performing the person's official duties; or
6. An insurance carrier or other third party payor authorized by a patient to receive such information.

C. A pharmacy shall provide written policies and procedures to prohibit the unauthorized disclosure of confidential records.

Board of Pharmacy Rule 291.28
Patient Access to Confidential Records

A. Access to Confidential Records. A pharmacy shall comply with the request of a patient or a patient's agent to inspect or obtain a copy of the patient's confidential records maintained by the pharmacy as defined in Section 551.003(10) of the Act. A pharmacy shall comply with all relevant state and federal laws regarding the release of confidential records to third party requestors.

B. Form of Request. The pharmacy may require a patient or a patient's agent or any authorized third party to make requests for confidential records in writing provided such a requirement has been communicated to the requestor.

C. Timely Action by Pharmacy. The pharmacy must respond to a request for confidential records in a timely manner.
1. The pharmacy must respond to a request for confidential records no later than 15 days after receipt of the request by providing a copy of the records or, with the consent of the patient or patient's agent, a summary or explanation of such information.
2. The pharmacy must provide confidential records as requested in a mutually agreed upon format.
3. Access to confidential records may be expedited at the request of a patient or a patient's agent if there is a medical emergency. The pharmacy must respond to a request for expedited access to confidential records within 24 hours if the records are maintained at the pharmacy or within 72 hours if the records are stored off-site. The pharmacy may charge a reasonable fee, in addition to the fees outlined in D. below, of no more than $25 for expediting a request for access to confidential records.

D. Fees. The pharmacy may charge a reasonable, cost-based fee for providing a copy of confidential records or a summary or explanation of such information requested by a patient or patient's agent or with the consent of the patient or patient's agent.

1. A reasonable fee shall be no more than $50 for the first 20 pages and $0.50 per page for every page thereafter. A reasonable fee shall include only the cost of:
   a. Copying including the cost of supplies for and labor of copying;
   b. Postage when the individual has requested the records be mailed; and
   c. Preparing an explanation or summary of the protected health information if appropriate and consented to by the patient or patient's agent.
2. If an affidavit is requested certifying that the information is a true and correct copy of the records, a reasonable fee of no more than $15 may be charged for executing the affidavit.
3. If an affidavit or questionnaire accompanies the request, the pharmacy may charge a reasonable fee of no more than $50 to complete the written response.

Board of Pharmacy Rule 291.29
Professional Responsibility of Pharmacists

A. A pharmacist shall exercise sound professional judgment with respect to the accuracy and authenticity of any prescription drug order dispensed. If the pharmacist questions the accuracy or authenticity of a prescription drug order, the pharmacist shall verify the order with the practitioner prior to dispensing.
B. A pharmacist shall make every reasonable effort to ensure that any prescription drug order, regardless of the means of transmission, has been issued for a legitimate medical purpose by a practitioner in the course of medical practice. A pharmacist shall not dispense a prescription drug if the pharmacist knows or should have known that the order for such a drug was issued without a valid pre-existing patient-practitioner relationship as defined by the Texas Medical Board Rule 190.8 (Violation Guidelines) or without a valid prescription order.
   1. A prescription drug order may not be dispensed or delivered by means of the Internet unless pursuant to a valid prescription that was issued for a legitimate medical purpose in the course of medical practice by a practitioner or practitioner covering for another practitioner.
   Note: The practice of telemedicine is legal in Texas and that type of practice may use an Internet-based or telephone consultation between the prescriber and the patient. As a result, such prescriptions issued in this situation may be valid, but pharmacists must still ensure that there is a valid practitioner-patient relationship. See Section 562.112 of the Act in Chapter D. Texas Medical Board rules specify two prohibitions on telemedicine:
      1. A practitioner-patient relationship is not present if a practitioner prescribes an abortifacient or any other drug or device that terminates a pregnancy and
      2. Treatment for chronic pain with controlled substances using telemedicine is not allowed. TSBP has a Telemedicine Frequently Asked Questions document on its website which provides more information for pharmacists about telemedicine.
   2. A prescription drug order may not be dispensed or delivered if the pharmacist has reason to suspect that the prescription drug order may have been authorized in the absence of a valid patient-practitioner relationship or otherwise in violation of the practitioner's standard of practice to include that a practitioner:
      a. Did not establish a diagnosis through the use of acceptable medical practices for the treatment of the patient's condition;
      b. Prescribed prescription drugs that were not necessary for the patient due to the lack of a valid medical need or the lack of a therapeutic purpose for the prescription drugs; or
      c. Issued the prescription outside the usual course of medical practice.

3. Notwithstanding the provisions of this Board rule and as authorized by the Texas Medical Board Rule 190.8, a pharmacist may dispense a prescription when a physician has not established a professional relationship with a patient if the prescription is for medications for:
    a. Sexually transmitted diseases for partners of the physician's established patient or
    b. A patient's family member if the patient has an illness determined to be a pandemic by the Centers for Disease Control and Prevention, the World Health Organization, or the Governor's office.

    Note: A standing order for naloxone may be another example although it is not included in this rule.

C. If a pharmacist has reasons to suspect that a prescription was authorized solely based on the results of a questionnaire and/or in the absence of a documented patient evaluation including a physical examination, the pharmacist shall ascertain if that practitioner's standard of practice allows that practitioner to authorize a prescription under such circumstances. (*Note: A legitimate telemedicine practice might be such a circumstance as mentioned in B.1. above.*) Reasons to suspect that a prescription may have been authorized in the absence of a valid patient-practitioner relationship or in violation of the practitioner's standard of practice include:
    1. The number of prescriptions authorized on a daily basis by the practitioner;
    2. A disproportionate number of patients of the prescriber receive controlled substances;
    3. The manner in which the prescriptions are authorized by the practitioner or received by the pharmacy;
    4. The geographical distance between the practitioner and the patient;
    5. Knowledge by the pharmacist that the prescription was issued solely based on answers to a questionnaire;
    6. Knowledge by the pharmacist that the pharmacy he or she works for directly or indirectly participates in or is otherwise associated with an Internet site that markets prescription drugs to the public without requiring the patient to provide a valid prescription order from his or her medical practitioner; or
    7. Knowledge by the pharmacist that the patient has exhibited doctor-shopping or pharmacy-shopping tendencies.

D. A pharmacist shall ensure that prescription drug orders for the treatment of chronic pain have been issued in accordance with the guidelines set forth by the Texas Medical Board Rule 170.3 (Guidelines) prior to dispensing or delivering such prescriptions.

E. A prescription drug order may not be dispensed or delivered if issued by a practitioner practicing at a pain management clinic that is not in compliance with the Texas Medical Board Rules 195.1–195.4 (Pain Management Clinics). A prescription drug order from a practitioner practicing at a certified pain management clinic is not automatically valid and does not negate a pharmacist's responsibility to determine that the prescription is valid and has been issued for a legitimate or appropriate medical purpose.

F. A pharmacist shall not dispense a prescription drug if the pharmacist knows or should know the prescription drug order is fraudulent or forged. A pharmacist shall make every reasonable effort to prevent inappropriate dispensing due to fraudulent, forged, invalid, or medically inappropriate prescriptions in violation of a pharmacist's corresponding responsibility. The following patterns (i.e., red flag factors) are relevant to preventing the nontherapeutic dispensing of controlled substances and shall be considered by evaluating the totality of the circumstances rather than any single factor.

Notes

Notes

1. The pharmacy dispenses a reasonably discernible pattern of substantially identical prescriptions for the same controlled substances potentially paired with other drugs for numerous persons, indicating a lack of individual drug therapy in prescriptions issued by the practitioner;
2. The pharmacy operates with a reasonably discernible pattern of overall low prescription dispensing volume maintaining relatively consistent 1:1 ratio of controlled substances to dangerous drugs and/or over-the-counter products dispensed as prescriptions;
3. Prescriptions by a prescriber presented to the pharmacy are routinely for controlled substances commonly known to be abused drugs including opioids, benzodiazepines, muscle relaxants, psychostimulants, cough syrups containing codeine, or any combination of these drugs;
4. Prescriptions for controlled substances by a prescriber presented to the pharmacy contain nonspecific or no diagnoses or lack the intended use of the drug;
5. Prescriptions for controlled substances are commonly for the highest strength of the drug and/or for large quantities (e.g., monthly supply), indicating a lack of individual drug therapy in prescriptions issued by the practitioner;
6. Dangerous drugs or over-the-counter products (e.g., multivitamins or laxatives) are consistently added by the prescriber to prescriptions for controlled substances presented to the pharmacy, indicating a lack of individual drug therapy in prescriptions issued by the practitioner;
7. Upon contacting the practitioner's office regarding a controlled substance prescription, the pharmacist is unable to engage in a discussion with the actual prescribing practitioner; the practitioner fails to appropriately address based on a reasonable pharmacist standard the pharmacist's concerns regarding the practitioner's prescribing practices with regard to the prescription; and/or the practitioner is unwilling to provide additional information, such as treatment goals and/or prognosis with prescribed drug therapy;
8. The practitioner's clinic is not registered as and not exempted from registration as a pain management clinic by the Texas Medical Board, despite prescriptions by the practitioner presented to the pharmacy indicating that the practitioner is mostly prescribing opioids, benzodiazepines, barbiturates, or carisoprodol, but not including suboxone, or any combination of these drugs;
9. The controlled substance(s) or the quantity of the controlled substance(s) prescribed are inconsistent with the practitioner's area of medical practice;
10. The Texas Prescription Monitoring Program indicates the person presenting the prescriptions is obtaining similar drugs from multiple practitioners and/or that the person is being dispensed similar drugs at multiple pharmacies;
11. Multiple persons with the same address present substantially similar controlled substance prescriptions from the same practitioner;
12. Persons consistently pay for controlled substance prescriptions with cash or cash equivalents more often than through insurance;
13. Persons presenting controlled substance prescriptions are doing so in such a manner that varies from the manner in which persons routinely seek pharmacy services (e.g., persons arriving in the same vehicle with prescriptions from the same practitioner; one person seeking to pick up prescriptions for multiple others; drugs referenced by street names);
14. The pharmacy charges and persons are willing to pay significantly more for controlled substances relative to nearby pharmacies;
15. The pharmacy routinely orders controlled substances from more than one drug supplier;
16. The pharmacy has been discontinued by a drug supplier related to controlled substance orders;

17. The pharmacy has a sporadic and inconsistent dispensing volume (including zero dispensing);
18. The pharmacy does not maintain normal operational hours each week from Monday through Friday; and
19. The pharmacy has been previously warned or disciplined by the Texas State Board of Pharmacy for inappropriate dispensing of controlled substances.

Note: Some of these factors are "red flags" that a pharmacist should consider when evaluating the legitimacy of a prescription while others appear to be factors that may indicate a pharmacy is engaged in nontherapeutic dispensing.

Board of Pharmacy Rule 291.125
Centralized Prescription Dispensing

A. Definitions.
   1. **Central fill pharmacy**—A Class A, Class A-S, Class C, Class C-S, Class E, or Class E-S pharmacy that prepares prescription drug orders for dispensing pursuant to a valid prescription transmitted to the central fill pharmacy by an outsourcing pharmacy.
   2. **Centralized prescription dispensing**—The dispensing or refilling of a prescription drug order by a Class A, Class C, or Class E pharmacy at the request of another Class A or Class C pharmacy and the return of the dispensed prescriptions to the outsourcing pharmacy for delivery to the patient or patient's agent or at the request of the outsourcing pharmacy for direct delivery to the patient.
   3. **Outsourcing pharmacy**—A Class A or Class C pharmacy that transmits a prescription drug order via facsimile or communicates prescription information electronically to a central fill pharmacy to be dispensed by the central fill pharmacy.
B. Class A or Class C pharmacies may outsource prescription drug order dispensing to a central fill pharmacy provided the pharmacies:
   1. Have the same owner or
   2. Have entered into a written contract or agreement which outlines the services to be provided and the responsibilities and accountabilities of each pharmacy.
C. The pharmacies must share a common electronic file or have appropriate technology to allow access to sufficient information necessary or required to dispense or process a prescription drug order.
D. The pharmacist-in-charge of the central fill pharmacy shall ensure that:
   1. The pharmacy maintains and uses adequate storage or shipment containers and shipping processes to ensure drug stability and potency. Such shipping processes shall include the use of appropriate packaging material and/or devices to ensure that the drug is maintained at an appropriate temperature range to maintain the integrity of the medication throughout the delivery process and
   2. The dispensed prescriptions are shipped in containers which are sealed in a manner as to show evidence of opening or tampering.
E. Prior to outsourcing prescription dispensing to a central fill pharmacy, a pharmacy must notify patients that their prescriptions may be outsourced and give the name of the central fill pharmacy. Such notice may be provided through a one-time written notification to the patient or a sign in the pharmacy.
F. If a prescription that is not for a controlled substance is delivered directly to the patient by the central fill pharmacy and not returned to the outsourcing pharmacy, the central fill pharmacy must place on the prescription container or on a separate sheet delivered with the prescription container, in both English and

Spanish, the local and, if applicable, the toll-free telephone number of the pharmacy and the statement: "Written information about this prescription has been provided for you. Please read this information before you take the medication. If you have questions concerning this prescription, a pharmacist is available during normal business hours to answer these questions at (insert the pharmacy's local and toll-free telephone numbers)." A prescription for a controlled substance may not be delivered directly to the patient by the central fill pharmacy.
Note: DEA rules do not permit a central fill pharmacy to send filled controlled substance prescriptions directly to the patient.

G. The central fill pharmacy shall place on the label the name and address of the outsourcing pharmacy and a unique identifier (i.e., the central fill pharmacy's DEA registration number). If the pharmacy does not have a DEA registration number, then the central fill pharmacy's Texas license number shall be indicated on the label showing that the prescription was dispensed by the central fill pharmacy. The central fill pharmacy must comply with all other labeling requirements.

H. A policy and procedure manual must be kept at both pharmacies meeting specific requirements listed in the rule.

I. The outsourcing pharmacy must maintain records including the date the request for dispensing was transmitted to the central fill pharmacy, the date the prescription was received from the central fill pharmacy including the method of delivery, and the name, address, license number, and unique identifier of the central fill pharmacy.

J. The central fill pharmacy must maintain records including the date the prescription was shipped to the outsourcing pharmacy or the patient if shipped directly to the patient; the name and address where the prescription was shipped; the method of delivery; and the name, address, and license number of the outsourcing pharmacy.

Board of Pharmacy Rule 291.123
Centralized Prescription Drug or Medication Order Processing

A. Allows Class A (community), Class C (institutional), and Class E (nonresident) pharmacies to provide central prescription drug order or medication order processing if they meet specific standards outlined in the rule.
Note: If the pharmacy is only providing these services, the pharmacy may be licensed as a Class G pharmacy. See Chapter J.

B. Central prescription drug or medication order processing allows one pharmacy to perform processing functions on behalf of another pharmacy. It does not include the dispensing of a prescription drug (*see Board Rule 291.37*) but may include activities such as:
   1. Receiving, interpreting, or clarifying prescription drug or medication drug orders;
   2. Data entering and transferring of prescription drug or medication order information;
   3. Performing drug regimen review;
   4. Obtaining refill and substitution authorizations;
   5. Interpreting clinical data for prior authorization for dispensing;
   6. Performing therapeutic interventions; and
   7. Providing drug information concerning a patient's prescription.

C. Class A, C, or E pharmacies may outsource prescription drug or medication order processing to another Class A, C, or E pharmacy provided the pharmacies have the same owner or have a written contract which outlines the services to be provided and the pharmacies share a common electronic file or have appropriate technology to allow sufficient information necessary to provide such services.

D. A facility established in Texas for the purpose of processing prescription drug or medication orders shall be licensed as a Class A pharmacy. However, an individual pharmacist employee is not prohibited from remotely accessing a pharmacy's electronic database from outside the pharmacy to process prescription drug orders or medication orders.
E. Pharmacies that outsource their prescription drug order processing must notify patients that the processing of their prescriptions may be outsourced to another pharmacy. This notification does not apply to patients in facilities where drugs are administered to patients by persons required to do so under Texas law (i.e., hospitals and nursing homes).
F. A policy and procedure manual must be maintained at all pharmacies involved in central processing and must meet specific requirements as outlined in the rule.
G. All pharmacies must maintain appropriate records which identify by prescription drug or medication order the name, initials, or identification code of each pharmacist or pharmacy technician who performs a processing function. Such records may be maintained separately by each pharmacy or in a common electronic file so long as the data processing system can produce a printout listing the functions performed by each pharmacy and pharmacist.

Board of Pharmacy Rule 291.129
Satellite Pharmacy

Note: This rule allows a Class A or C pharmacy to provide pharmacy services at a satellite location. This is not what is typically considered a "satellite pharmacy" in a hospital. This rule allows a pharmacy to operate a satellite location that is not separately licensed. Prescriptions may be dropped off and sent to the provider pharmacy to be filled and can then be sent back to the satellite location where the patient picks up the prescription. However, these satellite pharmacies cannot possess stock prescription drugs for dispensing.

A. Purpose. The purpose of this section is to create a new class of pharmacy for the provision of pharmacy services by a Class A or Class C pharmacy in a location that is not at the same location as a Class A or Class C pharmacy through a satellite pharmacy and to provide standards for the operation of this class of pharmacy established under Section 560.053 of the Texas Pharmacy Act.
B. Definitions.
The following words and terms shall have the following meanings unless the context clearly indicates otherwise. All other words and terms shall have the meanings defined in the Act or Board Rule 291.31.
   1. **Provider pharmacy**—The Class A or Class C pharmacy providing satellite pharmacy services.
   2. **Satellite pharmacy**—A facility not located at the same location as a Class A or Class C pharmacy at which satellite pharmacy services are provided.
   3. **Satellite pharmacy services**—The provision of pharmacy services including the storage and delivery of prescription drugs in an alternate location.
C. General Requirements.
   1. A Class A or Class C provider pharmacy may establish a satellite pharmacy in a location that is not at the same location as a Class A or Class C pharmacy.
   2. The pharmacist-in-charge of the provider pharmacy is responsible for all pharmacy operations involving the satellite pharmacy including supervision of satellite pharmacy personnel and compliance with this section.
   3. A satellite pharmacy may not store bulk drugs and may only store prescription medications that have been previously verified and dispensed by the provider pharmacy.
   4. A Class C pharmacy that is a provider pharmacy dispensing outpatient prescriptions for a satellite pharmacy shall comply with the provisions of Board

Rules 291.31–291.34 (Definitions, Personnel, Operational Standards, and Records for Class A pharmacies) and this rule.

5. The provider pharmacy and the satellite pharmacy must have:
   a. The same owner and
   b. Share a common electronic file or have appropriate technology to allow access to sufficient information necessary or required to process a non-dispensing function.

D. Personnel.
   1. All individuals working at the satellite pharmacy shall be employees of the provider pharmacy and must report their employment to the Board as such.
   2. A satellite pharmacy shall have sufficient pharmacists on duty to operate the satellite pharmacy competently, safely, and adequately to meet the needs of the patients of the pharmacy.
   3. Pharmacists are solely responsible for the direct supervision of pharmacy technicians and pharmacy technician trainees and for designating and delegating duties, other than those listed in 7. below, to pharmacy technicians and pharmacy technician trainees. Each pharmacist:
      a. Shall verify the accuracy of all acts, tasks, and functions performed by pharmacy technicians and pharmacy technician trainees and
      b. Shall be responsible for any delegated act performed by pharmacy technicians and pharmacy technician trainees under his or her supervision.
   4. A pharmacist shall be physically present to directly supervise a pharmacy technician or pharmacy technician trainee who is entering prescription data into the data processing system. Each prescription entered into the data processing system shall be verified at the time of data entry.
   5. All pharmacists while on duty shall be responsible for complying with all state and federal laws or rules governing the practice of pharmacy.
   6. A pharmacist shall ensure that the drug is dispensed and delivered safely and accurately as prescribed. A pharmacist shall ensure the safety and accuracy of the portion of the process the pharmacist is performing.
   7. Duties in a satellite pharmacy that may only be performed by a pharmacist are as follows:
      a. Receiving oral prescription drug orders and reducing these orders to writing either manually or electronically;
      b. Interpreting or clarifying prescription drug orders;
      c. Communicating to the patient or patient's agent information about the prescription drug or device which, in the exercise of the pharmacist's professional judgment, the pharmacist deems significant as specified in Board Rule 291.33(c);
      d. Communicating to the patient or the patient's agent requested information concerning any prescription drugs dispensed to the patient by the pharmacy;
      e. Assuring that a reasonable effort is made to obtain, record, and maintain patient medication records;
      f. Interpreting patient medication records and performing drug regimen reviews; and
      g. Performing a specific act of drug therapy management for a patient when delegated to a pharmacist by a written protocol from a physician licensed in this state in compliance with the Medical Practice Act.
   8. Pharmacy technicians and pharmacy technician trainees may not perform any of the duties listed in 7. above. However, a pharmacist may delegate to pharmacy technicians and pharmacy technician trainees any nonjudgmental technical duty associated with the preparation and distribution of prescription drugs provided:

a. A pharmacist verifies the accuracy of all acts, tasks, and functions performed by pharmacy technicians and pharmacy technician trainees and
b. Pharmacy technicians and pharmacy technician trainees are under the direct supervision of and responsible to a pharmacist.
9. Pharmacy technicians and pharmacy technician trainees in a satellite pharmacy may perform only nonjudgmental technical duties associated with the preparation and distribution of prescription drugs as follows:
   a. Initiating and receiving refill authorization requests;
   b. Entering prescription data into a data processing system; and
   c. Reconstituting medications.
10. In a satellite pharmacy, the ratio of pharmacists to pharmacy technicians/pharmacy technician trainees may be 1:3 provided at least one of the three is a pharmacy technician and not a pharmacy technician trainee.
11. All satellite pharmacy personnel shall wear identification tags or badges that bear the person's name and identifies him or her as a pharmacist, pharmacist intern, pharmacy technician, or pharmacy technician trainee.

E. Operational Requirements.
   1. Application for Permission to Provide Satellite Pharmacy Services.
      a. A Class A or Class C pharmacy shall make an application to the Board to provide satellite pharmacy services. The application shall include the following:
         (1) The name, address, and license number of the provider pharmacy;
         (2) The name and address of the facility where the satellite pharmacy will be located;
         (3) The anticipated date of opening and hours of operation; and
         (4) A copy of the lease agreement or, if the location of the satellite pharmacy is owned by the applicant, a notarized statement certifying such location ownership. Alternatively, a notarized statement signed by the lessee and lessor certifying the existence of a lease shall be provided.
      b. A renewal application shall be resubmitted every two years with the application for renewal of the provider pharmacy's license. The renewal application shall contain the documentation required in a. above.
      c. Upon approval of the application, the provider pharmacy will be sent a certificate which must be displayed at the satellite pharmacy.
   2. Notification Requirements.
      a. A provider pharmacy shall notify the Board in writing within ten days of a change of location, discontinuance of service, or closure of a satellite pharmacy that is operated by the pharmacy.
      b. A provider pharmacy shall comply with appropriate federal and state controlled substance registrations for each satellite pharmacy if controlled substances are maintained at the satellite pharmacy.
   3. Environment.
      a. The satellite pharmacy shall be arranged in an orderly fashion and kept clean. All required equipment shall be clean and in good operating condition.
      b. A satellite pharmacy shall contain an area which is suitable for confidential patient counseling.
         (1) Such counseling area shall:
            (a) Be easily accessible to both patient and pharmacists and not allow patient access to prescription drugs and
            (b) Be designed to maintain the confidentiality and privacy of the pharmacist/patient communication.

(2) In determining whether the area is suitable for confidential patient counseling and designed to maintain the confidentiality and privacy of the pharmacist/patient communication, the Board may consider factors such as the following:
   (a) The proximity of the counseling area to the checkout or cash register area;
   (b) The volume of pedestrian traffic in and around the counseling area;
   (c) The presence of walls or other barriers between the counseling area and other areas of the pharmacy; and
   (d) Any evidence of confidential information being overheard by persons other than the patient or patient's agent or the pharmacist or agents of the pharmacist.
   c. The satellite pharmacy shall be properly lighted and ventilated.
   d. The temperature of the satellite pharmacy shall be maintained within a range compatible with the proper storage of drugs in compliance with the provisions of Board Rule 291.33(f) including the requirements for temperature. The temperature of the refrigerator shall be maintained within a range compatible with the proper storage of drugs requiring refrigeration.
   e. Animals including birds and reptiles shall not be kept within the pharmacy and in immediately adjacent areas under the control of the pharmacy. This provision does not apply to fish in aquariums, guide dogs accompanying disabled persons, or animals for sale to the general public in a separate area that is inspected by local health jurisdictions.
4. Security.
   a. A satellite pharmacy shall be under the continuous physically present supervision of a pharmacist at all times the satellite pharmacy is open to provide pharmacy services.
   b. The satellite pharmacy shall be enclosed by walls, partitions, or other means of floor-to-ceiling enclosure. In addition to the security requirements outlined in Board Rule 291.33(b)(2), satellite pharmacies shall have adequate security and procedures to:
   (1) Prohibit unauthorized access;
   (2) Comply with federal and state regulations; and
   (3) Maintain patient confidentiality.
   c. Access to the satellite pharmacy shall be limited to pharmacists, pharmacy technicians, and pharmacy technician trainees employed by the provider pharmacy and who are designated in writing by the pharmacist-in-charge.
   d. The provider pharmacy shall have procedures that specify prescriptions may only be delivered to the satellite pharmacy by the provider pharmacy and shall:
   (1) Be delivered in a sealed container with a list of the prescriptions delivered;
   (2) Signed for on receipt by the pharmacist at the satellite pharmacy; and
   (3) Be checked by personnel designated by the pharmacist-in-charge to verify that the prescriptions sent by the provider pharmacy were actually received. The designated person who checks the order shall document the verification by signing and dating the list of prescriptions delivered.
5. Prescription Dispensing and Delivery. A satellite pharmacy shall comply with the requirements outlined in Board Rule 291.33(c) with regard to prescription dispensing and delivery.

6. Equipment and Supplies. A satellite pharmacy shall have the following equipment and supplies:
   a. Typewriter or comparable equipment;
   b. Refrigerator if storing drugs requiring refrigeration; and
   c. Metric-apothecary weight and measure conversion charts.
7. Library. A reference library shall be maintained by the satellite pharmacy that includes the following in hard copy or electronic format:
   a. Current copies of the following:
      (1) Texas Pharmacy Act and rules;
      (2) Texas Dangerous Drug Act and rules;
      (3) Texas Controlled Substances Act and rules; and
      (4) Federal Controlled Substances Act and rules (or official publication describing the requirements of the Federal Controlled Substances Act and rules);
   b. At least one current or updated reference from each of the following categories:
      (1) Patient information:
         (a) United States Pharmacopeia Dispensing Information, Volume II (Advice to the Patient) or
         (b) A reference text or information leaflets which provide patient information;
      (2) Drug interactions: A reference text on drug interactions such as *Drug Interaction Facts*. A separate reference is not required if other references maintained by the satellite pharmacy contain drug interaction information including information needed to determine severity or significance of the interaction and appropriate recommendations or actions to be taken;
      (3) A general information reference text such as:
         (a) Facts and Comparisons with current supplements;
         (b) United States Pharmacopeia Dispensing Information, Volume I (Drug Information for the Healthcare Provider);
         (c) Clinical Pharmacology;
         (d) American Hospital Formulary Service with current supplements; or
         (e) Remington's Pharmaceutical Sciences; and
   c. Basic antidote information and the telephone number of the nearest regional poison control center.

F. Records.
   1. Maintenance of Records.
      a. Every record required to be kept under Board Rule 291.34 and under this rule shall be:
         (1) Kept by the provider pharmacy and be available for at least two years from the date of such inventory or record for inspecting and copying by the Board or its representative and to other authorized local, state, or federal law enforcement agencies and
         (2) Supplied by the provider pharmacy within 72 hours if requested by an authorized agent of the Texas State Board of Pharmacy. If the pharmacy maintains the records in an electronic format, the requested records must be provided in an electronic format if specifically requested by the Board or its representative. Failure to provide the records set out in this section, either on-site or within 72 hours, constitutes prima facie evidence of failure to keep and maintain records and is in violation of the Act.

b. Records, except when specifically required to be maintained in original or hardcopy form, may be maintained in an alternative data retention system such as a data processing system or direct imaging system provided:
      (1) The records maintained in the alternative system contain all of the information required on the manual record and
      (2) The data processing system is capable of producing a hard copy of the record upon the request of the Board, its representative, or other authorized local, state, or federal law enforcement or regulatory agencies.
   c. Prescription drug orders shall be maintained by the provider pharmacy in the manner required by Board Rule 291.34(d) or (e).
2. Prescriptions.
   a. Prescription drug orders shall meet the requirements of Board Rule 291.34(b).
   b. The provider pharmacy must maintain appropriate records to identify the name(s) or initials, identification code(s), and specific activity(ies) of each pharmacist, pharmacy technician, or pharmacy technician trainee who performed any processing at the satellite pharmacy.
   c. A provider pharmacy shall keep a record of all prescriptions sent and returned between the pharmacies separate from the records of the provider pharmacy and from any other satellite pharmacy's records.
   d. A satellite pharmacy shall keep a record of all prescriptions received and returned between the pharmacies.

Destruction and Disposal of Dangerous Drugs and Controlled Substances
Chapter 303

Board of Pharmacy Rule 303.1
Destruction of Dispensed Drugs

A. Drugs Dispensed to Patients in Healthcare Facilities or Institutions.
   1. Destruction by the Consultant Pharmacist.
      A consultant pharmacist in good standing with the Board is authorized to destroy dangerous drugs dispensed to patients in healthcare facilities or institutions (nursing homes). A consultant pharmacist may destroy controlled substances as allowed to do so by federal laws or rules of the Drug Enforcement Administration. (*See Chapter B, Section XII. for requirements.*) Dangerous drugs may be destroyed provided the following conditions are met.
      a. A written agreement exists between the facility or institution and the consultant pharmacist.
      b. The drugs are inventoried and the inventory is verified by the consultant pharmacist. The inventory shall include:
         (1) Name and address of the facility or institution;
         (2) Name and pharmacist license number of the consultant pharmacist;
         (3) Date of drug destruction;
         (4) Date the prescription was dispensed;
         (5) Unique identification number assigned to the prescription by the pharmacy;
         (6) Name of dispensing pharmacy;

   (7) Name, strength, and quantity of drug;
   (8) Signature of consultant pharmacist destroying drugs;
   (9) Signature of the witness(es); and
   (10) Method of destruction.
  c. The signature of the consultant pharmacist and witness(es) to the destruction and the method of destruction specified in A.1.b. above may be on a cover sheet attached to the inventory and not on each individual inventory sheet, provided the cover sheet contains a statement indicating the number of inventory pages that are attached and each of the attached pages are initialed by the consultant pharmacist and witness(es).
  d. The drugs are destroyed in a manner to render the drugs unfit for human consumption and disposed of in compliance with all applicable state and federal requirements.
  e. The actual destruction of the drugs is witnessed by one of the following:
   (1) A commissioned peace officer;
   (2) An agent of the Texas State Board of Pharmacy;
   (3) An agent of the Texas Health and Human Services Commission as authorized by the Texas State Board of Pharmacy to destroy drugs;
   (4) An agent of the Texas Department of State Health Services as authorized by the Texas State Board of Pharmacy; or
   (5) Any two individuals working in the following capacities at the facility:
    (a) Facility administrator;
    (b) Director of nursing;
    (c) Acting director of nursing; or
    (d) Licensed nurse.
  f. If actual destruction of the drugs is conducted at a location other than the facility or institution, the consultant pharmacist and witness(es) shall retrieve the drugs from the facility, transport the drugs, and destroy the drugs at the other location.
2. Destruction by a Waste Disposal Service.
Note: This is not the same procedure as a transfer of drugs to a DEA registered reverse distributor for destruction.
A consultant pharmacist may use a waste disposal service to destroy dangerous drugs dispensed to patients in healthcare facilities or institutions. A consultant pharmacist may destroy controlled substances as allowed to do so by federal laws or rules of the Drug Enforcement Administration. (*See Chapter B, Section XII. for requirements.*) Dangerous drugs may be destroyed provided the following conditions are met.
  a. The waste disposal service is in compliance with applicable rules of the Texas Commission on Environmental Quality and the United States Environmental Protection Agency relating to waste disposal.
  b. The drugs are inventoried and such inventory is verified by the consultant pharmacist prior to placing the drugs in an appropriate container and sealing the container. The following information must be on this inventory:
   (1) Name and address of the facility or institution;
   (2) Name and pharmacist license number of the consultant pharmacist;
   (3) Date of packaging and sealing of the container;
   (4) Date the prescription was dispensed;
   (5) Unique identification number assigned to the prescription by the pharmacy;
   (6) Name of dispensing pharmacy;

(7) Name, strength, and quantity of drug;
(8) Signature of consultant pharmacist packaging and sealing the container; and
(9) Signature of the witness(es).
   c. The consultant pharmacist must seal the container of drugs in the presence of the facility administrator and the director of nursing or one of the other witnesses listed in A.1.e. above as follows:
      (1) Tamper-resistant tape is placed on the container in such a manner that any attempt to reopen the container will result in the breaking of the tape and
      (2) The signature of the consultant pharmacist is placed over the tape seal.
   d. The sealed container is maintained in a secure area at the facility or institution until transferred to the waste disposal service by the consultant pharmacist, the facility administrator, the director of nursing, or the acting director of nursing. A record of the transfer is maintained containing the following information:
      (1) Date of transfer;
      (2) Signature of person who transferred drugs to the waste disposal service;
      (3) Name and address of waste disposal service; and
      (4) Signature of employee of the waste disposal service who receives the container.
   e. The waste disposal service shall provide the facility with proof of destruction of the sealed container. Such proof of destruction shall contain the date, location, and method of destruction of the container and shall be attached to the inventory of drugs specified in b. above.
  3. Record Retention.
     All records required in this rule shall be maintained by the consultant pharmacist at the healthcare facility or institution for two years from the date of destruction. Such proof of destruction shall contain the date, location, and method of destruction of the container and shall be attached to the inventory of drugs specified in b. above.
B. Drugs Returned to a Pharmacy.
  1. Dangerous Drugs. A pharmacist in a pharmacy may accept and destroy dangerous drugs that have been previously dispensed to a patient and returned to a pharmacy by the patient or an agent of the patient. The following procedures shall be followed in destroying dangerous drugs.
     a. The dangerous drugs shall be destroyed in a manner to render the drugs unfit for human consumption and disposed of in compliance with all applicable state and federal requirements.
     b. Documentation shall be maintained that includes the following information:
        (1) Name and address of the dispensing pharmacy;
        (2) Unique identification number assigned to the prescription if available;
        (3) Name and strength of the dangerous drug; and
        (4) Signature of the pharmacist.
  2. Controlled Substances. Pharmacists in pharmacies are not generally allowed to take back controlled substances previously dispensed to patients. However, DEA now allows pharmacies to serve as "authorized collectors" which means that pharmacies can take back previously dispensed controlled substances provided they meet certain DEA rules. This is a voluntary program which is further explained in Chapter B, Section XII. (Disposal and Destruction of Controlled Substances).

Board of Pharmacy Rule 303.2
Destruction of Stock Prescription Drugs

These procedures apply to stock prescription drugs belonging to a pharmacy (drugs that are packaged in an original manufacturer's container or have been prepackaged by the pharmacy for internal distribution).
   A. Stock Dangerous Drugs.
      Pharmacists licensed by the Texas State Board of Pharmacy may destroy stock dangerous drugs if the drugs are destroyed in a manner to render the drugs unfit for human consumption (i.e., destroyed beyond reclamation) and disposed of in compliance with all applicable state and federal requirements.
   B. Stock Controlled Substances.
      See DEA rules for disposal of controlled substances in Chapter B, Section XII.

Board of Pharmacy Rule 303.3
Records

All inventory records and forms of disposed drugs shall be kept for two years from the date of transfer, disposal, or destruction and be available for inspection.

Confidentiality of Certain Information Regarding the Execution of a Convict

Subchapter C, Section 552.1081 of the Government Code creates an exception to the Texas Open Records Act to keep confidential the identifying information of any person who participates in an execution procedure, including a person who uses, supplies, or administers a substance during the execution and any person or entity that manufactures, transports, tests, procures, compounds, prescribes, dispenses, or provides a substance or supplies used in an execution.

Medication Synchronization

Medication synchronization is the process by which a pharmacist coordinates a patient's prescriptions and refills so that the patient can receive all of them on a single day each month. The Texas Insurance Code (Law) allows pharmacists to provide medication synchronization and eliminates some of the barriers to providing the service by requiring health plans to prorate any cost sharing amount charged for a prescription drug dispensed in a quantity less than the full prescribed amount. The law applies to medication that:
   1. Is covered under the patient's health benefit plan;
   2. Meets any prior authorization requirement;
   3. Is used for the treatment and management of a chronic illness;
   4. May be prescribed with refills;
   5. Is a formulation that can be effectively dispensed in accordance with the medication synchronization plan; and
   6. Is not a Schedule II controlled substance or a Schedule III controlled substance containing hydrocodone.

Note: See Chapter 1369 of the Texas Insurance Code for additional information.

CHAPTER E HIGHLIGHTS
Miscellaneous Texas Pharmacy and Drug Laws and Rules

1. Drug Therapy Management by a Pharmacist Under Written Protocol
   a. Allows pharmacists to perform specific drug therapy related tasks under a written protocol with a physician.
   b. May include the authority for pharmacists practicing in federally qualified health centers, hospitals, hospital-based clinics, or academic healthcare institutions to sign a prescription drug order for dangerous drugs.
2. Required Notifications for Pharmacies
   a. Change of location—Requires a new pharmacy application be filed no later than 30 days before the change.
   b. Change of pharmacy name—Requires a new pharmacy application be filed no later than 10 days before the change.
   c. Change of managing officers—Within 10 days.
   d. Change of ownership—Requires new pharmacy application.
   e. Change of pharmacist employment—Within 10 days.
   f. Change of pharmacist-in-charge—Within 10 days.
   g. Theft or significant loss of controlled substances or dangerous drugs—Immediately upon discovery.
   h. Fire or other disaster—Within 10 days.
3. Closing a Pharmacy
   a. At least 14 days prior to closing, the pharmacist-in-charge must post a closing notice at the pharmacy.
   b. On the day of closing, the pharmacist-in-charge must take a closing inventory, remove all prescription drugs, and transfer prescription files.
   c. Within 10 days of the closing date, the pharmacist-in-charge must forward written notice of closing and return licenses/registrations to TSBP and DEA.
4. Prescription Drug Recalls
   a. Pharmacies must have a written policy and procedure for the proper management of drug recalls.
   b. The pharmacist-in-charge must ensure that a recalled drug has been removed from inventory no more than 24 hours after the receipt of a recall notice.
5. Return of Prescriptions Drugs
   a. It is generally illegal to accept a return of a prescription drug after it has been dispensed and left the control of the pharmacy for purposes of resale or redispensing.
   b. Exceptions apply for a voluntary drug donation program under specific conditions and for certain unused drugs in healthcare facilities (primarily nursing homes) if specific conditions are met.
6. Inventory Requirements
   a. The pharmacist-in-charge is responsible for taking all required inventories.
   b. Inventories include all controlled substances on hand in a pharmacy.
   c. Required inventories include initial inventory, closing inventory, annual inventory, change of ownership (constitutes closing inventory for the seller and initial inventory for the buyer), and change of pharmacist-in-charge inventory.
   d. All inventories except the initial inventory and change of pharmacist-in-charge inventory must be signed by the pharmacist-in-charge and dated with the date the inventory was taken. The signature must be notarized within three days of the day the inventory was taken.
   e. Perpetual inventories of all controlled substances are required in remote pharmacy practice sites, Class C Ambulatory Care Facility pharmacies, and Class F (Freestanding Emergency Medical Facility) pharmacies. A perpetual inventory of Schedule II controlled substances is required in Class C (institutional) pharmacies.
7. Centralized Prescription Dispensing
   a. Allows the dispensing or filling of a prescription drug order by a Class A, C, or E pharmacy at the request of a Class A or Class C pharmacy (the outsourcing pharmacy).

- b. Dispensed prescriptions are returned to the outsourcing pharmacy for delivery to patients or delivered directly to the patient by the central fill pharmacy.
- c. Requires notification to patients and the prescription label must have a code to indicate that the prescription was filled at the central fill pharmacy.
8. Centralized Prescription Drug or Medication Order Processing
   a. Allows Class A, C, and E pharmacies to perform prescription or medication order processing functions on behalf of another pharmacy.
   b. Includes activities such as data entry, drug regimen review, claim adjudication, etc., but does not include dispensing.
9. Satellite Pharmacy
   a. A Class A or C pharmacy is allowed to operate a satellite location that is not separately licensed.
   b. Prescriptions may be dropped off at the satellite location and sent to the provider pharmacy where they are dispensed and then sent back to the satellite location where the patient picks them up and counseling is performed for new prescriptions.
   c. The satellite pharmacy may not store bulk drugs and may only store filled prescriptions that have been dispensed by the provider pharmacy.
10. Disposal and Destruction of Drugs
    a. Dangerous drugs dispensed to patients in healthcare facilities such as nursing homes may be destroyed by the consultant pharmacist following specific requirements including having a witness. The consultant pharmacist may use a waste disposal service following specific procedures that include taking an inventory of the drugs and sealing the drugs before delivery to the waste disposal service.
    b. Dangerous drugs returned to a pharmacy by a patient and stock dangerous drugs may be destroyed by a pharmacist as long as the drugs are rendered unfit for human consumption. In addition, the destruction must be conducted in compliance with all state and federal laws and proper documentation must be kept.
    c. Stock controlled substances may only be destroyed in compliance with DEA requirements. (*See Chapter B.*)
    d. Pharmacies may not accept controlled substances returned by patients for destruction unless the pharmacies meet DEA requirements to serve as an authorized collector. (*See Chapter B.*)
11. Telemedicine
    a. The practice of telemedicine is a legal practice in Texas. This allows for the use of an Internet-based or telephone consultation between the practitioner and the patient, but a valid physician-patient relationship must still be established.
    b. *See TSBP website for Telemedicine Frequently Asked Questions.*

CHAPTER F

Complaints, Inspections, Disciplinary Actions, and Procedures

Chapter 555 Public Interest Information and Complaint Procedures

CHAPTER F

Complaints, Inspections, Disciplinary Actions, and Procedures

Chapter 555 Public Interest Information and Complaint Procedures

Section 555.001 Public Interest Information
A. The Board shall prepare information of public interest describing the functions of the Board and procedures by which complaints are filed with and resolved by the Board.
B. The Board shall make the information available to the public and appropriate state agencies.
C. The Board shall provide on its website a list of all Internet pharmacies licensed by the Board and shall provide information about each pharmacy including the pharmacy's name, license number, and state of physical location. An Internet pharmacy is a pharmacy physically located in this state or another state that:
   1. Dispenses a prescription drug or device under a prescription drug order in response to a request received by way of the Internet to dispense the drug or device and
   2. Delivers the drug or device to a patient in this state by United States mail, common carrier, or delivery service.
D. Information regarding the home address or home telephone number of a person licensed or registered under this subtitle including a pharmacy owner is confidential and not subject to disclosure under Chapter 552, Government Code (Texas Public Information Act). However, each person licensed or registered must provide the Board with a business address or address of record that is subject to disclosure under Chapter 552 and that may be posted on the Board's Internet site or in the Board's licensure verification database.

Section 555.002 Complaints
A. The Board by rule shall establish methods by which consumers and service recipients are notified of the name, mailing address, and telephone number of the Board for the purpose of directing complaints to the Board. The Board may provide for that notice:
   1. On each registration form, application, or written contract for services of a person regulated by the Board;
   2. On a sign prominently displayed in the place of business of each person regulated by the Board;
   3. On an electronic messaging system in a font specified by Board rule that is prominently displayed in the place of business of each person regulated by the Board; or
   4. In a bill for service provided by a person regulated by the Board.
B. The Board shall list with its regular telephone number any toll-free telephone number established under another state law that may be called to present a complaint about a health professional.
C. Any person who has knowledge relating to an action or omission of a pharmacist or pharmacy licensed by the Board that constitutes a ground for disciplinary action under Section 565.001 or 565.002 of the Act or a rule adopted under one of those sections may provide relevant records, report relevant information, or provide assistance to the Board.

D. A complaint directed to the Board under this section may be made through the Internet.

Note: The Board has established the following rules to implement this section of the Act.

Board of Pharmacy Rule 291.3(h)(1)
Notification to Consumers Regarding
Filing a Complaint (For Licensed Pharmacies)

A. Every licensed pharmacy shall provide notification to consumers of the name, mailing address, Internet site address, and telephone number of the Board for the purpose of directing complaints concerning the practice of pharmacy to the Board. The notification shall be as follows:
   1. If the pharmacy serves walk-in customers, the pharmacy shall either:
      a. Post in a prominent place that is in clear public view where prescription drugs are dispensed:
         (1) A sign which notifies the consumer how complaints may be filed with the Board and lists the Board's name, mailing address, Internet site address, telephone number, and a toll-free telephone number for filing complaints or
         (2) An electronic messaging system in a type size no smaller than 10-point Times Roman which notifies the consumer that complaints concerning the practice of pharmacy may be filed with the Board and lists the Board's name, mailing address, Internet site address, telephone number, and a toll-free number for filing complaints or
      b. Provide with each dispensed prescription a written notification in type size no smaller than 10-point Times Roman which states: "Complaints concerning the practice of pharmacy may be filed with the Texas State Board of Pharmacy at: (list the mailing address, Internet site address, telephone number of the Board, and a toll-free telephone number for filing complaints)."
   2. If prescriptions are delivered to patients at their residence or another designated location, the pharmacy shall provide with each dispensed prescription written notification in type size no smaller than 10-point Times Roman which states: "Complaints concerning the practice of pharmacy may be filed with the Texas State Board of Pharmacy at: (list the mailing address, Internet site address, telephone number of the Board, and a toll-free telephone number for filing complaints)." If multiple prescriptions are delivered to the same location, only one notice is required.
   3. The provisions of this paragraph do not apply to prescriptions for patients where drugs are administered to patients by a person required to do so by the laws of the state (e.g., nursing homes).
B. A pharmacy that maintains a generally accessible site on the Internet and that is located in Texas or sells or distributes prescription drugs through this site to residents of this state shall post the following information on the pharmacy's initial home page and on the page where a sale of prescription drugs occurs:
   1. Information on the ownership of the pharmacy to include at a minimum the:
      a. Owner's name or, if the owner is a partnership or corporation, the partnership or corporation's name and the name of the chief operating officer;
      b. Owner's address;
      c. Owner's telephone number; and
      d. Year the owner began operating pharmacies in the United States.

2. The Internet address and toll-free telephone number that a consumer may use to:
   a. Report medication/device problems to the pharmacy and
   b. Report business compliance problems.
3. Information about each pharmacy that dispenses prescriptions for this site to include at a minimum the:
   a. Pharmacy's name, address, and telephone number;
   b. Name of the pharmacist responsible for the operation of the pharmacy;
   c. Texas pharmacy license number for the pharmacy and a link to the Internet site maintained by the Texas State Board of Pharmacy; and
   d. The names of all other states in which the pharmacy is licensed, the license number in that state, and a link to the Internet site of the entity that regulates pharmacies in that state if available.
4. A pharmacy whose Internet site has been verified by the National Association of Boards of Pharmacy to be in compliance with the laws of this state, as well as all other states the pharmacy is licensed in, shall be in compliance with B. above.

C. Pharmacy Profile.
The Board maintains a profile on every pharmacy with specific information including ownership, names and addresses of all pharmacists working at a location, and disciplinary history.

Board of Pharmacy Rule 295.11
Notification to Consumers Regarding
Filing a Complaint (For Licensed Pharmacists)

A. Every pharmacist who practices pharmacy other than in a licensed pharmacy shall provide notification to consumers of the name, mailing address, Internet site address, and telephone number of the Board for the purpose of filing a complaint with the Board. The notification shall be as follows:
1. If the pharmacist maintains an office and provides pharmacy services to patients who come to the office, the pharmacist shall either:
   a. Post in a prominent place that is in clear public view where pharmacy services are provided:
      (1) A sign which notifies the consumer how complaints may be filed with the Board and lists the Board's name, mailing address, Internet site address, telephone number, and a toll-free telephone number for filing complaints or
      (2) An electronic messaging system in a type size no smaller than 10-point Times Roman which notifies the consumer that complaints concerning the practice of pharmacy may be filed with the Board and list the Board's name, mailing address, Internet site address, and a toll-free number for filing complaints or
   b. Provide to the patient each time pharmacy services are provided a written notification in type size no smaller than 10-point Times Roman which states: "Complaints concerning the practice of pharmacy may be filed with the Texas State Board of Pharmacy at: (list the mailing address, Internet site address, telephone number of the Board, and a toll-free telephone number for filing complaints)."
2. If the pharmacist provides pharmacy services (clinical, consulting, etc.) to patients not at the pharmacist's office, the pharmacist shall provide to the patient each time pharmacy services are provided written notification in type size no smaller than 10-point Times Roman which states: "Complaints

concerning the practice of pharmacy may be filed with the Texas State Board of Pharmacy at: (list the mailing address, Internet site address, telephone number of the Board, and a toll-free telephone number for filing complaints)." Such notification shall be included in each written contract for pharmacist services or on each bill for services provided by the pharmacist.
   3. The notification provisions do not apply for patients in facilities where drugs are administered by a person required to do so by law (e.g., nursing homes).
   B. Pharmacist Profile.
   The Board maintains a profile on each pharmacist with specific information including educational background, licensure status, work location, and disciplinary history.

TSBP Complaint Process
   A. Complaints are received from:
      1. Patients (or their family);
      2. Physicians or other practitioners;
      3. Pharmacists;
      4. Law enforcement agencies (e.g., DEA, DPS, or local); and
      5. Other state and federal regulatory agencies (e.g., FDA, Texas Department of Health and Human Services, Texas Department of State Health Services, and Texas Medical Board).
   B. Upon receipt, the complaint is reviewed. If the complaint alleges a violation over which the Board has jurisdiction, the complaint is assigned to the Enforcement Division of the Texas State Board of Pharmacy.

Section 555.003 Complaint Form
The Board shall provide reasonable assistance to a person who wants to file a complaint with the Board.

Section 555.005 Records of Complaints
For each complaint received by the Board, the Board shall maintain information about parties to the complaint including the complainant's identity, the subject matter of the complaint, a summary of the results of the review or investigation of the complaint, and the disposition of the complaint.

Section 555.006 Notification Concerning Complaint
   A. The Board shall notify the complainant no later than the 30th day after the date the Board receives the complaint and shall provide an estimated time for resolution of the complaint.
   B. If a written complaint is filed with the Board that the Board has the authority to resolve, the Board, at least every four months and until final disposition of the complaint, shall notify the parties to the complaint of the status of the complaint unless the notice would jeopardize an undercover investigation.

Section 555.007 General Rules Regarding Complaints
   A. The Board shall adopt policies and procedures concerning the investigation of a complaint filed with the Board. The policies and procedures must:
      1. Determine the seriousness of the complaint;
      2. Ensure that a complaint is not closed without appropriate consideration;
      3. Ensure that a letter is sent to the person who filed the complaint explaining the action taken on the complaint;
      4. Ensure that the person who filed the complaint has an opportunity to explain the allegations made in the complaint;
      5. Prescribe guidelines concerning the types of complaints that require the use of a private investigator and the procedures for the Board to obtain the services of a private investigator; and

      6. Allow appropriate employees of the Board to dismiss a complaint if an investigation shows that:
         a. No violation occurred or
         b. The subject of the complaint is outside the Board's jurisdiction.
  B. The Board shall:
      1. Dispose of a complaint in a timely manner and
      2. Establish a schedule for conducting each phase of the investigation or disposition that is under the control of the Board.
  C. At each public meeting of the Board, the executive director shall report to the Board each complaint dismissed under A.6. above since the Board's last public meeting.
  D. The Board may not consider or act on a complaint involving a violation alleged to have occurred more than seven years before the date the complaint is received by the Board.

Section 555.008 Notice to the Board Concerning Complaints
  A. The executive director shall notify the Board of the number of complaints that are unresolved two years after the date of the filing of the complaint. The executive director shall provide the Board with an explanation of the reason that a complaint has not been resolved.
  B. The executive director shall provide the notice and explanation required under A. above periodically at regularly scheduled Board meetings.

Section 555.009 Public Participation
  A. The Board shall develop and implement policies that provide the public with a reasonable opportunity to appear before the Board and to speak on an issue under the Board's jurisdiction.
  B. The Board shall prepare and maintain a written plan that describes how a person who does not speak English may be provided reasonable access to the Board's programs.

Section 555.010 Confidentiality
The identity of a person who reports to or assists the Board under Section 555.002(c) of the Act and a document that could disclose the identity of that person are confidential and are not considered public information for the purposes of Chapter 552 of the Act.

Section 555.011 Immunity
  A. A person who provides information or assistance under Section 555.002(c) of the Act is immune from civil liability arising from providing the information or assistance.
  B. A. above shall be liberally construed to accomplish the purposes of the Act, and the immunity provided under that subsection is in addition to any other immunity provided for by law.
  C. A person who provides information or assistance to the Board under this chapter is presumed to have acted in good faith. A person who alleges a lack of good faith has the burden of proof on that issue.

Section 555.012 Counterclaim or Suit
  A. A person who provides information or assistance under Section 555.002C. of the Act and who is named as a defendant in a civil action filed as a result of the information or assistance may file a counterclaim in a pending action or may prove a cause of action in a subsequent suit to recover defense costs. These costs include court costs, attorney's fees, and damages incurred as a result of the civil action if the plaintiff's original suit is determined to be frivolous, unreasonable, without foundation, or brought in bad faith.

B. A Board employee or member or an agent of the Board who is named as a defendant in a civil action filed as a result of an action taken in the person's official capacity or in the course and scope of employment may file a counterclaim in a pending action or may prove a cause of action in a subsequent suit to recover defense costs. These costs include court costs, attorney's fees, and damages incurred as a result of the civil action if the plaintiff's original suit is determined to be frivolous, unreasonable, without foundation, or brought in bad faith.

Chapter 556 Administrative Inspections and Warrants
SUBCHAPTER A. General Provisions

Section 556.001 Definition
In this chapter, "facility" means a place:
1. For which an application has been made for a pharmacy license under this Act;
2. At which a pharmacy licensed under this Act is located;
3. At which a pharmacy is being operated in violation of this Act; or
4. Where the practice of pharmacy occurs.

SUBCHAPTER B. Inspections

Section 556.051 Authorization to Enter and Inspect
A. The Board or a representative of the Board may enter and inspect a facility relative to the following:
   1. Drug storage and security;
   2. Equipment;
   3. Components used in compounding, finished and unfinished products, containers, and labeling of any item;
   4. Sanitary conditions;
   5. Records, reports, or other documents required to be kept or made under this Act, Chapter 481 (TCSA) or 483 (TDDA), Health and Safety Code, or the Comprehensive Drug Abuse Prevention and Control Act of 1970 (FCSA); and
   6. Subject to B. below, financial records relating to the operation of the facility.
B. The Board or a representative of the Board may inspect financial records under A.6. above only in the course of the investigation of a specific complaint. The inspection is subject to Section 565.055 of the Act (Confidentiality of Investigative Information).
Note: This inspection of financial records by TSBP is different from DEA which does not have the authority to inspect financial records without the consent of the registrant.

Section 556.052 Requirements Before Entry and Inspection
A. Before an entry and inspection of the facility, the person authorized to represent the Board must:
   1. State the purpose for the inspection and
   2. Present to the owner, pharmacist, or agent in charge of the facility:
      a. Appropriate credentials and
      b. Written notice of the authority for the inspection.
B. If an inspection is required by or is supported by an administrative inspection warrant, the warrant is the notice for purposes of A.2.b. above.

Section 556.053 Extent of Inspection
Except as otherwise provided in an inspection warrant, the person authorized to represent the Board may:

1. Inspect and copy documents including records or reports required to be kept or made under this Act, the TCSA, the TDDA, the FCSA, or rules adopted under one of those laws;
2. Inspect within reasonable limits and in a reasonable manner a facility's storage, equipment, security, prescription drugs or devices, components used in compounding, finished and unfinished products, or records; or
3. Perform an inventory of any stock of prescription drugs or devices, components used in compounding, or finished and unfinished products in a facility and obtain samples of those substances.

Section 556.054 Confidentiality of Certain Information

The following information obtained by the Board during an inspection of a facility is confidential and not subject to disclosure under Chapter 552, Government Code (Texas Public Information Act).
1. Financial data;
2. Sales data other than shipment data; or
3. Pricing data.

Section 556.055 Inspections with a Warning Notice

Before a complaint may be filed with the Board as the result of a written warning notice that is issued during an inspection authorized by this chapter and that lists a specific violation of this Act or a rule adopted under this Act, the license holder must be given a reasonable time as determined by the Board to comply.

Board of Pharmacy Rule 291.18
Time Limit for Filing a Complaint

The Board determines that a "reasonable time" is to be no less than 10 days from the date of an inspection giving rise to a possible complaint. However, in situations presenting imminent danger to the public health and safety, the Board may obtain an injunction to restrain or enjoin a person from continuing to violate the Act or rules without waiting the 10-day period.

Board of Pharmacy Rule 291.19
Administrative Actions as a Result of a Compliance Inspection

A. An agent of the Board may issue a written report of areas of noncompliance that need improvement.
B. An agent of the Board may issue a written warning notice listing specific violations to which the licensee shall respond in writing to the Board by a specified date which states that the violations specified in the warning notice will be corrected (in most instances, 30 days is allowed for a response to a warning notice).
C. An agent of the Board may recommend instituting disciplinary action against a licensee if:
   1. Previously cited violations are continuing to occur or
   2. Violations observed are of a nature that written notice of noncompliance or a written warning notice would not be in the best interest of the public.
D. If violations pose imminent peril to the public, an agent of the Board may recommend to the director of compliance instituting action by a district court in Travis County, Texas to restrain or enjoin a licensee from continuing the violation. This action would be in addition to recommending the disciplinary action against a licensee in C. above.

Section 556.0551 Inspection of a Licensed Nonresident Pharmacy
See Chapter J of this book.

Section 556.056 Code of Professional Responsibility
Requires the Board to establish a code of professional responsibility to regulate the conduct of Board representatives authorized to inspect pharmacies.

Section 556.057 Inspection of Pharmacist Records
A pharmacist shall provide to the Board on request the records of the pharmacist's practice that occur outside of a pharmacy. The pharmacist shall provide the records at a time specified by Board rule.

SUBCHAPTER C. Warrants

Section 556.101 Warrant Not Required
A warrant is not required under this chapter to:
1. Inspect books or records under an administrative subpoena issued under this Act or
2. Enter a facility or conduct an administrative inspection of a facility if:
   a. The owner, pharmacist, or agent in charge of the facility consents to the inspection;
   b. The situation presents imminent danger to the public health and safety;
   c. The situation involves inspection of a conveyance if there is reasonable cause to believe that the mobility of the conveyance makes it impracticable to obtain a warrant; or
   d. Any other exceptional situation or emergency exists involving an act of God or natural disaster in which time or opportunity to apply for a warrant is lacking.

Section 556.102 Compliance with Chapter
An administrative inspection warrant may be issued and executed only in accordance with this chapter.

Section 556.103 Issuance of Warrant

Section 556.104 Contents of Warrant

Section 556.105 Execution and Return of Warrant

Section 556.106 Filing with District Court

Section 556.107 Destruction of Seized Property

Chapter 565 Disciplinary Actions and Procedures; Reinstatement of License
SUBCHAPTER A. Grounds for Discipline of an Applicant or a License Holder

Section 565.001 Applicant for or Holder of a License to Practice Pharmacy (Pharmacist)
A. The Board may discipline an applicant for or the holder of a current or expired license to practice pharmacy if the Board finds that the applicant or license holder has:
   1. Violated this Act or a Board rule adopted under this Act;
   2. Engaged in unprofessional conduct as defined by Board rule;

Board of Pharmacy Rule 281.7.A.
Unprofessional Conduct

Unprofessional conduct is defined as engaging in behavior or committing an act that fails to conform with the standards of the pharmacy profession including, but not limited to, criminal activity or activity involving moral turpitude, dishonesty, or corruption. This conduct includes but is not limited to:

1. Dispensing a forged, altered, or fraudulent prescription;
2. Dispensing a prescription drug pursuant to a prescription from a practitioner as follows:
   a. Dispensing of a prescription drug order not issued for a legitimate medical purpose or in the usual course of professional practice shall include the following:
      (1) Dispensing controlled substances or dangerous drugs to an individual or individuals in quantities, dosages, or for periods of time which grossly exceed standards of practice, approved labeling of the federal Food and Drug Administration, or the guidelines published in professional literature or
      (2) Dispensing controlled substances or dangerous drugs when the pharmacist knows or reasonably should have known that the controlled substances or dangerous drugs are not necessary or required for the patient's valid medical needs or for a valid therapeutic purpose.
   b. The provisions of A.2.a.(1) and A.2.a.(2) above are not applicable for prescriptions dispensed to persons with intractable pain in accordance with the requirements of the Intractable Pain Treatment Act or to a narcotic drug dependent person in accordance with the requirements of Title 21, Code of Federal Regulations, 1306.07 and the Regulation of Narcotic Drug Treatment Programs Act;
3. Delivering or offering to deliver a prescription drug in violation of the Texas Pharmacy Act, the Controlled Substances Act, the Dangerous Drug Act, or rules adopted under these Acts;
4. Acquiring or possessing or attempting to acquire or possess prescription drugs in violation of the Texas Pharmacy Act, the Controlled Substances Act, the Dangerous Drug Act, or rules adopted under these Acts;
5. Distributing prescription drugs to a practitioner or pharmacy not in the usual course of professional practice or in violation of the Texas Pharmacy Act, Controlled Substances Act, Dangerous Drug Act, or any rule adopted under these Acts;
6. Refusing or failing to keep/maintain/furnish any record, notification, or information required by the Texas Pharmacy Act, Controlled Substances Act, Dangerous Drug Act, or any rule adopted under these Acts;
7. Refusing an inspection;
8. Making false or fraudulent claims to third parties for reimbursement for pharmacy services (e.g., Medicaid or health insurance);
9. Operating a pharmacy in an unsanitary manner;
10. Making false or fraudulent claims concerning any drug;
11. Persistently and flagrantly overcharging for dispensing controlled substances;
12. Dispensing prescription drugs in a manner not consistent with the public health and welfare;
13. Failing to practice pharmacy in an acceptable manner consistent with the public health and welfare;
14. Refilling a prescription which authorized "prn" refills for over one year from the date of issuance;

15. Engaging in a conspiracy resulting in a restraint of trade, coercion, or monopoly in the practice of pharmacy;
16. Sharing or offering to share with a practitioner compensation from an individual who is provided pharmacy services by a pharmacist;
17. Obstructing a Board employee in the lawful performance of his or her duties;
18. Engaging in conduct that subverts or attempts to subvert any examination (e.g., NAPLEX or MPJE) or examination process required for a license to practice pharmacy. Conduct that subverts or attempts to subvert the pharmacist licensing examination process includes but is not limited to:
    a. Copying, retaining, repeating, or transmitting in any manner the questions contained in any examination administered by the Board or questions contained in a question pool of any examination administered by the Board;
    b. Copying or attempting to copy another candidate's answers to any questions on any examination required for a license to practice pharmacy;
    c. Obtaining or attempting to obtain confidential examination materials compiled by testing services or the Board;
    d. Impersonating or acting as a proxy for another in any examination required for a license to practice pharmacy;
    e. Requesting or allowing another to impersonate or act as a proxy in any examination required for a license to practice pharmacy; or
    f. Violating or attempting to violate the security of examination materials or the examination process in any manner;
19. Violating the provisions of an Agreed Board Order or Board Order;
20. Dispensing a prescription drug while not acting in the usual course of professional pharmacy practice;
21. Failing to provide or providing false or fraudulent information on any application, notification, or other document required under the Texas Pharmacy Act, Dangerous Drug Act, Controlled Substances Act, or rules under these Acts;
22. Demonstrating abusive, intimidating, or threatening behavior toward a Board member or employee during the performance of such person's lawful duties;
23. Failing to establish or maintain effective controls against the diversion or loss of controlled substances or dangerous drugs, loss of controlled substance records, or failure to ensure that controlled substances or dangerous drugs are dispensed in compliance with state and federal laws or rules by a pharmacist who is:
    a. A pharmacist-in-charge;
    b. A sole proprietor or individual owner of a pharmacy;
    c. A partner in the ownership of a pharmacy;
    d. A managing officer of a corporation, association, or joint-stock company owning a pharmacy; or
    e. A pharmacist listed in 23.b.–d. above is equally responsible with the pharmacist-in-charge to ensure the employee pharmacists and the pharmacy are in compliance with all laws relating to controlled substances or dangerous drugs;
24. Failing to correct the issues identified in a warning notice by the specified time;
25. Being the subject of civil fines imposed by a court as a result of violating the Controlled Substances Act or Dangerous Drug Act;
26. Selling, purchasing, trading, or offering to sell, purchase, or trade prescription drug samples; provided, however, this paragraph does not apply to:

a. Prescription drugs provided by a manufacturer as starter prescriptions or as replacements for such manufacturer's outdated drugs;
b. Prescription drugs provided by a manufacturer in replacement for such manufacturer's drugs that were dispensed pursuant to written starter prescriptions; or
c. Prescription drug samples possessed by a pharmacy of a healthcare entity which provides health care primarily to indigent or low-income patients at no or reduced cost and if:
   (1) The samples are possessed in compliance with the Prescription Drug Marketing Act of 1987;
   (2) The pharmacy is owned by a charitable organization described in the Internal Revenue Code of 1986, 501(c)(3) or by a city, state, or county government; and
   (3) The samples are for dispensing or provision at no charge to patients of such a healthcare entity;
27. Selling, purchasing, trading, or offering to sell, purchase, or trade prescription drugs:
    a. Sold for export use only;
    b. Purchased by a public or private hospital or other healthcare entity;
    c. Donated or supplied at a reduced price to a charitable organization described in the Internal Revenue Code of 1986, 501(c)(3); or
    d. Provided that 27.a.–c. above do not apply to:
       (1) The purchase or other acquisition by a hospital or other healthcare entity which is a member of a group purchasing organization or from other hospitals or healthcare entities which are members of such an organization;
       (2) The sale, purchase, or trade of a drug or an offer to sell, purchase, or trade a drug by an organization described in 27.c. above to a nonprofit affiliate of the organization to the extent otherwise permitted by law;
       (3) The sale, purchase, or trade of a drug or an offer to sell, purchase, or trade a drug among hospitals or other healthcare entities which are under common control;
       (4) The sale, purchase, or trade of a drug or an offer to sell, purchase, or trade a drug for emergency medical reasons including the transfer of a drug between pharmacies to alleviate temporary shortages of the drug arising from delays in or interruptions of regular distribution schedules; or
       (5) The dispensing of a prescription drug pursuant to a valid prescription drug order to the extent otherwise permitted by law;
28. Selling, purchasing, or trading or offering to sell, purchase, or trade:
    a. Misbranded prescription drugs or
    b. Prescription drugs beyond the manufacturer's expiration date;
29. Failing to respond and to provide all requested records within the time specified in an audit of continuing education records under Board Rule 295.8 (Continuing Education Requirements); or
30. Allowing an individual whose license to practice pharmacy either as a pharmacist or a pharmacist intern or a pharmacy technician or a pharmacy technician trainee whose registration has been disciplined by the Board resulting in the license or registration being revoked, retired, surrendered, denied, or suspended to have access to prescription drugs in a pharmacy.

(Continued from Section 565.001A.)
3. Engaged in gross immorality as defined by Board rule;

Board of Pharmacy Rule 281.7.B. Gross Immorality

Gross immorality includes but is not limited to:
1. Conduct which is willful, flagrant, and shameless and which shows moral indifference to community standards;
2. Engaging in an act which is a felony;
3. Engaging in an act that constitutes sexually deviant behavior; or
4. Being required to register with the Department of Public Safety as a sex offender under Chapter 62, Code of Criminal Procedure.

(Continued from Section 565.001A.)
4. Developed an incapacity that prevents or could prevent the applicant or license holder from practicing pharmacy with reasonable skill, competence, and safety to the public;
5. Engaged in fraud, deceit, or misrepresentation as defined by Board rule in practicing pharmacy or in seeking a license to practice pharmacy;

Board of Pharmacy Rule 281.7.C. Fraud, Deceit, or Misrepresentation

1. Fraud means an intentional perversion of truth for the purpose of inducing another in reliance upon it to part with some valuable thing belonging to him or her or to surrender a legal right or to issue a license. Fraud also means a false representation of a matter of fact whether by words or conduct, by false or misleading allegations, or by concealment of that which should have been disclosed which deceives or is intended to deceive another.
2. Deceit means the assertion as a fact of that which is not true by any means whatsoever to deceive or defraud another.
3. Misrepresentation means a manifestation by words or other conduct which is a false representation of a matter of fact.

(Continued from Section 565.001A.)
6. Been convicted of or placed on deferred adjudication community supervision or deferred disposition or the applicable federal equivalent for:
    a. A misdemeanor
        (1) Involving moral turpitude or
        (2) Under the Texas Dangerous Drug Act, Texas Controlled Substances Act, or Federal Controlled Substances Act or
    b. A felony;
7. Used alcohol or drugs in an intemperate manner that in the Board's opinion could endanger a patient's life;
8. Failed to maintain records required by this Act or failed to maintain complete and accurate records of purchases or disposals of drugs listed in Chapter 481 (TCSA) or 483 (TDDA), Health and Safety Code, or the Comprehensive Drug Abuse Prevention and Control Act of 1970 (FCSA);
9. Violated any provision of:
    a. Chapter 481 (TCSA) or 483 (TDDA), Health and Safety Code, or the Comprehensive Drug Abuse Prevention and Control Act of 1970 (FCSA) or rules relating to one of those laws;
    b. Sections 485.031, 485.032, 485.033, 485.034, or 485.035 (Abusable Volatile Chemicals), Health and Safety Code; or
    c. A rule adopted under Section 485.011 (Sale of Abusable Volatile Chemicals), Health and Safety Code;

10. Aided or abetted an unlicensed person in the practice of pharmacy if the pharmacist knew or reasonably should have known that the person was unlicensed at the time;
11. Refused entry into a pharmacy for an inspection authorized by this Act if the pharmacist received notification from which the pharmacist knew or reasonably should have known that the attempted inspection was authorized;
12. Violated any pharmacy or drug statute or rule of this state, another state, or the United States;
13. Been negligent in the practice of pharmacy;
14. Failed to submit to an examination after hearing and being ordered to do so by the Board under Section 565.052 of the Act;
15. Dispensed a prescription drug while acting outside the usual course and scope of professional practice;
16. Been disciplined by the regulatory board of another state for conduct substantially equivalent to conduct described under this Act;
17. Violated a disciplinary order including a confidential order or contract under the program to aid impaired pharmacists and pharmacy students under Chapter 564 of the Act;
18. Failed to adequately supervise a task delegated to a pharmacy technician or pharmacy technician trainee;
19. Inappropriately delegated a task to a pharmacy technician or a pharmacy technician trainee;
20. Been responsible for a drug audit shortage; or
21. Been convicted or adjudicated of a criminal offense that requires registration as a sex offender under Chapter 62, Code of Criminal Procedure.

Note: Although it is not included in this section of the Act and rules, another law requires all Texas licensing agencies (including TSBP) to suspend a person's license for failure to pay child support.

(Continued from Section 565.001)
B. A certified copy of the record of the state taking action described by A.16. above is conclusive evidence of the action taken by that state.

Section 565.002 Applicant for or Holder of a Pharmacy License
A. The Board may discipline an applicant for or the holder of a pharmacy license, including a Class E license subject to Section 565.003 of the Act, if the Board finds that the applicant or license holder has:
1. Been convicted of or placed on deferred adjudication community supervision or deferred disposition or the applicable federal equivalent for
   a. A misdemeanor
      (1) Involving moral turpitude or
      (2) Under Chapter 481 (TCSA) or 483 (TDDA), Health and Safety Code, or the Comprehensive Drug Abuse Prevention and Control Act of 1970 (FCSA) or
   b. A felony;
2. Advertised a prescription drug or device in a deceitful, misleading, or fraudulent manner;
3. Violated any provision of this Act or any rule adopted under this Act or an owner or employee of a pharmacy has violated any provision of this Act or any rule adopted under this Act;
4. Sold without legal authorization a prescription drug or device to a person other than:
   a. A pharmacy licensed by the Board;
   b. A practitioner;

Notes

      c. A person who procures a prescription drug or device for lawful research, teaching, or testing and not for resale;
      d. A manufacturer or wholesaler licensed by the Commissioner of Public Health as required by Chapter 431 (Texas Food, Drug, and Cosmetic Act), Health and Safety Code; or
      e. A carrier or warehouseman;
5. Allowed an employee who is not a pharmacist to practice pharmacy;
6. Sold an adulterated or misbranded prescription or nonprescription drug; or
7. Failed to engage in or ceased to engage in the business described in the application for a license;

Board of Pharmacy Rule 291.11
Operation of a Pharmacy

      a. "Failure to engage in the business described in the application for a license" means the holder of a pharmacy license has not commenced operating the pharmacy within six months of the date of issuance of the license.
      b. "Ceased to engage in the business described in the application for a license" means the holder of a pharmacy license, once it has been in operation, discontinues operating the pharmacy for a period of 30 days or longer unless the pharmacy experiences a fire or disaster, in which case the pharmacy must comply with Board Rule 291.3(f) (Notifications).
      c. "Operating the pharmacy" means the pharmacy shall demonstrate observable pharmacy business activity on a regular, routine basis including a sufficient number of transactions of receiving, processing, or dispensing prescription drug orders or medication drug orders.
      d. No person may operate a pharmacy in a personal residence.

(Continued from Section 565.002)

8. Failed to maintain records as required by this Act, Chapter 481 or 483, Health and Safety Code, the Comprehensive Drug Abuse Prevention and Control Act of 1970, or any rule adopted under this Act or Chapter 483, Health and Safety Code;
9. Failed to establish and maintain effective controls against diversion of prescription drugs into other than a legitimate medical, scientific, or industrial channel as provided by this Act, another state law or rule, or a federal law or rule;
10. Engaged in fraud, deceit, or misrepresentation as defined by Board rule in:
    a. Operating a pharmacy;
    b. Applying for a license to operate a pharmacy; or
    c. Dispensing drugs for nontherapeutic purposes;
11. Violated a disciplinary order;
12. Been responsible for a drug audit shortage;
13. Been disciplined by the regulatory board of another state for conduct substantially equivalent to conduct described under this subsection; or
14. Waived, discounted, or reduced or offered to waive, discount, or reduce a patient copayment or deductible for a compounded drug in the absence of:
    a. A legitimate, documented financial hardship of the patient or
    b. Evidence of a good faith effort to collect the copayment or deductible from the patient.

B. This subsection applies only to an applicant or license holder that is a legal business entity. The Board may discipline an applicant for or the holder of a pharmacy license including a Class E (nonresident) pharmacy license if the Board

finds that a managing officer of the applicant or license holder has been convicted of or placed on deferred adjudication community supervision or deferred disposition or the applicable federal equivalent for:
1. A misdemeanor
   a. Involving moral turpitude or
   b. Under Chapter 481 or 483, Health and Safety Code, or the Comprehensive Drug Abuse Prevention and Control Act of 1970 or
2. Any felony.
C. A certified copy of the record of the state taking action described by A.13. above is conclusive evidence of the action taken by that state.

Board of Pharmacy Rule 281.8
Grounds for Discipline for a Pharmacy License

A. A pharmacy license is subject to discipline if a pharmacy fails to establish and maintain effective controls against diversion of prescription drugs due to:
   1. Inadequate security or procedures to prevent unauthorized access to prescription drugs and
   2. Inadequate security or procedures to prevent diversion of prescription drugs.
B. It is grounds for discipline for a pharmacy license when:
   1. During the time an individual's license to practice pharmacy either as a pharmacist or an intern or a pharmacy technician's registration has been disciplined by the Board resulting in the license or registration being revoked, retired, surrendered, denied, or suspended, the pharmacy employs or allows that individual access to prescription drugs.
   2. The pharmacy possesses or engages in the sale, purchase, or trade or the offer to sell, purchase, or trade prescription drug samples. (B.2. does not apply to prescription drugs provided by a manufacturer as starter prescriptions or to samples possessed by healthcare entities that provide indigent care as long as the pharmacy is owned by a charitable organization and samples are dispensed at no charge.)
   3. The pharmacy possesses or engages in the sale, purchase, or trade or the offer to sell, purchase, or trade prescription drugs in violation of the Prescription Drug Marketing Act (i.e., drugs sold for export only, drugs purchased by a public or private hospital or other healthcare entity, or drugs donated or supplied at a reduced price to charitable organizations).
   4. The pharmacy engages in the sale, purchase, or trade or the offer to sell, purchase, or trade of misbranded products or prescription drugs beyond the manufacturer's expiration date.
   5. The owner or managing officer has previously been disciplined by the Board.
   6. A nonresident pharmacy fails to reimburse the Board or its designee for all expenses including travel incurred by the Board in inspecting the nonresident pharmacy as specified in Section 556.0551 of the Act.
   7. The owner, managing officer(s), or other pharmacy employee(s) displays abusive, intimidating, or threatening behavior toward a Board member or employee during the performance of such member's or employee's lawful duties.
   8. The pharmacy waived, discounted, or reduced or offered to waive, discount, or reduce a patient copayment or deductible for a compounded drug in the absence of:
      a. A legitimate, documented financial hardship of the patient or
      b. Evidence of a good faith effort to collect the copayment or deductible from the patient.

Chapter 568 Pharmacy Technicians
(Selected Disciplinary Provisions)

Section 568.003 Grounds for Disciplinary Action

A. The Board may take disciplinary action under Section 568.0035 of the Act against an applicant for or the holder of a current or expired pharmacy technician or pharmacy technician trainee registration if the Board determines that the applicant or registrant has:
1. Violated this Act or a rule adopted under this Act;
2. Engaged in gross immorality as that term is defined by the rules of the Board;
3. Engaged in any fraud, deceit, or misrepresentation as those terms are defined by the rules of the Board in seeking a registration to act as a pharmacy technician or pharmacy technician trainee;
4. Been convicted of or placed on deferred adjudication community supervision or deferred disposition or the applicable federal equivalent for:
   a. A misdemeanor
      (1) Involving moral turpitude or
      (2) Under Chapter 481 or 483, Health and Safety Code, or the Comprehensive Drug Abuse Prevention and Control Act of 1970; or
   b. Any felony;
5. Developed an incapacity that prevents the applicant or registrant from practicing as a pharmacy technician or pharmacy technician trainee with reasonable skill, competence, and safety to the public;
6. Violated
   a. Chapter 481 (Controlled Substances Act) or 483 (Dangerous Drug Act), Health and Safety Code, or rules relating to those chapters;
   b. Sections 485.031–485.035 (Abusable Volatile Chemicals), Health and Safety Code; or
   c. A rule adopted under Section 485.011 (Sale of Abusable Volatile Chemicals), Health and Safety Code;
7. Violated the pharmacy or drug laws or rules of this state, another state, or the United States;
8. Performed duties in a pharmacy that only a pharmacist may perform as defined by the rules of the Board;
9. Used alcohol or drugs in an intemperate manner that in the Board's opinion could endanger a patient's life;
10. Engaged in negligent, unreasonable, or inappropriate conduct when working in a pharmacy;
11. Violated a disciplinary order;
12. Been convicted or adjudicated of a criminal offense that requires registration as a sex offender under Chapter 62, Code of Criminal Procedure; or
13. Been disciplined by a pharmacy or other health regulatory board of this state or another state for conduct substantially equivalent to conduct described by this Act.

B. A certified copy of the record of a state taking action described by A.13. above is conclusive evidence of the action taken by the state.

Board of Pharmacy Rule 281.9
Grounds for Discipline for a Pharmacy Technician
or a Pharmacy Technician Trainee

A. Pharmacy technicians and pharmacy technician trainees shall be subject to all disciplinary grounds set forth in Section 568.003 of the Act.

B. For the purpose of Section 568.003A.10. of the Act, "negligent, unreasonable, or inappropriate conduct" shall include but not be limited to:
   1. Delivering or offering to deliver a prescription drug or device in violation of this Act, the Controlled Substances Act, the Dangerous Drug Act, or rules under these Acts;
   2. Acquiring or possessing or attempting to acquire or possess prescription drugs in violation of this Act, the Controlled Substances Act, the Dangerous Drug Act, or rules adopted pursuant to these Acts;
   3. Failing to perform the duties of a pharmacy technician or pharmacy technician trainee in an acceptable manner consistent with the public health and welfare which contributes to a prescription not being dispensed or delivered accurately;
   4. Obstructing a Board employee in the lawful performance of his or her duties of enforcing the Act;
   5. Violating the provisions of an Agreed Board Order or Board Order including accessing prescription drugs with a revoked or suspended pharmacy technician or pharmacy technician trainee registration;
   6. Demonstrating abusive, intimidating, or threatening behavior toward a Board member or employee during the performance of such person's lawful duties; or
   7. Failing to respond and to provide all requested records within the time specified in an audit of continuing education records under Board Rule 297.8 (Continuing Education Requirements).
C. For the purpose of Section 568.003A.2. of the Act, the term "gross immorality" shall include but not be limited to:
   1. Demonstrating conduct which is willful, flagrant, or shameless and which shows a moral indifference to standards of the community;
   2. Engaging in an act that constitutes sexually deviant behavior; or
   3. Being required to register with the Department of Public Safety as a sex offender under Chapter 62, Code of Criminal Procedure.
D. For the purpose of Section 568.003A.3. of the Act, the terms "fraud," "deceit," or "misrepresentation" shall apply to an individual seeking a registration as a pharmacy technician, as well as making an application to any entity that certifies or registers pharmacy technicians, and shall be defined as follows:
   1. "Fraud" means an intentional perversion of truth for the purpose of inducing the Board in reliance upon it to issue a registration; a false representation of a matter of fact, whether by words or by conduct, by false or misleading allegations or by concealment of that which should have been disclosed which deceives or is intended to deceive the Board.
   2. "Deceit" means the assertion as a fact of that which is not true by any means whatsoever to deceive or defraud the Board.
   3. "Misrepresentation" means a manifestation by words or other conduct which is a false representation of a matter of fact.

Section 568.0035 Discipline Authorized and Effect on a Pharmacy Technician Trainee
A. On a determination that a ground for discipline exists under Section 568.003 of the Act, the Board may:
   1. Suspend the person's registration;
   2. Revoke the person's registration;
   3. Restrict the person's registration to prohibit the person from performing certain acts or from practicing as a pharmacy technician or a pharmacy technician trainee in a particular manner for a term and under conditions determined by the Board;
   4. Impose an administrative penalty under Chapter 566 of the Act;
   5. Refuse to issue or renew the person's registration;

6. Place the offender's registration on probation and require supervision by the Board for a period determined by the Board and impose a requirement that the registrant:
    a. Report regularly to the Board on matters that are the basis of the probation;
    b. Limit practice to the areas prescribed by the Board;
    c. Continue or review professional education until the registrant attains a degree of skill satisfactory to the Board in each area that is the basis of the probation; or
    d. Pay the Board a probation fee to defray the costs of monitoring the registrant during the period of probation;
7. Reprimand the person;
8. Retire the person's registration as provided by Board rule; or
9. Impose more than one of the sanctions listed in this section.

B. A disciplinary action affecting the registration of a pharmacy technician trainee remains in effect if the trainee obtains registration as a pharmacy technician.

Section 568.0036 Submission to a Mental or Physical Examination
A. This section applies to a pharmacy technician, pharmacy technician applicant, pharmacy technician trainee, or pharmacy technician trainee applicant.
B. In enforcing Section 568.003A.5. or 7. of the Act, the Board or an authorized agent of the Board, on probable cause as determined by the Board or agent, may request a person subject to this section to submit to a mental or physical examination by a physician or other healthcare professional designated by the Board.
C. If the person refuses to submit to the examination, the Board or the executive director of the Board shall:
    1. Issue an order requiring the person to show cause why the person will not submit to the examination and
    2. Schedule a hearing before a panel of three members of the Board appointed by the president of the Board on the order no later than the 30th day after the date notice of the order is served on the person under D. below.
D. The person shall be notified by either personal service or certified mail with return receipt requested.
E. At the hearing, the person and the person's counsel may present testimony or other evidence to show why the person should not be required to submit to the examination. The person has the burden of proof to show why the person should not be required to submit to the examination.
F. After the hearing, as applicable, the panel shall by order:
    1. Require the person to submit to the examination no later than the 60th day after the date of the order or
    2. Withdraw the request for examination.

Section 568.0037 Temporary Suspension or Restriction of Registration
A. The president of the Board shall appoint a disciplinary panel consisting of three Board members to determine whether a registration under this chapter should be temporarily suspended or restricted. If a majority of the panel determines from evidence or information presented to the panel that the registrant by continuation in practice as a pharmacy technician or pharmacy technician trainee would constitute a continuing threat to the public welfare, the panel shall temporarily suspend or restrict the registration as provided by B. below.
B. A disciplinary panel may temporarily suspend or restrict the registration:
    1. After a hearing conducted by the panel after the 10th day after the date notice of the hearing is provided to the registrant or
    2. Without notice or hearing if, at the time the suspension or restriction is ordered, a hearing before the panel is scheduled to be held no later than the

14th day after the date of the temporary suspension or restriction to determine whether the suspension or restriction should be continued.
C. No later than the 90th day after the date of the temporary suspension or restriction, the Board shall initiate a disciplinary action under this chapter, and a contested case hearing shall be held by the State Office of Administrative Hearings. If the State Office of Administrative Hearings does not hold the hearing in the time required, the suspended or restricted registration is automatically reinstated.
D. Notwithstanding Chapter 551, Government Code (Texas Open Meetings Act), the disciplinary panel may hold a meeting by telephone conference call if immediate action is required and if convening the panel at one location is inconvenient for any member of the disciplinary panel.

SUBCHAPTER B. Disciplinary Actions and Procedures

Section 565.051 Discipline Authorized

On a determination that a ground for discipline exists under Subchapter A or that a violation of this Act or a rule adopted under this Act has been committed by a license holder or applicant for a license or renewal of a license, the Board may:
1. Suspend the person's license;
2. Revoke the person's license;
3. Restrict the person's license to prohibit the person from performing certain acts or from practicing pharmacy or operating a pharmacy in a particular manner for a term and under conditions determined by the Board;
4. Impose an administrative penalty (fine) under Chapter 566 of the Act;
5. Refuse to issue or renew the person's license;
6. Place the offender's license on probation and supervision by the Board for a period determined by the Board and impose a requirement that the license holder:
    a. Report regularly to the Board on matters that are the basis of the probation;
    b. Limit practice to the areas prescribed by the Board;
    c. Continue or review professional education until the license holder attains a degree of skill satisfactory to the Board in each area that is the basis of the probation; or
    d. Pay the Board a probation fee to defray the costs of monitoring the license holder during the period of probation;
7. Reprimand the person;
8. Retire the person's license as provided by Board rule; or
9. Impose more than one of the sanctions listed in this Act.

Board of Pharmacy Rule 281.61
Definitions of Discipline Authorized

For the purpose of Section 565.051 (applies to Pharmacists and Pharmacies) and Section 568.003 and 568.0035 (apply to Pharmacy Technicians and Pharmacy Technician Trainees) of the Act:
1. "Probation" means a period of supervision by the Board imposed against a license or registration for a term and under conditions as determined by the Board including a probation fee.
2. "Reprimand" means a public and formal censure against a license or registration.
3. "Restrict" means to limit, confine, abridge, narrow, or restrain a license or registration for a term and under conditions determined by the Board.
4. "Revoke" means a license or registration is void and may not be reissued provided, however, upon the expiration of 12 months from and after the

effective date of the order revoking a license or registration, the license or registration may be reinstated by the Board upon the successful completion of any requirements by the Board.
5. "Suspend" means a license or registration is of no further force and effect for a period of time as determined by the Board.
6. "Retire" means a license or registration has been withdrawn and is of no further force and effect.
7. "Administrative Penalty" means a fine.

Section 565.052 Submission to a Mental or Physical Examination
A. In enforcing Section 565.001A.4. or 7. of the Act, the Board or an authorized agent of the Board on probable cause, as determined by the Board or agent, shall request a pharmacist, pharmacist applicant, pharmacist intern, or pharmacist intern applicant to submit to a mental or physical examination by a physician or other healthcare professional designated by the Board.
B. If the pharmacist, pharmacist applicant, pharmacist intern, or pharmacist intern applicant refuses to submit to the examination, the Board or the executive director of the Board shall issue an order requiring the pharmacist, pharmacist applicant, pharmacist intern, or pharmacist intern applicant to show cause why the pharmacist, pharmacist applicant, pharmacist intern, or pharmacist intern applicant will not submit to the examination. In addition, the Board or the executive director of the Board shall schedule a hearing before a panel of three members of the Board appointed by the president of the Board on the order no later than the 30th day after the date notice is served on the pharmacist, pharmacist applicant, pharmacist intern, or pharmacist intern applicant. The pharmacist, pharmacist applicant, pharmacist intern, or pharmacist intern applicant shall be notified by either personal service or certified mail with return receipt requested.
C. At the hearing, the pharmacist, pharmacist applicant, pharmacist intern, or pharmacist intern applicant and an attorney are entitled to present testimony or other evidence to show why the pharmacist, pharmacist applicant, pharmacist intern, or pharmacist intern applicant should not be required to submit to the examination. The pharmacist, pharmacist applicant, pharmacist intern, or pharmacist intern applicant has the burden of proof to show why the pharmacist, pharmacist applicant, pharmacist intern, or pharmacist intern applicant should not be required to submit to the examination.
D. After the hearing, the panel shall by order require the pharmacist, pharmacist applicant, pharmacist intern, or pharmacist intern applicant to submit to the examination no later than the 60th day after the date of the order or withdraw the request for examination as applicable.

Board of Pharmacy Rule 281.6
Mental or Physical Examination

For the purposes of Sections 565.001A.4., 565.052, 568.003A.5., and 568.0036 of the Act, the following shall be applied.
1. The Board may discipline an applicant, licensee, or registrant if the Board finds that the applicant, licensee, or registrant has developed a mental or physical incapacity that in the estimation of the Board would prevent a pharmacist from engaging in the practice of pharmacy or a pharmacy technician or pharmacy technician trainee from practicing with a level of skill and competence that ensures the public health, safety, and welfare.
2. Upon a finding of probable cause as determined by the Board or an authorized agent of the Board that the applicant, licensee, or registrant has

developed an incapacity that in the estimation of the Board would prevent a pharmacist from engaging in the practice of pharmacy or a pharmacy technician or pharmacy technician trainee from practicing with a level of skill and competence that ensures the public health, safety, and welfare, the following is applicable:

  a. The executive director, legal counsel of the agency, or other representative of the agency as designated by the executive director shall request the applicant, licensee, or registrant to submit to a mental or physical examination by a physician or other healthcare professional designated by the Board. The individual providing the examination shall be approved by the Board. Such examination shall be coordinated through the entity that contracts with the Board to aid impaired pharmacists and pharmacy students. The applicant, licensee, or registrant shall follow the procedures of such entity for each examination conducted as follows:
     (1) Provide the entity with written notice of the appointment at least three days prior to the appointment;
     (2) Execute and return to the entity an authorization for release of relevant information on the form required by the entity within ten days of receipt of request for the release from the entity; and
     (3) Follow all other procedures of the entity for each examination.
  b. The applicant, licensee, or registrant shall be notified in writing by either personal service or certified mail with return receipt requested of the request to submit to the examination.
  c. The applicant, licensee, or registrant shall submit to the examination within 30 days of the date of the receipt of the request.
  d. The applicant, licensee, or registrant shall authorize the release of the results of the examination, and the results shall be submitted to the Board within 15 days of the date of the examination.
3. If the applicant, licensee, or registrant does not comply with the provisions of 2. above, the following is applicable.
  a. The executive director shall cause to be issued an order requiring the applicant, licensee, or registrant to show cause why he or she will not submit to the examination.
  b. The executive director shall schedule a hearing on the order before a panel of three members of the Board appointed by the president of the Board within 30 days after notice is served on the applicant, licensee, or registrant.
  c. The applicant, licensee, or registrant shall be notified of the hearing by either personal service or certified mail with return receipt requested.
  d. At the hearing, the applicant, licensee, or registrant has the burden of proof once probable cause has been established by the Board as required by Section 565.062 of the Act to rebut the probable cause. The applicant, licensee, or registrant and, if applicable, the applicant's, licensee's, or registrant's attorney are entitled to present testimony and other evidence to show why probable cause has not been established requiring the applicant, licensee, or registrant to submit to the examination. An evaluation that has not been approved by the Board and coordinated by the entity that contracts with the Board to aid impaired pharmacists and pharmacy students according to its procedure cannot be admitted at the hearing in lieu of one that has been properly approved and coordinated.
  e. After the hearing, the panel shall issue an order either requiring the applicant, licensee, or registrant to submit to the examination no later than the 60th day after the date of the order or withdrawing the request for examination, as applicable.

Section 565.055 Confidentiality of Information Relating to an Investigation
A. The Board or the Board's authorized representative may investigate and gather evidence concerning any alleged violation of this Act or a Board rule.
B. Information or material compiled by the Board in connection with an investigation including an investigative file of the Board is confidential and not subject to:
   1. Disclosure under Chapter 552, Government Code (Texas Public Information Act) or
   2. Any means of legal compulsion for release including disclosure, discovery, or subpoena to anyone other than the Board or a Board employee or a Board agent involved in the discipline of a license holder.
C. Notwithstanding B. above, information or material compiled by the Board in connection with an investigation may be disclosed:
   1. During any proceeding conducted by the State Office of Administrative Hearings to the Board or a panel of the Board or in a subsequent trial or appeal of a Board action or order;
   2. To a person providing a service to the Board related to a disciplinary proceeding against an applicant or license holder or in a subsequent trial or appeal, if the information is necessary for preparation for or a presentation in the proceeding;
   3. To an entity in another jurisdiction that licenses or disciplines pharmacists or pharmacies or registers or disciplines pharmacy technicians or pharmacy technician trainees;
   4. To a pharmaceutical or pharmacy peer review committee as described under Chapter 564 of the Act;
   5. To a law enforcement agency;
   6. To a person engaged in bona fide research if all information identifying a specific individual has been deleted; or
   7. To an entity that administers a Board-approved pharmacy technician certification examination.

Section 565.0551 Surety Bond
A. The executive director of the Board may require a license holder to submit a surety bond to the Board in an amount as prescribed by Board rule not to exceed $25,000.
B. The Board may use a pharmacy's surety bond to secure the payment of a fine, fee, or penalty imposed on the pharmacy or costs incurred by the Board in conducting an investigation of the pharmacy only under Section 565.002A.7. or 10. if the pharmacy fails to pay the fine, fee, penalty, or cost as prescribed by Board rule.

Section 565.057 Monitoring of a License Holder
A. The Board shall develop a policy and procedure for monitoring a license holder's compliance with this Act.
B. A policy or procedure adopted under this section must include a procedure to:
   1. Monitor for compliance a license holder who is ordered by the Board to perform a certain act and
   2. Identify and monitor a license holder who represents a risk to the public.

Section 565.058 Subpoena Authority
A. The Board or an officer of the Board may:
   1. Issue subpoenas ad testificandum to compel the attendance of witnesses or subpoenas duces tecum to compel the production of items including books, records, or documents;
   2. Administer oaths; and
   3. Take testimony concerning matters in the Board's or officer's jurisdiction.
B. A person designated in the subpoena may serve the subpoena.

Board of Pharmacy Rule 281.23
Subpoenas

A. A subpoena issued by the executive director under the authority of Section 565.058 of the Act is considered by the Board to be a ministerial act. Such a subpoena shall be used to obtain information and testimony at the request of Board staff.

B. If a subpoena is requested by an applicant, licensee, or registrant under Chapter 2001.089 of the Texas Administrative Procedures Act, a showing of good cause shall be made to the executive director. Such a showing shall be by submission of a written request for the subpoena indicating the purpose of the subpoena and indicating that the subpoena is not requested in bad faith. In addition, the requesting party shall aver (i.e., assert or represent) that the subpoena:
   1. Does not request information that is privileged;
   2. Requests information relevant to the contested case;
   3. Is not an undue burden; and
   4. Is sufficiently specific.

C. Once the requesting party has complied with the requirements in B. above, the executive director may issue the subpoena.

D. If the requesting party, the subpoenaed party, any other party to the contested case, or any person or entity affected by the subpoena objects, a challenge to the subpoena shall be filed with an Administrative Law Judge at the State Office of Administrative Hearings.

Section 565.059 Temporary Suspension or Restriction of a License

A. The president of the Board shall appoint a three-member disciplinary panel consisting of Board members to determine whether a license under this Act should be temporarily suspended or restricted. If a majority of the disciplinary panel determines from evidence or information presented to the panel that the holder of a license by continuation in the practice of pharmacy or in the operation of a pharmacy would constitute a continuing threat to the public welfare, the panel shall temporarily suspend or restrict the license as provided by B. below.

B. The disciplinary panel may temporarily suspend or restrict the license:
   1. After a hearing conducted by the panel after the 10th day after the date of notice of the hearing is provided to the license holder or
   2. Without notice or hearing if, at the time the suspension or restriction is ordered, a hearing before the panel is scheduled to be held no later than the 14th day after the date of the temporary suspension or restriction to determine whether the suspension or restriction should be continued.

C. No later than the 90th day after the date of the temporary suspension or restriction, the Board shall initiate a disciplinary action against the license holder, and a contested case hearing shall be held by the State Office of Administrative Hearings. If the State Office of Administrative Hearings does not hold the hearing in the time required by the Act, the suspended or restricted license is automatically reinstated.

D. Notwithstanding Chapter 551 (Open Records Act), Government Code, the disciplinary panel may hold a meeting by telephone conference call if immediate action is required and convening of the panel at one location is inconvenient for any member of the disciplinary panel.

Section 565.0591 Revocation of Pharmacy License for Failure to Operate

A. On discovery by the Board that a pharmacy licensed under Chapter 560 has ceased to operate for a period of 30 days or longer, the Board shall notify the pharmacy that the license will be revoked.

B. The notice must:
   1. Include a statement that the pharmacy license is being revoked for failing to engage in or ceasing to engage in the business described in the application for a license and
   2. Inform the license holder of the license holder's right to a hearing to contest the revocation.
C. No later than the 20th day after the date the license holder receives the notice of revocation under this section, the license holder may submit a written request for a hearing to contest the revocation.
D. If the license holder does not request a hearing within the period prescribed by C. above, the Board shall:
   1. Enter an order revoking the license and
   2. Notify the license holder of the order.
E. If the license holder requests a hearing within the period prescribed by C. above, a panel of three Board members appointed by the president of the Board shall conduct the hearing. At the hearing, the panel shall determine whether the license holder has violated Section 565.002A.7. of the Act (failing to engage or ceasing to engage in the business described in the application for a license).
F. If the panel determines that the license holder committed the violation, the Board shall promptly:
   1. Enter an order revoking the license and
   2. Notify the license holder of the order.
G. The Texas Administrative Procedures Act (Chapter 2001, Government Code) does not apply to a determination under E. above.

Section 565.060 Remedial Plan
A. The Board may issue and establish the terms of a remedial plan to resolve the investigation of a complaint relating to this Act.
B. A remedial plan may not be imposed to resolve a complaint:
   1. Concerning
      a. A death;
      b. A hospitalization;
      c. The commission of a felony; or
      d. Any other matter designated by Board rule or
   2. In which the appropriate resolution may involve a restriction on the manner in which a license holder practices pharmacy.
C. The Board may not issue a remedial plan to resolve a complaint against a license holder if the license holder has entered into a remedial plan with the Board in the preceding 24 months for the resolution of a different complaint relating to this Act.
D. If a license holder complies with and successfully completes the terms of a remediation plan, the Board shall remove all records of the remedial plan from the Board's records at the end of the state fiscal year in which the fifth anniversary of the date the Board issued the terms of the remedial plan occurs.
E. The Board may assess a fee against a license holder participating in a remedial plan in the amount necessary to recover the costs of administering the plan.
F. The Board shall adopt rules necessary to implement this section.

Board of Pharmacy Rule 281.68
Remedial Plan

Note: A remedial plan is not considered disciplinary action, but it is public information. A remedial plan is removed from a licensee's or registrant's record after five years.

A. The Board may issue a remedial plan by agreement with the respondent to resolve the investigation of a complaint relating to the Act unless the complaint involves:
   1. A death;
   2. A hospitalization;
   3. The commission of a felony;
   4. The unlicensed practice of a licensee or registrant;
   5. Audit shortages;
   6. Diversion of controlled substances;
   7. Impairment by chemical abuse or mental or physical illness of a licensee or registrant;
   8. Unauthorized dispensing of a prescription drug;
   9. Gross immorality as defined by the Board;
   10. Engaging in fraud, deceit, or misrepresentation as defined by Board rule;
   11. Disciplinary action by another regulatory board of this state or another state; or
   12. Any other matter determined by the Board.
B. The Board shall not impose a remedial plan if the appropriate resolution of the complaint involves a restriction on the manner in which a license holder practices pharmacy.
C. The Board may not issue a remedial plan to resolve a complaint against a license holder if the license holder has entered into a remedial plan with the Board in the preceding 24 months for the resolution of a different complaint relating to this Act.
D. If a license holder complies with and successfully completes the terms of a remedial plan, the Board shall remove all records of the remedial plan from the Board's records at the end of the state fiscal year in which the fifth anniversary of the date the Board issued the terms of the remedial plan occurs.
E. The Board may assess a fee against a license holder participating in a remedial plan in an amount of $1000 to recover the costs of administering the plan.

Section 565.061 Administrative Procedure
A. Except as provided by Chapter 564 of the Act, a disciplinary action taken by the Board or on the basis of a ground for discipline under this Act is governed by Chapter 2001, Government Code (Texas Administrative Procedures Act), and the rules of practice and procedure before the Board.
B. A final decision of the Board under this chapter is subject to judicial review under Chapter 2001, Government Code (Texas Administrative Procedures Act).

Section 565.062 Burden of Proof
A. In a proceeding under this Act, including a trial or hearing, the state is not required to negate an exemption or exception set forth by this Act in a pleading, including in a complaint, information, or indictment.
B. The burden of going forward with the evidence with respect to an exemption or exception is on the person claiming the benefit of the exemption or exception.
C. In the absence of proof that a person is the authorized holder of an appropriate license issued under this Act, the person is presumed not to be the holder of the license. The presumption is subject to rebuttal by a person charged with an offense under this Act.

Board of Pharmacy Rule 281.31
Burden of Proof

A. In a contested case hearing at the State Office of Administrative Hearings involving grounds for disciplinary action, the Board has the burden to prove

that grounds to discipline the respondent exist. However, the party that claims any exemption or exception, including mitigating factors as specified in Board Rule 281.62, has the burden to prove that the exemption or exception should be applied.
- B. In a contested case hearing at the State Office of Administrative Hearings involving a petition for reinstatement or removal of restriction, the petitioner has the burden to prove that the license should be reinstated or that a restriction on the license should be removed in accordance with Board Rule 281.66.
- C. In a show cause order hearing before a panel of the Board involving an applicant, licensee, or registrant who has been previously ordered by the Board to submit to a mental or physical examination under Section 565.052 or Section 568.0036 of the Act, the applicant, licensee, or registrant has the burden to prove that the applicant, licensee, or registrant should not be required to submit to the examination.

Section 565.063 Liability

This Act does not impose liability on an authorized Board employee or person acting under the supervision of a Board employee or on a state, county, or municipal officer engaged in the lawful enforcement of this Act.

Board of Pharmacy Rule 281.12
Rules Governing Cooperating Practitioners

For the purpose of Section 565.063 of the Act, a person acting under the supervision of a Board employee engaged in the lawful enforcement of the Act shall include, but not be limited to, a practitioner who provides prescriptions for the use in investigations of licensees when such prescriptions are issued by a practitioner at the request of and under the supervision of a Board investigator.

Section 565.064 Construction

This Act does not bar a criminal prosecution for a violation of this Act if the violation is a criminal offense under another law of this state or a law of the United States.

SUBCHAPTER C. Petition for Reinstatement of a License or Removal of a Restriction

Section 565.101 Petition for Reinstatement
- A. A person whose pharmacy license, license to practice pharmacy, pharmacy technician registration, or pharmacy technician trainee registration in this state has been revoked or restricted under this Act, whether voluntarily or by Board action, may, after the first anniversary of the effective date of the revocation or restriction, petition the Board for reinstatement or removal of the restriction of the license or registration.
- B. The petition must be in writing and in the form prescribed by the Board.
- C. A person petitioning for reinstatement has the burden of proof.

Board of Pharmacy Rule 281.66
Application for the Reissuance or Removal of Restrictions of a License or Registration
---

- A. A person whose pharmacy license, pharmacy technician registration, or license or registration to practice pharmacy has been revoked or restricted, whether

voluntary or by action of the Board, may, after 12 months from the effective date of the revocation or restriction, apply to the Board for reinstatement or removal of the restriction of the license or registration.
   1. The application shall be given under oath and on the form prescribed by the Board.
   2. A person applying for reinstatement or removal of restrictions may be required to meet all requirements necessary for the Board to access the criminal history record information including submitting fingerprint information and being responsible for all associated costs.
   3. A person applying for reinstatement or removal of restrictions has the burden of proof.
   4. On an investigation and in a hearing, the Board may in its discretion grant or deny the application or it may modify its original finding to reflect any circumstances that have changed sufficiently to warrant the modification.
   5. If such application is denied by the Board, a subsequent application may not be considered by the Board until 12 months from the date of denial of the previous application.
   6. The Board in its discretion may require a person to pass an examination or examinations to reenter the practice of pharmacy.
B. In reinstatement cases not involving criminal offenses, the Board can consider the following items in determining the reinstatement of a previously revoked or canceled license or registration:
   1. Moral character in the community;
   2. Employment history;
   3. Financial support to his or her family;
   4. Participation in continuing education;
   5. Criminal history;
   6. Offers of employment in a pharmacy;
   7. Involvement in public service;
   8. Failure to comply with Board Order provisions;
   9. Action by other state or federal regulatory agencies;
   10. Any impairment;
   11. Gravity of the offense which resulted in action against the license or registration;
   12. Length of time since license or registration was sanctioned and whether the time period has been sufficient for rehabilitation to occur;
   13. Competency to engage in the practice of pharmacy; and
   14. Other rehabilitation actions taken by the applicant.
C. If a reinstatement case involves criminal offenses, the sanctions specified in Board Rule 281.64 apply.

Section 565.102 Action by the Board
A. On investigation and review of a petition under this Act, the Board may grant or deny the petition or may modify the Board's original finding to reflect a circumstance that has changed sufficiently to warrant the modification.
B. If the Board denies the petition, the Board may not consider a subsequent petition from the petitioner until the first anniversary of the date of denial of the previous petition.

Section 565.103 Condition for Reinstatement or Removal of a Restriction
The Board may require a person to pass one or more examinations to reenter the practice of pharmacy.

Chapter 566 Penalties and Enforcement Provisions
SUBCHAPTER A. Administrative Penalty (Fine)

Section 566.001 Imposition of a Penalty

The Board may impose an administrative penalty (fine) on:
A. A person licensed or regulated under this Act who violates this Act or a rule or order adopted under this Act and
B. An applicant who fails to submit a sworn disclosure statement with an application if required by Section 560.052B.3.
Note: See Chapter D for applicants who must provide a sworn disclosure statement with the application for a pharmacy license.

Section 566.002 Amount of a Penalty

A. The amount of the administrative penalty may not exceed $5,000 for each violation including a violation involving the diversion of a controlled substance.
B. Each day a violation continues or occurs is a separate violation for purposes of imposing the penalty.
C. The amount to the extent possible shall be based on:
   1. The seriousness of the violation, including the nature, circumstances, extent, and gravity of any prohibited act, and the hazard or potential hazard created to the health, safety, or economic welfare of the public;
   2. The economic harm to property or the environment caused by the violation;
   3. The history of previous violations;
   4. The amount necessary to deter a future violation;
   5. Efforts to correct the violation; and
   6. Any other matter that justice may require.
D. The Board by rule shall adopt an administrative penalty schedule for violations of this Act or Board rules to ensure that the amounts of penalties imposed are appropriate to the violation.

Section 566.003 Notice of a Violation

A. If the Board by order determines that a violation occurred and imposes an administrative penalty, the Board shall give notice of the Board's order to the person found to have committed the violation.
B. The notice must include a statement of the person's right to judicial review of the order.

Section 566.004 Options Following a Decision: Pay or Appeal

A. No later than the 30th day after the date the Board's order becomes final, the person shall:
   1. Pay the administrative penalty;
   2. Pay the penalty and file a petition for judicial review contesting the fact of the violation, the amount of the penalty, or both; or
   3. Without paying the penalty, file a petition for judicial review contesting the fact of the violation, the amount of the penalty, or both.
B. Within the 30-day period, a person who acts under A.3. above may:
   1. Stay enforcement of the penalty by:
      a. Paying the penalty to the court for placement in an escrow account or
      b. Paying to the court a supersedeas bond (defendant's appeal bond) that is approved by the court and that:
         (1) Is for the amount of the penalty and
         (2) Is effective until judicial review of the Board's order is final or

2. Request the court to stay enforcement of the penalty by:
   a. Filing with the court a sworn affidavit of the person stating that the person is financially unable to pay the penalty and is financially unable to give the supersedeas bond and
   b. Giving a copy of the affidavit to the executive director by certified mail.
C. If the executive director receives a copy of an affidavit under B.2. above, the executive director may file with the court a contest to the affidavit no later than the fifth day after the date the copy is received.
D. The court shall hold a hearing on the facts alleged in the affidavit as soon as practicable and shall stay the enforcement of the penalty on finding that the alleged facts are true. The person who files an affidavit has the burden of proving that the person is financially unable to pay the penalty and to give a supersedeas bond.

Section 566.005 Collection of a Penalty

If the person does not pay the administrative penalty and the enforcement of the penalty is not stayed, the executive director may refer the matter to the attorney general for collection of the penalty.

Section 566.006 Determination by Court

A. If the court sustains the determination that a violation occurred on appeal, the court may uphold or reduce the amount of the administrative penalty and order the person to pay the full or reduced penalty.
B. If the court does not sustain the determination that a violation occurred, the court shall order that a penalty is not owed.

Section 566.007 Remittance of a Penalty and Interest

A. If after judicial review the administrative penalty is reduced or is not upheld by the court, the court after the judgment becomes final shall:
   1. Order that the appropriate amount plus accrued interest be remitted to the person if the person paid the penalty or
   2. Order the release of the bond in full if the penalty is not upheld or order the release of the bond after the person pays the penalty imposed if the person gave a supersedeas bond.
B. The interest paid under A.1. above is the rate charged on loans to depository institutions by the New York Federal Reserve Bank. The interest shall be paid for the period beginning on the date the penalty is paid and ending on the date the penalty is remitted.

Section 566.008 Effect of Subchapter (Act)

This Act does not limit the Board's ability to impose an administrative penalty under a consent order entered in accordance with Board rules and requirements adopted under Section 565.056 of the Act.

Section 566.009 Administrative Procedure

A. The Board by rule shall prescribe procedures consistent with the provisions of Chapter 2001 (Texas Administrative Procedures Act), Government Code, relating to contested cases by which the Board may impose an administrative penalty.
B. Chapter 2001, Government Code, applies to a proceeding under this Act.

SUBCHAPTER B. Injunctive Relief

Section 566.051 Injunctive Relief

A. The attorney general at the request of the Board may petition a district court for an injunction to prohibit a person who is violating this Act from continuing the violation.
B. Venue in a suit for injunctive relief is in Travis County.

C. After application and a finding that a person is violating this Act, the district court shall grant the injunctive relief that the facts warrant.

Section 566.052 Cease and Desist Order
A. If it appears to the Board that a person is engaging in an act or practice that constitutes the practice of pharmacy without a license or registration under this Act, the Board, after notice and opportunity for a hearing, may issue a cease and desist order prohibiting the person from engaging in the activity.
B. A violation of an order issued under this section constitutes grounds for imposing an administrative penalty under Subchapter A. of Chapter 566 of the Act.

SUBCHAPTER C. Civil Penalty

Section 566.101 Civil Penalty
A. A person who violates the license requirements of this Act is liable to the state for a civil penalty not to exceed $1,000 for each day the violation continues.
B. A person found by the Board to have unlawfully engaged in the practice of pharmacy or unlawfully operated a pharmacy is subject to a civil penalty under this section.

Section 566.102 Collection by the Attorney General
At the request of the Board, the attorney general shall institute an action to collect a civil penalty from a person who has violated this Act or any rule adopted under this Act.

Section 566.103 Collection by District, County, or City Attorney
A. If the attorney general fails to take action before the 31st day after the date of referral from the Board under Section 566.102 of the Act, the Board shall refer the case to the local district attorney, county attorney, or city attorney.
B. The district attorney, county attorney, or city attorney shall file suit in a district court to collect and retain the penalty.

Section 566.104 Venue
Venue for a suit under this Act is in Travis County.

SUBCHAPTER D. Criminal Offenses

Section 566.151 Offenses; Criminal Penalty
A. A person commits an offense if the person violates this Act or any rule adopted under this Act relating to unlawfully engaging in the practice of pharmacy or unlawfully operating a pharmacy.
B. A person commits an offense if the person knowingly violates the licensing requirements of this Act or Sections 558.001, 558.002, or 560.002 of the Act.
C. A person commits an offense if the person violates Section 560.001 or Section 560.003 of the Act.
D. Each day of violation under B. or C. above is a separate offense.
E. An offense under this section is a Class A misdemeanor. The penalty is up to one year in a county jail and/or a fine of up to $4000.

Summary of Texas Pharmacy Administrative Practice and Rules of Procedure
Chapter 281 (Board Rules 281.1–281.68)

Note: The following is a summary of the pertinent processes, procedures, and rules governing the TSBP disciplinary process. For the complete language and rule, see Chapter 281 on the TSBP website.

Four state laws affect TSBP disciplinary procedures, rulemaking procedures, meeting procedures, and availability of records.
- A. Administrative Procedures Act (APA) (Chapter 2001, Texas Government Code). All disciplinary action and rulemaking must be conducted in compliance with the provisions of this law.
- B. Texas Open Meetings Act (Chapter 551, Texas Government Code). All meetings and hearings are open to the public except for:
  1. Executive sessions authorized by the Open Meetings Act;
  2. TSBP deliberations relative to licensee disciplinary actions (however, the Board must vote and announce its decision in open session); and
  3. TSBP disciplinary hearings relating to impaired pharmacists or pharmacy students.
- C. Texas Public Information Act (Chapter 552, Texas Government Code). All records of hearings or meetings are open records except for records relating to executive sessions, impaired pharmacists, licensure information, Board investigative records or complaints, and identity of complainants.
- D. Texas Pharmacy Act and rules. This Act sets out TSBP responsibilities, practice standards, pharmacy standards, and disciplinary grounds and procedures.

Adjudication Procedures to Discipline a Licensee
- A. Institution of Contested Case Proceedings (anytime TSBP initiates disciplinary action against a license).
  1. The Board sends the licensee a Preliminary Notice Letter of the Board's intent to institute disciplinary action, a listing of the alleged violations, and a notice of the licensee's right to schedule a non-public Informal Conference consisting of the following individuals:
     - a. The executive director of the Board;
     - b. Any other staff of the agency that the executive director deems necessary;
     - c. The legal counsel of the Board;
     - d. An assistant attorney general assigned to the Board;
     - e. The affected licensee and/or the authorized representative;
     - f. One Board member (who will recuse himself or herself if the case is heard by an administrative law judge and such judge's decision will be subject to Board consideration); and
     - g. The complainant if he or she wants to be in attendance.

     Note: The Informal Conference is not open to the public. It gives the licensee the opportunity to show compliance with the law. However, the complainant must be provided the opportunity to be heard at the Informal Conference.
  2. Default Order. The Preliminary Notice Letter should never be ignored because failure to respond to the allegations in the Board's Preliminary Notice Letter either by personal appearance at the informal conference or in writing results in the allegations being admitted as true and the recommended sanctions made at the informal conference will be granted by default.

B. Informal Conference.
  1. If an Informal Conference is scheduled by the licensee, the alleged violations may be:
     a. Dismissed with no action taken if compliance with the law can be shown or
     b. Settled by the licensee who consents to an informal disposition of the case by accepting a proposed Agreed Board Order (ABO) which is presented to the Board members.
        (1) If the Board accepts the proposed ABO, the case is settled, and the ABO is in full force and effect. An ABO is a "consent order"; the licensee consents to sanctions but neither admits nor denies guilt.
        (2) If the Board rejects the proposed ABO, the case is scheduled for a formal disciplinary hearing before an Administrative Law Judge (ALJ) of the State Office of Administrative Hearings (SOAH).
        (3) Staff cannot settle a case; they can only make a recommendation.
     (*See procedures for Informal Conferences below.*)
  2. Because an ABO is a consent order (i.e., the licensee agreed to it), it cannot be appealed through the courts.

TSBP Disciplinary Process

Note: The following written communication is sent to licensees and/or their legal counsel prior to an Informal Conference being conducted at the Board's office. This communication explains all aspects of the TSBP disciplinary process.

I. **Informal Conference.**
   The Informal Conference is conducted as follows:
   A. You and/or your attorney will meet with a Board panel including a Board member, the Executive Director, and the Director of Enforcement. The General Counsel will serve as the Board panel's legal counsel.
   B. The General Counsel will explain the procedures of the Informal Conference.
   C. The Board's attorney (i.e., the attorney who sent the Preliminary Notice Letter) will:
      1. Present the allegations set forth in the Preliminary Notice Letter and the supporting documentary evidence that would be introduced in a public hearing if scheduling a hearing is necessary and
      2. Answer any questions that the Board panel may have regarding the allegations against you and/or the supporting documentary evidence.
   D. Any complainant who chooses to attend the Informal Conference will be given an opportunity to speak to the Board panel.
   E. You and/or your attorney will be given the opportunity to discuss any matter relating to the case and to show your compliance with the law. In this regard, the following is applicable:
      1. If compliance with the law is shown, no further action is taken by the Board concerning this matter and the case is dismissed or
      2. If compliance is not shown, you are presented an opportunity to discuss informal disposition.
   F. The Board panel will deliberate to make a recommendation for resolution of the case in accordance with the discipline authorized by the Texas Pharmacy Act such as denial of licensure, reprimand, administrative penalty, restriction, probation, suspension, revocation, or retirement.

II. **Informal Settlement (proposed Agreed Board Order).**
At the conclusion of the Informal Conference, you will be notified of the panel's recommendation for resolution. You may either accept or reject the panel's recommendation for informal settlement.
   A. If you reject the recommendation of the Board panel, the matter will be scheduled for a public hearing at the State Office of Administrative Hearings before an Administrative Law Judge.
   B. If you accept the recommendation of the Board panel, the following is applicable:
      1. A proposed Agreed Board Order (ABO) will be drafted and mailed to you and/or your attorney for review and approval. If you sign and return the proposed ABO, Board staff will present the proposed ABO to the Board (for approval or rejection) at its next scheduled meeting.
      2. If the proposed ABO is approved by the Board, the matter is settled. However, if the proposed ABO is rejected by the Board, the matter will be scheduled for a public hearing.

Note: All proposed ABOs are considered by the Board in open meetings except ABOs concerning pharmacists who are impaired by chemical abuse or mental or physical illness and certain ABOs involving applications for pharmacy and pharmacist licensure. (The Board considers ABOs relating to impaired pharmacists in a non-public Executive Session under the confidentiality provisions in the Texas Pharmacy Act. The executive director has authority to approve certain applicant ABOs according to guidelines set by the Board.)

You should understand that:
   1. It is your choice to attend an Informal Conference.
   2. It is your choice to accept or reject the recommendation of the Board panel at the Informal Conference.
   3. It is the decision of the Board itself whether to accept or reject any proposed resolution.
   4. The Board panel has the authority only to recommend a proposed resolution. The panel may not enter an Order resolving the case.
   5. You have the right to terminate the Informal Conference at any time and the right to appear in a public hearing. The results of any informal disposition (Agreed Board Order or Default Order) or formal disposition (Board Order entered as a result of a public hearing) is public information. Results of an informal or formal disposition will appear in the Board's newsletter and on the Board's website. The only exception is an Order concerning a pharmacist impaired by chemical abuse or mental or physical illness.
   6. A Default Order, based upon the allegations set out in the Preliminary Notice Letter, will be entered by the Board if you do not respond to this letter either by your attendance at the Informal Conference or in writing.
   7. The case will be scheduled for a public hearing if one of the following occurs:
      a. You inform the Board in writing that you decline to schedule an Informal Conference;
      b. You reject the recommendation of the Board panel after the Informal Conference; or
      c. The proposed ABO is rejected by the Board.

III. **Alternative Dispute Resolution (ADR).**
The State Office of Administrative Hearings (SOAH) offers Alternative Dispute Resolution (ADR) such as mediation to resolve TSBP disciplinary cases if recommended by SOAH or if requested by and agreed upon by the licensee and TSBP. ADR is used on a case-by-case basis depending on the facts of the case and the likelihood that

a mediation would result in an outcome agreeable to TSBP and the licensee. The ADR process occurs during the interim period following an Informal Conference (when an agreement could not be reached) and prior to a Formal Disciplinary Hearing. A SOAH Administrative Law Judge conducts the ADR/mediation process. If an agreement is reached through mediation, then the case is considered settled pending approval by the Board. If an agreement cannot be reached through this process, then the case will proceed to a Formal Disciplinary Hearing.
See TSBP Rule 281.16 for details on Alternative Dispute Resolution.

IV. Formal Disciplinary Hearing (Public Hearing).
A. A formal disciplinary hearing is similar to a trial, but it is held at the State Office of Administrative Hearings (SOAH) before an Administrative Law Judge (ALJ) and not before the Board as in many other states.
B. TSBP is represented by the Board's legal counsel and an assistant attorney general who serves as the prosecutor.
C. The licensee is the defendant and may be represented by legal counsel.
D. After the hearing, the ALJ issues Findings of Facts and Conclusions of Law and recommends sanctions against the licensee. If the ALJ finds in favor of the defendant, he or she may recommend no sanctions.
E. The ALJ's recommendations are then presented to the Board, and the Board can accept, modify, or reject the recommendations by issuing a Board Order (BO).
F. A Board Order is appealable through the courts.

V. Confidentiality.
A. Impaired pharmacist or pharmacy technician hearings are not open to the public, and ABOs and BOs pertaining to an impaired pharmacist or pharmacy technician are confidential. However, under the Pharmacy Act, the Board may disclose that the license of a pharmacist (or registration of a pharmacy technician) who is the subject of an order of the Board deemed confidential due to the licensee being impaired is suspended, revoked, restricted, or retired or that the licensee is in any manner otherwise limited. However, the Board may not disclose the nature of the impairment or other information that resulted in such action.
B. The Board may conduct deliberations relative to licensee disciplinary action in hearings (i.e., deliberations and sanctions) in executive session but must vote and announce its decision in public.
C. Records and proceedings of the Board (i.e., hearings and ABOs or BOs) not pertaining to impaired pharmacists are public.

VI. Reporting of Disciplinary Action.
A. TSBP submits reports regarding all disciplinary actions taken against pharmacists, pharmacies, pharmacist interns, and pharmacy technicians to the Healthcare Integrity and Protection Data Bank (HIPDB).
B. The HIPDB is a national healthcare fraud and abuse data collection program established as part of HIPAA.

Board of Pharmacy Rule 281.60
General Guidance

A. This rule is promulgated to:
1. Promote consistency and guidance in the exercise of sound discretion by the agency in licensure and disciplinary matters;
2. Provide notice as to the types of conduct that constitute violations of the Act and as to the disciplinary action that may be imposed; and
3. Provide a framework of analysis for administrative law judges in making recommendations in licensure and disciplinary matters.

B. Board's Role.

The Board shall render the final decision in a contested case and has the responsibility to assess sanctions against licensees who are found to have violated the Act. The Board welcomes recommendations of administrative law judges as to the sanctions to be imposed, but the Board is not bound by such recommendations. A sanction should be consistent with sanctions imposed in other similar cases and should reflect the Board's determination of the seriousness of the violation and the sanction required to deter future violations. A determination of the appropriate sanction is reserved for the Board. The appropriate sanction is not a proper finding of fact or conclusion of law. This rule shall be construed and applied so as to preserve Board member discretion in the imposition of sanctions and remedial measures pursuant to the Administrative Procedures Act and the Pharmacy Act's provisions related to types of discipline and administrative penalties. This rule shall be further construed and applied so as to be consistent with the Act and shall be limited to the extent as otherwise prohibited by law and Board rule.

C. Purpose of Guidelines.

These guidelines are designed to provide guidance in assessing sanctions for violations of the Act. The ultimate purpose of disciplinary sanctions is to protect and inform the public, deter future violations, offer opportunities for rehabilitation (if appropriate), punish violators, and deter others from violations. These guidelines are intended to promote consistent sanctions for similar violations, facilitate timely resolution of cases, and encourage settlements.

1. The standard sanctions outlined in the rule apply to cases involving a single violation of the Act and in which there are no aggravating factors that apply. The Board may impose more restrictive sanctions when there are multiple violations of the Act. In cases which do not have standard sanctions outlined in the rule, the Board may consider any aggravating and/or mitigating factors listed in Board Rule 281.62 (Aggravating and Mitigating Factors) that are found to apply in a particular case.
2. The standard and minimum sanctions outlined in the rule are applicable to first time violators. The Board shall consider revoking the person's license if the person is a repeat offender.
3. The maximum sanction in all cases is revocation of the licensee's license which may be accompanied by an administrative penalty of up to $5,000 per violation. Each day the violation continues is a separate violation.
4. Each statutory violation constitutes a separate offense even if arising out of a single act.

Board of Pharmacy Rule 281.62
Aggravating and Mitigating Factors

The following factors may be considered in determining disciplinary sanctions imposed by the Board if the factors are applicable to the factual situation alleged. The factors are not applicable in situations involving criminal actions (in which case Board Rule 281.63 (Considerations for Criminal Offenses) applies).

1. Aggravation. The following may be considered as aggravating factors so as to merit an increase in the severity of disciplinary sanction(s) to be imposed:
   a. Extent and gravity of personal, economic, or public damage or harm;
   b. Vulnerability of the patient(s);
   c. Willful or reckless conduct as a result of a knowingly made professional omission, as opposed to negligent conduct;
   d. Pattern of misconduct that serves as a basis of discipline;

e. Prior disciplinary action(s);
f. Attempted concealment of the conduct which serves as a basis for disciplinary action under the Act; and
g. Violation of a Board Order.
2. Extenuation and Mitigation. The following may be considered as extenuating and mitigating factors so as to merit a reduction in the severity of disciplinary sanction(s) to be imposed:
a. Isolated incident that serves as a basis for disciplinary action;
b. Remorse for conduct;
c. Interim implementation of remedial measures to correct or mitigate harm from the conduct which serves as a basis for disciplinary action under the Act;
d. Remoteness of misconduct when not based on a delay attributable to actions by the respondent;
e. Extent to which respondent cooperated with Board investigation;
f. Treatment and/or monitoring of an impairment;
g. Self-reported and voluntary admissions of the conduct which serve as a basis for disciplinary action under Section 565.001A.4. and 7. of the Act; and
h. If acting as pharmacist-in-charge, respondent did not personally engage either directly or indirectly in the conduct that serves as the basis for disciplinary action; did not permit or encourage either by professional oversight or extreme negligence the conduct that serves as the basis for disciplinary action; promptly reported the conduct to the Board or other state or federal regulatory authorities or law enforcement upon identifying the conduct that serves as the basis for disciplinary action; and took all reasonable steps to mitigate or remediate the conduct that serves as the basis for disciplinary action.

Board of Pharmacy Rule 281.63
Considerations for Criminal Offenses

A. The purpose of this section is to establish guidelines and criteria on the eligibility of persons with criminal backgrounds to obtain a license or registration from the Board and on the disciplinary actions taken by the Board. The section applies to criminal convictions and to deferred adjudication community supervisions or deferred dispositions as authorized by the Act for all types of licenses and registrations.
B. The Board may suspend, revoke, or impose other authorized disciplinary action on a current license or registration, disqualify a person from receiving a license or registration, or deny to a person the opportunity to be examined for a license or registration because of a person's conviction or deferred adjudication of a crime which serves as a ground for discipline action under the Act and that directly relates to the duties and responsibilities of a licensee, a registrant, or an owner of a pharmacy. This rule applies to persons who are not imprisoned at the time the Board considers the conviction or deferred adjudication. (*See Board Rule 281.63 for further details.*)

Board of Pharmacy Rule 281.64
Sanctions for Applicants with Criminal Offenses

A. The guidelines for disciplinary sanctions apply to criminal convictions and to deferred adjudication community supervisions or deferred dispositions as authorized by the Act for all types of licensees and registrants including applicants for

such licenses and registrations issued by the Board. The Board considers criminal behavior to be highly relevant to an individual's fitness to engage in pharmacy practice and has determined that the sanctions imposed by these guidelines promote the intent of Section 551.002 of the Act. The "date of disposition," when referring to the number of years used to calculate the application of disciplinary sanctions, refers to the date a conviction, a deferred adjudication, or a deferred disposition is entered by the court. The use of the term "currently on probation" is construed to refer to individuals currently serving community supervision or any other type of probationary term imposed by an order of a court for a conviction, deferred adjudication, or deferred disposition.
B. The sanctions imposed by the guidelines can be used with other types of disciplinary actions including administrative penalties as outlined in this rule. In addition to the guidelines, the Board is required by statute to deny an application or immediately revoke a license or registration for certain serious criminal offenses. (*See Board Rule 281.64 for further details.*)

Board of Pharmacy Rule 281.65
Schedule of Administrative Penalties
(Fines for Pharmacies, Pharmacists, and Pharmacy Technicians)

This rule sets forth the schedule for administrative penalties (fines) that may be assessed by the Board for various violations. (*See Board Rule 281.65 for specific fine amounts.*)

Board of Pharmacy Rule 281.67
Sanctions for Out-of-State Disciplinary Actions

A. When determining the appropriate sanction for a disciplinary action taken by a regulatory board of another state under Section 565.001A.16., Section 565.002A.13., or Section 568.003A.13. of the Act, the Board has determined that the following shall be applicable for all types of licensees and registrants for such licenses and registrations issued by the Board.
   1. If the other state's disciplinary action resulted in the license or registration being restricted, suspended, revoked, or surrendered, the appropriate sanction shall be the same as the sanction imposed by the other state such that the licensee or registrant has the same restriction against practice in Texas.
   2. If the license or registration is subject to any other type of disciplinary sanctions, the appropriate sanction shall be equivalent to or less than that imposed by the other state unless contrary to Board policy.
B. The sanctions imposed by this rule can be used with other types of disciplinary actions including administrative penalties as outlined in this chapter.
C. When a licensee or registrant has additional violations of the Texas Pharmacy Act, the Board shall consider imposing more severe types of disciplinary sanctions as deemed necessary.

CHAPTER F HIGHLIGHTS
Complaints, Inspections, Disciplinary Actions, and Procedures

1. Notifications
    a. Every licensed pharmacy and every pharmacist who works at a location other than a pharmacy must provide notification to consumers of the name, mailing address, Internet site address, and telephone number of the Board for the purpose of directing complaints concerning the practice of pharmacy to the Board.
    b. This notification can be done by posting a sign in the pharmacy or work location of the pharmacist with specific language or by providing notice with each dispensed prescription or patient bill or invoice.
2. Inspections
    a. The Board may enter and inspect a facility relative to drug storage and security, equipment, components used in compounding, sanitary conditions, records, reports or other documents, and financial records in the course of the investigation of a specific complaint.
    b. Financial data, sales data (other than shipment data), and pricing data obtained by the Board during an inspection of a facility is confidential and not subject to disclosure under the Texas Open Records Act.
3. Summary of Grounds for Discipline of Pharmacists
    a. Violated the Texas Pharmacy Act or Board rule adopted under the Act.
    b. Engaged in unprofessional conduct such as committing an act that fails to conform to the standards of the pharmacy profession. Board Rule 281.7.A. lists specific violations that are considered unprofessional conduct.
    c. Engaged in gross immorality as defined by Board Rule 281.7.B.
    d. Developed an incapacity that prevents or could prevent the applicant or license holder from practicing pharmacy with reasonable skill, competence, and safety to the public.
    e. Engaged in fraud, deceit, or misrepresentation as defined by Board Rule 281.7.C. in practicing pharmacy or in seeking a license to practice pharmacy.
    f. Been convicted of or placed on deferred adjudication community supervision or deferred disposition for certain misdemeanors and any felony.
    g. Used alcohol or drugs in an intemperate manner.
    h. Failed to maintain records required.
    i. Violated any provision of the Texas Dangerous Drug Act, Texas Controlled Substances Act, Federal Controlled Substances Act, or rules relating to one of those laws.
    j. Aided or abetted an unlicensed person in the practice of pharmacy.
    k. Refused entry into a pharmacy for an authorized inspection.
    l. Violated any state (including other states) or federal pharmacy or drug law.
    m. Been negligent in the practice of pharmacy.
    n. Failed to submit to a physical or mental examination as ordered.
    o. Dispensed a prescription drug outside the usual course and scope of professional practice.
    p. Been disciplined by the regulatory board of another state for conduct substantially equivalent to conduct described under Texas law.
    q. Violated a disciplinary order including a confidential order or contract under the program to aid impaired pharmacists and pharmacy students.
    r. Failed to adequately supervise a task delegated to a pharmacy technician.
    s. Inappropriately delegated a task to a pharmacy technician.
    t. Been responsible for a drug audit shortage.
    u. Been convicted or adjudicated of a criminal offense that requires registration as a sex offender.
4. Grounds for discipline of pharmacy technicians are substantially similar to those for pharmacists but also include performing duties in a pharmacy that only a pharmacist may perform.

5. Summary of Grounds for Discipline of a Pharmacy
   a. Failing to establish and maintain effective controls against the diversion of drugs.
   b. Employing an individual or permitting access to drugs to an individual whose license is or registration is revoked, retired, surrendered, denied, or suspended.
   c. Possessing or engaging in the sale, purchase, or trade of prescription drug samples.
   d. Engaging in the sale, purchase, or trade of misbranded drugs beyond the manufacturer's expiration date.
   e. Displaying abusive, intimidating, or threatening behavior on the part of an owner or managing officer toward a Board member or employee.
6. The Board may take any of the following actions or combination of these actions against a pharmacist. a pharmacy, a pharmacy technician, a pharmacy technician trainee, or an applicant for a pharmacist or pharmacy license or pharmacy technician or pharmacy technician trainee registration:
   a. Revocation
   b. Suspension
   c. Restriction
   d. Fine (Administrative Penalty)
   e. Refusal to issue or renew a license or registration
   f. Probation and supervision
   g. Reprimand
   h. Retire
7. Disciplinary action may be handled through an informal settlement resulting in an Agreed Board Order (ABO) which cannot be appealed or a formal disciplinary process resulting in a Board Order (BO) which may be appealed.
8. A licensee or registrant must wait a minimum of 12 months before seeking to remove a restriction on a license/registration or to have a license/registration reinstated.
9. The Board may issue a remedial plan to resolve certain complaints. A remedial plan is not considered discipline, but it is public information that is removed from a licensee's or registrant's record after five years.

CHAPTER G

Community Pharmacy (Class A) Rules

CHAPTER G

Community Pharmacy (Class A) Rules

Note: Class C pharmacies must comply with these rules if they operate an outpatient pharmacy.

Board of Pharmacy Rule 291.31
Definitions

1. **Accurately as prescribed**—Dispensing, delivering, and/or distributing a prescription drug order:
   a. To the correct patient (or agent of the patient) for whom the drug was prescribed;
   b. With the correct drug in the correct strength, quantity, and dosage form ordered by the practitioner; and
   c. With the correct labeling (including directions for use) as ordered by the practitioner provided, however, that nothing herein shall prohibit pharmacist substitution if substitution is conducted in strict accordance with applicable laws and rules.
2. **Act**—The Texas Pharmacy Act, Chapters 551–569, Occupations Code.
3. **Advanced practice registered nurse**—A registered nurse licensed by the Texas State Board of Nurse Examiners to practice as an advanced practice registered nurse on the basis of completion of an advanced education program. The term includes a nurse practitioner, a nurse midwife, a nurse anesthetist, and a clinical nurse specialist and is synonymous with advanced nurse practitioner.
4. **Automated checking device**—A device that confirms that the correct drug and strength have been labeled with the correct label for the correct patient prior to delivery of the drug to the patient.
5. **Automated counting device**—An automated device that is loaded with bulk drugs and counts and/or packages (i.e., fills a vial or other container) a specified quantity of dosage units of a designated drug product.
6. **Automated pharmacy dispensing system**—A system that automatically performs operations or activities, other than compounding or administration, relative to the storage, packaging, counting, and labeling for dispensing and delivery of medications and that collects, controls, and maintains all transaction information. "Automated pharmacy dispensing system" does not mean "Automated counting device" or "Automated medication supply device."
7. **Beyond-use date**—The date beyond which a product should not be used.
8. **Board**—Texas State Board of Pharmacy.
9. **Confidential record**—Any health-related record that contains information that identifies an individual and that is maintained by a pharmacy or pharmacist such as a patient medication record, prescription drug order, or medication order.
10. **Controlled substance**—A drug, immediate precursor, or other substance listed in Schedules I–V or Penalty Groups 1–4 of the Texas Controlled Substances Act, as amended, or a drug, immediate precursor, or other substance included in Schedules I, II, III, IV, or V of the Federal Comprehensive Drug Abuse Prevention and Control Act of 1970, as amended (Public Law 91-513).
11. **Dangerous drug**—A drug or device that is not included in penalty group I–IV of the Controlled Substances Act and is unsafe for self-medication or is required to bear the legend: "Caution: federal law prohibits dispensing without prescription" or "Rx only" or "Caution: federal law restricts this drug to use by or on the order of a licensed veterinarian."

Notes

12. **Data communication device**—An electronic device that receives electronic information from one source and transmits or routes it to another (e.g., bridge, router, switch, or gateway).
13. **Deliver or delivery**—The actual, constructive, or attempted transfer of a prescription drug or device or controlled substance from one person to another, whether or not for a consideration.
14. **Designated Agent**—
    a. An individual including a licensed nurse, physician assistant, or pharmacist designated by a practitioner and authorized to communicate a prescription drug order to a pharmacist and for whom the practitioner assumes legal responsibility;
    b. A licensed nurse, physician assistant, or pharmacist employed in a healthcare facility to whom the practitioner communicates a prescription drug order;
    c. An advanced practice registered nurse or physician assistant authorized by a practitioner to prescribe or order drugs or devices under Chapter 157 of the Medical Practice Act; or
    d. A person who is a licensed vocational nurse or has an education equivalent to or greater than that required for a vocational nurse designated by the practitioner to communicate prescriptions for an advanced practice registered nurse or physician assistant authorized by the practitioner to sign prescription drug orders.
15. **Dispense**—Preparing, packaging, compounding, or labeling for delivery a prescription drug or device in the course of professional practice to an ultimate user or his or her agent by or pursuant to the lawful order of a practitioner.
16. **Dispensing error**—An action committed by a pharmacist or other pharmacy personnel that causes the patient or patient's agent to take possession of a dispensed prescription drug and the individual subsequently discovers that the patient has received an incorrect drug product, which includes incorrect strength, incorrect quantity, incorrect dosage form, and/or incorrect directions for use.
17. **Dispensing pharmacist**—The pharmacist responsible for the final check of the dispensed prescription before delivery to the patient.
18. **Distribute**—The delivery of a prescription drug or device other than by administering or dispensing.
19. **Downtime**—Period of time during which a data processing system is not operable.
20. **Drug regimen review**—An evaluation of prescription drug orders and patient medication records for:
    a. Known allergies;
    b. Rational therapy-contraindications;
    c. Reasonable dose and route of administration;
    d. Reasonable directions for use;
    e. Duplication of therapy;
    f. Drug-drug interactions;
    g. Drug-food interactions;
    h. Drug-disease interactions;
    i. Adverse drug reactions; and
    j. Proper utilization including overutilization or underutilization.
21. **Electronic prescription drug order**—A prescription drug order that is generated on an electronic application and transmitted as an electronic data file.
22. **Electronic signature**—A unique security code or other identifier which specifically identifies the person entering information into a data processing system. A facility which utilizes electronic signatures must:

a. Maintain a permanent list of the unique security codes assigned to persons authorized to use the data processing system and
b. Have an ongoing security program which is capable of identifying misuse and/or unauthorized use of electronic signatures.
23. **Electronic verification process**—An electronic verification, bar code verification, weight verification, radio frequency identification (RFID), or similar electronic process or system that accurately verifies that medication has been properly dispensed and labeled by or loaded into an automated pharmacy dispensing system.
24. **Full-time pharmacist**—A pharmacist who works in a pharmacy from 30 to 40 hours per week or, if the pharmacy is open fewer than 60 hours per week, one-half of the time the pharmacy is open.
25. **Hard copy**—A physical document that is readable without the use of a special device.
26. **Hot water**—The temperature of water from the pharmacy's sink maintained at a minimum of 105 degrees F (41 degrees C).
27. **Medical Practice Act**—The Texas Medical Practice Act, Subtitle B, Occupations Code, as amended.
28. **Medication order**—A written order from a practitioner or a verbal order from a practitioner or his or her authorized agent for administration of a drug or device.
29. **New prescription drug order**—A prescription drug order that has not been dispensed to the patient in the same strength and dosage form by this or a pharmacy within the last year.
30. **Original prescription**—
    a. Original written prescription drug order or
    b. Original verbal or electronic prescription drug order reduced to writing either manually or electronically by the pharmacist.
31. **Part-time pharmacist**—A pharmacist who works less than full time.
32. **Patient counseling**—Communication by the pharmacist of information to the patient or patient's agent to improve therapy by ensuring proper use of drugs and devices.
33. **Patient med pack**—A package prepared by a pharmacist for a specific patient comprised of a series of containers and containing two or more prescribed solid oral dosage forms. The patient med pack is so designed or each container is so labeled as to indicate the day and time or period of time that the contents within each container are to be taken.
34. **Pharmaceutical care**—The provision of drug therapy and other pharmaceutical services intended to assist in the cure or prevention of a disease, elimination or reduction of a patient's symptoms, or arresting or slowing of a disease process.
35. **Pharmacist-in-charge (PIC)**—The pharmacist designated on a pharmacy license as the pharmacist who has the authority or responsibility for a pharmacy's compliance with laws and rules pertaining to the practice of pharmacy.
36. **Pharmacy technician**—An individual who is registered with the Board as a pharmacy technician and whose responsibility in a pharmacy is to provide technical services that do not require professional judgment regarding preparing and distributing drugs and who works under the direct supervision of and is responsible to a pharmacist.
37. **Pharmacy technician trainee**—An individual who is registered with the Board as a pharmacy technician trainee and is authorized to participate in a pharmacy's technician training program.
38. **Physician assistant**—A physician assistant recognized by the Texas Medical Board as having the specialized education and training required under the Medical Practice Act and who has been issued an identification number by the Texas State Board of Medical Examiners.

Notes

39. **Practitioner**—
    a. A person licensed or registered to prescribe, distribute, administer, or dispense a prescription drug or device in the course of professional practice in this state, including a physician, dentist, podiatrist, or veterinarian but excluding a person licensed under this Act;
    b. A person licensed by another state, Canada, or the United Mexican States in a health field in which, under the law of this state, a license holder in this state may legally prescribe a dangerous drug;
    c. A person practicing in another state and licensed by another state as a physician, dentist, veterinarian, or podiatrist, who has a current federal Drug Enforcement Administration registration number, and who may legally prescribe a Schedule II, III, IV, or V controlled substance as specified under Chapter 481, Health and Safety Code, in that other state; or
    d. An advanced practice registered nurse or physician assistant to whom a physician has delegated the authority to prescribe or order a drug or device under the Texas Medical Practice Act or, for the purposes of this Act, a pharmacist who practices in a hospital, hospital-based clinic, or an academic healthcare institution and a physician has delegated the authority to sign a prescription for a dangerous drug under Chapter 157.101 (Texas Medical Practice Act).
40. **Prepackaging**—The act of repackaging and relabeling quantities of drug products from a manufacturer's original commercial container into a prescription container, unit-dose packaging, or multi-compartment container for dispensing by a pharmacist to the ultimate consumer, including dispensing through the use of an automated pharmacy dispensing system or automated checking device.
41. **Prescription department**—The area of a pharmacy that contains prescription drugs.
42. **Prescription drug**—
    a. A substance for which federal or state law requires a prescription before the substance may be legally dispensed to the public or
    b. A drug or device that under federal law is required before being dispensed or delivered to be labeled with the statement:
        (1) "Caution: federal law prohibits dispensing without prescription" or "Rx only" or another legend that complies with federal law;
        (2) "Caution: federal law restricts this drug to use by or on the order of a licensed veterinarian"; or
        (3) A drug or device that is required by federal or state statute or regulation to be dispensed on prescription or that is restricted to use by a practitioner only.
43. **Prescription drug order**—
    a. A written order from a practitioner or a verbal order from a practitioner or his or her authorized agent to a pharmacist for a drug or device to be dispensed or
    b. A written order or a verbal order pursuant to the Medical Practice Act (regarding carrying out or signing prescriptions by physician assistants and advanced practice registered nurses).
44. **Prospective drug use review**—A review of the patient's drug therapy and prescription drug order or medication order prior to dispensing or distributing the drug.
45. **State**—One of the 50 United States of America, a U.S. territory, or the District of Columbia.
46. **Texas Controlled Substances Act**—The Texas Controlled Substances Act, Health and Safety Code, Chapter 481, as amended.

47. **Written protocol**—A physician's order, standing medical order, standing delegation order, or other order or protocol as defined by rule of the Texas Medical Board under the Texas Medical Practice Act.

Board of Pharmacy Rule 291.32
Personnel

A. Pharmacist-in-Charge (PIC).
   1. General.
      a. Each Class A pharmacy shall have one pharmacist-in-charge who is employed on a full-time basis and who may be the pharmacist-in-charge for only one such pharmacy provided, however, such pharmacist-in-charge may be the pharmacist-in-charge of:
         (1) More than one Class A pharmacy, if the additional Class A pharmacies are not open to provide pharmacy services simultaneously or
         (2) During an emergency, up to two Class A pharmacies open simultaneously if the pharmacist-in-charge works at least 10 hours per week in each pharmacy for no more than a period of 30 consecutive days.
      b. The pharmacist-in-charge must comply with controlled substance inventory requirements. (*See Board Rule 291.17.*)
      c. The pharmacist-in-charge of a Class A pharmacy may not serve as the pharmacist-in-charge of a Class B pharmacy or a Class C pharmacy with 101 beds or more.
   2. Responsibilities.
      a. Educating and training of pharmacy technicians and pharmacy technician trainees;
      b. Supervising a system to assure appropriate procurement of prescription drugs and devices and other products dispensed from the pharmacy;
      c. Disposing of and distributing drugs from the pharmacy;
      d. Storing all materials including drugs, chemicals, and biologicals;
      e. Maintaining records of all transactions of the pharmacy necessary to maintain accurate control over and accountability for all pharmaceutical materials required by applicable state and federal laws and sections;
      f. Supervising a system to ensure establishment and maintenance of effective controls against the theft or diversion of prescription drugs and records for such drugs;
      g. Adhering to policies and procedures regarding the maintenance of records in a data processing system such that the data processing system is in compliance with Class A (Community) pharmacy requirements;
      h. Legally operating the pharmacy including meeting all inspection and other requirements of all state and federal laws or rules governing the practice of pharmacy; and
      i. If the pharmacy uses an automated pharmacy dispensing system, shall be responsible for the following:
         (1) Reviewing and approving all policies and procedures for system operation, safety, security, accuracy and access, patient confidentiality, prevention or unauthorized access, and malfunction;
         (2) Inspecting medications in the automated pharmacy dispensing system at least monthly for expiration date, misbranding, physical integrity, security, and accountability;
         (3) Assigning, discontinuing, or changing personnel access to the automated pharmacy dispensing system;

(4) Ensuring that pharmacy technicians, pharmacy technician trainees, and licensed healthcare professionals performing any services in connection with an automated pharmacy dispensing system have been properly trained on the use of the system and can demonstrate comprehensive knowledge of the written policies and procedures for operation of the system; and

(5) Ensuring that the automated pharmacy dispensing system is stocked accurately and an accountability record is maintained in accordance with the written policies and procedures of operation.

B. Owner. The owner of a Class A pharmacy shall have responsibility for all administrative and operational functions of the pharmacy. The pharmacist-in-charge may advise the owner on administrative and operational concerns. If the owner is not a Texas licensed pharmacist, the owner shall consult with the pharmacist-in-charge or another Texas licensed pharmacist. The owner shall have responsibility for, at a minimum, the following:
1. Establishing policies for procurement of prescription drugs and devices and other products dispensed from the Class A pharmacy;
2. Establishing policies and procedures for the security of the prescription department including the maintenance of effective controls against the theft or diversion of prescription drugs;
3. If the pharmacy uses an automated pharmacy dispensing system, reviewing and approving all policies and procedures for system operation, safety, security, accuracy and access, patient confidentiality, prevention of unauthorized access, and malfunction;
4. Providing the pharmacy with the necessary equipment and resources commensurate with its level and type of practice; and
5. Establishing policies and procedures regarding maintenance, storage, and retrieval of records in a data processing system so that the system is in compliance with state and federal requirements.

C. Pharmacists (applies to pharmacists-in-charge and staff pharmacists).
1. General.
   a. A pharmacist-in-charge shall be assisted by a sufficient number of additional licensed pharmacists as may be required to operate the pharmacy competently, safely, and adequately to meet the needs of the patients of the pharmacy.
   b. Pharmacists are to assist the pharmacist-in-charge in meeting responsibilities in ordering, dispensing, and accounting for prescription drugs.
   c. Pharmacists are solely responsible for the direct supervision of pharmacy technicians and pharmacy technician trainees and for designating and delegating duties, other than those listed in D.2. below, to pharmacy technicians and pharmacy technician trainees. Each pharmacist shall be responsible for any delegated act performed by pharmacy technicians and pharmacy technician trainees under his or her supervision.
   d. Pharmacists shall directly supervise pharmacy technicians and pharmacy technician trainees who are entering prescription data into a pharmacy's data processing system by one of the following methods:
      (1) Physically present supervision. A pharmacist shall be physically present to directly supervise a pharmacy technician or pharmacy technician trainee who is entering prescription data into the data processing system. Each prescription entered into the data processing system shall be verified at the time of data entry. If the pharmacist is not physically present due to a temporary absence as allowed by Board Rule 291.33B.3., on return from such temporary absence the pharmacist must:

(a) Conduct a drug regimen review for prescription data entered during the temporary absence as specified in Board Rule 291.33(c)(2) and
(b) Verify that prescription data entered during the temporary absence was entered accurately prior to delivery of the prescription to the patient or the patient's agent.
(2) Electronic supervision. A pharmacist may electronically supervise a pharmacy technician or a pharmacy technician trainee who is entering prescription data into the data processing system provided the pharmacist:
   (a) Has the ability to immediately communicate directly with the pharmacy technician and the pharmacy technician trainee;
   (b) Has immediate access to any original document containing prescription information or other information related to the dispensing of the prescription. Such access may be through imaging technology provided the pharmacist has the ability to review the original hardcopy documents if needed for clarification; and
   (c) Verifies the accuracy of the data entered prior to the release of the information to the system for storage and/or generation of the prescription label.
(3) Electronic verification of data entry by pharmacy technicians or pharmacy technician trainees. A pharmacist may electronically verify the data entry of prescription information into a data processing system provided:
   (a) The pharmacist has the ability to immediately communicate directly with the pharmacy technician and the pharmacy technician trainee;
   (b) The pharmacist electronically conducting the verification is either a:
      (i) Texas licensed pharmacist or
      (ii) Pharmacist employed by a Class E pharmacy that
         (I) Has the same owner as the Class A pharmacy where the pharmacy technicians and the pharmacy technician trainees are located or
         (II) Has entered into a written contract or agreement with the Class A pharmacy, which outlines the services to be provided and the responsibilities and accountabilities of each pharmacy in compliance with federal and state laws and regulations;
   (c) The pharmacy establishes controls to protect the privacy and security of confidential records; and
   (d) The pharmacy keeps permanent records of prescriptions electronically verified for a period of two years.
e. All pharmacists while on duty shall be responsible for the legal operation of the pharmacy and for complying with all state and federal laws or rules governing the practice of pharmacy.
f. A dispensing pharmacist shall be responsible for and ensure that drugs are dispensed and delivered safely and accurately as prescribed, unless the pharmacy's data processing system can record the identity of each pharmacist involved in a specific portion of the dispensing processing. If the system can track the identity of each pharmacist involved in the dispensing process, each pharmacist involved in the dispensing process shall be responsible for and ensure that the portion of the process the pharmacist is performing results in the safe and accurate dispensing and delivery of

the drug as prescribed. The dispensing process shall include, but not be limited to, drug regimen review and verification of accurate prescription data entry including data entry of prescriptions placed on hold, packaging, preparation, compounding, transferring, labeling, and performance of the final check of the dispensed prescription. An intern has the same responsibilities described in this subparagraph as a pharmacist but must perform his or her duties under the supervision of a pharmacist.
2. Pharmacist Duties. Duties which may only be performed by a pharmacist are as follows:
    a. Receiving oral prescription drug orders and reducing these orders to writing either manually or electronically;
    b. Interpreting prescription drug orders;
    c. Selecting drug products;
    d. Performing the final check of the dispensed prescription before delivery to the patient to ensure that the prescription has been dispensed accurately as prescribed;
    e. Communicating to the patient or patient's agent information about the prescription drug or device which in the exercise of the pharmacist's professional judgment the pharmacist deems significant, as specified in Board Rule 291.33(C)(1) (Patient Counseling);
    f. Communicating to the patient or the patient's agent on his or her request information concerning any prescription drugs dispensed to the patient by the pharmacy;
    g. Assuring that a reasonable effort is made to obtain, record, and maintain patient medication records;
    h. Interpreting patient medication records and performing drug regimen reviews;
    i. Performing a specific act of drug therapy management for a patient delegated to a pharmacist by a written protocol from a physician licensed in this state in compliance with the Texas Medical Practice Act;
    j. Verifying that controlled substances listed on invoices are received by clearly recording his or her initials and the date of receipt of the controlled substances; and
    k. Transferring or receiving a transfer of original prescription information on behalf of a patient.

Note: While most of the duties listed above may only be performed by a pharmacist, these duties may also be performed by an intern working under a preceptor. The duty in 2.k. above requires a pharmacist's involvement. Transferring prescriptions from an intern to a pharmacist or from a pharmacist to an intern is allowed, but transfers between two interns is not permitted. (See Transfer of Prescription Drug Order Information later in this chapter.)

3. Special Requirements for Compounding. All pharmacists engaged in compounding nonsterile preparations shall meet the training requirements specified in Board Rule 291.131 (Pharmacies Compounding Nonsterile Preparations).

    Note: There are also training requirements for pharmacists engaged in sterile compounding, but because Class A pharmacies that are compounding sterile products are licensed as Class A-S pharmacies, those requirements are found in the Class A-S rule.

D. Pharmacy Technicians and Pharmacy Technician Trainees.
    1. General.
        a. All pharmacy technicians and pharmacy technician trainees shall meet the training requirements specified in Board Rule 297.6 (Pharmacy Technician and Pharmacy Technician Trainee Training).

b. Special requirements for compounding. All pharmacy technicians and pharmacy technician trainees engaged in compounding nonsterile preparations shall meet the training requirements specified in Board Rule 291.131.
Note: There are also training requirements for pharmacy technicians engaged in sterile compounding, but because Class A pharmacies that are compounding sterile products are licensed as Class A-S pharmacies, those requirements are found in the Class A-S rule.

2. Duties.
    a. Pharmacy technicians and pharmacy technician trainees may not perform any of the duties listed in C.2 above.
    Note: There is no difference between the duties that a pharmacy technician and a pharmacy technician trainee can perform in a Class A pharmacy.
    b. A pharmacist may delegate to pharmacy technicians and pharmacy technician trainees any nonjudgmental technical duty associated with the preparation and distribution of prescription drugs provided:
        (1) Unless otherwise provided under Board Rule 291.33, a pharmacist verifies the accuracy of all acts, tasks, and functions performed by pharmacy technicians and pharmacy technician trainees;
        (2) Pharmacy technicians and pharmacy technician trainees are under the direct supervision of and responsible to a pharmacist; and
        (3) Only pharmacy technicians and pharmacy technician trainees who have been properly trained on the use of an automated pharmacy dispensing system and can demonstrate comprehensive knowledge of the written policies and procedures for the operation of the system may be allowed access to the system.
    c. Pharmacy technicians and pharmacy technician trainees may perform only nonjudgmental technical duties associated with the preparation and distribution of prescription drugs as follows:
        (1) Initiating and receiving refill authorization requests;
        (2) Initiating electronic transfer requests between pharmacies electronically sharing a common prescription database;
        Note: This is allowed by Board Rule 291.34 in this chapter. Although not specifically listed in this part of the rules, it was added here for completeness.
        (3) Entering prescription data into a data processing system;
        (4) Selecting a stock container from the shelf for a prescription;
        (5) Preparing and packaging prescription drug orders (e.g., counting tablets/capsules and measuring liquids and/or placing them into the prescription container);
        (6) Affixing prescription labels and auxiliary labels to the prescription container;
        (7) Reconstituting medications;
        (8) Prepackaging and labeling prepackaged drugs;
        (9) Loading bulk unlabeled drugs into an automated dispensing system provided a pharmacist verifies that the system is properly loaded prior to use;
        (10) Loading prepackaged containers previously verified by a pharmacist or manufacturer's unit-of-use packages into an automated dispensing system;
        (11) Compounding nonsterile prescription drug orders; and
        (12) Compounding bulk nonsterile preparations.

E. Ratio of Onsite Pharmacists to Pharmacy Technicians.
    1. The ratio of onsite pharmacists to pharmacy technicians and pharmacy technician trainees in a Class A pharmacy may be 1:4 provided that at least

one of the four technicians is a pharmacy technician and not a pharmacy technician trainee. The ratio of pharmacists to pharmacy technician trainees may not exceed 1:3.
      2. There is a special statutory exception in Section 568.006 of the Act that allows a ratio of 1:5 for pharmacies that dispense no more than 20 different prescription drugs. This type of pharmacy is extremely rare.
   F. Identification of Pharmacy Personnel.
      1. Pharmacy technicians must wear an identification tag or badge that bears their name and identifies them as a pharmacy technician or a certified pharmacy technician if the technician maintains current certification with the Pharmacy Technician Certification Board or any other entity providing an examination approved by the Board.
      2. Pharmacy technician trainees must wear an identification tag or badge that bears the person's name and identifies him or her as a pharmacy technician trainee.
      3. Pharmacist interns must wear an identification tag or badge that bears their name and identifies them as a pharmacist intern.
      4. Pharmacists must wear an identification tag or badge that bears their name and identifies them as a pharmacist.

Class A Pharmacy Technician/Trainee Duties

Tasks Pharmacy Technicians/Trainees MAY NOT Perform

Certain tasks must be performed by a pharmacist or pharmacist intern and not be performed by pharmacy technicians or pharmacy technician trainees. Tasks which pharmacy technicians and pharmacy technician trainees MAY NOT perform include:
   A. Providing drug information to the patient or patient's agent (patient counseling);
   B. Transferring (via telephone or facsimile) prescriptions between pharmacies;
   C. Interpreting patient profiles and performing prospective drug use reviews;
   D. Receiving oral prescription drug orders and reducing these orders to writing either manually or electronically (includes transcribing from a telephone answering machine);
   E. Interpreting prescription drug orders;
   F. Selecting drug products (i.e., brand versus generic equivalent); and
   G. Verifying receipt of controlled substances by initialing and dating invoices of controlled substances received in the pharmacy.

Tasks Pharmacy Technicians/Trainees MAY Perform

With proper training and under pharmacist supervision, pharmacy technicians and pharmacy technician trainees MAY perform nonjudgmental technical duties associated with the preparation of a prescription drug order. These duties may include:
   A. Creating or updating patient medication records;
   B. Preparing prescription labels;
   C. Affixing labels to the prescription containers;
   D. Affixing auxiliary labels if indicated;
   E. Entering prescription drug order information into a computer system or typing a label in a manual system;
   F. Entering patient specific information into a patient medication record;
   G. Selecting the correct stock bottle for a prescription and accurately counting or pouring the appropriate quantity of the drug product;
   H. Reconstituting medications;
   I. Initiating and receiving refill authorization requests;
   J. Initiating electronic transfer requests between pharmacies electronically that share a common prescription database;

K. Bulk compounding;
L. Prepackaging drugs and loading bulk unlabeled drugs into automated drug dispensing systems;
M. Compounding sterile pharmaceuticals if proper training is completed; and
N. Compounding nonsterile prescription drug orders if proper training is completed. (*See Chapter H in this book.*)

Other Pharmacy Personnel

Any duty which is not required to be performed by pharmacists or by persons designated, trained, and supervised as pharmacy technicians or pharmacy technician trainees may be performed by other employees of the pharmacy. Examples of duties which may be performed by persons other than pharmacists or pharmacy technicians or pharmacy technician trainees include:
A. Completing charge and delivery receipts;
B. Selling nonprescription drugs in their original containers;
C. Stocking or cleaning pharmacy shelves;
D. Ordering pharmacy stock;
E. Delivering prescriptions to a patient's home or place of business;
F. Soliciting information from the patient to complete a patient medication record; and
G. Taking refill numbers from patients.

Board of Pharmacy Rule 291.33
Operational Standards

A. Licensing Requirements.
  1. The pharmacy shall be licensed annually or biennially in compliance with Board Rule 291.1 (Pharmacy License Application).
  2. A Class A pharmacy which changes ownership shall notify the Board within ten days of the change of ownership and apply for a new and separate license as specified in Board Rule 291.3 (Required Notifications).
  3. A Class A pharmacy which changes location and/or name shall notify the Board as specified in Board Rule 291.3 (Required Notifications).
     Note: The Board requires notification no later than 30 days prior to the date for a change in location and within 10 days for a change of name.
  4. A Class A pharmacy owned by a partnership or corporation which changes managing officers shall notify the Board in writing of the names of the new managing officers within ten days of the change following the procedures in Board Rule 291.3 (Required Notifications).
  5. A Class A pharmacy shall notify the Board in writing within ten days of closing following the procedures as specified in Board Rule 291.5.
  6. A separate license is required for each principal place of business, and only one pharmacy license may be issued to a specific location.
  7. A fee as specified in Board Rule 291.6 will be charged for the issuance and renewal of a license and the issuance of an amended license.
  8. A Class A pharmacy, which also operates another type of pharmacy which would otherwise be required to be licensed as a Class B pharmacy, is NOT required to secure a Class B pharmacy license. However, the Class A pharmacy shall comply with the provisions of Class B (Nuclear Pharmacy) rules to the extent such rules are applicable to the operation of the pharmacy.
  9. A Class A pharmacy engaged in the compounding of nonsterile preparations shall comply with the provisions of Board Rule 291.131.
  10. A Class A pharmacy shall not compound sterile preparations unless it is licensed as a Class A-S pharmacy.

11. A Class A pharmacy engaged in the provision of remote pharmacy services including storage and dispensing of prescription drugs shall comply with the provisions of Board Rule 291.121.
    Note: This includes remote pharmacy services using automated systems, emergency medication kits, telepharmacy services, and automated storage and delivery systems.
12. A Class A pharmacy engaged in centralized prescription dispensing and/or prescription drug or medication order processing shall comply with the provisions of Board Rule 291.125 (Centralized Prescription Dispensing) and/or Board Rule 291.123 (Centralized Prescription Drug or Medication Order Processing).

B. Environment.
   1. General Requirements.
      a. Pharmacies shall be orderly and clean, and required equipment shall be clean and in good operating condition.
      b. Pharmacies shall have a sink with hot and cold running water within the pharmacy, exclusive of restroom facilities, available to all pharmacy personnel and maintained in a sanitary condition.
      c. Class A pharmacies which serve the general public shall contain an area which is suitable for confidential patient counseling. The counseling area shall:
         (1) Be easily accessible to both patients and pharmacists and not allow patient access to prescription drugs and
         (2) Be designed to maintain the confidentiality and privacy of the pharmacist/patient communication. In determining whether the area is suitable for confidential patient counseling and designed to maintain the confidentiality and privacy of the pharmacist/patient communication, the Board may consider factors such as the following:
            (a) The proximity of the counseling area to the check-out or cash register area;
            (b) The volume of pedestrian traffic in and around the counseling area;
            (c) The presence of walls or other barriers between the counseling area and other areas of the pharmacy; and
            (d) Any evidence of confidential information being overheard by persons other than the patient or patient's agent or the pharmacist or agents of the pharmacist.
      d. Pharmacies shall be properly lighted and ventilated.
      e. Temperature of the pharmacy and the refrigerator shall be maintained within a range compatible with the proper storage of drugs.
      f. Animals including birds and reptiles shall not be kept within the pharmacy and in immediate adjacent areas under the control of the pharmacy. This provision does not apply to fish in aquariums, service animals accompanying disabled persons, or animals for sale to the general public in a separate area that is inspected by local health jurisdictions.
      g. If the pharmacy has flammable materials, the pharmacy shall have a designated area for the storage of flammable materials. Such area shall meet the requirements set by local and state fire laws.
   2. Security.
      Note: Pharmacies that do not possess or dispense prescription drugs (e.g., central processing or call centers) do not have to comply with these security requirements.
      a. Each pharmacist on duty is responsible for the security of the prescription department including provisions for effective control against theft or diversion of prescription drugs and records.

b. The prescription department shall be locked by key, combination, or other mechanical or electronic means to prohibit unauthorized access when a pharmacist is not on-site except as provided in 2.c., 2.d., and 3. below. The following is applicable:
   (1) If the prescription department is closed at any time when the rest of the facility is open, the prescription department must be physically or electronically secured. The security may be accomplished by means such as floor to ceiling walls; walls, partitions, or barriers at least 9 feet 6 inches high; electronically monitored motion detectors; pull down sliders; or other systems or technologies that will secure the pharmacy from unauthorized entrance when the pharmacy is closed. Pharmacies licensed prior to June 1, 2009 shall be exempt from this provision unless the pharmacy changes location. Change of location shall include the relocation of the pharmacy within the licensed address. A pharmacy licensed prior to June 1, 2009 that files a change of ownership but does not change location shall be exempt from these provisions.
   (2) The pharmacy's key, combination, or other mechanical or electronic means of locking the pharmacy may not be duplicated without the authorization of the pharmacist-in-charge or owner.
   (3) At a minimum, the pharmacy must have a basic alarm system with off-site monitoring and perimeter and motion sensors. The pharmacy may have additional security by video surveillance camera systems.
c. Prior to authorizing individuals to enter the prescription department, the pharmacist-in-charge or owner may designate persons who may enter the prescription department to perform functions other than dispensing functions or prescription processing documented by the pharmacist-in-charge, including access to the prescription department by other pharmacists, pharmacy personnel, and other individuals. The pharmacy must maintain written documentation of authorized individuals other than individuals employed by the pharmacy who accessed the prescription department when a pharmacist is not on-site.
d. The pharmacist-in-charge must put in writing that only persons designated either by name or by title, including such titles as "relief" or "floater" pharmacist, may unlock the prescription department except in emergency situations. An additional key to the prescription department may be maintained in a secure location outside the prescription department for use during an emergency or as designated by the pharmacist-in-charge.
e. Written policies and procedures for the pharmacy's security shall be developed and implemented by the pharmacist-in-charge and/or the owner of the pharmacy. Such policies and procedures may include quarterly audits of controlled substances commonly abused or diverted; perpetual inventories for the comparison of the receipt, dispensing, and distribution of controlled substances; monthly reports from the pharmacy's wholesaler(s) of controlled substances purchased by the pharmacy; opening and closing procedures; product storage and placement; and central management oversight.

3. Temporary Absence of Pharmacist.
   a. On-site supervision by a pharmacist.
      (1) If a pharmacy is staffed by only one pharmacist, the pharmacist may leave the prescription department for short periods of time without closing the prescription department and removing pharmacy

technicians, pharmacy technician trainees, and other pharmacy personnel from the prescription department provided the following conditions are met:
   (a) At least one pharmacy technician remains in the prescription department;
   (b) The pharmacist remains on-site at the licensed location of the pharmacy and is immediately available;
   (c) The pharmacist reasonably believes that the security of the prescription department will be maintained in his or her absence. If in the professional judgment of the pharmacist a determination is made that the prescription department should close during his or her absence, then the pharmacist shall close the prescription department and remove the pharmacy technicians, pharmacy technician trainees, and other pharmacy personnel from the prescription department during his or her absence; and
   (d) A notice is posted which includes the following information:
      (i) The pharmacist is on a break and the time the pharmacist will return and
      (ii) Pharmacy technicians may begin the processing of prescription drug orders or refills brought in during the pharmacist's absence, but the prescription or refill may not be delivered to the patient or the patient's agent until the pharmacist verifies the accuracy of the prescription.
(2) During the time the pharmacist is absent from the prescription department, only pharmacy technicians who have completed the pharmacy's training program may perform the following duties, provided a pharmacist verifies the accuracy of all acts, tasks, and functions performed by the pharmacy technicians prior to the delivery of the prescription to the patient or the patient's agent:
   (a) Initiating and receiving refill authorization requests;
   (b) Entering prescription data into a data processing system;
   (c) Taking a stock bottle from the shelf for a prescription;
   (d) Preparing and packaging prescription drug orders (i.e., counting tablets/capsules and measuring liquids and placing them in the prescription container);
   (e) Affixing prescription labels and auxiliary labels to the prescription container; and
   (f) Prepackaging and labeling prepackaged drugs.
(3) Upon return to the prescription department, the pharmacist shall:
   (a) Conduct a drug regimen review as specified in C.2. below and
   (b) Verify the accuracy of all acts, tasks, and functions performed by the pharmacy technicians prior to delivery of the prescription to the patient or the patient's agent.
(4) An agent of the pharmacist may deliver a previously verified prescription to the patient or his or her agent provided a record of the delivery is maintained in a log or record containing the following information:
   (a) Date of the delivery;
   (b) Unique identification number of the prescription drug order;
   (c) Patient's name;
   (d) Patient's phone number or the phone number of the person picking up the prescription; and
   (e) Signature of the person picking up the prescription.

(5) Any prescription delivered to a patient when a pharmacist is not in the prescription department must meet the requirements for a prescription delivered to a patient as described in C.1.f. below.
(6) During the times a pharmacist is absent from the prescription department, a pharmacist intern shall be considered a registered pharmacy technician and may perform only the duties of a registered pharmacy technician.
(7) In pharmacies with two or more pharmacists on duty, the pharmacists shall stagger their breaks and meal periods so that the prescription department is not left without a pharmacist on duty.

  b. Pharmacist is off-site.
(1) The prescription department must be secured with procedures for entry during the time that a pharmacy is not under the continuous on-site supervision of a pharmacist and the pharmacy is not open for pharmacy services.
(2) Pharmacy technicians and pharmacy technician trainees may not perform any duties of a pharmacy technician or pharmacy technician trainee during the time that the pharmacist is off-site.
(3) A pharmacy may use an automated storage and delivery device for pick-up of a previously verified prescription by a patient or patient's agent. *See Remote Services Rule 291.121(d) in Chapter D.*
(4) An agent of the pharmacist may deliver a previously verified prescription to a patient or patient's agent during short periods of time when a pharmacist is off-site provided the following conditions are met:
    (a) Short periods of time may not exceed two consecutive hours in a 24-hour period;
    (b) A notice is posted which includes the following information:
        (i) The pharmacist is off-site and not present in the pharmacy;
        (ii) No new prescriptions may be prepared at the pharmacy, but previously verified prescriptions may be delivered to the patient or the patient's agent; and
        (iii) The date/time when the pharmacist will return;
    (c) The pharmacy must maintain documentation of the absences of the pharmacist(s); and
    (d) The prescription department is locked and secured to prohibit unauthorized entry.
(5) During the time a pharmacist is absent from the prescription department and is off-site, a log or record of prescriptions delivered must be maintained and contain the following information:
    (a) Date and time of the delivery;
    (b) Unique identification number of the prescription drug order;
    (c) Patient's name;
    (d) Patient's phone number or the phone number of the person picking up the prescription; and
    (e) Signature of the person picking up the prescription.
(6) Any prescription delivered to a patient when a pharmacist is not on-site at the pharmacy must meet the requirements for a prescription delivered to a patient as described in C.1.f. below.

C. Prescription Dispensing and Delivery.
  1. Patient Counseling and Provision of Drug Information.
Note: This rule applies to all patients. Therefore, it satisfies federal OBRA 90 requirements which only apply to Medicaid patients.
    a. To optimize drug therapy, a pharmacist shall communicate to the patient or the patient's agent information about the prescription drug or

device which, in the exercise of the pharmacist's professional judgment, the pharmacist deems significant such as the following:
(1) The name and description of the drug or device;
(2) Dosage form, dosage, route of administration, and duration of drug therapy;
(3) Special directions and precautions for preparation, administration, and use by the patient;
(4) Common severe side or adverse effects or interactions and therapeutic contraindications that may be encountered, including their avoidance, and the action required if they occur;
(5) Techniques for self-monitoring of drug therapy;
(6) Proper storage;
(7) Refill information; and
(8) Action to be taken in the event of a missed dose.
  b. Such communication:
  (1) Shall be provided to new and existing patients of a pharmacy with each new prescription drug order. A new prescription drug order is one that has not been dispensed to the patient by the pharmacy in the same strength and dosage form within the last year;
  Note: While a patient may refuse counseling, there is no such thing as an "offer to counsel" in Texas. Counseling is required for all new prescription drug orders.
  (2) Shall be provided for any prescription drug order dispensed by the pharmacy on the request of the patient or patient's agent;
  (3) Shall be communicated orally in person unless the patient or patient's agent is not at the pharmacy or a specific communication barrier prohibits such oral communication;
  (4) Shall be documented by recording the name of the patient, date of counseling, prescription number, and initials or identification code of the pharmacist providing the counseling in the prescription dispensing record as follows:
    (a) On the original hardcopy prescription provided the counseling pharmacist clearly records his or her initials on the prescription for the purpose of identifying who provided the counseling;
    (b) In the pharmacy's data processing system (computer);
    (c) In an electronic logbook; or
    (d) In a hardcopy log; and
  (5) Shall be reinforced with written information relevant to the prescription and provided to the patient or patient's agent. The following is applicable concerning this written information.
    (a) Written information must be in plain language designed for the patient and printed in an easily readable font comparable but not smaller than 10-point Times Roman. This information may be provided in an electronic format such as email if the patient or patient's agent requests an electronic format and the pharmacy documents the request.
    (b) When a compounded preparation is dispensed, information shall be provided for the major active ingredient(s) if available.
    (c) For new drug entities, if no written information is initially available, the pharmacist is not required to provide information until such information is available, provided that:
      (i) The pharmacist informs the patient or the patient's agent that the product is a new drug entity and written information is not available;

(ii) The pharmacist documents the fact that no written information was provided; and

(iii) If the prescription is refilled after written information is available, such information is provided to the patient or patient's agent.

(d) The written information accompanying the prescription or the prescription label shall contain the statement "Do not flush unused medications or pour down a sink or drain." A drug product on a list of medicines developed by the FDA recommended for disposal by flushing is not required to bear this statement.

c. Only a pharmacist may verbally provide drug information to a patient or patient's agent and answer questions concerning prescription drugs. Non-pharmacist personnel and/or the pharmacy's computer system may not ask questions of a patient or patient's agent which are intended to screen and/or limit interaction with the pharmacist.

d. Nothing herein shall be construed as requiring a pharmacist to provide consultation when a patient or patient's agent refuses such consultation. The pharmacist shall document such refusal for consultation.

e. *Note: This section (e.) describes how patient counseling is provided to a patient when a prescription is delivered "at the pharmacy" and the pharmacist is not present, which is allowed under the Temporary Absence of Pharmacist rule in B.3. above. Notice that it requires complying with f. below which is the rule for providing counseling (written information) when prescriptions are delivered to a patient at his or her home or other designated location.*

In addition to the requirements of C.1.a.-d. above, if a prescription drug order is delivered to the patient at the pharmacy, the following is applicable:

(1) So that a patient will have access to information concerning his or her prescription, a prescription may not be delivered to a patient unless a pharmacist is in the pharmacy except as provided under the Temporary Absence of Pharmacist rule in B.3. above.

(2) Any prescription delivered to a patient when a pharmacist is not in the pharmacy (under the Temporary Absence of Pharmacist rule in B.3. above) must meet the requirements described in f. below.

f. *Note: This section (f.) describes procedures for providing drug information if a prescription is delivered to a patient at his or her home or any other location.*

In addition to the requirements of C.1.a.-c. above, if a prescription drug order is delivered to the patient or his or her agent at the patient's residence or other designated location, the following is applicable:

(1) The information specified in C.1.a. above shall be delivered with the dispensed prescription in writing.

(2) If prescriptions are routinely delivered outside the area covered by the pharmacy's local telephone service, the pharmacy shall provide a toll-free telephone number which is answered during normal hours to enable communication between the patient and a pharmacist.

(3) The pharmacist shall place on the prescription container or on a separate sheet delivered with the prescription container in both English and Spanish the local and, if applicable, toll-free telephone number of the pharmacy and the statement: "Written information about this prescription has been provided for you. Please read this information before you take the medication. If you have questions concerning this prescription, a pharmacist is available during normal business hours to answer these questions at (insert phone number)."

(4) The pharmacy shall maintain and use adequate storage or shipment containers and use shipping processes to ensure drug stability and potency. Such shipping processes shall include the use of appropriate packaging material and/or devices to ensure that the drug is maintained at an appropriate temperature range to maintain the integrity of the medication throughout the delivery process.
(5) The pharmacy shall use a delivery system which is designed to ensure that the drugs are delivered to the appropriate patient.
g. The provisions of C. above do not apply to patients in facilities where drugs are administered to patients by a person required to do so by the laws of Texas (i.e., nursing homes or hospital inpatients).
2. Pharmaceutical Care Services.
a. Drug Regimen Review (DRR). For the purpose of promoting therapeutic appropriateness, a pharmacist shall prior to or at the time of dispensing a prescription drug order review the patient's medication record. Such review shall at a minimum identify clinically significant:
(1) Known allergies;
(2) Rational therapy-contraindications;
(3) Reasonable dose and route of administration;
(4) Reasonable directions for use;
(5) Duplication of therapy;
(6) Drug-drug interactions;
(7) Drug-food interactions;
(8) Drug-disease interactions;
(9) Adverse drug reactions; and
(10) Proper utilization including overutilization or underutilization.
b. Upon identifying any clinically significant conditions, situations, or items listed above, the pharmacist shall take appropriate steps to avoid or resolve the problem including consultation with the prescribing practitioner. The pharmacist shall document such occurrences.
c. Documentation of consultation. When a pharmacist consults with a prescriber as described in b. above, the pharmacist shall document on the prescription or in the pharmacy's data processing system associated with the prescription such occurrences and shall include the following information:
(1) Date the prescriber was consulted;
(2) Name of the person communicating the prescriber's instructions;
(3) Any applicable information pertaining to the consultation; and
(4) Initials or identification code of the pharmacist performing the consultation clearly recorded for the purpose of identifying the pharmacist who performed the consultation.
d. The drug regimen review may be conducted by remotely accessing the pharmacy's electronic data base from outside the pharmacy by:
(1) An individual Texas licensed pharmacist who is an employee of the pharmacy provided the pharmacy establishes controls to protect the privacy of the patient and the security of confidential records or
(2) A pharmacist employed by a Class E pharmacy provided the pharmacies have entered into a written contract or agreement which outlines the services to be provided and the responsibilities and accountabilities of each pharmacy in compliance with federal and state laws and regulations.
e. Prior to dispensing, any questions regarding a prescription drug order must be resolved with the prescriber, and written documentation of these discussions must be made and maintained as specified in 2.c. above.

f. Other pharmaceutical care services which may be provided by pharmacists include but are not limited to the following:
   (1) Managing drug therapy as delegated by a practitioner as allowed under the provisions of the Texas Medical Practice Act;
   (2) Administering immunizations and vaccinations under written protocol of a physician;
   (3) Managing patient compliance programs;
   (4) Providing preventative healthcare services; and
   (5) Providing case management of patients who are being treated with high-risk or high-cost drugs or who are considered "high risk" due to their age, medical condition, family history, or a related concern.

3. Generic Substitution. (*See Chapter 309 in Chapter D of this book.*)
4. Substitution of Dosage Form. (*See Chapter 309 in Chapter D of this book.*)
5. Therapeutic Drug Interchange.
   A switch to a drug providing a similar therapeutic response to the one prescribed shall not be made without prior approval of the prescribing practitioner. This paragraph does not apply to generic substitution as described in Chapter 309 of Chapter D in this book.
   a. The patient shall be notified of the therapeutic drug interchange prior to or upon delivery of the dispensed prescription to the patient. Such notification shall include:
      (1) A description of the change;
      (2) The reason for the change;
      (3) Whom to contact with questions concerning the change; and
      (4) Instructions for return of the drug if not wanted by the patient.
   b. The pharmacy shall maintain documentation of the patient's notification of the therapeutic interchange which shall include:
      (1) The date of the notification;
      (2) The method of notification;
      (3) A description of the change; and
      (4) The reason for the change.
   c. The provisions of 5.a. and 5.b. above do not apply to prescriptions for patients in facilities where drugs are administered to patients by a person required to do so by the laws of this state, if the practitioner issuing the prescription has agreed to the use of a formulary that includes a listing of therapeutic interchanges that the practitioner has agreed to allow. The pharmacy must maintain a copy of the formulary including a list of the practitioners that have agreed to the formulary and the signature of these practitioners.

6. Notification on Safe Disposal of Schedule II Controlled Substances.
   a. Unless exempted per b. or c. below, a pharmacy that dispenses a Schedule II controlled substance prescription must provide the patient a notification on the safe disposal of controlled substances. The notice must provide information on locations where Schedule II controlled substances are accepted for safe disposal or provide an Internet address specified by the Board that provides a searchable database of such locations. *See Board Rule 315.3(a)(5) for details.*
   b. A pharmacy that is registered with DEA as an "authorized collector" of controlled substances and regularly accepts controlled substances for safe disposal does not have to provide the notice in a. above.
   c. A pharmacy that provides to the patient at the time of dispensing and at no cost to the patient either a mail-in pouch for surrendering unused controlled substances or chemicals to render any unused controlled

substances unusable or non-retrievable does not have to provide the notification in a. above.

D. Prescription Containers.
1. A drug shall be dispensed in a child-resistant container unless:
   a. The patient or the practitioner requests the prescription not be dispensed in a child-resistant container or
   b. The product is exempted from requirements of the Poison Prevention Packaging Act of 1970.
2. A drug shall be dispensed in an appropriate container as specified on the manufacturer's container.
3. Prescription containers or closures shall not be reused. However, if a patient or patient's agent has difficulty reading or understanding a prescription label, a prescription container may be reused provided:
   a. The container is designed to provide audio-recorded information about the proper use of the prescription medication;
   b. The container is reused for the same patient;
   c. The container is cleaned; and
   d. A new safety closure is used each time the prescription container is reused.

E. Labeling.
1. At the time of delivery of the drug, the dispensing container shall bear a label in plain language and printed in an easily readable font size, unless otherwise specified, with at least the following information:
   a. Name, address, and phone number of the pharmacy;
   b. Unique identification number of the prescription that is printed in an easily readable font size comparable to but no smaller than 10-point Times Roman;
   c. Date dispensed;
   d. Initials or identification code of the dispensing pharmacist;
      Note: This is not required if maintained in a computer system. See 3. below.
   e. Name of prescribing practitioner;
   f. If the prescription was signed by a pharmacist, the name of the pharmacist who signed the prescription for a dangerous drug under delegated authority of a physician as specified in the Texas Medical Practice Act;
   g. Name of the patient or, if such drug was prescribed for an animal, the species of the animal and the name of the owner that is printed in an easily readable font size comparable to but no smaller than 10-point Times Roman. The name of the patient's partner or family member is not required to be on the label of a drug prescribed for a partner for a sexually transmitted disease or for a patient's family member if the patient has an illness determined to be a pandemic by the Centers for Disease Control and Prevention, the World Health Organization, or the Governor's office;
   h. Instructions for use that are printed in an easily readable font size comparable to but no smaller than 10-point Times Roman;
   i. Quantity dispensed;
   j. Appropriate ancillary instructions such as storage instructions or cautionary statements such as warnings of potential harmful effects of combining the drug product with any product containing alcohol;
   k. If a CII-IV, federal transfer caution statement "Caution: Federal law prohibits the transfer of this drug to any person other than the patient for whom it was prescribed";

l. If the pharmacist has selected a generically equivalent drug pursuant to the provisions of Chapter 562 of the Act, the statement "Substituted for Brand Prescribed" or "Substituted for 'Brand Name'" where "Brand Name" is the actual name of the brand name product prescribed;

m. Name and strength of the actual drug product dispensed that is printed in an easily readable size comparable to but no smaller than 10-point Times Roman, unless otherwise directed by the prescribing practitioner.
   (1) The name shall be either:
      (a) The brand name or
      (b) If no brand name, then the generic name and name of the manufacturer or distributor of such generic drug. (The name of the manufacturer or distributor may be reduced to an abbreviation or initials, provided the abbreviation or initials are sufficient to identify the manufacturer or distributor. For combination drug preparations or nonsterile compounded drug products having no brand name, the principal active ingredients shall be indicated on the label).
   (2) Except as provided in (1)(a) above, the brand name of the prescribed drug shall not appear on the prescription container label unless it is the drug product actually dispensed;

n. Beyond-use date. The beyond-use date is the date beyond which a product should not be used. If the drug is dispensed in the original manufacturer's container, the beyond-use date (expiration date) is the one specified on the manufacturer's container. If the drug is dispensed in a container other than the manufacturer's original container, unless otherwise specified by the manufacturer, the beyond-use date shall be one year from the date the drug is dispensed or the manufacturer's expiration date, whichever is earlier. The beyond-use date may be placed on the prescription label or on a flag label attached to the bottle. A beyond-use date is not required on the label of a prescription dispensed to a person at the time of release from prison or jail if the prescription is for no more than a 10-day supply of medication; and

o. Either on the prescription label or the written information accompanying the prescription shall contain the statement "Do not flush unused medications or pour down a sink or drain." A drug product on a list of medicines developed by FDA recommended for disposal by flushing is not required to bear this statement.

2. If the prescription label required as specified in E.1. above is printed in a type size smaller than 10-point Times Roman, the pharmacy shall provide the patient written information containing the information specified in E.1. above in an easily readable font size comparable to but no smaller than 10-point Times Roman.

3. The label is not required to include the initials or identification code of the dispensing pharmacist specified in E.1. above if the identity of the dispensing pharmacist is recorded in the pharmacy's data processing system. The record of the identity of the dispensing pharmacist shall not be altered in the pharmacy's data processing system.

4. The dispensing container is not required to bear the label specified in E.1. above if all of the following provisions are met:
   a. The drug is prescribed for administration to an ultimate user who is institutionalized in a licensed healthcare institution (e.g., nursing home or hospital);
   b. No more than a 90-day supply is dispensed at one time;

c. The drug is not in the possession of the ultimate user prior to administration;
d. The pharmacist-in-charge has determined that the institution:
   (1) Maintains medication administration records which include adequate directions for use for the drug(s) prescribed;
   (2) Maintains records of ordering, receiving, and administering the drug(s); and
   (3) Provides for appropriate safeguards for the control and storage of the drug(s); and
e. The dispensing container bears a label that adequately:
   (1) Identifies the:
       (a) Pharmacy by name and address;
       (b) Unique identification number of the prescription;
       (c) Name and strength of the drug dispensed;
       (d) Name of the patient; and
       (e) Name of the prescribing practitioner or, if applicable, the advance practice registered nurse, physician assistant, or pharmacist who signed the prescription drug order.
   (2) Beyond-use date. The beyond-use date is the date beyond which a product should not be used. If the drug is dispensed in the original manufacturer's container, the beyond-use date (expiration date) is the one specified on the manufacturer's container. If the drug is dispensed in a container other than the manufacturer's original container, unless otherwise specified by the manufacturer, the beyond-use date shall be one year from the date the drug is dispensed or the manufacturer's expiration date, whichever is earlier. The beyond-use date may be placed on the prescription label or on a flag label attached to the bottle. A beyond-use date is not required on the label of a prescription dispensed to a person at the time of release from prison or jail if the prescription is for no more than a 10-day supply of medication.
   (3) Sets forth the directions for use and cautionary statements if any contained on the prescription drug order or required by law.

F. Returning Undelivered Medication to Stock.
   1. As specified in Section 431.021(w) of the Texas Food, Drug, and Cosmetic Act, a pharmacist may not accept an unused prescription or drug in whole or in part for the purpose of resale or redispensing to any person after the prescription or drug has been originally dispensed or sold except as provided in Board Rule 291.8 (Return of Prescription Drugs). Prescriptions that have not been picked up by or delivered to the patient or patient's agent may be returned to the pharmacy's stock for dispensing.
   2. A pharmacist shall evaluate the quality and safety of the prescriptions to be returned to stock.
   3. Prescriptions returned to stock for dispensing shall not be mixed with the manufacturer's container.
   4. Prescriptions returned to stock for dispensing should be used as soon as possible and stored in the dispensing container. The expiration date of the medication shall be the lesser of one year from the dispensing date on the prescription label or the manufacturer's expiration date if dispensed in the manufacturer's original container.
   5. At the time of dispensing, the prescription medication shall be placed in a new prescription container and not dispensed in the previously labeled container unless the label can be completely removed. However, if the medication is in the manufacturer's original container, the pharmacy label must be removed so that no confidential patient information is released.

Label Requirements for Dispensed Prescriptions

REQUIRED INFORMATION	FDA	DEA	TSBP
Name & address of the pharmacy	X	X	X
Phone number of the pharmacy			X
Prescription number & date	X	X	X
Name, initials, or identification code of dispensing pharmacist*			X
Name of practitioner	X	X	X
Name of patient	X	X	X
Quantity dispensed			X
Directions or instructions for use and cautionary statements, if any contained in Rx	X	X	X
Appropriate ancillary instructions such as for storage or cautionary statements, such as potential harmful effects of drug or alcohol combination.			X
If CII-IV, the statement: "CAUTION: FEDERAL LAW PROHIBITS THE TRANSFER OF THIS DRUG TO ANY PERSON OTHER THAN THE PATIENT FOR WHOM IT WAS PRESCRIBED."		X	X
If a generically equivalent drug is dispensed, the statement: "SUBSTITUTED FOR BRAND PRESCRIBED OR SUBSTITUTED FOR 'BRAND NAME' WHERE BRAND NAME IS THE ACTUAL NAME OF THE BRAND NAME PRODUCT PRESCRIBED."			X
Name & strength of actual drug dispensed, unless otherwise directed by prescriber. Name shall be brand name or, if no brand name, the generic name & name of the manufacturer.			X
Beyond-use date			X
The prescription label or the written information accompanying the prescription shall contain the statement "Do not flush unused medications or pour down a sink or drain." A drug product on a list developed by the Federal Food and Drug Administration of medicines recommended for disposal by flushing is not required to bear this statement.			X

*Not required on label if stored in computer.

Note: The dispensing container is not required to bear the label specified above, if the drug is prescribed for administration to an ultimate user who is institutionalized in a licensed healthcare institution.

G. Equipment and Supplies.
   1. Data processing system (computer) including a printer or comparable equipment;
   2. Refrigerator;
   3. Child-resistant, light-resistant, tight, and if applicable, glass containers;
   4. Prescription, poison, and other applicable labels;
   5. Equipment necessary for the proper preparation of prescriptions; and
   6. Metric/apothecary weight and measure conversion charts.
H. Library. Current copies (in hard copy or electronic format) of:
   1. Laws/Rules.
      a. Texas Pharmacy Act and rules;
      b. Texas Dangerous Drug Act and rules;
      c. Texas Controlled Substances Act and rules; and
      d. Federal Controlled Substances Act and rules (or official publication describing the requirements of the Federal Controlled Substances Act and rules).
   2. At least one current or updated reference from each of the following categories:
      a. Patient prescription drug information reference text or leaflets which are designed for the patient and must be available to the patient;
      b. At least one current or updated general drug information reference which is required to contain drug interaction information including information needed to determine severity or significance of the interaction and appropriate recommendations or actions to be taken; and
      c. If the pharmacy dispenses veterinary prescriptions, a general reference text on veterinary drugs.
   3. Basic antidote information and the telephone number of the nearest regional poison control center.
I. Drugs.
   1. Procurement and Storage.
      a. The pharmacist-in-charge is responsible for procurement and storage.
      b. Prescription drugs and devices shall be stored within the prescription department or a locked storage area.
      c. All drugs shall be stored at the proper temperature as defined in the USP/NF and Board Rule 291.15 (Storage of Drugs).
   2. Out-of-date drugs or devices shall not be dispensed beyond the expiration date, shall be removed from dispensing stock, and shall be quarantined until disposed of properly.
      Note: Stock should be checked regularly to ensure no expired drugs or devices are on the shelf of the pharmacy.
   3. Nonprescription C-Vs.
      Note: This rule sets forth the requirements for selling certain nonprescription Schedule V products. However, there are no commercially available products available that can be sold as a nonprescription product in Texas, so the rule language is not included in the book. See Chapter B.
   4. Class A pharmacies may not sell, purchase, trade, or possess prescription drug samples unless the pharmacy meets the requirements as specified in Board Rule 291.16 (Samples).
J. Prepackaging of Drugs (only for internal distribution by the pharmacy).
   1. Drugs may be prepackaged in quantities suitable for internal distribution only by a pharmacist or by pharmacy technicians or pharmacy technician trainees under the direction and direct supervision of a pharmacist.
      Note: These prepackaged drugs cannot be distributed to another pharmacy or to a practitioner.

2. The label of a prepackaged unit shall indicate:
   a. Brand name, strength, and dosage form of the drug; if no brand name, then indicate the generic name, strength, dosage form, and name of the manufacturer or distributor;
   b. Facility's lot number (the pharmacy's control number);
   c. Facility's (pharmacy's) beyond-use date; and
   d. Quantity of the drug if the quantity is greater than one.
3. Records of prepackaging shall be maintained to show:
   a. Name of the drug, strength, and dosage form;
   b. Pharmacy's lot number;
   c. Manufacturer or distributor;
   d. Manufacturer's lot number;
   e. Manufacturer's expiration date;
   f. Quantity per prepackaged unit;
   g. Number of prepackaged units;
   h. Date packaged;
   i. Name or initials of the prepacker; and
   j. Signature of the responsible pharmacist.
4. Stock packages, repackaged units, and control records shall be quarantined together until checked/released by the pharmacist.

K. Customized Patient Medication Packages.
1. Purpose.
   Instead of dispensing two or more prescribed drug products in separate containers, a pharmacist may with the consent of the patient, the patient's caregiver, or the prescriber provide a customized patient medication package (patient med pack).
2. Label.
   The patient med pack shall bear a label stating:
   a. Patient name;
   b. Unique identification number of patient med pack and a separate unique identifying number for each prescription drug;
   c. Name, strength, physical description or identification, and total quantity of each drug product contained in the med pack;
   d. Directions for use and cautionary statements for each drug product;
   e. If applicable, a warning of the potential harmful effect of combining any form of alcoholic beverage with any drug product contained therein;
   f. Storage instructions or cautionary statements required by the official compendia;
   g. Prescriber's name for each product;
   h. Date of preparation;
   i. Name, address, and telephone number of the pharmacy;
   j. Initials of the dispensing pharmacist;
   Note: This is not required on the label if recorded in the computer.
   k. The date after which the prescription should not be used or beyond-use date. Unless otherwise specified by the manufacturer, the beyond-use date shall be one year from the date the med pack is dispensed or the earliest manufacturer's expiration date for a product contained in the med pack if it is less than one year from the date dispensed. The beyond-use date may be placed on the prescription label or on a flag label attached to the bottle. A beyond-use date is not required on the label of a prescription dispensed to a person at the time of release from prison or jail if the prescription is for no more than a 10-day supply of medication;
   l. The prescription label or the written information accompanying the prescription shall contain the statement "Do not flush unused medications

or pour down a sink or drain." A drug product on a list of medicines developed by FDA recommended for disposal by flushing is not required to bear this statement;

m. Any other information required; and

n. If the patient med pack allows the removal or separation of intact containers, each shall bear a label for the product contained.

3. The dispensing container is not required to bear the label specified in K.2. above if:

a. The drug is prescribed for administration to an ultimate user who is institutionalized in a licensed healthcare institution (e.g., nursing home or hospital);

b. No more than a 90-day supply is dispensed at one time;

c. The drug is not in the possession of the ultimate user prior to administration;

d. The pharmacist-in-charge has determined that the institution:

(1) Maintains medication administration records which include adequate directions for the use of the drug(s) prescribed;

(2) Maintains records of ordering, receiving, and administering the drug(s); and

(3) Provides for appropriate safeguards for the control and storage of the drug(s); and

e. The dispensing container bears a label that adequately:

(1) Identifies the:

(a) Pharmacy name and address;

(b) Name and strength of each drug product dispensed;

(c) Name of the patient; and

(d) Name of the prescribing practitioner of each drug product or the pharmacist who signed the prescription drug order;

(2) Sets forth a beyond-use date; and

(3) For each drug product, sets forth the directions for use and cautionary statements, if any, contained on the prescription drug order or required by law.

4. Labeling.

The patient package insert for each drug dispensed is required or the drug information may be combined into one sheet.

5. Packaging.

It is the responsibility of the dispensing pharmacist when preparing a patient med pack to take into account any applicable compendial requirements or guidelines as well as the physical and chemical compatibility of the dosage forms placed within each container. Also, any therapeutic incompatibilities that may occur in the simultaneous administration of the drugs should be taken into account.

6. Guidelines.

It is the responsibility of the dispensing pharmacist to take into account physical and chemical compatibility of the drugs in each container and therapeutic incompatibility when drugs are administered simultaneously.

7. Recordkeeping.

In addition to regular filing requirements, a record of each patient med pack shall be made and filed containing:

a. Name and address of patient;

b. Serial number of the prescription order for each drug product contained therein;

c. Name of manufacturer or labeler and lot number of each drug;

d. Information describing the design so that a subsequent identical med pack can be prepared;

  e. Date of preparation and expiration date;
  f. Any special labeling instructions; and
  g. Name or initial of the pharmacist who prepared the med pack.
 L. Automated Devices and Systems in a Pharmacy.
  1. Automated Counting Devices. If a pharmacy uses automated counting devices:
   a. The pharmacy shall have a method to calibrate and verify the accuracy of the automated counting device and document the calibration and verification on a routine basis;
   b. The device may be loaded with bulk drugs only by a pharmacist or by a pharmacy technician under the direction and direct supervision of a pharmacist;
   c. The label of an automated counting device container containing a bulk drug shall indicate the brand name and strength of the drug. If no brand name, then the generic name, strength, and name of the manufacturer or distributor shall be indicated;
   d. Records of loading bulk drugs into an automated counting device shall be maintained to show:
    (1) Name of the drug, strength, and dosage form;
    (2) Manufacturer or distributor;
    (3) Manufacturer's lot number;
    (4) Manufacturer's expiration date;
    (5) Quantity added to the automated counting device;
    (6) Date of loading;
    (7) Name, initials, or electronic signature of the person loading the automated counting device; and
    (8) Name, initials, or electronic signature of the responsible pharmacist; and
   e. The automated counting device shall not be used until a pharmacist verifies that the system is properly loaded and affixes his or her name, initials, or electronic signature to the record specified in d. above.
  2. Automated Pharmacy Dispensing Systems.
   a. Authority to use automated pharmacy dispensing systems. A pharmacy may use an automated pharmacy dispensing system to fill prescription drug orders provided that:
    (1) The pharmacist-in-charge is responsible for the supervision of the system's operation;
    (2) The automated pharmacy dispensing system has been tested by the pharmacy and found to dispense accurately. The pharmacy shall make the results of such testing available to the Board upon request; and
    (3) The pharmacy will make the automated pharmacy dispensing system available for inspection by the Board for the purpose of validating the accuracy of the system.
   b. Automated pharmacy dispensing systems may be stocked or loaded by a pharmacist or by a pharmacy technician or pharmacy technician trainee under the supervision of a pharmacist.
   c. Quality assurance program.
   A pharmacy which uses an automated pharmacy dispensing system to fill prescription drug orders shall operate according to a quality assurance program of the automated pharmacy dispensing system which:
    (1) Requires continuous monitoring of the automated pharmacy dispensing system and
    (2) Establishes mechanisms and procedures to test the accuracy of the automated pharmacy dispensing system at least every twelve months

and whenever any upgrade or change is made to the system. Each activity must be documented.
  d. Policies and procedures of operation.
    (1) When an automated pharmacy dispensing system is used to fill prescription drug orders, it shall be operated according to written policies and procedures of operation. The policies and procedures of operation shall:
      (a) Provide for a pharmacist's review, approval, and accountability for the transmission of each original or new prescription drug order to the automated pharmacy dispensing system before the transmission is made;
      (b) Provide for access to the automated pharmacy dispensing system for stocking and retrieval of medications which is limited to licensed healthcare professionals or pharmacy technicians acting under the supervision of a pharmacist;
      (c) Require that a pharmacist checks, verifies, and documents that the correct medication and strength of bulk drugs, prepackaged containers, or manufacturer's unit-of-use packages were properly stocked, filled, and loaded in the automated pharmacy dispensing system prior to initiating the fill process. Alternatively, an electronic verification system may be used for verification of manufacturer's unit-of-use packages or prepacked medication previously verified by a pharmacist;
      (d) Provide for an accountability record to be maintained that documents all transactions relative to stocking and removing medications from the automated pharmacy dispensing system;
      (e) Require a prospective drug regimen review is conducted; and
      (f) Establish and make provisions for documentation of a preventative maintenance program for the automated pharmacy dispensing system.
    (2) A pharmacy that uses an automated pharmacy dispensing system to fill prescription drug orders shall at least annually review its written policies and procedures, revise them if necessary, and document the review.
  e. Recovery plan.
    A pharmacy that uses an automated pharmacy dispensing system to fill prescription drug orders shall maintain a written plan for recovery from a disaster or any other situation which interrupts the ability of the automated pharmacy dispensing system to provide services necessary for the operation of the pharmacy. The written plan for recovery shall include:
    (1) Planning and preparation for maintaining pharmacy services when an automated pharmacy dispensing system is experiencing downtime;
    (2) Procedures for response when an automated pharmacy dispensing system is experiencing downtime; and
    (3) Procedures for the maintenance and testing of the written plan for recovery.
  f. Final check of the prescriptions dispensed using an automated pharmacy dispensing system. A pharmacist must perform the final check of all prescriptions prior to delivery to the patient to ensure that the prescription is dispensed accurately as prescribed.
    (1) This final check shall be considered accomplished if:
      (a) A check of the final product is conducted by a pharmacist after the automated pharmacy dispensing system has completed the prescription and prior to delivery to the patient or

(b) The following checks are conducted:
  (i) If the automated pharmacy dispensing system contains bulk stock drugs, a pharmacist verifies that those drugs have been accurately stocked as specified in 2.d.(1)(c) above;
  (ii) If the automated pharmacy dispensing system contains manufacturer's unit-of-use packages or prepackaged medication previously verified by a pharmacist, an electronic verification system has confirmed that the medications have been accurately stocked as specified in 2.d.(1)(c) above;
  (iii) A pharmacist checks the accuracy of the data entry of each original or new prescription drug order entered into the automated dispensing system; and
  (iv) An electronic verification process is used to verify the proper prescription label has been affixed to the correct medication container, prepackaged medication, or manufacturer's unit-of-use package for the correct patient.
(2) If the final check is accomplished as specified in f.(1)(b) above, the following additional requirements must be met.
  (a) The dispensing process must be fully automated from the time the pharmacist releases the prescription to the automated pharmacy dispensing system until a completed, labeled prescription ready for delivery to the patient is produced.
  (b) The pharmacy has conducted initial testing and has a continuous quality assurance program which documents that the automated pharmacy dispensing system dispenses accurately as prescribed.
  (c) The automated pharmacy dispensing system documents and maintains:
    (i) The name(s), initials, or identification code(s) of each pharmacist responsible for the checks outlined in f.(1)(b) above (verification of stocking bulk drugs, electronic verification of manufacturer's unit-of-use or prepackaged drugs, and data entry for prescription drug orders) and
    (ii) The name(s), initials, or identification code(s) and specific activity(ies) of each pharmacist, pharmacy technician, or pharmacy technician trainee who performs any other portion of the dispensing process.
  (d) The pharmacy establishes mechanisms and procedures to test the accuracy of the automated pharmacy dispensing system at least every month rather than every twelve months.
3. Automated Checking Device.
  a. An automated checking device is a fully automated device which confirms after dispensing but prior to delivery to the patient that the correct drug and strength have been labeled with the correct label for the correct patient.
  b. The final check of a dispensed prescription shall be considered accomplished using an automated checking device provided a check of the final product is conducted by a pharmacist prior to delivery to the patient or the following checks are performed:
    (1) The drug used to fill the order is checked through the use of an automated checking device which verifies that the drug is labeled and packaged accurately and
    (2) A pharmacist checks the accuracy of each original or new prescription drug order and is responsible for the final check of the order through the automated checking device.

c. If the final check is accomplished as specified using an automated checking device, the following additional requirements must be met.
   (1) The pharmacy has conducted initial testing of the automated checking device and has a continuous quality assurance program which documents that the automated checking device accurately confirms that the correct drug and strength have been labeled with the correct label for the correct patient.
   (2) The pharmacy documents and maintains the name(s), initials, or identification code(s) of each pharmacist responsible for the checks outlined in 3.b.(1) and (2) above and the name(s), initials, or identification code(s) and specific activity(ies) of each pharmacist, pharmacy technician, or pharmacy technician trainee who performs any other portion of the dispensing process.
   (3) The pharmacy establishes mechanisms and procedures to test the accuracy of the automated checking device at least monthly.
   (4) The pharmacy establishes procedures to ensure that errors identified by the automated checking device may not be overridden by a pharmacy technician and must be reviewed and corrected by a pharmacist.

Questions and Answers
Automation in Class A (Community) Pharmacies

Q1. What automated devices are recognized in the rules for Class A Pharmacies?
Answer: There are three types of automated devices that may be used in a Class A pharmacy:
1. Automated counting devices;
2. Automated pharmacy dispensing systems; and
3. Automated checking devices.

Q2. How are these three devices defined?
Answer:
1. **Automated counting device**—An automated device that is loaded with bulk drugs and counts and/or packages (i.e., fills a vial or other container) a specified quantity of dosage units of a designated drug product.
   Note: These devices contain bulk drugs which are counted. A common example used in a Class A pharmacy is a Baker cell or similar device.
2. **Automated pharmacy dispensing system**—A system that automatically performs operations or activities other than compounding or administration relative to the storing, packaging, counting, and labeling for dispensing and delivery of medications and that collects, controls, and maintains all transaction information.
   Note: These devices perform all of the mechanical aspects of preparing a prescription.
3. **Automated checking device**—A fully automated device which confirms, after dispensing but prior to delivery to the patient, that the correct drug and strength have been labeled with the correct label for the correct patient.
   Note: These devices use technology (e.g., barcoding) to check a final prescription after it has been dispensed.

Q3. What about automated storage and delivery devices such as kiosks for patients to pick up dispensed prescriptions?
Answer: A Class A pharmacy may use an automated storage and delivery device to deliver dispensed prescriptions to patients at a remote site with Board approval. However,

since these devices are located outside of the pharmacy, the rules for these systems are found in Board Rule 291.121 (Remote Services). *See Chapter D.*

Automated Counting Devices

Q4. Can an automated counting device be loaded by a pharmacy technician?
Answer: Yes. These devices must be loaded by a pharmacist or by a pharmacy technician under the direction and direct supervision of a pharmacist. In addition, the device has to be labeled with the brand name of the drug and the strength. If there is no brand name, it must be labeled with the generic name of the drug, strength, and the manufacturer or distributor. A record of loading the device must be made which contains the:
1. Name of the drug, strength, and dosage form;
2. Name of manufacturer or distributor;
3. Manufacturer's lot number;
4. Expiration date;
5. Date of loading;
6. Name, initials, or electronic signature of the person loading the automated counting device; and
7. Name, initials, or electronic signature of the responsible pharmacist.

Q5. Once the automated counting device has been loaded and labeled by a technician and a proper record made, is the device ready for use?
Answer: Not yet. A pharmacist must verify that the system was properly loaded and affix his or her name, initials, or electronic signature to the record indicated in the answer to Q4. Now the device is ready for use in the dispensing process.

Automated Pharmacy Dispensing Systems

Q6. Under what conditions can an automated pharmacy dispensing system be used?
Answer: An automated pharmacy dispensing system may only be used if the pharmacist-in-charge is responsible for the supervision of the system's operation. Before the first prescription is dispensed, the device has to be thoroughly tested and found to dispense accurately. There must also be an ongoing quality assurance program that continuously monitors the system and tests the accuracy of the system at least every twelve months and whenever an upgrade to the system is made.

Q7. Should an automated pharmacy dispensing system be operated according to formalized policies and procedures?
Answer: Yes. Board rules require the pharmacy to establish written requirements for operation of the device and describe policies and procedures that:
1. Include a description of the policies and procedures of operation;
2. Provide for a pharmacist's review, approval, and accountability for the transmission of each original or new prescription drug order to the automated pharmacy dispensing system before the transmission is made;
3. Provide for access to the automated pharmacy dispensing system for stocking and retrieval of medications which is limited to licensed healthcare professionals or pharmacy technicians acting under the supervision of a pharmacist;
4. Require prior to use that a pharmacist checks, verifies, and documents that the automated pharmacy dispensing system has been accurately filled each time the system is stocked;
5. Provide for an accountability record to be maintained which documents all transactions relative to stocking and removing medications from the automated pharmacy dispensing system;
6. Require a prospective drug regimen review; and

Notes

7. Establish and make provisions for documentation of a preventative maintenance program for the automated pharmacy dispensing system. In addition, the policies and procedures must be reviewed annually and updated if needed.

Q8. Since a properly tested and maintained automated pharmacy dispensing system is so accurate, is a pharmacist required to conduct a final check of a prescription dispensed by the device?

Answer: Yes. If a pharmacy uses an automated pharmacy dispensing system, the final check shall be considered accomplished if:

1. A check of the final product is conducted by a pharmacist after the automated system has completed the prescription and prior to delivery to the patient or
2. The following checks are conducted by a pharmacist:
   a. If the automated pharmacy dispensing system contains bulk stock drugs, a pharmacist verifies that those drugs have been accurately stocked as specified in the answer to Q7 and
   b. A pharmacist checks the accuracy of the data entry of each original or new prescription drug order entered into the automated pharmacy dispensing system.

If the final check is performed in the manner indicated in 2. above, the following additional requirements must be met.

1. The dispensing process is fully automated from the time the pharmacist releases the prescription to the automated system until a completed, labeled prescription ready for delivery to the patient is produced.
2. The pharmacy has conducted initial testing and has a continuous quality assurance program which documents that the automated pharmacy dispensing system dispenses accurately.
3. The automated pharmacy dispensing system documents and maintains:
   a. The name(s), initials, or identification code(s) of each pharmacist responsible for verifying drugs were accurately stocked in the device and for checking the accuracy of the data entry of prescription information and specific activity(ies) into the system and
   b. The name(s), initials, or identification code(s) of each pharmacist or pharmacy technician who performs any other portion of the dispensing process.
4. The pharmacy establishes mechanisms and procedures to test the accuracy of the automated pharmacy dispensing system at least every month rather than every twelve months.

Automated Checking Devices

Q9. Since an automated checking device and an automated pharmacy dispensing system can both be used to conduct a final check of a dispensed prescription, what is the difference between the two systems?

Answer: In an automated pharmacy dispensing system, the device is actually filling prescriptions while checking for accuracy. With the automated checking device, completed prescriptions are checked for accuracy using technology such as barcoding.

Q10. Can an automated checking device be used to complete the final check of a dispensed prescription?

Answer: Yes. If using an automated checking device, the final check shall be considered accomplished if:

1. A check of the final product is conducted by a pharmacist prior to delivery to the patient or the following checks are performed:
   a. The drug used to fill the order is checked through the use of an automated checking device which verifies that the drug is labeled and packaged accurately and

b. A pharmacist checks the accuracy of each original or new prescription drug order and is responsible for the final check of the order through the automated checking device.
2. The following additional requirements must be met when using an automated checking device to perform the final check.
   a. The pharmacy has conducted initial testing of the automated checking device and has a continuous quality assurance program which documents that the automated checking device accurately confirms that the correct drug and strength have been labeled with the correct label for the correct patient.
   b. The pharmacy documents and maintains the name(s), initials, or identification code(s) of each pharmacist responsible for the checks above and the name(s), initials, or identification code(s) and specific activity(ies) of each pharmacist, pharmacy technician, or pharmacy technician trainee who performs any other portion of the dispensing process.
   c. The pharmacy establishes mechanisms and procedures to test the accuracy of the automated checking device at least monthly.
   d. The pharmacy establishes procedures to ensure that errors identified by the automated checking device may not be overridden by a pharmacy technician and must be reviewed and corrected by a pharmacist.

Board of Pharmacy Rule 291.34
Records

A. Maintenance of Records.
   1. Every inventory or other record required to be kept by a community pharmacy (Class A) shall be:
      a. Kept by the pharmacy at the pharmacy's licensed location and be available for at least two years from the date of such inventory or record for inspecting and copying by the Board or its representatives and to other authorized local, state, or federal law enforcement agencies and
      b. Supplied by the pharmacy within 72 hours if requested by an authorized agent of the Texas State Board of Pharmacy. If the pharmacy maintains the records in an electronic format, the requested records must be provided in a mutually agreeable electronic format if specifically requested by the Board or its representative. Failure to provide the records set out in this rule either on-site or within 72 hours constitutes prima facie evidence of failure to keep and maintain records in violation of the Act.
   2. Schedule II records shall be maintained separately from all other records.
   3. Schedule III, IV, and V records, other than prescriptions, shall be maintained separately or readily retrievable from all other records of the pharmacy. Readily retrievable means that the controlled substances records shall be asterisked, redlined, or in some other manner readily identifiable apart from all other items appearing on the record.
   4. Records, except when specifically required to be maintained in original or hardcopy form, may be maintained in a data processing system or direct imaging system provided:
      a. The records maintained in the alternative system contain all of the information required on the manual record and
      b. The data processing system is capable of producing a hard copy of the record upon the request of the Board or other authorized agencies.
B. Prescriptions.
   1. Professional Responsibility.
      a. Pharmacists shall exercise sound professional judgment with respect to the accuracy and authenticity of any prescription drug order they

dispense. If the pharmacist questions the accuracy or authenticity of a prescription drug order, he or she shall verify the order with a practitioner prior to dispensing.
   b. Prior to dispensing a prescription, pharmacists shall determine in the exercise of sound professional judgment that the prescription is a valid prescription. A pharmacist may not dispense a prescription drug unless the pharmacist complies with the requirements of Section 562.056 and 562.112 of the Act and Board Rule 291.29 (Professional Responsibility of Pharmacists). *(See Chapter E in this book.)*
   Note: This extends the concept of the pharmacist's "corresponding responsibility" to ensure that controlled substance prescriptions are written for a legitimate medical purpose and in the usual course of professional practice to all prescriptions, both controlled substances and dangerous drugs.
   c. This rule does not prohibit a pharmacist from dispensing a prescription when a valid patient-practitioner relationship is not present in an emergency situation (e.g., a practitioner on call for the patient's regular practitioner).
   d. The owner of a Class A pharmacy shall have responsibility for ensuring his or her agents and employees engage in appropriate decisions regarding dispensing of valid prescriptions as set forth in Section 562.112 of the Texas Pharmacy Act (regarding a valid practitioner-patient relationship).
   e. The practice of telemedicine/telehealth is a "legal" practice in the state of Texas. The Texas Medical Practice Act allows for the use of an Internet-based or telephone consultation between the prescriber and a patient. Prescriptions issued in these circumstances may be valid, but pharmacists must still ensure that there is a valid practitioner-patient relationship. Texas Medical Board rules specify two prohibitions on telemedicine:
      (1) A practitioner-patient relationship is not present if a practitioner prescribes an abortifacient or any other drug or device that terminates a pregnancy and
      (2) Treatment for chronic pain with controlled substances using telemedicine is not allowed.
      TSBP has a *Telemedicine Frequently Asked Questions* document on its website which provides more information on telemedicine for pharmacists.
2. Written Prescriptions.
   a. Practitioner's signature.
      (1) Dangerous drug prescription orders. Written prescription drug orders shall be manually signed by the practitioner or electronically signed by the practitioner using a system that electronically replicates the practitioner's manual signature on the written prescription provided:
         (a) The security features of the system require the practitioner to authorize each use and
         (b) The prescription is printed on paper that is designed to prevent unauthorized copying of a completed prescription and to prevent the erasure or modification of information written on the prescription by the prescribing practitioner. (For example, the prescription paper contains security provisions against copying that result in some indication on the copy that it is a copy and, therefore, renders the prescription null and void.)
      (2) Controlled substance prescription orders. Prescription drug orders for Schedules II, III, IV, or V controlled substances shall be manually signed by the practitioner. Prescription drug orders for Schedule II

controlled substances shall be issued on an official prescription form as required by Section 481.075 of the Texas Controlled Substances Act.
- (3) Other provisions for a practitioner's signature.
  - (a) A practitioner may sign a prescription drug order in the same manner as he or she would sign a check or legal document (e.g., J.H. Smith or John H. Smith).
  - (b) Rubber stamped signatures may not be used.
  - (c) A practitioner's agent may prepare a prescription for the signature of a practitioner but may not sign the prescription.

b. Prescriptions written by practitioners in another state.
- (1) Dangerous drug prescriptions may be dispensed in the same manner as are prescriptions issued by practitioners in Texas.
- (2) C-III-V prescriptions. A pharmacist may dispense prescription drug orders for controlled substances in Schedules III, IV, or V issued by a physician, dentist, veterinarian, or podiatrist in another state provided:
  - (a) The prescription drug order is issued by a person practicing in another state and licensed by another state as a physician, dentist, veterinarian, or podiatrist who has a current federal DEA registration number and who may legally prescribe Schedule III, IV, or V controlled substances in such other state;
  - (b) The prescription drug order is not dispensed or refilled more than six months from the initial date of issuance and may not be refilled more than five times; and
  - (c) If there are no refill instructions on the original prescription drug order (which shall be interpreted as no refills authorized) or if all refills authorized on the original prescription drug order have been dispensed, a new prescription drug order is obtained from the prescribing practitioner prior to dispensing any additional quantities of controlled substances.
- (3) C-II prescriptions may not be dispensed from out-of-state practitioners unless:
  - (a) The prescription is filled in compliance with Board Rule 315.9 including having a written plan approved by the Texas State Board of Pharmacy;
  - (b) An original written prescription is required;
  - (c) The prescription is issued by a physician, dentist, veterinarian, or podiatrist having a current DEA registration and who may legally prescribe Schedule II controlled substances in such other state; and
  - (d) The prescription is not dispensed beyond 21 days from the date the prescription was issued.

Note: Controlled substance prescriptions from out-of-state nurse practitioners or physician assistants are not valid in Texas and cannot be filled by Texas pharmacies.

c. Prescription drug orders written by practitioners in Mexico or Canada.
- (1) Controlled substance prescriptions may not be dispensed.
- (2) Prescriptions issued for dangerous drugs by a person licensed in Canada or Mexico as a physician, dentist, veterinarian, or podiatrist may be dispensed provided:
  - (a) The prescription is an original written prescription and
  - (b) If there are no refill instructions on the original written prescription or if all refills authorized on the original written

prescription drug order have been dispensed, a new written prescription drug order shall be obtained.
   d. Prescription drug orders issued by an advanced practice registered nurse (APRN) or physician assistant (PA) or signed by a pharmacist.
      (1) A pharmacist may dispense a prescription drug order issued by an APRN or PA if the APRN or PA is practicing in accordance with Chapter 157 of the Texas Medical Practice Act. Additionally, a prescription drug order for a dangerous drug signed by a pharmacist under delegated authority in accordance with the Texas Medical Practice Act may also be dispensed by a pharmacist.
      (2) Each practitioner must designate in writing the name of each APRN or PA authorized to prescribe or order a prescription, maintain the list in the physician's usual place of business, and furnish the list to a pharmacist upon request.
   e. Prescriptions for Schedule II controlled substances.
      Except in "emergency situations," written Schedule II prescriptions may not be dispensed without an official prescription form as required by the Texas Controlled Substances Act.
3. Verbal Prescription Drug Orders.
   a. A verbal prescription drug order from a practitioner or his or her designated agent may only be taken by a pharmacist or pharmacist intern under direct supervision of a pharmacist.
   b. A practitioner shall designate in writing the name of each agent authorized by the practitioner to communicate prescriptions verbally for the practitioner. The practitioner shall maintain at the practitioner's usual place of business a list of the designated agents and shall provide a copy of the list upon the request of a pharmacist.
   c. Verbal prescriptions for a dangerous drug or a controlled substance issued by a practitioner licensed in Canada or Mexico may not be dispensed unless the practitioner is also licensed in Texas.
4. Electronic Prescription Drug Orders.
   Note: This section does not apply to faxed prescriptions. See 5. below for rules on faxed prescriptions.
   a. Dangerous drug prescription orders.
      (1) An electronic prescription for a dangerous drug may be transmitted by a practitioner or his or her designated agent directly to a pharmacy.
      (2) Another alternative is through the use of a data communication device provided the confidential prescription information is not altered during transmission and confidential patient information is not accessed or maintained by the operator of the data communication device other than for legal purposes under federal and state law.
   b. Controlled substance prescription orders.
      A pharmacist may only dispense an electronic prescription drug order for a Schedule II, III, IV, or V controlled substance in compliance with federal and state laws and the rules of the Drug Enforcement Administration and the Texas State Board of Pharmacy.
   c. Prescriptions issued by a practitioner licensed in Canada or Mexico.
      A pharmacist may not dispense an electronic prescription drug order for a dangerous drug or controlled substance issued by a practitioner licensed in the Dominion of Canada or the United Mexican States unless the practitioner is also licensed in Texas.
5. Facsimile (faxed) Prescription Drug Orders.
   a. A pharmacist may dispense a prescription drug order for a dangerous drug transmitted to the pharmacy by facsimile.

b. A pharmacist may dispense a prescription drug order for a Schedule III, IV, or V controlled substance transmitted to the pharmacy by facsimile provided the prescription is manually signed by the practitioner and not electronically signed using a system that electronically replicates the practitioner's manual signature on the prescription drug order.
c. A pharmacist may not dispense a prescription drug order for a Schedule II controlled substance transmitted to the pharmacy by facsimile except for limited situations (i.e., injectable narcotics, Schedule II prescriptions for long term care facility residents, and narcotic Schedule II prescriptions for hospice patients). *(See Chapter B in this book.)*
d. A pharmacist may not dispense a facsimile prescription drug order for a dangerous drug or a controlled substance issued by a practitioner licensed in Canada or Mexico unless the practitioner is also licensed in Texas.

6. Original Prescription Drug Order Records.
   a. Original prescriptions may be dispensed only in accordance with the prescriber's authorization as indicated on the original prescription drug order.
   b. Notwithstanding a. above, a pharmacist may dispense a quantity less than indicated on the original prescription drug order at the request of the patient or patient's agent.
   c. Original prescriptions shall be maintained in numerical order and remain legible for a period of two years from the date of filling or the date of the last refill dispensed. "Original prescriptions" means:
      (1) Original written prescriptions or
      (2) Original verbal or electronic prescriptions reduced to writing either manually or electronically by the pharmacist.
   d. If an original prescription drug order is changed, the prescription shall be invalid. If additional drugs are to be dispensed, a new prescription with a new and separate number is required. However, an original prescription drug order for a dangerous drug may be changed in accordance with 9. below (Accelerated Refills).
   e. Original prescriptions shall be maintained in three separate files:
      (1) Schedule II;
      (2) Schedule III–V; and
      (3) Dangerous drugs and nonprescription drugs.
   f. Original prescription records, other than prescriptions for Schedule II controlled substances, may be stored in a system that is capable of producing a direct image of the original prescription provided:
      (1) Refills recorded on the original prescription must also be stored in this system;
      (2) Original prescription records must be maintained in numerical order and separated in three files as previously indicated; and
      (3) The pharmacy must provide immediate access to equipment necessary to render the records easily readable.

   Note: Although TSBP rules permit imaging of Schedule III–V controlled substance prescriptions, DEA requires the original prescription to be kept for two years for all controlled substance prescriptions.

7. Prescription Drug Order Information (prescriptions issued by practitioners).
   a. All original prescriptions issued by practitioners shall bear:
      (1) Name of the patient; if such drug is for an animal, the species of such animal and the name of the owner;
      (2) Address of the patient provided, however, a dangerous drug prescription is not required to bear the address of the patient if such

address is readily retrievable on another pharmacy record (e.g., medication records) or in the pharmacy's computer system;
(3) Name, address, and telephone number legibly printed or stamped of the practitioner's usual place of business and, if for a controlled substance, the DEA registration number of the practitioner;
(4) Name and strength of the drug prescribed;
(5) Quantity prescribed numerically and if for a controlled substance:
   (a) Numerically, followed by the number written as a word if the prescription is written;
   (b) Numerically if the prescription is electronic; or
   (c) If the prescription is communicated orally or by telephone, as transcribed by the receiving pharmacist;
(6) Directions for use;
(7) Intended use for the drug unless the practitioner determines the furnishing of this information is not in the best interest of the patient;
(8) Date of issuance;
(9) If a faxed prescription:
   (a) A statement that the prescription has been faxed (e.g., faxed to) and
   (b) If transmitted by a designated agent, the full name of the designated agent;
(10) If electronically transmitted:
   (a) The date the prescription drug order was electronically transmitted to the pharmacy if different from the date of issuance of the prescription and
   (b) If transmitted by a designated agent, the full name of the designated agent;
(11) If issued by an advanced practice registered nurse (APRN) or physician assistant (PA), the:
   (a) Name, address, telephone number, and, if the prescription is for a controlled substance, the DEA number of the supervising practitioner and
   (b) The address and telephone number of the clinic where the prescription drug order was prescribed; and
(12) If communicated orally or telephonically:
   (a) The initials or identification code of the transcribing pharmacist and
   (b) The name of the prescriber or prescriber's agent communicating the prescription information.
b. At the time of dispensing, a pharmacist is responsible for documenting the following information on either the original hardcopy prescription or in the pharmacy's data processing system:
   (1) Unique identification number of the prescription;
   (2) Initials or identification code of the dispensing pharmacist;
   (3) Initials or identification code of the pharmacy technician or pharmacy technician trainee performing data entry of the prescription if applicable;
   (4) Quantity dispensed if different from the quantity prescribed;
   (5) Date of dispensing if different from the date of issuance; and
   (6) Brand name or manufacturer of the drug or biological product actually dispensed if the drug was prescribed by generic name or interchangeable biological name or if a drug or interchangeable biological product other than the one prescribed was dispensed pursuant to provisions of the Act, Chapters 562 and 563.

c. Prescription drug orders may be utilized as authorized in Title 40, Part 1, Chapter 231 of the Texas Administrative Code (Nursing Facility Requirements for Licensure and Medicaid Certification).

Note: This rule allows nursing facilities to use a chart order as the prescription drug order for dangerous drugs. The rule does not apply to controlled substance prescriptions.

  (1) A prescription drug order for a dangerous drug is not required to bear the information listed above in 7.a. if the dangerous drug is prescribed for administration to an ultimate user who is institutionalized in a licensed healthcare institution (e.g., nursing home, hospice, or hospital). Such prescription drug orders must contain the following information:
     (a) The full name of the patient;
     (b) The date of issuance;
     (c) The name, strength, and dosage form of the drug prescribed;
     (d) Directions for use; and
     (e) The signature(s) of the prescriber as required by Rule 19.1506, Texas Administrative Code (drug order rule for nursing facilities).
  (2) Prescription drug orders for dangerous drugs shall not be dispensed following one year after the date of issuance unless the authorized prescriber renews the prescription drug order.
  (3) Controlled substances shall not be dispensed pursuant to a prescription drug order under this rule.

8. Refills.
   a. General information.
      (1) Refills may be dispensed only in accordance with the prescriber's authorization on the original prescription except as authorized in 9. below (Accelerated Refills).
      (2) If there are no refill instructions on the original prescription (which shall be interpreted as no refills authorized) or if all refills authorized on the original prescription have been dispensed, authorization from the practitioner shall be obtained and documented prior to dispensing any refills.
   b. Refills of prescriptions for dangerous drugs or nonprescription drugs.
      (1) Prescriptions for dangerous drugs or nonprescription drugs (including PRN refill prescriptions) may not be refilled after one year from the date of issuance.
      (2) If one year has expired from the date of issuance, authorization shall be obtained from the practitioner prior to dispensing any additional quantities of the drug.
   c. Refills of prescription drug orders for Schedule III–V controlled substances.
      (1) May not be refilled more than five times or after six months from the date of issuance of the original prescription drug order, whichever occurs first.
      (2) If a prescription drug order for a Schedule III, IV, or V controlled substance has been refilled a total of five times or if six months have expired from the date of issuance, whichever occurs first, a new prescription shall be obtained from the prescribing practitioner prior to dispensing any additional quantities of controlled substances.
   d. Emergency refills (unable to contact prescriber—72-Hour Rule).
      If a pharmacist is unable to contact the prescribing practitioner after a reasonable effort, a pharmacist may exercise his or her professional judgment in refilling a prescription drug order for a drug other than a

controlled substance listed in Schedule II without the authorization of the prescribing practitioner provided:
(1) Failure to refill the prescription might result in an interruption of a therapeutic regimen or create patient suffering;
(2) The quantity of the prescription drug dispensed does not exceed a 72-hour supply;
Note: If the prescription drug is in a unit-of-use package or is a product such as an inhaler or eye drops, TSBP allows dispensing of the entire package or product which may be more than a 72-hour supply.
(3) The pharmacist informs the patient or the patient's agent at the time of dispensing that the refill is being provided without such authorization and that authorization of the practitioner is required for future refills;
(4) The pharmacist informs the practitioner of the emergency refill at the earliest reasonable time;
(5) The pharmacist maintains a record of the emergency refill containing the information required to be maintained on a prescription as specified in this rule;
(6) The pharmacist affixes a label to the dispensing container as specified in Board Rule 291.33(c)(7) (Operational Standards); and
(7) If the prescription was initially filled at another pharmacy, the pharmacist may exercise his or her professional judgment in refilling the prescription provided:
  (a) The patient has the prescription container, label, receipt, or other documentation from the other pharmacy that contains the essential information;
  (b) After a reasonable effort, the pharmacist is unable to contact the other pharmacy to transfer the remaining prescription refills or there are no refills remaining on the prescription;
  (c) The pharmacist in his or her professional judgment determines that such a request for an emergency refill is appropriate and meets the requirements of (1) and (2) above; and
  (d) The pharmacist complies with the requirements of (3)-(5) above.
e. Emergency refills (governor declared state of disaster—30-Day Rule).
If a natural or manmade disaster occurs that prohibits a pharmacist from being able to contact a practitioner, a pharmacist may exercise his or her professional judgment in refilling a prescription drug order for a drug other than a controlled substance listed in Schedule II without the authorization of the prescribing practitioner provided:
(1) Failure to refill the prescription might result in an interruption of a therapeutic regimen or create patient suffering;
(2) The quantity of the prescription drug dispensed does not exceed a 30-day supply;
Note: If the prescription drug is in a unit-of-use package or is a product such as an inhaler or eye drops, TSBP allows dispensing of the entire package or product which may be more than a 72-hour supply.
(3) The governor has declared a state of disaster;
(4) The Board through the executive director has notified pharmacies in this state that pharmacists may dispense up to a 30-day supply of prescription drugs;
(5) The pharmacist informs the patient or the patient's agent at the time of dispensing that the refill is being provided without such authorization and that authorization of the practitioner is required for future refills;

(6) The pharmacist informs the practitioner of the emergency refill at the earliest reasonable time;
(7) The pharmacist maintains a record of the emergency refill containing the information required to be maintained on a prescription as specified in this rule;
(8) The pharmacist affixes a label to the dispensing container as specified in Board Rule 291.33(c)(7) (Operational Standards); and
(9) If the prescription was initially filled at another pharmacy, the pharmacist may exercise his or her professional judgment in refilling the prescription provided:
  (a) The patient has the prescription container, label, receipt, or other documentation from the other pharmacy that contains the essential information;
  (b) After a reasonable effort, the pharmacist is unable to contact the other pharmacy to transfer the remaining prescription refills or there are no refills remaining on the prescription;
  (c) The pharmacist in his or her professional judgment determines that such a request for an emergency refill is appropriate and meets the requirements of (1) and (2) above; and
  (d) The pharmacist complies with the requirements of (3)-(5) above.
f. Auto-refill programs. A pharmacy may use a program that automatically refills prescriptions that have existing refills available to improve patient compliance with and adherence to prescribed medication therapy. The following is applicable in order to enroll patients into an auto-refill program:
  (1) Notice of availability of an auto-refill program shall be given to the patient or the patient's agent, and the patient or the patient's agent must affirmatively indicate that they wish to enroll in such a program. The pharmacy shall document such indication.
  (2) The patient or patient's agent shall have the option to withdraw from such a program at any time.
  (3) Auto-refill programs may be used for refills of dangerous drugs and Schedule IV and V controlled substances. Schedule II and III controlled substances may not be dispensed by an auto-refill program. *Note: Refills for Schedule II prescriptions are not allowed.*
  (4) As is required for all prescriptions, a drug regimen review shall be completed on all prescriptions filled as a result of an auto-refill program. Special attention shall be noted for drug regimen review warnings of duplication of therapy, and all such conflicts shall be resolved with the prescribing practitioner prior to refilling the prescription.
9. Accelerated Refills. In accordance with Section 562.0545 of the Act, a pharmacist may dispense up to a 90-day supply of a dangerous drug pursuant to a valid prescription that specifies the dispensing of a lesser amount followed by periodic refills of that amount if:
  a. The total quantity of dosage units dispensed does not exceed the total quantity of dosage units authorized by the prescriber on the original prescription including refills;
  b. The patient consents to the dispensing of up to a 90-day supply, and the physician has been notified electronically or by telephone;
  c. The physician has not specified on the prescription that dispensing the prescription in an initial amount followed by periodic refills is medically necessary;
  d. The dangerous drug is not a psychotropic drug; and
  e. The patient is at least 18 years of age.

10. Records Relating to Dispensing Errors.

    If a dispensing error occurs, the following is applicable.
    a. Original prescription drug orders:
        (1) Shall not be destroyed and must be maintained in accordance with Board Rule 291.34A. above and
        (2) Shall not be altered. Altering includes placing a label or any other item over any of the information on the prescription drug order (e.g., a dispensing tag or label that is affixed to the back of a prescription drug order must not be affixed on top of another dispensing tag or label in such a manner as to obliterate the information relating to the error).
    b. Prescription drug order records maintained in a data processing system:
        (1) Shall not be deleted and must be maintained in accordance with Board Rule 291.34A. above;
        (2) May be changed only in compliance with E.2.b. below; and
        (3) If the error involved incorrect data entry into the pharmacy's data processing system, this record must be either voided or cancelled in the data processing system so that the incorrectly entered prescription drug order may not be dispensed.

C. Patient Medication Records (PMR).
   1. A patient medication record system shall be maintained by the pharmacy for patients to whom prescription drug orders are dispensed and must be used to perform a drug regimen review (DRR).
   2. The PMR system shall provide for the immediate retrieval of information for the previous 12 months that is necessary for the dispensing pharmacist to conduct a prospective drug regimen review at the time a prescription drug order is presented for dispensing.
   3. The pharmacist-in-charge shall assure that a reasonable effort is made to obtain and record in the PMR at least the following information:
      a. Full name of the patient for whom the drug is prescribed;
      b. Address and telephone number of the patient;
      c. Patient's age or date of birth;
      d. Patient's gender;
      e. Any known allergies, drug reactions, idiosyncrasies, and chronic conditions or disease states of the patient and the identity of any other drugs currently being used by the patient which may relate to the prospective drug review;
      f. Pharmacist's comments relevant to the individual's drug therapy including any other information unique to the specific patient or drug; and
      g. A list of all prescription drug orders dispensed (new and refill) to the patient by the pharmacy during the last two years. Such list shall contain the following information:
         (1) Date dispensed;
         (2) Name, strength, and quantity of the drug dispensed;
         (3) Prescribing practitioner's name;
         (4) Unique identification number of the prescription; and
         (5) Name or initials of the dispensing pharmacist.
   4. A PMR shall be maintained in the pharmacy for two years. If patient medication records are maintained in a data processing system, all of the information specified in this rule shall be maintained in a retrievable form for two years and information for the previous 12 months shall be maintained online. A PMR must contain documentation of any modification, change, or manipulation to a patient profile.

5. Nothing herein shall be construed as requiring a pharmacist to obtain, record, and maintain patient information other than prescription drug order information when a patient or patient's agent refuses to provide the necessary information for such patient medication records.

D. Prescription Drug Order Records Maintained in a Manual System.
   1. Original (written or verbal) prescriptions shall be maintained in three separate files as previously indicated.
   2. Refills.
      a. A record of refilling shall be made:
         (1) On the back of the prescription: date of dispensing, the written initials or identification code of the dispensing pharmacist, the initials or identification code of the pharmacy technician or pharmacy technician trainee preparing the prescription label, if applicable, and the amount dispensed. (If the pharmacist merely initials and dates the back of the prescription drug order, he or she shall be deemed to have dispensed a refill for the full face amount of the prescription drug order) or
         (2) On another readily retrievable record such as medication records that indicates by patient name the:
            (a) Unique identification number of the prescription;
            (b) Name and strength of the drug dispensed;
            (c) Date of each dispensing;
            (d) Quantity dispensed at each dispensing;
            (e) Initials or identification code of the dispensing pharmacist;
            (f) Initials or identification code of the pharmacy technician or pharmacy technician trainee preparing the prescription label if applicable; and
            (g) Total number of refills for the prescription.
      b. Refill records for CIII-V drugs shall be maintained separately from refill records of dangerous drugs and nonprescription drugs.
   3. Authorization of refills shall be noted on the original prescription in addition to the documentation of dispensing the refill.
   4. Each time a modification, change, or manipulation is made to a record of dispensing, documentation of such change shall be recorded on the back of the prescription or another appropriate, uniformly maintained readily retrievable record such as a medication record. The documentation of any modification, change, or manipulation to a record of dispensing shall include the identification of the individual responsible for the alteration.

E. Records Maintained in a Data Processing System (computer system).
   1. General Requirements for Records Maintained in a Data Processing System.
      a. If a Class A pharmacy's data processing system is not in compliance with these data processing system rules, records must be maintained in a manual recordkeeping system as set out in D. above (Prescription Drug Order Records Maintained in a Manual System).
      b. Original (written, electronic, faxed, or verbal) prescriptions shall be maintained as indicated in Board Rule 291.34B.6. above.
      c. Requirements for backup systems.
         (1) Maintain a backup copy of information stored in a data processing system using a disk, tape, or other electronic backup system and update the backup copy at least monthly.
         (2) Data processing systems shall have a workable (electronic) data retention system that can produce an audit trail of drug usage for the preceding two years as specified in E.2.b. below.

Notes

    d. Change or discontinuance of a data processing system.
       (1) Records of dispensing.
           (a) Transfer the records of dispensing to the new data processing system or
           (b) Purge the records of dispensing to a printout containing the same information required on the daily printout. The information on this hardcopy printout shall be printed by prescription number and list chronologically each dispensing for this prescription.
       (2) Other records.
           (a) Transfer the records to the new data processing system or
           (b) Purge the records to a printout containing all of the information required on the original document.
       (3) Maintenance of purged records.
       Information purged from a data processing system must be maintained by the pharmacy for two years from the date of initial entry into the data processing system.
    e. Loss of data.
    The pharmacist-in-charge shall report to the Board in writing any significant loss of information from the data processing system within 10 days of the discovery of the loss.

2. Records of Dispensing (data entry of prescriptions into a computer system).
    a. Each time a prescription drug order is filled or refilled, a record of dispensing shall be entered into the system.
    b. Each time a modification, change, or manipulation is made to a record of a dispensing, documentation of such change shall be recorded in the data processing system. The documentation of any modification, change, or manipulation to a record of dispensing shall include the identification of the individual responsible for the alteration. Should the data processing system not be able to record a modification, change. or manipulation to a record of dispensing, the information should be clearly documented on the hardcopy prescription.
    c. The system shall have the capacity to produce a daily hardcopy printout of all original prescriptions dispensed and refilled. This printout shall contain the following information:
    (1) Unique identification number of the prescription;
    (2) Date of dispensing;
    (3) Patient name;
    (4) Practitioner's name and the supervising physician's name if the prescription was issued by an advanced practice registered nurse, physician assistant, or pharmacist;
    (5) Name and strength of the drug product actually dispensed; if for a generic product, the brand name or manufacturer of the drug dispensed;
    (6) Quantity dispensed;
    (7) Initials or an identification code of the dispensing pharmacist;
    (8) Initials or identification code of the pharmacy technician or pharmacy technician trainee performing data entry of the prescription if applicable;
    (9) If not immediately retrievable via computer display, the following shall also be included on the hardcopy printout:
       (a) Patient's address;
       (b) Prescribing practitioner's address;
       (c) Practitioner's DEA registration number if the prescription is for a controlled substance;

(d) Quantity dispensed if different from the quantity prescribed;
(e) Date of issuance of the prescription drug order if different from the date of dispensing; and
(f) Total number of refills dispensed to date for that prescription drug order; and
(10) Any changes made to a record of dispensing.
   d. The daily hardcopy printout shall be produced within 72 hours of the date on which the prescription drug orders were dispensed and be maintained in a separate file at the pharmacy. Records of controlled substances shall be readily retrievable from noncontrolled substances.
   e. Each individual pharmacist who dispenses or refills a prescription shall verify the data on the daily hardcopy printout by dating and signing within seven days from the date of dispensing.
   f. Instead of the printout described in 2.c. above, the pharmacy shall maintain a logbook in which each individual pharmacist using the system shall sign a statement each day that the information entered into the data processing system has been reviewed and is correct. The logbook shall be maintained at the pharmacy for two years after the date of dispensing.
      (1) Even if using a logbook, the computer system must be able to produce the printout described above on demand by an agent of the Board or DEA.
      (2) If the printer is not on-site, the printout must be available within 72 hours with a certification by the individual providing the printout stating it is correct as of the date of entry and that the information has not been changed.
   g. The pharmacist-in-charge is responsible for the proper maintenance of records, that the data processing system can produce the records, and that the system is in compliance with Board rules.
   h. A hardcopy printout of an audit trail for all dispensings (original and refills) of any specified strength and dosage form of a drug (by either brand or generic name or both) during a specified time period must be producible by the system within 72 hours and contain the information described in 2.c., above.
   i. Failure to provide the records described in this section (Records Maintained in a Data Processing System) either on-site or within 72 hours for whatever reason constitutes prima facie evidence of failure to keep and maintain records.
   j. The audit trail shall be supplied by the pharmacy within 72 hours if requested by authorized agents of the Board.
   k. The system shall provide online retrieval (via computer display or hardcopy printout) of the information described in b. and c. above of:
      (1) The original controlled substance prescription drug orders currently authorized for refilling and
      (2) The current refill history for Schedule III, IV, and V controlled substances for the immediately preceding six-month period.
   l. For system downtime, auxiliary procedures:
      (1) Shall ensure that refills are authorized and the maximum number of refills have not been exceeded.
      (2) Shall ensure that data be retained for entry when the system is available for use.
3. Authorization of Refills.
   Practitioner authorization for additional refills shall be noted in one of the following methods:
   a. On the hardcopy prescription drug order;

b. On the daily hardcopy printout; or
c. Via the computer display.
F. Limitation to One Type of Recordkeeping System.
When filing prescription drug order information, a pharmacy may use only one of the two systems described above: manual system or data processing system but not a combination of the two systems.
G. Transfer of Prescription Drug Order Information.
For the purposes of initial or refill dispensing, the transfer of original prescription drug order information is permissible between pharmacies subject to the following requirements:
1. The transfer of original prescription drug order information for controlled substances listed in Schedule III, IV, or V for the purpose of refill dispensing but not for initial dispensing is permissible between pharmacies on a one-time basis only. However, pharmacies electronically sharing a real-time, on-line database may transfer up to the maximum number of refills permitted by law.
2. The transfer of original prescription drug order information for dangerous drugs is permissible between pharmacies without limitation up to the number of originally authorized refills.
3. The transfer is communicated orally or by telephone or via facsimile directly by a pharmacist to another pharmacist, by a pharmacist to a pharmacist intern, or by a pharmacist intern to another pharmacist.
Note: The transfer of prescriptions between interns is not allowed.
4. Both the original and the transferred prescription drug orders are maintained for a period of two years from the date of the last refill.
5. The individual transferring the prescription drug order information shall ensure the following occurs:
    a. The word "void" is written on the face of the invalidated prescription or the prescription is voided in the computer system;
    b. Record the name, address, DEA registration number of the pharmacy to which it is transferred (if for a controlled substance), and the name of the individual on the reverse side of the invalidated prescription or store with the invalidated prescription drug record in the data processing system;
    c. Record the date of the transfer and the name of the individual transferring the information; and
    d. If the prescription is transferred electronically, provide the following:
        (1) Date of original dispensing and prescription number;
        (2) Number of refills remaining and the date(s) and location(s) of previous refills;
        (3) Name, address, and, if for a controlled substance, the DEA registration number of the transferring pharmacy;
        (4) Name of the individual transferring the prescription; and
        (5) If for a controlled substance, the name, address, DEA registration number, and prescription number from the pharmacy that originally dispensed the prescription if different.
6. The individual receiving the prescription drug order information shall:
    a. Write the word "transfer" on the prescription or the prescription record in the computer system indicating the prescription was a transfer;
    b. Reduce to writing all of the information required to be on a prescription as specified in B.7 (Prescriptions) above including the following information:
        (1) Date of issuance and prescription number;
        (2) Original number of refills authorized on the original prescription drug order;
        (3) Date of original dispensing;

  (4) Number of valid refills remaining and date(s) and location(s) of previous refills;
  (5) Name, address, and, if for a controlled substance, the DEA registration number of the transferring pharmacy; and
  (6) Name of the individual transferring the prescription. If for a controlled substance, the name, address, DEA registration number, and prescription number from the pharmacy that originally dispensed the prescription if different; or
 c. If the prescription is transferred electronically, an electronic record must be created for the prescription that includes the receiving pharmacist's name and all of the information required to be on a prescription as specified in B.7 (Prescriptions) above including the following information:
  (1) Date of original dispensing;
  (2) Number of refills remaining and the date(s) and location(s) of previous refills;
  (3) Name, address, and, if for a controlled substance, the DEA registration number;
  (4) Name of the individual transferring the prescription; and
  (5) If for a controlled substance, the name, address, and DEA registration number of the pharmacy that originally dispensed the prescription.
7. Both the individual transferring the prescription and the individual receiving the prescription must engage in confirmation of the prescription information by means such as:
 a. The transferring of individual faxes of the hardcopy prescription to the receiving individual or
 b. The receiving individual repeats the verbal information from the transferring individual and the transferring individual verbally confirms the repeated information is correct.
8. Pharmacies transferring a prescription electronically shall comply with the following.
 a. Prescription drug orders may not be transferred by nonelectronic means during periods of downtime except on consultation with and authorization by a prescribing practitioner. However, during downtime, a hard copy of a prescription drug order may be made available for only informational purposes to the patient, a pharmacist, or pharmacist intern. Also, the prescription may be read to a pharmacist or pharmacist intern by telephone.
 b. The original prescription drug order shall be invalidated in the data processing system for purposes of filling or refilling but shall be maintained in the data processing system for refill history purposes.
 c. If the data processing system does not have the capacity to store all the information as specified in 5. and 6. above, the pharmacist is required to record this information on the original or transferred prescription drug order.
 d. The data processing system shall have a mechanism to prohibit the transfer or refilling of controlled substance prescription drug orders which have been previously transferred.
 e. Pharmacies electronically accessing the same prescription drug order records may electronically transfer prescription information if the following requirements are met.
  (1) The original prescription is voided, and the pharmacies' data processing systems shall store all the information as specified in 5. and 6 above.

(2) Pharmacies not owned by the same entity may electronically access the same prescription drug order records provided the owner or chief executive officer of each pharmacy signs an agreement allowing such access to such prescription drug order records.

(3) An electronic transfer between pharmacies may be initiated by a pharmacist intern, pharmacy technician, or pharmacy technician trainee acting under the direct supervision of a pharmacist.

9. An individual may not refuse to transfer original prescription information to another pharmacist or pharmacist intern who is acting on behalf of a patient and who is making a request for this information as specified above. Transfer of original prescription information must be completed within four business hours of the request.

10. When transferring a compounded prescription, a pharmacy is required to provide all of the information regarding the compounded preparation including the formula unless the formula is patented or otherwise protected. If that is the case, the transferring pharmacy shall at a minimum provide the quantity or strength of all of the active ingredients of the compounded preparation.

11. The electronic transfer of multiple or bulk prescription records between two pharmacies is permitted provided:
    a. A record of the transfer as specified in 5. above is maintained by the transferring pharmacy;
    b. The information specified in 6. above is maintained by the receiving pharmacy; and
    c. If the patient or patient's agent is unaware of the transfer of the prescription drug order record, the transferring pharmacy must notify the patient or patient's agent of the transfer and must provide the patient or patient's agent with the telephone number of the pharmacy receiving the multiple or bulk prescription drug order records.

H. Distribution of Prescription Drugs to Another Registrant.
Note: This Board rule is similar to the DEA 5% rule for controlled substance distributions. However, this TSBP rule applies to all prescription drugs not just controlled substances.

A pharmacy may distribute prescription drugs to a practitioner, another pharmacy, or other registrant without having to be registered as a "distributor" under the following conditions.

1. If the distribution is for a controlled substance, the registrant to whom the controlled substance is to be distributed is registered under the Controlled Substances Act to possess that controlled substance.

2. The total number of dosage units of prescription drugs distributed by a pharmacy may not exceed 5% of all prescription drugs dispensed and distributed by the pharmacy during the 12-month period in which the pharmacy is registered. If at any time it does exceed 5%, the pharmacy is required to obtain an additional registration as a wholesaler from TDSHS to distribute prescription drugs.

3. If the distribution is for a dangerous drug, a record shall be maintained that indicates:
    a. Date of distribution;
    b. Name, strength, and quantity of the dangerous drug distributed;
    c. Name and address of the distributing pharmacy; and
    d. Name and address of the pharmacy, practitioner, or other registrant to whom the dangerous drugs are distributed.

4. If the distribution is for a Schedule III, IV, or V controlled substance, a record shall be maintained that indicates:
    a. Date of distribution;

b. Name, strength, and quantity of controlled substances distributed;
c. Name, address, and DEA registration number of the distributing pharmacy; and
d. Name, address, and DEA registration number of the pharmacy, practitioner, or other registrant to whom the controlled substances are distributed.
5. If the distribution is for a Schedule II controlled substance, the following is applicable.
   a. The pharmacy, practitioner, or other registrant who is receiving the controlled substances shall issue Copy 1 and Copy 2 of a DEA Form 222 to the distributing pharmacy.
   b. The distributing pharmacy shall:
      (1) Complete the area on DEA Form 222 titled "To Be Filled in by Supplier";
      (2) Maintain Copy 1 of DEA Form 222 at the pharmacy for two years; and
      (3) Forward Copy 2 of DEA Form 222 to the Divisional Office of the Drug Enforcement Administration.

I. Other Records.
Other records to be maintained by a pharmacy are as follows:
1. A log of the unique initials or identification codes must be available within the data processing system which will identify each pharmacist, pharmacist intern, pharmacy technician, or pharmacy technician trainee involved in the dispensing process. The initials or identification code shall be unique to ensure that each individual can be identified (i.e., identical initials or identification code shall not be used). The log shall be maintained at the pharmacy for a minimum of seven years from the date of the transaction;
2. Copy 3 of completed DEA Forms 222 that have been properly dated, initialed, and filed, all copies of each unaccepted or defective DEA Form 222, and any attached statements or other documents. When ordering Schedule II controlled substances using the DEA Controlled Substance Ordering System (CSOS), the original signed order and all linked orders for that order must be maintained;
3. A copy of the power of attorney to sign DEA Forms 222 (if applicable);
4. Suppliers' invoices of dangerous drugs and controlled substances on which are recorded the actual date of receipt of the controlled substances and the initials of the pharmacist who verified that the controlled substances listed on the invoices were actually received;
5. Suppliers' credit memos;
6. A copy of the controlled substance inventories required by Board Rule 291.17 (Controlled Substances Inventory Requirements);
7. Reports of surrender or destruction of controlled substances (DEA Form 41) and/or dangerous drugs;
8. Records of distribution of drugs to other pharmacies, practitioners or registrants; and
9. A copy of any notification required by the Act or rules including but not limited to:
   a. Reports of theft or significant loss of controlled substances (DEA Form 106);
   b. Notifications of a change in the pharmacist-in-charge; and
   c. Reports of a fire or other disaster that may affect the strength, purity, or labeling of drugs, medications, or devices.

J. Permission to Maintain Central Records.
See Chapter B.

K. Ownership of Pharmacy Records.
A pharmacy is the only entity which may legally own and maintain prescription drug records.
L. Documentation of Consultation With a Prescriber.
When a pharmacist consults a prescriber, the pharmacist shall document on the prescription hard copy or in the pharmacy's data processing system each consultation and shall include the following information:
1. Date the prescriber was consulted;
2. Name of the person communicating the prescriber's instructions;
3. Any applicable information pertaining to the consultation; and
4. Initials or identification code of the pharmacist performing the consultation clearly recorded for the purpose of identifying the pharmacist who performed the consultation.

Board of Pharmacy Rule 291.36
Pharmacies Compounding Sterile Preparations (Class A-S)

Note: This rule requires all Class A pharmacies that are engaged in compounding sterile preparations to obtain a Class A-S license. This designation provides the Board information on which pharmacies are performing sterile compounding. However, Class A-S pharmacies are still subject to all other Class A rules.

Licensing Requirements. A community pharmacy engaged in the compounding of sterile preparations shall be designated as a Class A-S pharmacy.
1. A Class A-S pharmacy shall register annually or biennially with the Board on a pharmacy license application provided by the Board following the procedures as specified in Board Rule 291.1 (Pharmacy License Application). A Class A-S license may not be issued unless the pharmacy has been inspected by the Board to ensure the pharmacy meets the requirements as specified in Board Rule 291.133 (Pharmacies Compounding Sterile Preparations).
2. A Class A-S pharmacy may not renew a pharmacy license unless the pharmacy has been inspected by the Board within the last renewal period.
3. A Class A-S pharmacy which changes ownership shall notify the Board within ten days of the change of ownership and apply for a new and separate license as specified in Board Rule 291.3 (Required Notifications).
4. A Class A-S pharmacy which changes location shall file for an amended license no later than 30 days before the date of the change of location as specified in Board Rule 291.3 (Required Notifications).
5. A Class A-S pharmacy owned by a partnership or corporation which changes managing officers shall notify the Board in writing of the names of the new managing officers within ten days of the change following the procedures as specified in Board Rule 291.3 (Required Notifications).
6. A Class A-S pharmacy shall notify the Board in writing within ten days after the date of closing following the procedures as specified in Board Rule 291.5 (Closing a Pharmacy).
7. A separate license is required for each principal place of business, and only one pharmacy license may be issued to a specific location.
8. A fee as specified in Board Rule 291.6 (Pharmacy License Fees) will be charged for the issuance and renewal of a license and the issuance of an amended license.
9. A Class A-S pharmacy which would otherwise be required to be licensed under Section 560.051A.1. of the Act concerning a Class A pharmacy is required to comply with the provisions of Board Rule 291.31 (Definitions), Board Rule 291.32 (Personnel), Board Rule 291.33 (Operational Standards), Board Rule 291.34 (Records), Board Rule 291.35 (Official Prescription

Requirements), and Board Rule 291.133 (Pharmacies Compounding Sterile Preparations).
10. A Class A-S pharmacy engaged in the compounding of nonsterile preparations shall comply with the provisions of Board Rule 291.131 (Pharmacies Compounding Nonsterile Preparations).
11. A Class A-S pharmacy engaged in the provision of remote pharmacy services including storage and dispensing of prescription drugs shall comply with the provisions of Board Rule 291.121 (Remote Pharmacy Services).
12. A Class A-S pharmacy engaged in centralized prescription dispensing and/or prescription drug or medication order processing shall comply with the provisions of Board Rule 291.123 (Centralized Prescription Drug or Medication Order Processing) and/or Board Rule 291.125 (Centralized Prescription Dispensing).

Records Pharmacists Should be Able to Locate in a Class A Pharmacy

If a TSBP compliance inspection or investigation audit of a Class A pharmacy occurs, the pharmacist-in-charge or the pharmacist on duty should be able to locate the following records for the previous two years:
1. Annual inventories;
2. Executed DEA Forms 222;
3. Controlled substance invoices;
4. Theft and loss reports;
5. Drug destruction reports;
6. All prescriptions;
7. DEA registration certificate if it is not posted;
8. Daily dispensing printouts or dispensing logs;
9. Prepackaging records if applicable; and
10. Technician training manual and documentation of technician training.

CHAPTER G HIGHLIGHTS
Class A (Community) Pharmacy Rules

1. Pharmacist-in-Charge (PIC)
   a. With a few exceptions, each Class A pharmacy must have one PIC who is employed on a full-time basis who may be the PIC for only one such pharmacy.
   b. The PIC has a broad range of responsibilities including legally operating the pharmacy, meeting inspection and other requirements of all state and federal laws or rules governing the practice of pharmacy, training the pharmacy technicians and pharmacy technician trainees, and maintaining records.
2. Pharmacists
   a. Each pharmacist shall be responsible for any delegated act performed by pharmacy technicians and pharmacy technician trainees under his or her supervision. Supervision of pharmacy technicians and pharmacy technician trainees who are entering prescription data into a pharmacy's data processing system may be done either by physically present supervision or electronic supervision which may be done on-site or off-site if specific conditions are met.
   b. While on duty, pharmacists are responsible for the legal operation of the pharmacy and for complying with all state and federal laws or rules governing the practice of pharmacy.
3. Duties of a Pharmacist (and Intern) and a Pharmacy Technician
   a. Only a pharmacist or intern may perform certain functions including:
      (1) Receiving verbal prescription drug orders;
      (2) Interpreting prescription drug orders;
      (3) Interpreting patient profiles and performing prospective drug use reviews;
      (4) Performing the final check of the dispensed prescription before delivery to the patient to ensure that the prescription has been dispensed accurately as prescribed;
      (5) Patient counseling; and
      (6) Verifying receipt of controlled substances (only a pharmacist).
   b. Pharmacy technicians can perform nonjudgmental tasks including:
      (1) Initiating and receiving refill authorization requests;
      (2) Creating or updating patient medication records;
      (3) Preparing prescription labels;
      (4) Entering prescription data into a data processing system;
      (5) Selecting a stock container from the shelf for a prescription;
      (6) Preparing and packaging prescription drug orders; and
      (7) Compounding sterile and nonsterile products with proper training.
4. The ratio of onsite pharmacists to pharmacy technicians and pharmacy technician trainees in a Class A pharmacy may be 1:4 provided that at least one of the four technicians is a pharmacy technician and not a pharmacy technician trainee. The ratio of pharmacists to pharmacy technician trainees may not exceed 1:3.
5. Class A pharmacies which serve the general public shall contain an area which is suitable for confidential patient counseling.
6. Security
   a. The prescription department shall be locked by key, combination, or other mechanical or electronic means to prohibit unauthorized access when a pharmacist is not on-site except as authorized under the temporary absence of pharmacist rules.
   b. The PIC or owner may designate persons who may enter the prescription department to perform functions other than dispensing or prescription processing functions.
   c. Written policies and procedures for the pharmacy's security shall be developed and implemented by the PIC and/or the owner of the pharmacy.
   d. If a pharmacy does not possess prescription drugs (e.g., call center or central processing), it does not have to meet the security requirements.

7. Temporary Absence of Pharmacist
   a. A pharmacist may leave the prescription department to take breaks, and the prescription department may remain open. Pharmacy technicians and trainees, pharmacist interns, and other personnel may remain in the pharmacy and perform specific functions as long as at least one pharmacy technician (not a technician trainee) remains in the prescription department.
   b. If a pharmacist leaves the premises, the prescription department must be secured and closed. Pharmacy technicians may not remain in the prescription department, but patients may pick up previously filled and verified prescriptions using an automated storage and distribution device. Also, the pharmacist may designate an agent to deliver a previously verified prescription to a patient or patient's agent during short periods not to exceed two consecutive hours in a 24-hour period.
8. Patient Counseling
   a. There is no offer to counsel in Texas. A pharmacist must provide verbal counseling (unless refused by the patient) on each new prescription drug order. A new prescription drug order is one that has not been dispensed to the patient by the pharmacy in the same strength and dosage form within the last year.
   b. Verbal counseling must be reinforced with written information.
   c. If a prescription is delivered either to a patient's home or in the pharmacy during the temporary absence of the pharmacist (see above), written information on the drug must be provided along with a toll-free number and notice that a pharmacist is available during normal business hours to answer questions.
9. A pharmacist must perform a drug regimen review for each new and refill prescription.
10. A prescription must be labeled with specific information including, among other things, a beyond-use date and the initials or identification code of the dispensing pharmacist if that information is not maintained in a computer system.
11. Three types of automated devices and systems may be used in a Class A pharmacy:
    a. Automated counting device—An automated device that is loaded with bulk drugs and counts and/or packages (i.e., fills a vial or other container) a specified quantity of dosage units of a designated drug product.
    b. Automated pharmacy dispensing system—A system that automatically performs operations or activities other than compounding or administration relative to the storing, packaging, counting, and labeling for dispensing and delivery of medications and that collects, controls, and maintains all transaction information.
    c. Automated checking device—A device that confirms that the correct drug and strength have been labeled with the correct label for the correct patient prior to delivery of the drug to the patient.
    Note: A Class A pharmacy may also use an automated storage and delivery system to deliver dispensed prescriptions at a remote site with Board approval.
12. Original written prescriptions shall be maintained in three separate files:
    a. Schedule II;
    b. Schedules III–V; and
    c. Dangerous drugs and nonprescription drugs.
13. Auto-Refill Programs—A pharmacy may use a program that automatically refills prescriptions for dangerous drugs and Schedule IV and V drugs (not Schedule III) that have existing refills available to improve patient compliance with and adherence to prescribed medication therapy.
    a. Patients must affirmatively indicate that they wish to enroll in such a program, and the pharmacy shall document such indication.
    b. The patient or patient's agent shall have the option to withdraw from such a program at any time.
14. Emergency Refills—Pharmacists may provide a 72-hour supply of an emergency refill of dangerous drugs and Schedule III–V controlled substances if failure to refill the prescription might result in an interruption of a therapeutic regimen or create patient suffering and either a natural or manmade disaster has occurred which prohibits the pharmacist from being able to contact the practitioner or if the pharmacist is unable to contact the practitioner after reasonable effort. The quantity may be extended to a 30-day supply under certain circumstances.

15. Accelerated Refills—Pharmacists may dispense up to a 90-day supply of a dangerous drug (not controlled substance) prescription written for a lesser amount with refills provided the patient consents and is at least 18 years old, the prescriber is notified, and the prescription is not for a psychotropic drug.
16. A patient medication record system containing specific information must be maintained by the pharmacy for patients to whom prescription drug orders are dispensed and must be used to perform drug regimen review.
17. Transfers
    a. For dangerous drugs, the transfer of original prescription drug order information to another pharmacy for initial filling or for refills is permitted.
    b. For Schedule III–V controlled substances, the transfer of original prescription drug order information to another pharmacy for refills only (not for initial filling) is permitted on a one-time basis only unless the pharmacies electronically share a real-time, on-line database.
    c. Transfers may be communicated electronically, orally, by telephone, or by facsimile directly by a pharmacist to another pharmacist or intern (not an intern trainee) or from an intern to a pharmacist.
    d. Transfers cannot be made from intern to intern.
    e. The original prescription must be voided either manually or in the pharmacy's computer system.
    f. Transfers requested must be provided within four hours of the request.
18. A pharmacy may distribute prescription drugs to a practitioner, another pharmacy, or other registrant without having to be registered as a "distributor" with TDSHS if the total number of dosage units of prescription drugs distributed by a pharmacy does not exceed 5% of all prescription drugs dispensed and distributed by the pharmacy during the 12-month period in which the pharmacy is registered.
19. All Class A pharmacies that are engaged in compounding sterile preparations must obtain a Class A-S license. This provides the Board information about which pharmacies are performing sterile compounding. However, Class A-S pharmacies are still subject to all other Class A rules.

CHAPTER H

Compounding Laws and Rules

CHAPTER H

Compounding Laws and Rules

Major annotations to this chapter provided by:
E. Paul Holder, Pharm.D., M.S., FTSHP
Assistant Professor of Pharmacy Practice
Texas A&M Rangel College of Pharmacy

I. History of Compounding Regulation
   A. The distinction between compounding and manufacturing is sometimes difficult to make. However, it is important because the manufacturing of drugs is primarily regulated by the FDA while compounding is generally considered part of the practice of pharmacy and is regulated by the states.
   B. In the 1990s, the FDA became concerned about some pharmacies whose compounding practices began to resemble drug manufacturing operations. To address these concerns, the FDA issued a Compliance Policy Guideline (CPG) in 1992 that set forth the factors that the FDA would use to determine if a pharmacy's practices constituted manufacturing. The CPG included a statement that the FDA considered all compounded drugs to be "new drugs" requiring a New Drug Application, but that the agency would exercise "enforcement discretion" and only take action against pharmacies that appeared to be acting as manufacturers.
   C. The Food and Drug Administration Modernization Act of 1997 (FDAMA) included provisions that attempted to clarify the distinction between manufacturing and compounding. FDAMA created Section 503A of the FDCA which set forth several conditions that would allow a pharmacy's compounding activities to be exempt from most FDA regulations. Among these conditions was a restriction that a pharmacy could not advertise the compounded products.
   D. A group of pharmacists sued the FDA challenging the constitutionality of the advertising restrictions as a violation of free speech. In 2001, the 9th Circuit Court of Appeals held that the advertising restrictions were a violation of commercial free speech and also held that the advertising restrictions could not be separated from the other nonadvertising portions of Section 503A, thus invalidating all of Section 503A. The Supreme Court affirmed the 9th Circuit Court's ruling in 2002 but did not comment on whether the advertising provision could be separated from the rest of Section 503A.
   E. With Section 503A invalidated, FDA responded in 2002 by issuing a new Compliance Policy Guideline (CPG) on pharmacy compounding listing factors the agency will consider in determining when a pharmacy's activities may be considered manufacturing. The new guideline included most of the nonadvertising factors that were in Section 503A.
   F. Later the distinction between compounding and manufacturing became even more complex when the 5th Circuit Court of Appeals disagreed with the 9th Circuit's ruling and held that the nonadvertising provisions of Section 503A could be separated and are still valid.
   G. Fungal Meningitis Outbreak and Passage of the 2013 Compounding Quality Act.
      1. On September 21, 2012, the Tennessee Department of Health notified the Centers for Disease Control (CDC) that a patient developed meningitis 19 days after being injected with an epidural steroid at a Tennessee ambulatory care facility. Four days later the New England Compounding Center

(NECC), a pharmacy in Massachusetts, recalled three lots of preservative-free methylprednisolone acetate. Within a week there were 25 meningitis cases reported in Tennessee with three deaths and other cases reported in five other states. NECC later expanded its recall to all products and then shut down operations as over 750 meningitis cases were eventually reported in 20 states with over 60 deaths.

2. This incident brought the issue of the distinction between pharmacy compounding and pharmaceutical manufacturing to the forefront. Investigations following the tragedy placed blame on both state and federal regulators. In testimony before Congress, FDA argued it needed new authority to regulate entities that compound sterile drug products in advance of or without a prescription and ship them interstate.

3. In response to this tragedy, Congress passed the Compounding Quality Act as part of the Drug Product Quality and Security Act in late 2013. The Act attempts to distinguish between pharmacies that are performing traditional compounding for specific patients based on individual prescriptions from pharmacies that are compounding large quantities of drugs that are not based on individual prescriptions. The Act creates a new type of FDA registrant called an "Outsourcing Facility" under Section 503B of the Act. While registration with FDA as an outsourcing facility is voluntary, facilities that register and meet the Act's requirements are permitted to compound sterile products without obtaining patient-specific prescriptions. Outsourcing facilities are exempt from the new drug provisions (Section 505), adequate directions for use (Section 505(f)(1)), and the new track and trace provisions (Section 582) of the FDCA. However, they are not exempt from FDA's CGMP requirements and also must meet other specific requirements in the Act. An outsourcing facility does not have to be a licensed pharmacy unless it is also compounding individual prescriptions, but all outsourcing facilities must be under direct supervision of a licensed pharmacist.

4. The Compounding Quality Act also resolved the conflict between the 9th Circuit and the 5th Circuit as to whether the remaining portions of the compounding provisions in FDAMA (Section 503A) were still in effect. The 2013 Act removed the provisions in Section 503A related to advertising and promotion that were found to be unconstitutional but retained the other provisions in Section 503A. This means that pharmacies compounding under Section 503A are exempt from the new drug requirements, adequate directions for use, and CGMP requirements. However, they must meet the requirements of Section 503A including that they are compounding preparations for an identified individual patient based on receipt of a valid prescription or in limited quantities based on a history of receiving prescriptions for the preparation. There is no provision under Section 503A that allows a pharmacy to compound for a physician's office use unless it is for an identified patient. Larger scale compounders of sterile preparations have to register with FDA as an outsourcing facility under Section 503B or risk being considered a full-scale manufacturer by FDA subject to the new drug requirements.

5. Only compounders of sterile preparations are allowed to register with FDA as outsourcing facilities under Section 503B. Pharmacies compounding non-sterile preparations are subject to Section 503A, and there are no provisions in Section 503A that allow "office use compounding" which many states, including Texas, specifically allow. Because the 2013 Compounding Quality Act appears to preempt state laws, there is a valid legal argument that TSBP's office use compounding laws and regulations are now invalid. However, because the Texas laws and rules on office use compounding are still

in the Act and rules and there has been no court or Texas Attorney General opinion that has found they are invalid, they are included in this chapter.

6. Under the Compounding Quality Act, pharmacies that compound under Section 503A may only compound drug products using bulk drug substances that:
   a. Comply with an applicable United States Pharmacopeia (USP) or National Formulary (NF) monograph if one exists and the USP chapter on pharmacy compounding;
   b. Are components of FDA-approved drug products if an applicable USP or NF monograph does not exist; or
   c. Appear on FDA's list of bulk drug substances that can be used in compounding (the 503A bulk drug list) if such a monograph does not exist and the substance is not a component of an FDA-approved drug product.

   In addition, bulk drug substances for 503A facilities must be accompanied by a valid certificate of analysis and must have been manufactured by an establishment registered with FDA under Section 510 of the FD&C Act.

7. Similarly, outsourcing facilities operating under section 503B may not compound a drug product that includes a bulk drug substance unless:
   a. The bulk drug substance appears on a list established by the Secretary of HHS identifying bulk drug substances for which there is a clinical need (the 503B bulk drug list) or
   b. The drug product compounded from such bulk drug substance appears on FDA's drug shortage list at the time of compounding, distribution, and dispensing.

   Bulk drug substances for 503B facilities must be accompanied by a valid certificate of analysis and must have been manufactured by an establishment registered with FDA under Section 510 of the FD&C Act. In addition, if an applicable United States Pharmacopeia (USP) or National Formulary monograph exists, bulk drug substances must comply with the monograph.

8. A detailed explanation of the federal regulations on compounding is beyond the scope of this book. Since passage of the Drug Compounding Quality Act, FDA has issued more than 30 notices, guidance documents, and rules on compounding and outsourcing facilities. See the compounding page on the FDA website for more information.

II. Texas Pharmacy Act Compounding Provisions (Chapter 562 Subchapter D)

Section 562.151 Definitions

A. **Office use**—Means the provision and administration of a compounded drug to a patient by a practitioner in the practitioner's office or by the practitioner in a healthcare facility or treatment setting, including a hospital, ambulatory surgical center, or pharmacy in accordance with Chapter 563.

B. **Prepackaging**—The act of repackaging and relabeling quantities of drug products from a manufacturer's original container into unit-dose packaging or a multiple dose container for distribution within a facility licensed as a Class C pharmacy or to other pharmacies under common ownership for distribution within those facilities. The term as defined does not prohibit the prepackaging of drug products for use within other pharmacy classes.

C. **Reasonable quantity**—With reference to drug compounding, reasonable quantity means an amount of a drug that:
   1. Does not exceed the amount a practitioner anticipates may be used in the practitioner's office before the expiration date of the drug;
   2. Is reasonable considering the intended use of the compounded drug and the nature of the practitioner's practice; and

3. For any practitioner and all practitioners as a whole, is not greater than an amount the pharmacy is capable of compounding in compliance with pharmaceutical standards for identity, strength, quality, and purity of the compounded drug that are consistent with United States Pharmacopeia guidelines and accreditation practices.

Section 562.152 Compounding for Office Use

A pharmacy may dispense and deliver a reasonable quantity of a compounded drug to a practitioner for office use by the practitioner in accordance with this chapter.

Section 562.153 Requirements for Office Compounding

To dispense and deliver a compounded drug under Section 562.152, a pharmacy must:
A. Verify the source of the raw materials to be used in a compounded drug;
B. Comply with applicable United States Pharmacopeia guidelines, including the testing requirements, and the Health Insurance Portability and Accountability Act of 1996;
C. Comply with all applicable competency and accrediting standards as determined by the Board; and
D. Comply with Board rules, including rules regarding the reporting of adverse events by practitioners and recall procedures for compounded products.

Note: These provisions for office use compounding in these sections of the Texas Pharmacy Act should be read with the federal law on compounding, including Section 503B of the Federal Food, Drug, and Cosmetic Act (FDCA) (21 U.S.C. 353b) and the Drug Compounding Quality Act. There are concerns that the Texas law may be in conflict with federal law as mentioned in the History of Compounding Regulation above.

Section 562.154 Distribution of Compounded and Prepackaged Products to Certain Pharmacies

A. A Class A pharmacy licensed under Chapter 560 is not required to register or be licensed under Chapter 431, Health and Safety Code (Wholesale Distributors), to distribute compounded pharmaceutical products to a Class C pharmacy licensed under Chapter 560.
B. A Class C pharmacy licensed under Chapter 560 is not required to register or be licensed under Chapter 431, Health and Safety Code (Wholesale Distributors), to distribute compounded and prepackaged pharmaceutical products that the Class C pharmacy has compounded or prepackaged to other Class C pharmacies licensed under Chapter 560 and under common ownership.

Note: In simple terms, a Class A pharmacy may compound for a Class C pharmacy and a Class C pharmacy may compound for another Class C pharmacy under common ownership. However, this section does not allow one Class A pharmacy to compound for another Class A pharmacy.

Section 562.155 Compounding Service and Compounded Products

A compounding pharmacist or pharmacy may advertise or promote:
1. Nonsterile prescription compounding services provided by the pharmacist or pharmacy and
2. Specific compounded drug products that the pharmacy or pharmacist dispenses or delivers.

All classes of pharmacies engaged in nonsterile compounding must meet the requirements of Board Rule 291.131, and all pharmacies engaged in sterile compounding must meet the requirements of Board Rule 291.133.

Note: There is not a specific pharmacy license class designation for a "compounding pharmacy" that compounds nonsterile products. Most "compounding pharmacies" will be either licensed as a Class A or Class C pharmacy and must follow all rules of the class for which it is licensed.

Section 562.156 Compounded Sterile Preparation; Notice to Board

A. A pharmacy may not compound and dispense a sterile preparation unless the pharmacy holds a license as required by Board rule.

Note: Effective September 1, 2014, all pharmacies compounding sterile preparations must have obtained a designation of either A-S, C-S, or E-S (as appropriate) and must be inspected by TSBP prior to beginning the compounding of sterile preparations and annually thereafter.

B. A pharmacy that compounds a sterile preparation shall notify the Board:
   1. Immediately of any adverse effects reported to the pharmacy or that are known by the pharmacy to be potentially attributable to a sterile preparation compounded by the pharmacy and
   2. No later than 24 hours after the pharmacy issues a recall for a sterile preparation compounded by the pharmacy.

III. **TSBP Rule on Nonsterile Compounding**

Note: There was some uncertainty whether the compounding of nasal sprays was required to be sterile or nonsterile. TSBP has determined that such products are considered nonsterile preparations.

Board of Pharmacy Rule 291.131
Pharmacies Compounding Nonsterile Preparations

(a) Purpose. Pharmacies compounding nonsterile preparations, prepackaging pharmaceutical products, and distributing those products shall comply with all requirements for their specific license classification and this rule. The purpose of this rule is to provide standards for the:

  (1) Compounding of nonsterile preparations pursuant to a prescription or medication order for a patient from a practitioner in Class A (Community), Class C (Institutional), and Class E (Nonresident) pharmacies;

  (2) Compounding, dispensing, and delivery of a reasonable quantity of a compounded nonsterile preparation in Class A (Community), Class C (Institutional), and Class E (Nonresident) pharmacies to a practitioner's office for office use by the practitioner;

  (3) Compounding and distribution of compounded nonsterile preparations by a Class A (Community) pharmacy for a Class C (Institutional) pharmacy; and

  (4) Compounding of nonsterile preparations by a Class C (Institutional) pharmacy and the distribution of the compounded preparations to other Class C (Institutional) pharmacies under common ownership.

(b) Definitions. In addition to the definitions for specific license classifications, the following words and terms shall have the following meanings, unless the context clearly indicates otherwise.

  (1) **Beyond-use date**—The date or time after which the compounded nonsterile preparation shall not be stored or transported or begin to be administered to a patient. The beyond-use date is determined from the date or time when the preparation was compounded.
  Note: The beyond-use date for a compounded preparation is similar to the expiration date on a manufactured product and is determined from the date or time when the preparation was compounded.

  (2) **Component**—Any ingredient intended for use in the compounding of a drug preparation, including those that may not appear in such preparation.

  (3) **Compounding**—The preparation, mixing, assembling, packaging, or labeling of a drug or device:

(A) As the result of a practitioner's prescription drug or medication order, based on the practitioner-patient-pharmacist relationship in the course of professional practice;

(B) For administration to a patient by a practitioner as the result of a practitioner's initiative based on the practitioner-patient-pharmacist relationship in the course of professional practice;

(C) In anticipation of prescription drug or medication orders based on routine, regularly observed prescribing patterns; or

(D) For or as an incident to research, teaching, or chemical analysis and not for sale or dispensing, except as allowed under Section 562.154 of the Act.

(4) **Hot water**—The temperature of water from the pharmacy's sink maintained at a minimum of 105 degrees F (41 degrees C).

Note: TSBP chose to define hot water as 105 degrees F (41 degrees C) to coincide with the definitions used by some other healthcare regulatory agencies. However, it is important to remember that some potentially pathogenic microorganisms grow at this temperature.

(5) **Reasonable quantity**—An amount of a compounded drug that:

(A) Does not exceed the amount a practitioner anticipates may be used in the practitioner's office or facility before the beyond-use date of the drug;

(B) Is reasonable considering the intended use of the compounded drug and the nature of the practitioner's practice; and

(C) For any practitioner and all practitioners as a whole is not greater than an amount the pharmacy is capable of compounding in compliance with pharmaceutical standards for identity, strength, quality, and purity of the compounded drug that are consistent with United States Pharmacopeia guidelines and accreditation practices.

(6) **SOPs**—Standard operating procedures.

(7) **USP/NF**—The current edition of the United States Pharmacopeia/National Formulary.

(c) Personnel.

(1) Pharmacist-in-Charge. In addition to the responsibilities for the specific class of pharmacy, the pharmacist-in-charge shall have the responsibility for, at a minimum, the following concerning nonsterile compounding:

(A) Determining that all personnel involved in nonsterile compounding possess the education, training, and proficiency necessary to properly and safely perform compounding duties undertaken or supervised;

(B) Determining that all personnel involved in nonsterile compounding obtain continuing education appropriate for the type of compounding done by the personnel;

(C) Assuring that the equipment used in compounding is properly maintained;

(D) Maintaining an appropriate environment in areas where nonsterile compounding occurs; and

(E) Assuring that effective quality control procedures are developed and followed.

(2) Pharmacists. Special requirements for nonsterile compounding.

(A) All pharmacists engaged in compounding shall:

(i) Possess the education, training, and proficiency necessary to properly and safely perform compounding duties undertaken or supervised and

(ii) Obtain continuing education appropriate for the type of compounding done by the pharmacist.

Note: Even if a pharmacist only occasionally verifies the final preparation compounded by a pharmacy technician, he or she must meet this requirement.

(B) A pharmacist shall inspect and approve all components, drug product containers, closures, labeling, and any other materials involved in the compounding process.

(C) A pharmacist shall review all compounding records for accuracy and conduct in-process and final checks to ensure that errors have not occurred in the compounding process.

(D) A pharmacist is responsible for the proper maintenance, cleanliness, and use of all equipment used in the compounding process.

Note: (B), (C), and (D) above mean that a pharmacist must verify all components used in a compound before a pharmacy technician begins compounding a preparation, at some point (defined by pharmacy policy) during the compounding of a preparation, and after the technician completes the preparation. This does not mean that a pharmacist must oversee every act performed by a technician during the compounding process. However, a compounding pharmacy must have in its policies a mechanism for conducting an in-process check and must follow that policy.

(3) Pharmacy Technicians and Pharmacy Technician Trainees. All pharmacy technicians and pharmacy technician trainees engaged in nonsterile compounding shall:

(A) Possess the education, training, and proficiency necessary to properly and safely perform compounding duties undertaken;

(B) Obtain continuing education appropriate for the type of compounding done by the pharmacy technician or pharmacy technician trainee; and

(C) Perform compounding duties under the direct supervision of and be responsible to a pharmacist.

Note: All compounding by a pharmacy technician must be under the direct supervision of a pharmacist. If no pharmacist is on duty, a pharmacy technician may not compound a preparation and then quarantine it for later review and approval when the pharmacist returns to the pharmacy.

(4) Training.

(A) All training activities shall be documented and covered by appropriate SOPs as outlined in subsection (d)(8)(A) of this section.

(B) All personnel involved in nonsterile compounding shall be well trained and must participate in continuing relevant training programs.

(d) Operational Standards.

(1) General Requirements.

(A) Nonsterile drug preparations may be compounded in licensed pharmacies:

(i) Upon presentation of a practitioner's prescription drug or medication order based on a valid pharmacist/patient/prescriber relationship;

(ii) In anticipation of future prescription drug or medication orders based on routine, regularly observed prescribing patterns; or

(iii) In reasonable quantities for office use by a practitioner and for use by a veterinarian.

(B) Nonsterile compounding in anticipation of future prescription drug or medication orders must be based upon a history of receiving valid prescriptions issued within an established pharmacist/patient/prescriber relationship, provided that in the pharmacist's professional judgment the quantity prepared is stable for the anticipated shelf time.
  (i) The pharmacist's professional judgment shall be based on the criteria used to determine a beyond-use date outlined in (5)(C) (Labeling) below.
  (ii) Documentation of the criteria used to determine the stability for the anticipated shelf time must be maintained and be available for inspection.
  (iii) Any preparation compounded in anticipation of future prescription drug or medication orders shall be labeled. Such label shall contain:
    (I) Name and strength of the compounded preparation or list of the active ingredients and strengths;
    (II) Facility's lot number;
    (III) Beyond-use date as determined by the pharmacist using appropriate documented criteria as outlined in paragraph (5)(C) (Labeling) below; and
    (IV) Quantity or amount in the container.
(C) Commercially available products may be compounded for dispensing to individual patients provided the following conditions are met:
  (i) The commercial product is not reasonably available from normal distribution channels in a timely manner to meet the patient's needs;
  (ii) The pharmacy maintains documentation that the product is not reasonably available due to a drug shortage or unavailability from the manufacturer; and
  (iii) The prescribing practitioner has requested that the drug be compounded as described in (D) below.
  Note: A pharmacy cannot say that a commercial product is unavailable simply because its normal supplier is out of stock or no longer carries the product. If the product is readily available from an alternate supplier, then the product is commercially available. If a product becomes available again once a drug shortage no longer exists, then the pharmacy must not continue to compound the medication.
(D) A pharmacy may not compound preparations that are essentially copies of commercially available products (e.g., the preparation is dispensed in a strength that is only slightly different from a commercially available product) unless the prescribing practitioner specifically orders the strength or dosage form and specifies why the patient needs the particular strength or dosage form of the preparation. The prescribing practitioner shall provide documentation of a patient specific medical need and that the preparation produces a clinically significant therapeutic response (e.g., the physician requests an alternate product due to hypersensitivity to excipients or preservative in the FDA-approved product or the physician requests an effective alternate dosage form) or if the drug product is not commercially available. The unavailability of such drug product must be documented prior to compounding. The methodology

for documenting unavailability includes maintaining a copy of the wholesaler's notification showing backordered, discontinued, or out-of-stock items. This documentation must be available in hardcopy or electronic format for inspection by the Board.

(E) A pharmacy may enter into an agreement to compound and dispense prescription/medication orders for another pharmacy provided the pharmacy complies with the provisions of Board Rule 291.125 (Centralized Prescription Dispensing).

(F) Compounding pharmacies/pharmacists may advertise and promote that they provide nonsterile prescription compounding services, which may include specific drug products and classes of drugs.

(G) A pharmacy may not compound veterinary preparations for use in food-producing animals except in accordance with federal guidelines.

(H) A pharmacist may add flavoring to a prescription at the request of a patient or patient's agent provided the pharmacy has documentation of testing provided by the manufacturer of the flavoring product, documentation of testing from appropriate literature sources, or documentation of direct testing to show that the addition of the flavoring does not alter the desired clinical outcomes and contains the same amount of active ingredient per dosage unit as the dosage prescribed for the patient. The pharmacy shall maintain such documentation in the pharmacy and make it available to agents of the Board. A pharmacist may not add flavoring to an over-the-counter product at the request of a patient or patient's agent unless the pharmacist obtains a prescription for the over-the-counter product from the patient's practitioner.

(2) Library. In addition to the library requirements of the pharmacy's specific license classification, a pharmacy shall maintain a current copy, in hardcopy or electronic format, of Chapter 795 of the USP/NF concerning Pharmacy Compounding Nonsterile Preparations.

(3) Environment.
(A) Pharmacies regularly engaging in compounding shall have a designated and adequate area for the safe and orderly compounding of nonsterile preparations, including the placement of equipment and materials. Pharmacies involved in occasional compounding shall prepare an area prior to each compounding activity which is adequate for safe and orderly compounding.
(B) Only personnel authorized by the responsible pharmacist shall be in the immediate vicinity of a drug compounding operation.
(C) A sink with hot and cold running water, exclusive of restroom facilities, shall be accessible to the compounding areas and be maintained in a sanitary condition. Supplies necessary for adequate washing shall be accessible in the immediate area of the sink and include:
    (i) Soap or detergent and
    (ii) Air dryers or single-use towels.
(D) If drug products which require special precautions to prevent contamination such as penicillin are involved in a compounding operation, appropriate measures, including dedication of equipment for such operations or the meticulous cleaning of contaminated equipment prior to its use for the preparation of other drug products, must be used to prevent cross-contamination.

Notes

(4) Equipment and Supplies. The pharmacy shall:
 (A) Have a Class A prescription balance or analytical balance and weights which shall be properly maintained and be subject to periodic inspection by the Texas State Board of Pharmacy and
 (B) Have equipment and utensils necessary for the proper compounding of prescription drug or medication orders. Such equipment and utensils used in the compounding process shall be:
  (i) Of appropriate design and capacity and be operated within designed operational limits;
  (ii) Of suitable composition so that surfaces that contact components, in-process material, or drug products shall not be reactive, additive, or absorptive to alter the safety, identity, strength, quality, or purity of the drug product beyond the desired result;
  (iii) Cleaned and sanitized immediately prior to and after each use; and
  (iv) Routinely inspected, calibrated (if necessary), or checked to ensure proper performance.

(5) Labeling. In addition to the labeling requirements of the pharmacy's specific license classification, the label dispensed or distributed pursuant to a prescription drug or medication order shall contain the following.
 (A) The generic name(s) or the official name(s) of the principal active ingredient(s) of the compounded preparation.
 (B) A statement that the preparation has been compounded by the pharmacy. (An auxiliary label may be used on the container to meet this requirement).
 (C) A beyond-use date after which the compounded preparation should not be used. The beyond-use date shall be determined as outlined in Chapter 795 of the USP/NF concerning Pharmacy Compounding Nonsterile Preparations including the following:
  (i) The pharmacist shall consider:
   (I) Physical and chemical properties of active ingredients;
   (II) Use of preservatives and/or stabilizing agents;
   (III) Dosage form;
   (IV) Storage containers and conditions; and
   (V) Scientific, laboratory, or reference data from a peer reviewed source and retained in the pharmacy. The reference data should follow the same preparation instructions for combining raw materials and packaged in a container with similar properties.
   Note: If a component of a specific compounded preparation differs significantly (e.g., a plastic storage container is used when the reference source used glass), then that reference source cannot be used as the standard for the specific compound.
  (ii) In the absence of stability information applicable for a specific drug or preparation, the following maximum beyond-use dates are to be used when the compounded preparation is packaged in tight, light-resistant containers and stored at controlled room temperatures:
   (I) Nonaqueous liquids and solid formulations (where the manufactured drug product is the source of active ingredient): 25% of the time remaining until the product's expiration date or six months, whichever is earlier.

(II) Water-containing formulations (prepared from ingredients in solid form): No later than 14 days when refrigerated between 2–8 degrees Celsius (36–46 degrees Fahrenheit).
(III) All other formulations: Intended duration of therapy or 30 days, whichever is earlier.
(iii) Beyond-use date limits may be exceeded when supported by valid scientific stability information for the specific compounded preparation.
(6) Written Drug Information. Written information about the compounded preparation or its major active ingredient(s) shall be given to the patient at the time of dispensing. A statement which indicates that the preparation was compounded by the pharmacy must be included in this written information. If there is no written information available, the patient should be advised that the drug has been compounded and how to contact a pharmacist and, if appropriate, the prescriber concerning the drug.
(7) Drugs, Components, and Materials Used in Nonsterile Compounding.
   (A) Drugs used in nonsterile compounding shall be USP/NF grade substances manufactured in an FDA-registered facility.
   (B) If USP/NF grade substances are not available or when food, cosmetics, or other substances are or must be used, the substance shall be of a chemical grade in one of the following categories:
      (i) Chemically Pure (CP);
      (ii) Analytical Reagent (AR);
      (iii) American Chemical Society (ACS); or
      (iv) Food Chemical Codex.
   (C) If a drug, component, or material is not purchased from an FDA-registered facility, the pharmacist shall establish purity and stability by obtaining a Certificate of Analysis from the supplier, and the pharmacist shall compare the monograph of drugs in a similar class to the Certificate of Analysis.
   (D) A manufactured drug product may be a source of an active ingredient. Only manufactured drugs from containers labeled with a batch control number and a future expiration date are acceptable as a potential source of active ingredients. When compounding with manufactured drug products, the pharmacist must consider all ingredients present in the drug product relative to the intended use of the compounded preparation.
   Note: Some manufactured drugs are shipped in containers with no batch control number or a future expiration date. Some containers may have one of these numbers but not the other. According to this rule, both a batch control number and a future expiration date must be on the container or the drug cannot be used as the source of an active ingredient.
   (E) All components shall be stored in properly labeled containers in a clean, dry area under proper temperatures.
   (F) Drug product containers and closures shall not be reactive, additive, or absorptive so as to alter the safety, identity, strength, quality, or purity of the compounded drug product beyond the desired result.
   Note: This rule is very important. Often pharmacies will receive a drug product in a glass container and later store part or all of the drug product in a plastic container. It cannot be assumed that the drug product will have the same reactivity, absorptivity, quality, or purity

if it is stored in a container made of different materials. Some drug products, especially those with strong ionic properties, will have very different absorptive properties in glass containers that these products have in plastic containers. Drug products used for compounding, if not stored in the original container(s), must be stored in containers made of the same material as the original container. Failure to do this can lead to altered drug products or loss of effectiveness of the drug product.

- (G) Components, drug product containers, and closures shall be rotated so that the oldest stock is used first.
- (H) Container closure systems shall provide adequate protection against foreseeable external factors in storage and use that can cause deterioration or contamination of the compounded drug product.
- (I) A pharmacy may not compound a preparation that contains ingredients appearing on a federal or state agency list of drug products withdrawn or removed from the market for safety reasons.

(8) Compounding Process.
- (A) All significant procedures performed in the compounding area shall be covered by written SOPs designed to ensure accountability, accuracy, quality, safety, and uniformity in the compounding process. At a minimum, SOPs shall be developed for:
  - (i) The facility;
  - (ii) Equipment;
  - (iii) Personnel;
  - (iv) Preparation evaluation;
  - (v) Quality assurance;
  - (vi) Preparation recall;
  - (vii) Packaging; and
  - (viii) Storage of compounded preparations.
- (B) Any compounded preparation with an official monograph in the USP/NF shall be compounded, labeled, and packaged in conformity with the USP/NF monograph for the drug.
  Note: This means that if a preparation to be compounded has an official USP/NF monograph, the preparation must be compounded according to that monograph.
- (C) Any person with an apparent illness or open lesion that may adversely affect the safety or quality of a drug product being compounded shall be excluded from direct contact with components, drug product containers, closures, any materials involved in the compounding process, and drug products until the condition is corrected.
- (D) Personnel engaged in the compounding of drug preparations shall wear clean clothing appropriate to the operation being performed. Protective apparel such as coats/jackets, aprons, hair nets, gowns, hand or arm coverings, or masks shall be worn as necessary to protect personnel from chemical exposure and drug preparations from contamination.
- (E) At each step of the compounding process, the pharmacist shall ensure that components used in compounding are accurately weighed, measured, or subdivided as appropriate to conform to the formula being prepared.
  Note: All checks made by the pharmacist as outlined in (E) above should be documented and signed or initialed (either manually or electronically) by the pharmacist.

(9) Quality Assurance.
    (A) Initial formula validation. Prior to routine compounding of a nonsterile preparation, a pharmacy shall conduct an evaluation that shows that the pharmacy is capable of compounding a product that contains the stated amount of active ingredient(s).
Note: In other words, a pharmacy must prove that a formula used for compounding a specific preparation actually results in the preparation it purports to produce.
    (B) Finished preparation checks. The prescription drug and medication orders, written compounding procedure, preparation records, and expended materials used to make compounded nonsterile preparations shall be inspected for accuracy of correct identities and amounts of ingredients, packaging, labeling, and expected physical appearance before the nonsterile preparations are dispensed.
Note: Texas State Board of Pharmacy (TSBP) inspectors may ask to inspect records of formula validations and finished preparation check. Failure to have these records available could result in citations from TSBP.

(10) Quality Control.
    (A) The pharmacy shall follow established quality control procedures to monitor the quality of compounded drug preparations for uniformity and consistency such as capsule weight variations, adequacy of mixing, clarity, or pH of solutions. When developing these procedures, pharmacy personnel shall consider the provisions of Chapter 795 (Pharmacy Compounding Nonsterile Preparations), Chapter 1075 (Good Compounding Practices), and Chapter 1160 (Pharmaceutical Calculations in Prescription Compounding) contained in the current USP/NF. These procedures shall be documented and be available for inspection.
Note: USP Chapter 1075 continues to be listed in this TSBP rule. However, it does not appear in the current version of USP/NF.
    (B) Compounding procedures that are routinely performed, including batch compounding, shall be completed and verified according to written procedures. The act of verification of a compounding procedure involves checking to ensure that calculations, weighing and measuring, order of mixing, and compounding techniques were appropriate and accurately performed.
    (C) Unless otherwise indicated or appropriate, compounded preparations are to be prepared to ensure that each preparation shall contain no less than 90.0 percent and no more than 110.0 percent of the theoretically calculated and labeled quantity of active ingredient per unit weight or volume and no less than 90.0 percent and no more than 110.0 percent of the theoretically calculated weight or volume per unit of the preparation.

Note: Paragraphs (9) Quality Assurance and (10) Quality Control list the minimum requirements set by rule. However, many pharmacies compounding nonsterile preparations will have Quality Assurance and Quality Control policies and procedures that exceed these minimum standards. Any pharmacist working in a pharmacy that performs substantial amounts of compounding should familiarize himself or herself with the pharmacy's policies and follow the more stringent policies and procedures even though these are not regulatory requirements of TSBP.

(e) Records.
   (1) Maintenance of Records. Every record required by this section shall be:
       (A) Kept by the pharmacy and be available for at least two years for inspecting and copying by the Board or its representative and to other authorized local, state, or federal law enforcement agencies and
       (B) Supplied by the pharmacy within 72 hours if requested by an authorized agent of the Board. If the pharmacy maintains the records in an electronic format, the requested records must be provided in an electronic format. Failure to provide the records set out in this section, either on-site or within 72 hours, constitutes prima facie evidence of failure to keep and maintain records in violation of the Act.
   (2) Compounding Records.
       (A) Compounding pursuant to patient specific prescription drug or medication orders. Compounding records for all compounded preparations shall be maintained by the pharmacy electronically or manually as part of the prescription drug or medication order, formula record, formula book, or compounding log and shall include:
           (i) The date of preparation;
           (ii) A complete formula including methodology and necessary equipment which includes the brand name(s) of the raw materials or, if no brand name, the generic name(s) and name(s) of the manufacturer(s) of the raw materials and the quantities of each;
           (iii) Signature or initials of the pharmacist or pharmacy technician or pharmacy technician trainee performing the compounding;
           (iv) Signature or initials of the pharmacist responsible for supervising pharmacy technicians or pharmacy technician trainees and conducting in-process and final checks of compounded preparations if pharmacy technicians or pharmacy technician trainees perform the compounding function;
           (v) The quantity in units of finished preparations or amount of raw materials;
           (vi) The container used and the number of units prepared; and
           (vii) A reference to the location of the following documentation which may be maintained with other records, such as quality control records:
               (I) The criteria used to determine the beyond-use date and
               (II) Documentation of performance of quality control procedures. Documentation of the performance of quality control procedures is not required if the compounding process is done pursuant to a patient specific order and involves the mixing of two or more commercially available oral liquids or commercially available preparations when the final product is intended for external use.
       (B) Compounding records when batch compounding or compounding in anticipation of future prescription drug or medication orders.
           (i) Master work sheet. A master work sheet shall be developed and approved by a pharmacist for preparations prepared in batch. Once approved, a duplicate of the master work sheet shall be used as the preparation work sheet from which each batch is prepared and on which all documentation for that batch occurs. The master work sheet shall contain at a minimum:
               (I) The formula;
               (II) The components;

(III) The compounding directions;
(IV) A sample label;
(V) Evaluation and testing requirements;
(VI) Specific equipment used during preparation; and
(VII) Storage requirements.
   (ii) Preparation work sheet. The preparation work sheet for each batch of preparations shall document the following:
   (I) Identity of all solutions and ingredients and their corresponding amounts, concentrations, or volumes;
   (II) Lot number of each component;
   (III) Component manufacturer/distributor or suitable identifying number;
   (IV) Container specifications;
   (V) Unique lot or control number assigned to batch;
   (VI) Beyond-use date of batch-prepared preparations;
   (VII) Date of preparation;
   (VIII) Name, initials, or electronic signature of the person(s) involved in the preparation;
   (IX) Name, initials, or electronic signature of the responsible pharmacist;
   (X) Finished preparation evaluation and testing specifications, if applicable; and
   (XI) Comparison of actual yield to anticipated or theoretical yield when appropriate.
(f) Office Use Compounding and Distribution of Compounded Preparations to Class C Pharmacies or Veterinarians in Accordance With Section 563.054 of the Act.
Note: Recall that Office Use Compounding may be in violation of the Federal Food, Drug, and Cosmetic Act unless the pharmacy is also registered with FDA as an outsourcing facility under Section 503B of the FDCA. In addition, DEA does not allow pharmacies to provide compounded controlled substances to practitioners for "office use." The pharmacy must have a valid prescription for an individual patient for the compounded controlled substance.
   (1) General.
      (A) A pharmacy may dispense and deliver a reasonable quantity of a compounded preparation to a practitioner for office use by the practitioner in accordance with this subsection.
      (B) A Class A (Community) pharmacy is not required to register or be licensed under Chapter 431, Health and Safety Code, to distribute nonsterile compounded preparations to a Class C (Institutional) pharmacy.
      (C) A Class C (Institutional) pharmacy is not required to register or be licensed under Chapter 431, Health and Safety Code, to distribute nonsterile compounded preparations that the Class C pharmacy has compounded for other Class C pharmacies under common ownership.
      (D) To dispense and deliver a compounded preparation under this subsection, a pharmacy must:
         (i) Verify the source of the raw materials to be used in a compounded drug;
         (ii) Comply with applicable United States Pharmacopeia guidelines, including the testing requirements, and the Health Insurance Portability and Accountability Act of 1996 (HIPAA);

Notes

non-sterile Compounded "Office use" agreement →

        (iii) Enter into a <u>written agreement</u> with a <u>practitioner</u> for the practitioner's office use of a compounded preparation;

        (iv) <u>Comply</u> with all applicable <u>competency</u> and <u>accrediting standards</u> as determined by the Board; and

        (v) <u>Comply</u> with the provisions of this subsection.

  (2) Written Agreement. A pharmacy that provides <u>nonsterile</u> compounded preparations <u>to practitioners</u> for <u>office use</u> or to another pharmacy shall enter into a <u>written agreement</u> with the practitioner or pharmacy. The written agreement shall:

    (A) Address acceptable standards of practice for a compounding pharmacy and a practitioner and receiving pharmacy that enter into the agreement, including a statement that the compounded preparations may only be administered to the patient and may not be dispensed to the patient or sold to any other person or entity except as authorized by Section 563.054 of the Act;

    (B) State that the practitioner or receiving pharmacy should include on a separate log or in a patient's chart, medication order, or medication administration record the lot number and beyond-use date of a compounded preparation administered to a patient; and

    (C) Describe the scope of services to be performed by the pharmacy and practitioner or receiving pharmacy, including a statement of the process for:

        (i) A patient to report an adverse reaction or submit a complaint and

        (ii) The pharmacy to recall batches of compounded preparations.

  (3) Recordkeeping.

    (A) Maintenance of records.

        (i) Records of orders and distribution of nonsterile compounded preparations to a practitioner for <u>office use or to a Class C</u> (Institutional) pharmacy for administration to a patient shall be:

           (I) Kept by the pharmacy and be available for at least <u>two years</u> from the date of the record for inspecting and copying by the Board or its representative and to other authorized local, state, or federal law enforcement agencies;

           (II) <u>Maintained separately</u> from the records of products dispensed pursuant to a prescription or medication order; and

           (III) <u>Supplied</u> by the pharmacy <u>within 72 hours,</u> if requested by an authorized agent of the Board or its representative. If the pharmacy maintains the records in an electronic format, the requested records must be provided in an electronic format. Failure to provide the records set out in this subsection, either on-site or within 72 hours for whatever reason, constitutes prima facie evidence of failure to keep and maintain records.

        (ii) Records may be maintained in an alternative data retention system, such as a data processing system or direct imaging system, provided the data processing system is capable of producing a hard copy of the record upon the request of the Board, its representative, or other authorized local, state, or federal law enforcement or regulatory agencies.

    (B) <u>Orders.</u> The pharmacy shall maintain a <u>record of all nonsterile compounded preparations ordered</u> by a practitioner for office use or by

a Class C pharmacy for administration to a patient. The record shall include the following information:
- (i) Date of the order;
- (ii) Name, address, phone number of the practitioner who ordered the preparation, and if applicable the name, address, and phone number of the Class C pharmacy ordering the preparation; and
- (iii) Name, strength, and quantity of the preparation ordered.

(C) Distributions. The pharmacy shall maintain a record of all nonsterile compounded preparations distributed pursuant to an order from a practitioner for office use or by a Class C pharmacy for administration to a patient. The record shall include the following information:
- (i) Date the preparation was compounded;
- (ii) Date the preparation was distributed;
- (iii) Name, strength, and quantity in each container of the preparation;
- (iv) Pharmacy's lot number;
- (v) Quantity of containers shipped; and
- (vi) Name, address, and phone number of the practitioner or Class C pharmacy to whom the preparation is distributed.

(D) Audit trail.
- (i) The pharmacy shall store the order and distribution records of preparations for all nonsterile compounded preparations ordered by and/or distributed to a practitioner for office use or by a Class C pharmacy for administration to a patient in such a manner as to be able to provide an audit trail for all orders and distributions of any of the following during a specified time period.
  - (I) Any strength and dosage form of a preparation (by either brand or generic name or both);
  - (II) Any ingredient;
  - (III) Any lot number;
  - (IV) Any practitioner;
  - (V) Any facility; and
  - (VI) Any pharmacy, if applicable.
- (ii) The audit trail shall contain the following information:
  - (I) Date of order and date of the distribution;
  - (II) Practitioner's name and address and name of the Class C pharmacy, if applicable;
  - (III) Name, strength, and quantity of the preparation in each container of the preparation;
  - (IV) Name and quantity of each active ingredient;
  - (V) Quantity of containers distributed; and
  - (VI) Pharmacy's lot number.

Note: All records listed in (f) (Office Use Compounding and Distribution of Compounded Preparations to Class C Pharmacies or Veterinarians in Accordance With Section 563.054 of the Act) above and (3) (Recordkeeping) above are of paramount importance. All records should be maintained in a complete and current manner as these will usually be requested by TSBP inspectors and by inspectors from other regulatory agencies. Any incomplete or missing records may result in sanctions to the pharmacy license and the license of the pharmacist-in-charge.

(4) Labeling. The pharmacy shall affix a label to the preparation containing the following information:
- (A) Name, address, and phone number of the compounding pharmacy;

(B) The statement: "For Institutional or Office Use Only—Not for Resale" or if the preparation is distributed to a veterinarian the statement: "Compounded Preparation";
(C) Name and strength of the preparation or list of the active ingredients and strengths;
(D) Pharmacy's lot number;
(E) Beyond-use date as determined by the pharmacist using appropriate documented criteria;
(F) Quantity or amount in the container;
(G) Appropriate ancillary instructions such as storage instructions or cautionary statements, including hazardous drug warning labels where appropriate; and
(H) Device-specific instructions where appropriate.

(g) Recall Procedures.
(1) The pharmacy shall have written procedures for the recall of any compounded nonsterile preparations provided to a patient, to a practitioner for office use, or to a pharmacy for administration. The recall procedures shall require:
(A) Notification to each practitioner, facility, and/or pharmacy to which the preparation was distributed;
(B) Notification to each patient to whom the preparation was dispensed;
(C) Quarantine of the product if there is suspicion of harm to a patient; and
(D) A recall if there is probable or confirmed harm to a patient.
(2) If the pharmacy identifies suspicion of, probable, or confirmed harm to a patient, the pharmacy shall immediately notify and provide information as required by the Board to the following:
(A) The Texas Department of State Health Services, Drugs and Medical Devices Group, if the preparation is distributed for office use and
(B) The Board.
(3) The Board may require a pharmacy to institute a recall if there is probable or confirmed harm to a patient.

IV. TSBP Rule on Sterile Compounding

Note: Pharmacies compounding sterile products that are not for identified individual patients pursuant to a valid prescription or order may also need to register with FDA as a 503B Outsourcing Facility or risk being considered a manufacturer by FDA. It is also important for pharmacists and pharmacy technicians to remember that compounding personnel are working in a clean environment, not a sterile environment. Therefore, the term "sterile compounding" is actually a misnomer. Compounding personnel are to use good aseptic technique so that sterile manufactured products are combined to form a final sterile preparation or that nonsterile starting materials are combined with either other nonsterile materials or with sterile manufactured products, then terminally sterilized to prepare a final sterile preparation. Thus, the correct term for preparing compounded sterile preparations (CSPs) is "aseptic compounding." This being said, the industrial standard term is, and probably will always be, "sterile compounding." However, a knowledge of the correct terminology may help compounders remember that they must be extremely careful when compounding CSPs.

Board of Pharmacy Rule 291.133
Pharmacies Compounding Sterile Preparations

(a) Purpose. Pharmacies compounding sterile preparations, prepackaging pharmaceutical products, and distributing those products shall comply with all requirements for their specific license classification and this section. The purpose of this section is to provide standards for the:
  (1) Compounding of sterile preparations pursuant to a prescription or medication order for a patient from a practitioner in Class A-S, Class B, Class C-S, and Class E-S pharmacies;
  (2) Compounding, dispensing, and delivery of a reasonable quantity of a compounded sterile preparation in Class A-S, Class B, Class C-S, and Class E-S pharmacies to a practitioner's office for office use by the practitioner;
  (3) Compounding and distribution of compounded sterile preparations by a Class A-S pharmacy for a Class C-S pharmacy; and
  (4) Compounding of sterile preparations by a Class C-S pharmacy and the distribution of the compounded preparations to other Class C or Class C-S pharmacies under common ownership.

Note: As was the case for Board Rule 291.131 (Nonsterile Compounding), a Class A-S pharmacy may compound for a Class C-S pharmacy and a Class C-S pharmacy may compound for another Class C-S pharmacy under common ownership. However, this section does not allow one Class A-S pharmacy to compound for another Class A-S pharmacy nor does it allow for a Class B or a Class E-S pharmacy to compound for either a Class A-S or a Class C-S pharmacy.

(b) Definitions. In addition to the definitions for specific license classifications, the following words and terms, when used in this section, shall have the following meanings, unless the context clearly indicates otherwise.
  (1) **ACPE**—Accreditation Council for Pharmacy Education.
  (2) **Airborne particulate cleanliness class**—The level of cleanliness specified by the maximum allowable number of particles per cubic meter of air as specified in the International Organization of Standardization (ISO) Classification Air Cleanliness (ISO 14644-1). For example:
    (A) ISO Class 5 (formerly Class 100) is an atmospheric environment that contains less than 3,520 particles 0.5 microns in diameter per cubic meter of air (formerly stated as 100 particles 0.5 microns in diameter per cubic foot of air);
    (B) ISO Class 7 (formerly Class 10,000) is an atmospheric environment that contains less than 352,000 particles 0.5 microns in diameter per cubic meter of air (formerly stated as 10,000 particles 0.5 microns in diameter per cubic foot of air); and
    (C) ISO Class 8 (formerly Class 100,000) is an atmospheric environment that contains less than 3,520,000 particles 0.5 microns in diameter per cubic meter of air (formerly stated as 100,000 particles 0.5 microns in diameter per cubic foot of air).

Note: Many pharmacists who have been in practice for a number of years will be more familiar with the older classification scheme for airborne particulate cleanliness. Therefore, it may be beneficial for younger pharmacists to have a way to convert between the two classification schemes. To make the conversion, take the new ISO Class number, subtract 3, and then raise 10 to the power of the remainder. For example, what was ISO Class 7 known as formerly? Take the ISO Class number 7 and subtract 3 to give a remainder of 4. Now raise 10 to the 4th power (10^4) to obtain 10,000. So, ISO Class 7 is equivalent to Class 10,000. Conversely, what is the ISO Class of the older Class 100,000? $100,000 = 10^5$. So, $5 + 3 = 8$. Thus, Class 100,000 is equivalent to ISO Class 8.

(3) **Ancillary supplies**—Supplies necessary for the preparation and administration of compounded sterile preparations.

(4) **Ante-area**—An ISO Class 8 or better area where personnel may perform hand hygiene and garbing procedures, staging of components, order entry, labeling, and other high-particulate generating activities. It is also a transition area that:

    (A) Provides assurance that pressure relationships are constantly maintained so that air flows from clean to dirty areas and

    (B) Reduces the need for the heating, ventilating, and air conditioning (HVAC) control system to respond to large disturbances.

Note: In clean rooms with physical separation between the ante-area and the buffer area (i.e., a buffer room), the ante-area may be either ISO Class 7 or 8. However, if there is no physical separation between the ante-area and the buffer area, the ante-area must be ISO Class 7.

(5) **Aseptic processing**—A mode of processing pharmaceutical and medical preparations that involves the separate sterilization of the preparation and of the package (containers-closures or packaging material for medical devices) and the transfer of the preparation into the container and its closure under at least ISO Class 5 conditions.

(6) **Automated compounding device**—An automated device that compounds, measures, and/or packages a specified quantity of individual components in a predetermined sequence for a designated sterile preparation.

(7) **Batch**—A specific quantity of a drug or other material that is intended to have uniform character and quality within specified limits and is produced during a single preparation cycle.

(8) **Batch preparation compounding**—Compounding of multiple sterile preparation units in a single discrete process by the same individual(s) and carried out during one limited time period. Batch preparation compounding does not include the preparation of multiple sterile preparation units pursuant to patient specific medication orders.

(9) **Beyond-use date**—The date or time after which the compounded sterile preparation shall not be stored or transported or begin to be administered to a patient. The beyond-use date is determined from the date or time the preparation is compounded.

(10) **Biological safety cabinet, Class II**—A ventilated cabinet for personnel, product or preparation, and environmental protection having an open front with inward airflow for personnel protection, downward HEPA filtered laminar airflow for product protection, and HEPA filtered exhausted air for environmental protection.

(11) **Buffer area**—An ISO Class 7 area where the primary engineering control device(s) is physically located. If it is a Class B pharmacy, the area must be ISO Class 8 or better. Activities that occur in this area include the preparation and staging of components and supplies used when compounding sterile preparations.

(12) **Clean room**—A room in which the concentration of airborne particles is controlled to meet a specified airborne particulate cleanliness class. Microorganisms in the environment are monitored so that a microbial level for air, surface, and personnel gear are not exceeded for a specified cleanliness class.

(13) **Component**—Any ingredient intended for use in the compounding of a drug preparation, including those that may not appear in such preparation.

(14) **Compounding**—The preparing, mixing, assembling, packaging, or labeling of a drug or device:
   (A) As the result of a practitioner's prescription drug or medication order based on the practitioner-patient-pharmacist relationship in the course of professional practice;
   (B) For administration to a patient by a practitioner as the result of a practitioner's initiative based on the practitioner-patient-pharmacist relationship in the course of professional practice;
   (C) In anticipation of prescription drug or medication orders based on routine, regularly observed prescribing patterns; or
   (D) For or as an incident to research, teaching, or chemical analysis and not for sale or dispensing, except as allowed under Section 562.154 of the Act.

(15) **Compounding aseptic isolator**—A form of barrier isolator specifically designed for compounding pharmaceutical ingredients or preparations. It is designed to maintain an aseptic compounding environment within the isolator throughout the compounding and material transfer processes. Air exchange into the isolator from the surrounding environment shall not occur unless it has first passed through a microbial retentive filter (HEPA minimum).

(16) **Compounding aseptic containment isolator**—A compounding aseptic containment isolator designed to provide worker protection from exposure to undesirable levels of airborne drugs throughout the compounding and material transfer processes and to provide an aseptic environment for compounding sterile preparations. Air exchange with the surrounding environment should not occur unless the air is first passed through a microbial retentive filter (HEPA minimum) system capable of containing airborne concentrations of the physical size and state of the drug being compounded. Where volatile hazardous drugs are prepared, the exhaust air from the isolator should be appropriately removed by properly designed building ventilation.

Note: A Compounding Aseptic Isolator (CAI) is not to be used for compounding hazardous drugs or chemotherapeutic agents as it does not protect the compounder from exposure to the hazardous substance(s). A Compounding Aseptic Containment Isolator (CACI) provides protection against exposure to hazardous drugs and chemicals for the compounding personnel. A CACI can be used for compounding nonhazardous drugs, but it must be dedicated to that purpose and not be used to compound both hazardous and nonhazardous drugs.

(17) **Compounding personnel**—A pharmacist, pharmacy technician, or pharmacy technician trainee who performs the actual compounding; a pharmacist who supervises pharmacy technicians or pharmacy technician trainees compounding sterile preparations; and a pharmacist who performs an intermediate or final verification of a compounded sterile preparation.

(18) **Critical area**—An ISO Class 5 environment.

(19) **Critical sites**—A location that includes any component or fluid pathway surfaces (e.g., vial septa, injection ports, or beakers) or openings (e.g., opened ampuls or needle hubs) exposed to and at risk of direct contact with air (e.g., ambient room or HEPA filtered), moisture (e.g., oral and mucosal secretions), or touch contamination. Risk of microbial particulate contamination of the critical site increases with the size of the openings and exposure time.

(20) **Device**—An instrument, apparatus, implement, machine, contrivance, implant, in-vitro reagent, or other similar or related article, including any

component part or accessory, that is required under federal or state law to be ordered or prescribed by a practitioner.

(21) **Direct compounding area**—A critical area within the ISO Class 5 primary engineering control where critical sites are exposed to unidirectional HEPA-filtered air, also known as first air.

(22) **Disinfectant**—An agent that frees from infection, usually a chemical agent but sometimes a physical one, and that destroys disease-causing pathogens or other harmful microorganisms but may not kill bacterial and fungal spores. It refers to substances applied to inanimate objects.

(23) **First air**—The air exiting the HEPA filter in a unidirectional air stream that is essentially particle free.

(24) **Hazardous drugs**—Drugs that when used in animal or human studies indicate that exposure to the drugs can potentially cause cancer, development or reproductive toxicity, or harm to organs.

(25) **Hot water**—The temperature of water from the pharmacy's sink maintained at a minimum of 105 degrees F (41 degrees C).

Note: As stated in the nonsterile compounding section of this chapter, TSBP chose to define hot water as 105 degrees F (41 degrees C) to coincide with the definitions used by some other healthcare regulatory agencies. However, it is important to remember that some potentially pathogenic microorganisms grow quite well at this temperature. Since potentially harmful organisms may grow in water of this temperature, there could be increased risk of contamination should any water contact a component of a sterile compound.

(26) **HVAC**—Heating, ventilation, and air conditioning.

(27) **Immediate use**—A sterile preparation that is not prepared according to USP 797 standards (i.e., outside the pharmacy and most likely not by pharmacy personnel) which shall be stored for no longer than one hour after completion of the preparation.

(28) **IPA**—Isopropyl alcohol (2-propanol).

(29) **Labeling**—All labels and other written, printed, or graphic matter on an immediate container of an article or preparation or on or in any package or wrapper in which it is enclosed, except any outer shipping container. The term "label" designates that part of the labeling on the immediate container.

(30) **Media-fill test**—A test used to qualify aseptic technique of compounding personnel or processes and to ensure that the processes used are able to produce a sterile preparation without microbial contamination. During this test, a microbiological growth medium such as Soybean-Casein Digest Medium is substituted for the actual drug preparation to simulate admixture compounding. The issues to consider in the development of a media-fill test are the following: media-fill procedures, media selection, fill volume, incubation, time and temperature, inspection of filled units, documentation, interpretation of results, and possible corrective actions required.

(31) **Multiple-dose container**—A multiple-unit container for articles or preparations intended for potential administration only and usually contains antimicrobial preservatives. The beyond-use date for an opened or entered (e.g., needle-punctured) multiple-dose container with antimicrobial preservatives is 28 days, unless otherwise specified by the manufacturer.

Note: Manufacturers often conduct tests to determine if a preservative added to a product will inhibit growth of microorganisms. Frequently, tests involve adding the product containing the preservative to a growth medium or an agar plate, as appropriate, followed by determination of any growth at 7, 14,

21, and 28 days. If no growth is determined after 28 days, the test is stopped. Thus, a product sold in a multi-dose vial has been tested for 28 days and the expiration of an opened or entered multi-dose container is 28 days. Pharmacy personnel may want to make the expiration 30 days because it is easier to determine the date on which the open vial expires, but there are usually no data to support antimicrobial preservative action beyond 28 days.

(32) **Negative pressure room**—A room that is at a lower pressure compared to adjacent spaces and, therefore, the net flow of air is into the room.

(33) **Office use**—The administration of a compounded drug to a patient by a practitioner in the practitioner's office or by the practitioner in a healthcare facility or treatment setting, including a hospital, ambulatory surgical center, or pharmacy in accordance with Chapter 562 of the Act, or for administration or provision by a veterinarian in accordance with Section 563.054 of the Act.

(34) **Pharmacy bulk package**—A container of a sterile preparation for potential use that contains many single doses. The contents are intended for use in a pharmacy admixture program and are restricted to the preparation of admixtures for infusion or, through a sterile transfer device, for the filling of empty sterile syringes. The closure shall be penetrated only one time after constitution with a suitable sterile transfer device or dispensing set, which allows measured dispensing of the contents. The pharmacy bulk package is to be used only in a suitable work area such as a laminar flow hood (or an equivalent clean air compounding area).

(35) **Prepackaging**—The act of repackaging and relabeling quantities of drug products from a manufacturer's original container into unit-dose packaging or a multiple-dose container for distribution within a facility licensed as a Class C pharmacy or to other pharmacies under common ownership for distribution within those facilities. The term as defined does not prohibit the prepackaging of drug products for use within other pharmacy classes.

(36) **Preparation or compounded sterile preparation**—A sterile admixture compounded in a licensed pharmacy or other healthcare-related facility pursuant to the order of a licensed prescriber. The components of the preparation may or may not be sterile products.

(37) **Primary engineering control**—A device or room that provides an ISO Class 5 environment for the exposure of critical sites when compounding sterile preparations. Such devices include, but may not be limited to, laminar airflow workbenches, biological safety cabinets, compounding aseptic isolators, and compounding aseptic containment isolators.

(38) **Product**—A commercially manufactured sterile drug or nutrient that has been evaluated for safety and efficacy by the U.S. Food and Drug Administration (FDA). Products are accompanied by full prescribing information which is commonly known as the FDA-approved manufacturer's labeling or product package insert.

(39) **Positive control**—A quality assurance sample prepared to test positive for microbial growth.

(40) **Quality assurance**—The set of activities used to ensure that the process used in the preparation of sterile drug preparations leads to preparations that meet predetermined standards of quality.

(41) **Quality control**—The set of testing activities used to determine that the ingredients, components (e.g., containers), and final compounded sterile preparations meet predetermined requirements with respect to identity, purity, non-pyrogenicity, and sterility.

Notes

(42) **Reasonable quantity**—An amount of a compounded drug that:
  (A) Does not exceed the amount a practitioner anticipates may be used in the practitioner's office or facility before the beyond-use date of the drug;
  (B) Is reasonable considering the intended use of the compounded drug and the nature of the practitioner's practice; and
  (C) For any practitioner and all practitioners as a whole is not greater than an amount the pharmacy is capable of compounding in compliance with pharmaceutical standards for identity, strength, quality, and purity of the compounded drug that are consistent with United States Pharmacopeia guidelines and accreditation practices.

(43) **Segregated compounding area**—Designated space, either a demarcated area or room, that is restricted to preparing low-risk level compounded sterile preparations with 12-hour or less beyond-use date. Such area shall contain a device that provides unidirectional airflow of ISO Class 5 air quality for preparation of compounded sterile preparations and shall be void of activities and materials that are extraneous to sterile compounding.

(44) **Single-dose container**—A single-unit container for articles or preparations intended for parenteral administration only. It is intended for a single use. A single-dose container is labeled as such. Examples of single-dose containers include prefilled syringes, cartridges, fusion-sealed containers, and closure-sealed containers when so labeled.
Note: Unlike multiple-dose containers (see above), single-dose containers generally have no preservative added to the container.

(45) **SOPs**—Standard operating procedures.

(46) **Sterilizing grade membranes**—Membranes that are documented to retain 100% of a culture of 107 microorganisms of a strain of Brevundimonas (Pseudomonas) diminuta per square centimeter of membrane surface under a pressure of no less than 30 psi (2.0 bar). Such filter membranes are nominally at 0.22-μm or 0.2-μm nominal pore size, depending on the manufacturer's practice.

(47) **Sterilization by filtration**—Passage of a fluid or solution through a sterilizing grade membrane to produce a sterile effluent.

(48) **Terminal sterilization**—The application of a lethal process (e.g., steam under pressure or autoclaving) to sealed final preparation containers for the purpose of achieving a predetermined sterility assurance level of usually less than 10–6 or a probability of less than one in one million of a nonsterile unit.

(49) **Unidirectional flow**—An airflow moving in a single direction in a robust and uniform manner and at sufficient speed to reproducibly sweep particles away from the critical processing or testing area.

(50) **USP/NF**—The current edition of the United States Pharmacopeia/National Formulary.

(c) Personnel.
  (1) Pharmacist-in-Charge.
    (A) General. The pharmacy shall have a pharmacist-in-charge in compliance with the specific license classification of the pharmacy.
    (B) Responsibilities. In addition to the responsibilities for the specific class of pharmacy, the pharmacist-in-charge shall have the responsibility for, at a minimum, the following concerning the compounding of sterile preparations:
      (i) Developing a system to ensure that all pharmacy personnel responsible for compounding and/or supervising the compounding of

sterile preparations within the pharmacy receive appropriate education and training and competency evaluation;
- (ii) Determining that all personnel involved in compounding sterile preparations obtain continuing education appropriate for the type of compounding done by the personnel;
- (iii) Supervising a system to ensure appropriate procurement of drugs and devices and storage of all pharmaceutical materials including pharmaceuticals, components used in the compounding of sterile preparations, and drug delivery devices;
- (iv) Ensuring that the equipment used in compounding is properly maintained;
- (v) Developing a system for the disposal and distribution of drugs from the pharmacy;
- (vi) Developing a system for bulk compounding or batch preparation of drugs;
- (vii) Developing a system for the compounding, sterility assurance, quality assurance, and quality control of sterile preparations; and
- (viii) If applicable, ensuring that the pharmacy has a system to dispose of hazardous waste in a manner so as not to endanger the public health.

(2) Pharmacists.
  (A) General and responsibilities.
    (i) A pharmacist is responsible for ensuring that compounded sterile preparations are accurately identified, measured, diluted, and mixed and are correctly purified, sterilized, packaged, sealed, labeled, stored, dispensed, and distributed.
    (ii) A pharmacist shall inspect and approve all components, drug preparation containers, closures, labeling, and any other materials involved in the compounding process.
    (iii) A pharmacist shall review all compounding records for accuracy and conduct periodic in-process checks as defined in the pharmacy's policies and procedures.
    (iv) A pharmacist shall review all compounding records for accuracy and conduct a final check.
    (v) A pharmacist is responsible for ensuring the proper maintenance, cleanliness, and use of all equipment used in the compounding process.
    (vi) A pharmacist shall be accessible at all times, 24 hours a day, to respond to patients' and other health professionals' questions and needs.
  (B) Initial training and continuing education.
    (i) All pharmacists who compound sterile preparations or supervise pharmacy technicians and pharmacy technician trainees compounding sterile preparations shall comply with the following:
      (I) Complete through a single course a minimum of 20 hours of instruction and experience in the areas listed in (4)(D) below. Such training shall be obtained through completion of a recognized course in an accredited college of pharmacy or a course sponsored by an ACPE accredited provider which provides 20 hours of instruction and experience in the areas listed in (4)(D) below;

Notes

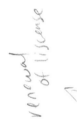 renewal of license

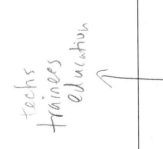 techs trainees education

        (II) Complete at their pharmacy a structured on-the-job didactic and experiential training program which provides sufficient hours of instruction and experience in the areas listed in (4)(D) below. Such training may not be transferred to another pharmacy unless the pharmacies are under common ownership and control and use a common training program; and

        (III) Possess knowledge about:
            (-a-) Aseptic processing;
            (-b-) Quality control and quality assurance as related to environmental, component, and finished preparation release checks and tests;
            (-c-) Chemical, pharmaceutical, and clinical properties of drugs;
            (-d-) Container, equipment, and closure system selection; and
            (-e-) Sterilization techniques.

    (ii) The required experiential portion of the training programs specified in this subparagraph must be supervised by an individual who is actively engaged in performing sterile compounding and is qualified and has completed training as specified in (2) above or (3) below.

Note: Clauses (i) and (ii) above apply to any pharmacist involved in sterile compounding in any manner, even if he or she only checks or verifies a compounded sterile product occasionally.

    (iii) To renew a license to practice pharmacy during the previous licensure period, a pharmacist engaged in sterile compounding shall complete a minimum of:
        (I) Two hours of ACPE accredited continuing education relating to the areas listed in (i)(II) above if the pharmacist is engaged in compounding low-risk and medium-risk sterile preparations or
        (II) Four hours of ACPE accredited continuing education relating to the areas listed in (i)(II) above if the pharmacist is engaged in compounding high-risk sterile preparations.

Note: Risk levels for sterile compounding are assigned based upon the risk to the patient when the final compounded preparation is administered. Therefore, most sterile chemotherapy compounding is low risk or medium risk. Seldom is high-risk compounding needed to prepare chemotherapy for IV administration.

(3) Pharmacy Technicians and Pharmacy Technician Trainees.
    (A) General. All pharmacy technicians and pharmacy technician trainees shall meet the training requirements specified in Board Rule 297.6 (Pharmacy Technician and Pharmacy Technician Trainee Training).
    (B) Initial training and continuing education.
        (i) Pharmacy technicians and pharmacy technician trainees may compound sterile preparations provided the pharmacy technicians and/or pharmacy technician trainees are supervised by a pharmacist who has completed the training specified in (4)(D) below, conducts in-process and final checks, and affixes his or her initials to the appropriate quality control records.

(ii) All pharmacy technicians and pharmacy technician trainees who compound sterile preparations for administration to patients shall:
  (I) Have initial training obtained either through the completion of:
    (-a-) A single course with a minimum of 40 hours of instruction and experience in the areas listed in (4)(D) below. Such training shall be obtained through completion of a course sponsored by an ACPE accredited provider which provides 40 hours of instruction and experience in the areas listed in (4)(D) below or
    (-b-) A training program which is accredited by the American Society of Health-System Pharmacists.
    Note: For pharmacy technicians and pharmacy technician trainees, the single course of training may be sponsored by an ACPE or ASHP accredited provider. However, for pharmacists, only an ACPE sponsored course is acceptable.
    Note: TSBP has determined that initial training courses for pharmacy technicians are not equivalent to initial training courses designed for pharmacists. Therefore, if a pharmacist completes an ACPE accredited initial training course designed for a pharmacy technician, the pharmacist has not met the requirements for initial training as specified in (B)(i)(I) above.
  (II) In addition, all pharmacy technicians and pharmacy technician trainees shall:
    (-a-) Complete at their pharmacy a structured on-the-job didactic and experiential training program which provides sufficient hours of instruction and experience in the facility's compounding policies and procedures. Such training may not be transferred to another pharmacy unless the pharmacies are under common ownership and control and use a common training program and
    (-b-) Possess knowledge about:
      (-1-) Aseptic processing;
      (-2-) Quality control and quality assurance as related to environmental, component, and finished preparation release checks and tests;
      (-3-) Chemical, pharmaceutical, and clinical properties of drugs;
      (-4-) Container, equipment, and closure system selection; and
      (-5-) Sterilization techniques.
(iii) Individuals enrolled in training programs accredited by the American Society of Health-System Pharmacists may compound sterile preparations in a licensed pharmacy provided the:
  (I) Compounding occurs only during times the individual is assigned to a pharmacy as a part of the experiential component of the American Society of Health-System Pharmacists training program;

Notes

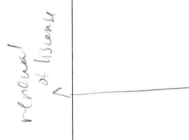
renewal of license

(II) Individual is under the direct supervision of and responsible to a pharmacist who has completed training as specified in (2) above;
(III) Supervising pharmacist conducts periodic in-process checks as documented in the pharmacy's policies and procedures; and
(IV) Supervising pharmacist conducts a final check.
 (iv) The required experiential portion of the training programs specified in this subparagraph must be supervised by an individual who is actively engaged in performing sterile compounding, is qualified, and has completed training as specified in (2) or (3) above.
 (v) To renew a registration as a pharmacy technician during the previous registration period, a pharmacy technician engaged in sterile compounding shall complete a minimum of:
(I) Two hours of ACPE accredited continuing education relating to the areas listed in (4)(D) below if the pharmacy technician is engaged in compounding low-risk and medium-risk sterile preparations or
(II) Four hours of ACPE accredited continuing education relating to the areas listed in (4)(D) below if the pharmacy technician is engaged in compounding high-risk sterile preparations.

Note: The continuing education requirements for the renewal of a pharmacy technician registration are the same as those required for a pharmacist license renewal.

(4) Evaluation and Testing Requirements.
 (A) All pharmacy personnel preparing sterile preparations shall be trained conscientiously and skillfully by expert personnel through multimedia instructional sources and professional publications in the theoretical principles and practical skills of aseptic manipulations, garbing procedures, aseptic work practices, achieving and maintaining ISO Class 5 environmental conditions, and cleaning and disinfection procedures before beginning to prepare compounded sterile preparations.

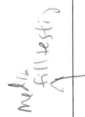
media fill testing

 (B) All pharmacy personnel shall perform didactic review and pass written and media-fill testing of aseptic manipulative skills initially followed by:
  (i) Every 12 months for low-risk and medium-risk level compounding and
  (ii) Every six months for high-risk level compounding.
 (C) Pharmacy personnel who fail written tests or whose media-fill tests result in gross microbial colonization shall:
  (i) Be immediately re-instructed and re-evaluated by expert compounding personnel to ensure correction of all aseptic practice deficiencies and
  (ii) Not be allowed to compound sterile preparations for patient use until passing results are achieved.
 (D) The didactic and experiential training shall include instruction, experience, and demonstrated proficiency in the following areas:
  (i) Aseptic technique;
  (ii) Critical area contamination factors;
  (iii) Environmental monitoring;

(iv) Structure and engineering controls related to facilities;
(v) Equipment and supplies;
(vi) Sterile preparation calculations and terminology;
(vii) Sterile preparation compounding documentation;
(viii) Quality assurance procedures;
(ix) Aseptic preparation procedures including proper gowning and gloving technique;
(x) Handling of hazardous drugs, if applicable;
(xi) Cleaning procedures; and
(xii) General conduct in the clean room.

(E) The aseptic technique of each person compounding or responsible for the direct supervision of personnel compounding sterile preparations shall be observed and evaluated by expert personnel as satisfactory through written and practical tests and media-fill challenge testing. Such evaluation must be documented. Compounding personnel shall not evaluate their own aseptic technique or results of their own media-fill challenge testing.

(F) Media-fill tests must be conducted at each pharmacy where an individual compounds low-risk and medium-risk sterile preparations. If pharmacies are under common ownership and control, the media-fill testing may be conducted at only one of the pharmacies provided each of the pharmacies is operated under equivalent policies and procedures and the testing is conducted under the most challenging or stressful conditions. In addition, each pharmacy must maintain documentation of the media-fill test. No preparation intended for patient use shall be compounded by an individual until the test of the on-site media-fill tests indicates that the individual can competently perform aseptic procedures. However, a pharmacist may temporarily compound sterile preparations and supervise pharmacy technicians compounding sterile preparations without media-fill tests provided the pharmacist completes the on-site media-fill tests within seven days of commencing work at the pharmacy.

(G) Media-fill tests must be conducted at each pharmacy where an individual compounds high-risk sterile preparations. No preparation intended for patient use shall be compounded by an individual until the on-site media-fill tests indicate that the individual can competently perform aseptic procedures, except that a pharmacist may temporarily compound sterile preparations and supervise pharmacy technicians compounding sterile preparations without media-fill tests provided the pharmacist completes the on-site media-fill tests within seven days of commencing work at the pharmacy.

(H) Media-fill testing procedures for assessing the preparation of specific types of sterile preparations shall be representative of the most challenging or stressful conditions encountered by the pharmacy personnel being evaluated and, if applicable, for sterilizing high-risk level compounded sterile preparations.

(I) Media-fill challenge tests simulating high-risk level compounding shall be used to verify the capability of the compounding environment and process to produce a sterile preparation.

(J) Commercially available sterile fluid culture media for low-risk and medium-risk level compounding or nonsterile fluid culture media for high-risk level compounding shall be able to promote exponential colonization of bacteria that are most likely to be transmitted to compounding sterile preparations from the compounding personnel and environment. Media-filled vials are generally incubated at 20 to 25 degrees Celsius or at 30 to 35 degrees Celsius for a minimum of 14 days. If two temperatures are used for incubation of media-filled samples, then these filled containers should be incubated for at least seven days at each temperature. Failure is indicated by visible turbidity in the medium on or before 14 days.

(K) The pharmacist-in-charge shall ensure continuing competency of pharmacy personnel through in-service education, training, and media-fill tests to supplement initial training. Personnel competency shall be evaluated:
  (i) During orientation and training prior to the regular performance of those tasks;
  (ii) Whenever the quality assurance program yields an unacceptable result;
  (iii) Whenever unacceptable techniques are observed; and
  (iv) At least on an annual basis for low-risk and medium-risk level compounding and every six months for high-risk level compounding.

(L) The pharmacist-in-charge shall ensure that proper hand hygiene and garbing practices of compounding personnel are evaluated prior to compounding, supervising, or verifying sterile preparations intended for patient use and whenever an aseptic media-fill is performed.
  (i) Sampling of compounding personnel glove fingertips shall be performed for all risk level compounding. If pharmacies are under common ownership and control, the gloved fingertip sampling may be conducted at only one of the pharmacies provided each of the pharmacies is operated under equivalent policies and procedures and the testing is conducted under the most challenging or stressful conditions. In addition, each pharmacy must maintain documentation of the gloved fingertip sampling of all compounding personnel.
  (ii) All compounding personnel shall demonstrate competency in proper hand hygiene and garbing procedures and in aseptic work practices (e.g., disinfection of component surfaces or routine disinfection of gloved hands).
  (iii) Sterile contact agar plates shall be used to sample the gloved fingertips of compounding personnel after garbing to assess garbing competency and after completing the media-fill preparation (without applying sterile 70% IPA).
  (iv) The visual observation shall be documented and maintained to provide a permanent record and long-term assessment of personnel competency.
  (v) All compounding personnel shall successfully complete an initial competency evaluation and gloved fingertip/thumb sampling procedure no fewer than three times before initially being allowed to compound sterile preparations for patient use. Immediately after the compounding personnel completes the hand hygiene and garbing procedure (i.e., after donning of sterile gloves and before any disinfecting with sterile 70% IPA), the evaluator will collect a gloved fingertip and thumb sample from both hands of the compounding personnel onto contact plates or swabs by having the individual lightly touching/

pressing each fingertip onto the testing medium. The contact plates or swabs will be incubated for the appropriate incubation period and at the appropriate temperature. Results of the initial gloved fingertip evaluations shall indicate zero Colony Forming Units (0 CFU) growth on the contact plates or swabs, or the test shall be considered a failure. In the event of a failed gloved fingertip test, the evaluation shall be repeated until the individual can successfully don sterile gloves and pass the gloved fingertip evaluation, defined as zero CFUs growth. No preparation intended for patient use shall be compounded by an individual until the results of the initial gloved fingertip evaluation indicate that the individual can competently perform aseptic procedures except that a pharmacist may temporarily physically supervise pharmacy technicians compounding sterile preparations before the results of the evaluation have been received for no more than three days from the date of the test.

(vi) Re-evaluation of all compounding personnel shall occur at least annually for compounding personnel who compound low-risk and medium-risk level preparations and every six months for compounding personnel who compound high-risk level preparations. Results of gloved fingertip tests conducted immediately after compounding personnel complete a compounding procedure shall indicate no more than 3 CFUs growth, or the test shall be considered a failure. In this case, the evaluation shall be repeated until an acceptable test can be achieved (i.e., the results indicate no more than 3 CFUs growth).

(M) The pharmacist-in-charge shall ensure surface sampling be conducted in all ISO classified areas on a periodic basis. Sampling shall be accomplished using contact plates or swabs at the conclusion of compounding. The sample area shall be gently touched with the agar surface by rolling the plate across the surface to be sampled.

(5) Documentation of Training. The pharmacy shall maintain a record of the training and continuing education of each person who compounds sterile preparations. The record shall contain at a minimum a written record of initial and in-service training and education and the results of written and practical testing and media-fill testing of pharmacy personnel. The record shall be maintained and available for inspection by the Board and contain the following information:

(A) Name of the person receiving the training or completing the testing or media-fill tests;
(B) Date(s) of the training, testing, or media-fill challenge testing;
(C) General description of the topics covered in the training or testing or of the process validated;
(D) Name of the person supervising the training, testing, or media-fill challenge testing; and
(E) Signature or initials of the person receiving the training or completing the testing or media-fill challenge testing and the pharmacist-in-charge or other pharmacist employed by the pharmacy and designated by the pharmacist-in-charge as responsible for training, testing, or media-fill challenge testing of personnel.

Note: The results of training and testing for each person involved in compounding CSPs must be maintained in the pharmacy in either hardcopy or electronic format for inspection by TSBP inspectors. Generally, inspectors will randomly select several personnel whose records will be reviewed during an inspection. Failure to have the appropriate records may result in sanctions against the pharmacy license, the PIC's license, and the individual's license or registration. *Test results shall be maintained for a minimum of two years.*

(d) Operational Standards.
   (1) General Requirements.
      (A) Sterile preparations may be compounded:
         (i) Upon presentation of a practitioner's prescription drug or medication order based on a valid pharmacist/patient/prescriber relationship;
         (ii) In anticipation of future prescription drug or medication orders based on routine, regularly observed prescribing patterns; or
         (iii) In reasonable quantities for office use by a practitioner and for use by a veterinarian.
      (B) Sterile compounding in anticipation of future prescription drug or medication orders must be based upon a history of receiving valid prescriptions issued within an established pharmacist/patient/prescriber relationship, provided that in the pharmacist's professional judgment the quantity prepared is stable for the anticipated shelf time.
         (i) The pharmacist's professional judgment shall be based on the criteria used to determine a beyond-use date outlined in (6)(H) below.
         (ii) Documentation of the criteria used to determine the stability for the anticipated shelf time must be maintained and be available for inspection.
         (iii) Any preparation compounded in anticipation of future prescription drug or medication orders shall be labeled. Such label shall contain:
            (I) Name and strength of the compounded preparation or list of the active ingredients and strengths;
            (II) Facility's lot number;
            (III) Beyond-use date as determined by the pharmacist using appropriate documented criteria as outlined in (6)(H) below;
            (IV) Quantity or amount in the container;
            (V) Appropriate ancillary instructions such as storage instructions or cautionary statements, including hazardous drug warning labels where appropriate; and
            (VI) Device-specific instructions where appropriate.
      (C) Commercially available products may be compounded for dispensing to individual patients or for office use provided the following conditions are met:
         (i) The commercial product is not reasonably available from normal distribution channels in a timely manner to meet an individual patient's needs;
         (ii) The pharmacy maintains documentation that the product is not reasonably available due to a drug shortage or unavailability from the manufacturer; and
         (iii) The prescribing practitioner has requested that the drug be compounded as described in (D) below.
      (D) A pharmacy may not compound preparations that are essentially copies of commercially available products (e.g., the preparation is

dispensed in a strength that is only slightly different from a commercially available product) unless the prescribing practitioner specifically orders the strength or dosage form and specifies why the individual patient needs the particular strength or dosage form of the preparation or why the preparation for office use is needed in the particular strength or dosage form of the preparation. The prescribing practitioner shall provide documentation of a patient's specific medical need and that the preparation produces a clinically significant therapeutic response (e.g., the physician requests an alternate preparation due to hypersensitivity to excipients or a preservative in the FDA-approved product, or the physician requests an effective alternate dosage form) or if the drug product is not commercially available. The unavailability of such drug product must be documented prior to compounding. The methodology for documenting unavailability includes maintaining a copy of the wholesaler's notification showing backordered, discontinued, or out-of-stock items. This documentation must be available in hardcopy or electronic format for inspection by the Board.

Note: A pharmacy cannot say that a commercial product is unavailable simply because its normal supplier is out of stock or no longer carries the product. If the product is readily available from an alternate supplier, then the product is commercially available. If a product becomes available again once a drug shortage no longer exists, then the pharmacy must not continue to compound the medication.

(E) A pharmacy may enter into an agreement to compound and dispense prescription/medication orders for another pharmacy provided the pharmacy complies with the provisions of Board Rule 291.125 (Centralized Prescription Dispensing).

(F) Compounding pharmacies/pharmacists may advertise and promote that they provide sterile prescription compounding services, which may include specific drug preparations and classes of drugs.

(G) A pharmacy may not compound veterinary preparations for use in food producing animals except in accordance with federal guidelines.

(H) Compounded sterile preparations, including hazardous drugs and radiopharmaceuticals, shall be prepared only under conditions that protect the pharmacy personnel in the preparation and storage areas.

(2) Microbial Contamination Risk Levels. Risk levels for sterile compounded preparations shall be as outlined in Chapter 797, Pharmacy Compounding—Sterile Preparations of the USP/NF as listed in this rule.

Note: It is important to remember that USP 797 risk levels are so designated due to the potential risk that the completed sterile preparation poses to the patient to whom it is administered. The risk level does not indicate the potential risk posed to the compounding personnel.

(A) Low-risk level compounded sterile preparations.
  (i) Low-risk conditions. Low-risk level compounded sterile preparations are those compounded under all of the following conditions.
    (I) The compounded sterile preparations are compounded with aseptic manipulations entirely within ISO Class 5 or better air quality using only sterile ingredients, products, components, and devices.
    (II) The compounding involves only transferring, measuring, and mixing manipulations using not more than three

commercially manufactured packages of sterile products and not more than two entries into any one sterile container or package (e.g., bag or vial) of sterile product or administration container/device to prepare the compounded sterile preparation.

Note: It must be remembered that the base solution into which commercial products are added counts as one of the three commercially manufactured products in the final sterile preparation. Therefore, the typical "banana bag" prepared in many hospitals and administered to alcoholic patients in the emergency room that contains injectable thiamine, folic acid, and multi-vitamins in a base solution (D5W or NS) would be a medium-risk preparation. This preparation involves four commercial ingredients and three entries into one administration container.

(III) Manipulations are limited to aseptically opening ampuls, penetrating disinfected stoppers on vials with sterile needles and syringes, and transferring sterile liquids in sterile syringes to sterile administration devices, package containers of other sterile products, and containers for storage and dispensing.

(IV) For a low-risk preparation in the absence of passing a sterility test, the storage periods cannot exceed the following periods: before administration the compounded sterile preparation is stored properly and is exposed for no more than 48 hours at controlled room temperature, for no more than 14 days if stored at a cold temperature, and for no more than 45 days if stored in a frozen state between minus 25 degrees Celsius and minus 10 degrees Celsius. For delayed activation device systems, the storage period begins when the device is activated.

(ii) Examples of low-risk compounding. Examples of low-risk compounding include the following:

(I) Single volume transfers of sterile dosage forms from ampuls, bottles, bags, and vials using sterile syringes with sterile needles, other administration devices, and other sterile containers. The solution content of ampules shall be passed through a sterile filter to remove any particles.

(II) Simple aseptic measuring and transferring with no more than three packages of manufactured sterile products, including an infusion or diluent solution to compound drug admixtures and nutritional solutions.

(B) Low-risk level compounded sterile preparations with 12-hour or less beyond-use date. Low-risk level compounded sterile preparations are those compounded pursuant to a physician's order for a specific patient under all of the following conditions.

(i) The compounded sterile preparations are compounded in a compounding aseptic isolator or a compounding aseptic containment isolator that does not meet the requirements described in (7)(C) or (D) (Primary Engineering Control Device) below, or the compounded sterile preparations are compounded in a laminar airflow workbench or a biological safety cabinet that cannot be located within the buffer area.

(ii) The primary engineering control device shall be certified and maintain ISO Class 5 for exposure of critical sites and shall be located in a segregated compounding area restricted to sterile compounding activities that minimizes the risk of contamination of the compounded sterile preparation.

(iii) The segregated compounding area shall not be in a location that has unsealed windows or doors that connect to the outdoors or high traffic flow or that is adjacent to construction sites, warehouses, or food preparation.

(iv) For a low-risk preparation compounded as described in (i), (ii), and (iii) above, administration of such compounded sterile preparations must commence within 12 hours of preparation or as recommended in the manufacturer's package insert, whichever is less. However, the administration of sterile radiopharmaceuticals with documented testing of chemical stability may be administered beyond 12 hours of preparation.

(C) Medium-risk level compounded sterile preparations.
   (i) Medium-risk conditions. Medium-risk level compounded sterile preparations are those compounded aseptically under low-risk conditions and one or more of the following conditions exist.
      (I) Multiple individual or small doses of sterile products are combined or pooled to prepare a compounded sterile preparation that will be administered either to multiple patients or to one patient on multiple occasions.
      Note: See Note under (2)(A)(II) above.
      (II) The compounding process includes complex aseptic manipulations other than the single-volume transfer.
      (III) The compounding process requires an unusually long duration such as that required to complete the dissolution or homogenous mixing (e.g., reconstitution of intravenous immunoglobulin or other intravenous protein products).
      (IV) The compounded sterile preparations do not contain broad spectrum bacteriostatic substances, and they are administered over several days (e.g., an externally worn infusion device).
      (V) For a medium-risk preparation in the absence of passing a sterility test, the storage periods cannot exceed the following time periods: before administration, the compounded sterile preparations are properly stored and are exposed for no more than 30 hours at controlled room temperature, for no more than 9 days at a cold temperature, and for no more than 45 days in a solid frozen state between minus 25 degrees Celsius and minus 10 degrees Celsius.
   (ii) Examples of medium-risk compounding include the following.
      (I) Compounding of total parenteral nutrition fluids using a manual or automated device during which there are multiple injections, detachments, and attachments of nutrient source products to the device or machine to deliver all nutritional components to a final sterile container.
      (II) Filling of reservoirs of injection and infusion devices with more than three sterile drug products and evacuations

of air from those reservoirs before the filled device is dispensed.
- (III) Filling of reservoirs of injection and infusion devices with volumes of sterile drug solutions that will be administered over several days at ambient temperatures between 25 and 40 degrees Celsius (77 and 104 degrees Fahrenheit).
- (IV) Transfer of volumes from multiple ampuls or vials into a single, final sterile container or product.

(D) High-risk level compounded sterile preparations.
- (i) High-risk conditions. High-risk level compounded sterile preparations are those compounded under any of the following conditions.
  - (I) Nonsterile ingredients, including manufactured products not intended for sterile routes of administration (e.g., oral), are incorporated or a nonsterile device is employed before terminal sterilization.
  - (II) Any of the following are exposed to air quality worse than ISO Class 5 for more than one hour:
    - (-a-) Sterile contents of commercially manufactured products;
    - (-b-) CSPs that lack effective antimicrobial preservatives; and
    - (-c-) Sterile surfaces of devices and containers for the preparation, transfer, sterilization, and packaging of CSPs.
  - (III) Compounding personnel are improperly garbed and gloved.
  - (IV) Nonsterile water-containing preparations are exposed no more than 6 hours before being sterilized.
  - (V) It is assumed and not verified by examination of labeling and documentation from suppliers or by direct determination that the chemical purity and content strength of ingredients meet their original or compendial specifications in unopened or in opened packages of bulk ingredients.
  - (VI) For a sterilized high-risk level preparation, in the absence of passing a sterility test, the storage periods cannot exceed the following time periods: before administration, the compounded sterile preparations are properly stored and are exposed for no more than 24 hours at controlled room temperature, for no more than 3 days at a cold temperature, and for no more than 45 days in solid frozen state between minus 25 degrees Celsius and minus 10 degrees Celsius.
  - (VII) All nonsterile measuring, mixing, and purifying devices are rinsed thoroughly with pyrogen-free or depyrogenated sterile water and then thoroughly drained or dried immediately before use for high-risk compounding. All high-risk compounded sterile solutions subjected to terminal sterilization are prefiltered by passing through a filter with a nominal pore size no larger than 1.2 micron preceding or during filling into their final containers to remove particulate matter. Sterilization of high-risk

level compounded sterile preparations by filtration shall be performed with a sterile 0.2 micrometer or 0.22 micrometer nominal pore size filter entirely within an ISO Class 5 or superior air quality environment.
- (ii) Examples of high-risk compounding include the following.
  - (I) Dissolving nonsterile bulk drug powders to make solutions which will be terminally sterilized.
  - (II) Exposing the sterile ingredients and components used to prepare and package compounded sterile preparations to room air quality worse than ISO Class 5 for more than one hour.
  - (III) Measuring and mixing sterile ingredients in nonsterile devices before sterilization is performed.
  - (IV) Assuming without appropriate evidence or direct determination that packages of bulk ingredients contain at least 95% by weight of their active chemical moiety and have not been contaminated or adulterated between uses.
- (3) Immediate Use Compounded Sterile Preparations. For the purpose of emergency or immediate patient care, such situations may include cardiopulmonary resuscitation, emergency room treatment, preparation of diagnostic agents, or critical therapy where the preparation of the compounded sterile preparation under low-risk level conditions would subject the patient to additional risk due to delays in therapy. Compounded sterile preparations are exempted from the requirements described in this paragraph for low-risk level compounded sterile preparations when all of the following criteria are met.

Note: As mentioned in (3) above, USP Chapter 797 states that the immediate use provision is intended only for those situations where there is a need for emergency or immediate patient administration of a CSP. Such situations may include cardiopulmonary resuscitation, emergency room treatment, preparation of diagnostic agents, or critical therapy where the preparation of the CSP under conditions described for low-risk level CSPs subjects the patient to additional risk due to delays in therapy. However, TSBP has allowed the immediate use provision to be used for a scheduled dose of a drug such as an antibiotic so that the nurse can mix the preparation in the hospital area where he or she is practicing.

- (A) Only simple aseptic measuring and transfer manipulations are performed with no more than three sterile nonhazardous commercial drug and diagnostic radiopharmaceutical drug products, including an infusion or diluent solution, from the manufacturers' original containers and no more than two entries into any one container or package of sterile infusion solution or administration container/device.
- (B) Unless required for the preparation, the compounding procedure occurs continuously without delays or interruptions and does not exceed one hour.
- (C) During preparation, aseptic technique is followed and, if not immediately administered, the finished compounded sterile preparation is under continuous supervision to minimize the potential for contact with nonsterile surfaces, introduction of particulate matter of biological fluids, mix-ups with other compounded sterile preparations, and direct contact with outside surfaces.
- (D) Administration begins no later than one hour following the completion of preparing the compounded sterile preparation.
- (E) When the compounded sterile preparation is not administered by the person who prepared it or its administration is not witnessed

by the person who prepared it, the compounded sterile preparation shall bear a label listing patient identification information such as the name and identification number(s), the names and amounts of all ingredients, the name or initials of the person who prepared the compounded sterile preparation, and the exact one-hour beyond-use time and date.
- (F) If administration has not begun within one hour following the completion of preparing the compounded sterile preparation, the compounded sterile preparation is promptly and safely discarded. Immediate use compounded sterile preparations shall not be stored for later use.
- (G) Hazardous drugs shall not be prepared as immediate use compounded sterile preparations.

(4) Single-Dose and Multiple-Dose Containers.
- (A) Opened or needle punctured single-dose containers such as bags, bottles, syringes, and vials of sterile products shall be used within one hour if opened in worse than ISO Class 5 air quality. Any remaining contents must be discarded.
- (B) Single-dose containers, including single-dose large volume parenteral solutions and single-dose vials, exposed to ISO Class 5 or cleaner air may be used up to six hours after initial needle puncture.
- (C) Opened single-dose fusion sealed containers shall not be stored for any time period.
- (D) Multiple-dose containers may be used up to 28 days after initial needle puncture unless otherwise specified by the manufacturer.

(5) Library. In addition to the library requirements of the pharmacy's specific license classification, a pharmacy shall maintain current or updated copies in hardcopy or electronic format of each of the following:
- (A) A reference text on injectable drug preparations such as *Handbook on Injectable Drug Products*;
- (B) A specialty reference text appropriate for the scope of pharmacy services provided by the pharmacy (e.g., if the pharmacy prepares hazardous drugs, a reference text on the preparation of hazardous drugs);
- (C) The United States Pharmacopeia/National Formulary containing USP Chapter 71, Sterility Tests; USP Chapter 85, Bacterial Endotoxins Test; USP Chapter 795, Pharmaceutical Compounding—Nonsterile Preparations; USP Chapter 797, Pharmaceutical Compounding—Sterile Preparations; and USP Chapter 1163, Quality Assurance in Pharmaceutical Compounding; and
- (D) Any additional USP/NF chapters applicable to the practice of the pharmacy (e.g., USP Chapter 800, Hazardous Drugs—Handling in Healthcare Settings and USP Chapter 823, Positron Emission Tomography Drugs for Compounding, Investigational, and Research Uses).

(6) Environment. Compounding facilities shall be physically designed and environmentally controlled to minimize airborne contamination from contacting critical sites.
- (A) Low-risk and medium-risk preparations. A pharmacy that prepares low-risk and medium-risk preparations shall have a clean room for the compounding of sterile preparations that is constructed to minimize the opportunities for particulate and microbial contamination. The clean room shall:

Note: The clean room is comprised of both the ante-area or anteroom and the buffer area or buffer room. The term "clean room" is often misinterpreted to mean only the buffer area or buffer room.

(i) Be clean, well lit, and of sufficient size to support sterile compounding activities;

(ii) Be maintained at a temperature of 20 degrees Celsius or cooler and at a humidity below 60%;

(iii) Be used only for the compounding of sterile preparations;

Note: Clause (iii) actually refers to the "buffer" area or room (see (xii) below). The buffer area is to be used only for sterile compounding and not for storing supplies such as needles, syringes, drugs, etc., that are needed for compounding sterile preparations. Supplies are permitted, in limited quantities, in the ante-area or ante room. Neither the buffer area or buffer room nor the ante-area or anteroom is to be used for general storage of supplies, even if the supplies are intended solely for compounding sterile preparations.

(iv) Be designed such that hand sanitizing and gowning occur outside the buffer area but allow hands-free access by compounding personnel to the buffer area;

(v) Have nonporous and washable floors or floor covering to enable regular disinfection;

(vi) Be ventilated in a manner to avoid disruption from the HVAC system and room cross-drafts;

(vii) Have walls, ceilings, floors, fixtures, shelving, counters, and cabinets that are smooth, impervious, free from cracks and crevices (e.g., coved), nonshedding, and resistant to damage by disinfectant agents;

Note: This is another area of the rule that causes confusion for many people. Often, cabinetry used in a clean room is constructed of pressed particle board or other forms of wood. Wood, especially pressed particle board, is not free from cracks and crevices and provides an excellent living environment for microorganisms and particulate matter that can compromise the air quality in the clean room. If wood shelving and cabinetry are used in the clean room, all surfaces must be sealed (using silicone caulking or similar materials) to ensure that all cracks and crevices in the material are covered and not exposed to air in the room. Additionally, the parenthetical expression (e.g., coved) has no real significance in (vii) above. It is used properly in (viii) below.

(viii) Have junctures of ceilings to walls coved or caulked to avoid cracks and crevices;

(ix) Have drugs and supplies stored on shelving areas above the floor to permit adequate floor cleaning;

(x) Contain only the appropriate compounding supplies and not be used for bulk storage for supplies and materials. Objects that shed particles shall not be brought into the clean room. A Class B pharmacy may use low-linting absorbent materials in the primary engineering control device;

(xi) Contain an ante-area that contains a sink with hot and cold running water that enables hands-free use with a closed system of soap dispensing to minimize the risk of extrinsic contamination. A Class B pharmacy may have a sink with hot and cold running water that enables hands-free use with a closed system of soap dispensing immediately outside the ante-area if antiseptic hand cleansing is performed using a waterless alcohol-based surgical hand scrub with persistent activity following manufacturers' recommendations once inside the ante-area; and

Note: In addition to a sink with hot and cold running water that enables hands-free use, the closed system of soap dispensing should be hands-free to minimize the risk of extrinsic contamination.

(xii) Contain a buffer area. The following is applicable for the buffer area.

(I) There shall be some demarcation designation that delineates the ante-area from the buffer area. The demarcation shall be such that it does not create conditions that could adversely affect the cleanliness of the area.

Note: In other words, the line of demarcation should not be created by placing tape on the floor. The line of demarcation could be different colored flooring on the ante-area side of the room from the floor coloring on the buffer side of the room, two points on walls on opposite sides of the room, etc.

(II) The buffer area shall be segregated from surrounding, unclassified spaces to reduce the risk of contaminants being blown, dragged, or otherwise introduced into the filtered unidirectional airflow environment. This segregation should be continuously monitored.

(III) A buffer area that is not physically separated from the ante-area shall employ the principle of displacement airflow as defined in Chapter 797, Pharmaceutical Compounding—Sterile Preparations, of the USP/NF, with limited access to personnel.

Note: In a clean room where the buffer area is not physically separated from the ante-area, the ISO classification of air must be ISO 7 in both the buffer area and the ante-area.

(IV) The buffer area shall not contain sources of water (i.e., sinks) or floor drains other than distilled or sterile water introduced for facilitating the use of heat block wells for radiopharmaceuticals.

Note: TSBP has determined that in older facilities where a clean room was created after completion of construction, buffer areas may have overhead sprinkler valves that were installed and are required to meet fire codes. It should also be noted that TSBP has determined that certain processes in Class B (Nuclear) pharmacies require the presence of a water source in the buffer area and has decided to allow such, when necessary, in Class B pharmacies.

(B) High-risk preparations.

(i) In addition to the requirements in (A) above, when high-risk preparations are compounded, the primary engineering control shall be located in a buffer area that provides a physical separation through the use of walls, doors, and pass-throughs and has a minimum differential positive pressure of 0.02 to 0.05 inches water column.

(ii) Presterilization procedures for high-risk level compounded sterile preparations such as weighing and mixing shall be completed in no worse than an ISO Class 8 environment.

(C) Automated compounding device.
  (i) General. If automated compounding devices are used, the pharmacy shall have a method to calibrate and verify the accuracy of automated compounding devices used in aseptic processing, document the calibration and verification on a daily basis based on the manufacturer's recommendations, and review the results at least weekly.
  (ii) Loading bulk drugs into automated compounding devices.
    (I) An automated compounding device may be loaded with bulk drugs only by a pharmacist or by pharmacy technicians or pharmacy technician trainees under the direction and direct supervision of a pharmacist.
    (II) The label of an automated compounding device container shall indicate the brand name and strength of the drug. If no brand name, then the generic name, strength, and name of the manufacturer or distributor shall be indicated.
    (III) Records of loading bulk drugs into an automated compounding device shall be maintained to show:
      (-a-) Name of the drug, strength, and dosage form;
      (-b-) Manufacturer or distributor;
      (-c-) Manufacturer's lot number;
      (-d-) Manufacturer's expiration date;
      (-e-) Quantity added to the automated compounding device;
      (-f-) Date of loading;
      (-g-) Name, initials, or electronic signature of the person loading the automated compounding device; and
      (-h-) Name, initials, or electronic signature of the responsible pharmacist.
    (IV) The automated compounding device shall not be used until a pharmacist verifies that the system is properly loaded and affixes his or her signature or electronic signature to the record specified in (III) above.
    Note: As with most records, records of calibration of automated compounding devices along with records for the labeling and loading of bulk drugs into automated compounding devices should be maintained in the pharmacy for a minimum of two years.
(D) Hazardous drugs. If the preparation is hazardous, the following is also applicable.
  (i) Hazardous drugs shall be prepared only under conditions that protect personnel during preparation and storage.
  (ii) Hazardous drugs shall be stored separately from other inventory in a manner to prevent contamination and personnel exposure.
  (iii) All personnel involved in the compounding of hazardous drugs shall wear appropriate protective apparel such as gowns, face masks, eye protection, hair covers, shoe covers or dedicated shoes, and appropriate gloving at all times when handling hazardous drugs, including receiving, distribution, stocking, inventorying, and preparation for administration and disposal.
  (iv) Appropriate safety and containment techniques for compounding hazardous drugs shall be used with aseptic techniques required for preparing sterile preparations.

[Handwritten note in margin: Chapter 800 is hazardous drugs]

- (v) Disposal of hazardous waste shall comply with all applicable local, state, and federal requirements.
- (vi) Prepared doses of hazardous drugs must be dispensed, labeled with proper precautions inside and outside, and distributed in a manner to minimize patient contact with hazardous agents. *Note: USP Chapter 800, which became effective on December 1, 2019, is an entire chapter in the USP/NF devoted to handling of hazardous drugs in healthcare settings. TSBP may elect to write and adopt a separate rule on hazardous drugs or may elect to harmonize the wording of Chapter 800 with that of Board Rule 291.133.*

(E) Blood-labeling procedures. When compounding activities require the manipulation of a patient's blood-derived material (e.g., radiolabeling a patient's or donor's white blood cells), the manipulations shall be performed in a ISO Class 5 biological safety cabinet located in a buffer area and clearly separated from routine material-handling procedures and equipment used in preparation activities to avoid any cross-contamination. The preparations shall not require sterilization.

(F) Cleaning and disinfecting the sterile compounding areas. The following cleaning and disinfecting practices and frequencies apply to direct and contiguous compounding areas, which include ISO Class 5 compounding areas for exposure of critical sites as well as buffer areas, ante-areas, and segregated compounding areas.
- (i) The pharmacist-in-charge is responsible for developing written procedures for cleaning and disinfecting the direct and contiguous compounding areas and assuring the procedures are followed.
- (ii) These procedures shall be conducted at the beginning of each work shift, before each batch preparation is started, when there are spills, and when surface contamination is known or suspected resulting from procedural breaches. In addition, these procedures shall be conducted every 30 minutes during continuous compounding of individual compounded sterile preparations, unless a particular compounding procedure requires more than 30 minutes to complete. If that is the case, the direct compounding area is to be cleaned immediately after the compounding activity is completed.
- (iii) Before compounding is performed, all items shall be removed from the direct and contiguous compounding areas and all surfaces shall be cleaned by removing loose material and residue from spills, followed by an application of a residue-free disinfecting agent (e.g., IPA) which is allowed to dry before compounding begins. In a Class B pharmacy, objects used in preparing sterile radiopharmaceuticals (e.g., dose calibrator) which cannot be reasonably removed from the compounding area shall be sterilized with an application of a residue-free disinfection agent.
Note: Clause (iii) provides minimum requirements for cleaning direct and contiguous compounding areas adopted by TSBP. However, USP Chapter 797 requires the use of STERILE isopropyl alcohol (IPA). Also, IPA has little or no sporicidal activity and proper cleaning of the contiguous compounding areas should include the use of a sporicidal agent such as 5% sodium

hypochlorite. If such an agent is used, the sporicidal agent should be used first to clean the surfaces followed by cleaning with sterile IPA.

(iv) Work surfaces in the buffer areas and ante-areas, as well as segregated compounding areas, shall be cleaned and disinfected at least daily. Dust and debris shall be removed when necessary from storage sites for compounding ingredients and supplies using a method that does not degrade the ISO Class 7 or 8 air quality.

(v) Floors in the buffer area, ante-area, and segregated compounding area are cleaned by mopping with a cleaning and disinfecting agent at least once daily when no aseptic operations are in progress. Mopping shall be performed by trained personnel using approved agents and procedures described in the written SOPs. It is incumbent on compounding personnel to ensure that such cleaning is performed properly.

(vi) In the buffer area, ante-area, and segregated compounding area, the walls, ceilings, and shelving shall be cleaned and disinfected monthly. Cleaning and disinfecting agents shall be used with careful consideration of compatibilities, effectiveness, and inappropriate or toxic residues.

(vii) All cleaning materials such as wipers, sponges, and mops shall be nonshedding and be dedicated to use in the buffer area, ante-area, and segregated compounding areas, and they shall not be removed from these areas except for disposal. Floor mops may be used in both the buffer area and ante-area but only in that order. If cleaning materials are reused, procedures shall be developed that ensure the effectiveness of the cleaning device is maintained and that repeated use does not add to the bio-burden of the area being cleaned.

Note: The statement "Floor mops may be used in both the buffer area and ante-area but only in that order" is important. Cleaning should proceed from the cleanest area to the dirtiest area to prevent movement of "dirt" from a dirty area to a clean area.

(viii) Supplies and equipment removed from shipping cartons must be wiped with a disinfecting agent such as sterile IPA. After the disinfectant is sprayed or wiped on a surface to be disinfected, the disinfectant shall be allowed to dry during which time the item shall not be used for compounding purposes. However, if sterile supplies are received in sealed pouches, the pouches may be removed as the supplies are introduced into the ISO Class 5 area without the need to disinfect the individual sterile supply items. No shipping or other external cartons may be taken into the buffer area or segregated compounding area.

(ix) Storage shelving emptied of all supplies, walls, and ceilings are cleaned and disinfected at planned monthly intervals, if not more frequently.

(x) Cleaning must be done by personnel trained in appropriate cleaning techniques.

(xi) Proper documentation and frequency of cleaning must be maintained and shall contain the following:
(I) Date and time of cleaning;
(II) Type of cleaning performed; and
(III) Name of individual who performed the cleaning.

Notes

Note: It is recommended that all cleaning procedures listed in (F) above be completed by pharmacy personnel with equipment dedicated to the clean room and stored in the clean room. Mops and other cleaning supplies used to clean the clean room should not be used to clean other areas of the pharmacy.

(G) Security requirements. In the absence of the pharmacist, the pharmacist-in-charge may authorize personnel to gain access to that area of the pharmacy containing dispensed sterile preparations for the purpose of retrieving dispensed prescriptions to deliver to patients. If the pharmacy allows such after-hours access, the area containing the dispensed sterile preparations shall be an enclosed and lockable area separate from the area containing undispensed prescription drugs. A list of the authorized personnel having such access shall be in the pharmacy's policy and procedure manual.

(H) Storage requirements and beyond-use dating.
  (i) Storage requirements. All drugs shall be stored at the proper temperature and conditions as defined in the USP/NF and in Board Rule 291.15 (Storage of Drugs).
  (ii) Beyond-use dating.
    (I) Beyond-use dates for compounded sterile preparations shall be assigned based on professional experience, which shall include careful interpretation of appropriate information sources for the same or similar formulations.
    (II) Beyond-use dates for compounded sterile preparations that are prepared strictly in accordance with manufacturer's product labeling must be those specified in that labeling or from appropriate literature sources or direct testing.
    (III) When assigning a beyond-use date, compounding personnel shall consult and apply drug-specific and general stability documentation and literature where available. They should consider the nature of the drug and its degradation mechanism, the container in which it is packaged, the expected storage conditions, and the intended duration of therapy.
    (IV) The sterility, storage, and stability beyond-use date for attached and activated container pairs of drug products for intravascular administration shall be applied as indicated by the manufacturer.

(7) Primary Engineering Control Device (PEC). The pharmacy shall prepare sterile preparations in a primary engineering control device, such as a laminar air flow hood, biological safety cabinet, compounding aseptic isolator (CAI), or compounding aseptic containment isolator (CACI), which is capable of maintaining at least ISO Class 5 conditions for 0.5 micrometer particles while compounding sterile preparations.

  (A) Laminar air flow hood. If the pharmacy is using a laminar air flow hood as its PEC, the laminar air flow hood shall:
    (i) Be located in the buffer area and placed in the buffer area in a manner as to avoid conditions that could adversely affect its operation such as strong air currents from opened doors, personnel traffic, or air streams from the heating, ventilating, and air condition system;
    (ii) Be certified for operational efficiency using certification procedures, such as those outlined in the Certification Guide for

Sterile Compounding Facilities (CAG-003-2006), which shall be performed by a qualified independent individual no less than every six months and whenever the device or room is relocated or altered or major service to the facility is performed;

Note: Recertification of a laminar air flow workbench (LAFW) or other PEC is required when the PEC is moved, not just if it is relocated to another area. If the PEC is moved for cleaning or for any other reason, the PEC should be recertified by a qualified independent contractor.

    (iii) Have pre-filters inspected periodically and replaced as needed, in accordance with written policies and procedures and the manufacturer's specification, and the inspection and/or replacement date documented; and

    (iv) Be located in a buffer area that has a minimum differential positive pressure of 0.02 to 0.05 inches water column. A buffer area that is not physically separated from the ante-area shall employ the principle of displacement airflow as defined in Chapter 797, Pharmaceutical Compounding—Sterile Preparations, of the USP/NF, with limited access to personnel.

(B) Biological safety cabinet (BCS).

    (i) If the pharmacy is using a biological safety cabinet as its PEC for the preparation of hazardous sterile compounded preparations, the biological safety cabinet shall be a Class II or III vertical flow biological safety cabinet located in an ISO Class 7 area that is physically separated from other preparation areas. The area for preparation of sterile chemotherapeutic preparations shall:

        (I) Have no less than 0.01 inches water column negative pressure to the adjacent positive pressure ISO Class 7 or better ante-area and

        (II) Have a pressure indicator that can be readily monitored for correct room pressurization.

    (ii) Pharmacies that prepare a low volume of hazardous drugs are not required to comply with the provisions of (i) above if the pharmacy uses a device that provides two tiers of containment (e.g., closed-system vial transfer device within a BSC).

Note: USP Chapter 800 became effective on December 1, 2019. TSBP may elect to adopt new rules that could result in the repeal of part or all of (B) (Biological Safety Cabinets) above.

    (iii) If the pharmacy is using a biological safety cabinet as its PEC for the preparation of nonhazardous sterile compounded preparations, the biological safety cabinet shall:

        (I) Be located in the buffer area and placed in the buffer area in a manner as to avoid conditions that could adversely affect its operation, such as strong air currents from opened doors, personnel traffic, or air streams from the heating, ventilating, and air condition system;

        (II) Be certified by a qualified independent contractor according to the International Organization of Standardization (ISO) Classification of Particulate Matter in Room Air (ISO 14644-1) for operational efficiency at least every six months and whenever the device or room is relocated or altered or major service to the facility is performed, in accordance with the manufacturer's specifications

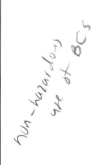

and test procedures specified in the Institute of Environmental Sciences and Technology (IEST) document IEST-RP-CC002.3;
- (III) Have pre-filters inspected periodically and replaced as needed, in accordance with written policies and procedures and the manufacturer's specification, and the inspection and/or replacement date documented; and
- (IV) Be located in a buffer area that has a minimum differential positive pressure of 0.02 to 0.05 inches water column.

(C) Compounding aseptic isolator (CAI).
- (i) If the pharmacy is using a compounding aseptic isolator as its PEC, the CAI shall provide unidirectional airflow within the main processing and antechambers and be placed in an ISO Class 7 buffer area unless the isolator meets all of the following conditions.
  - (I) The isolator must provide isolation from the room and maintain ISO Class 5 during dynamic operating conditions including transferring ingredients, components, and devices into and out of the isolator and during the preparation of compounded sterile preparations.
  - (II) Particle counts sampled approximately 6 to 12 inches upstream of the critical exposure site must maintain ISO Class 5 levels during compounding operations.
  - (III) The CAI must be certified for operational efficiency using certification procedures, such as those outlined in the Certification Guide for Sterile Compounding Facilities (CAG-003-2006), which shall be performed by a qualified independent individual no less than every six months and whenever the device or room is relocated or altered or major service to the facility is performed.
  - (IV) The pharmacy shall maintain documentation from the manufacturer that the isolator meets this standard when located in worse than ISO Class 7 environments.
- (ii) If the isolator meets the requirements in (i) above, the CAI may be placed in a non-ISO classified area of the pharmacy. However, the area shall be segregated from other areas of the pharmacy and shall:
  - (I) Be clean, well lit, and of sufficient size;
  - (II) Be used only for the compounding of low-risk and medium-risk nonhazardous sterile preparations;
  - (III) Be located in an area of the pharmacy with nonporous and washable floors or floor covering to enable regular disinfection; and
  - (IV) Be an area in which the CAI is placed in a manner as to avoid conditions that could adversely affect its operation.
- (iii) In addition to the requirements specified in (i) and (ii) above, if the CAI is used in the compounding of high-risk nonhazardous sterile preparations, the CAI shall be placed in an area or room with at least ISO 8 quality air so that high-risk powders weighed in at least ISO-8 air quality conditions, compounding utensils for measuring, and other compounding equipment are not exposed to lesser air quality prior to the completion of compounding and packaging of the high-risk preparation.

(D) Compounding aseptic containment isolator (CACI).
  (i) If the pharmacy is using a compounding aseptic containment isolator as its PEC for the preparation of low-risk and medium-risk hazardous drugs, the CACI shall be located in a separate room away from other areas of the pharmacy and shall:
   (I) Be vented to the outside of the building in which the pharmacy is located and provide at least 0.01 inches water column negative pressure compared to the other areas of the pharmacy and
   (II) Provide unidirectional airflow within the main processing and antechambers and be placed in an ISO Class 7 buffer area, unless the CACI meets all of the following conditions.
    (-a-) The isolator must provide isolation from the room and maintain ISO Class 5 environment during dynamic operating conditions including transferring ingredients, components, and devices into and out of the isolator and during preparation of compounded sterile preparations.
    (-b-) Particle counts sampled approximately 6 to 12 inches upstream of the critical exposure site must maintain ISO Class 5 levels during compounding operations.
    (-c-) The CACI must be certified for operational efficiency using certification procedures such as those outlined in the Certification Guide for Sterile Compounding Facilities (CAG-003-2006), which shall be performed by a qualified independent individual no less than every six months and whenever the device or room is relocated or altered or major service to the facility is performed.
    (-d-) The pharmacy shall maintain documentation from the manufacturer that the isolator meets this standard when located in worse than ISO Class 7 environments.
  (ii) If the CACI meets all conditions specified in (i) above, the CACI shall not be located in the same room as a CAI but shall be located in a separate room in the pharmacy that is not required to maintain ISO classified air. The room in which the CACI is located shall provide a minimum of 0.01 inches water column negative pressure compared with the other areas of the pharmacy and shall meet the following requirements:
   (I) Be clean, well lit, and of sufficient size;
   (II) Be maintained at a temperature of 20 degrees Celsius or cooler and a humidity below 60%;
   (III) Be used only for the compounding of hazardous sterile preparations;
   (IV) Be located in an area of the pharmacy with walls, ceilings, floors, fixtures, shelving, counters, and cabinets that are smooth, impervious, free from cracks and crevices, nonshedding, and resistant to damage by disinfectant agents; and
   (V) Have nonporous and washable floors or floor covering to enable regular disinfection.

(iii) If the CACI is used in the compounding of high-risk hazardous preparations, the CACI shall be placed in an area or room with at least ISO Class 8 quality air so that high-risk powders weighed in at least ISO Class 8 air quality conditions are not exposed to lesser air quality prior to the completion of compounding and packaging of the high-risk preparation.

(iv) Pharmacies that prepare a low volume of hazardous drugs are not required to comply with the provisions of (i) and (iii) above if the pharmacy uses a device that provides two tiers of containment (e.g., CACI that is located in a non-negative pressure room).

Note: A CACI used to compound hazardous preparations must be vented to the outside of the building and meet the conditions in either (ii) or (iii) above. This is also a requirement of USP Chapter 800.

(8) Additional Equipment and Supplies. Pharmacies compounding sterile preparations shall have the following equipment and supplies:

(A) A calibrated system or device (i.e., thermometer) to monitor the temperature to ensure that proper storage requirements are met if sterile preparations are stored in the refrigerator;

(B) A calibrated system or device to monitor the temperature where bulk chemicals are stored;

(C) A temperature-sensing mechanism suitably placed in the controlled temperature storage space to reflect accurately the true temperature;

(D) If applicable, a Class A prescription balance or analytical balance and weights. Such balance shall be properly maintained and subject to periodic inspection by the Texas State Board of Pharmacy;

Note: A Class A prescription balance or analytical balance is not required to be in the pharmacy if the pharmacy will not be weighing powders or other materials for compounding.

(E) Equipment and utensils necessary for the proper compounding of sterile preparations. Such equipment and utensils used in the compounding process shall be:
  (i) Of appropriate design, appropriate capacity, and be operated within designed operational limits;
  (ii) Of suitable composition so that surfaces that contact components, in-process material, or drug products shall not be reactive, additive, or absorptive so as to alter the safety, identity, strength, quality, or purity of the drug preparation beyond the desired result;
  (iii) Cleaned and sanitized immediately prior to and after each use; and
  (iv) Routinely inspected, calibrated (if necessary), or checked to ensure proper performance;

(F) Appropriate disposal containers for used needles, syringes, etc., and, if applicable, hazardous waste from the preparation of hazardous drugs and/or biohazardous waste;

(G) Appropriate packaging or delivery containers to maintain proper storage conditions for sterile preparations;

(H) Infusion devices, if applicable; and

(I) All necessary supplies including:
  (i) Disposable needles, syringes, and other supplies for aseptic mixing;

- (ii) Disinfectant cleaning solutions;
- (iii) Sterile 70% isopropyl alcohol;
- (iv) Sterile gloves for both hazardous and nonhazardous drug compounding;
- (v) Sterile alcohol-based or waterless alcohol-based surgical scrub;
- (vi) Handwashing agents with bactericidal action;
- (vii) Disposable, lint free towels or wipes;
- (viii) Appropriate filters and filtration equipment;
- (ix) Hazardous spill kits, if applicable; and
- (x) Masks, caps, coveralls or gowns with tight cuffs, shoe covers, and gloves as applicable.

(9) Labeling.
  (A) Prescription drug or medication orders. In addition to the labeling requirements for the pharmacy's specific license classification, the label dispensed or distributed pursuant to a prescription drug or medication order shall contain the following:
   (i) The generic name(s) or the official name(s) of the principal active ingredient(s) of the compounded sterile preparation;
   (ii) For outpatient prescription orders other than sterile radiopharmaceuticals, a statement that the compounded sterile preparation has been compounded by the pharmacy (an auxiliary label may be used on the container to meet this requirement); and
   (iii) A beyond-use date. The beyond-use date shall be determined as outlined in Chapter 797, Pharmacy Compounding—Sterile Preparations, of the USP/NF, and (8)(G) above.
  (B) Batch. If the sterile preparation is compounded in a batch, the following shall also be included on the batch label:
   (i) Unique lot number assigned to the batch;
   (ii) Quantity;
   (iii) Appropriate ancillary instructions such as storage instructions or cautionary statements, including hazardous drug warning labels where appropriate; and
   (iv) Device-specific instructions where appropriate.
  (C) Pharmacy bulk package. The label of a pharmacy bulk package shall:
   (i) State prominently "Pharmacy Bulk Package—Not for Direct Infusion";
   (ii) Contain or refer to information on proper techniques to help ensure safe use of the preparation; and
   (iii) Bear a statement limiting the time frame in which the container may be used once it has been entered, provided it is held under the labeled storage conditions.

(10) Written Drug Information for Prescription Drug Orders Only. Written information about the compounded preparation or its major active ingredient(s) shall be given to the patient at the time of dispensing a prescription drug order. A statement which indicates that the preparation was compounded by the pharmacy must be included in this written information. If there is no written information available, the patient shall be advised that the drug has been compounded and how to contact a pharmacist and, if appropriate, the prescriber concerning the drug. This paragraph does not apply to the preparation of radiopharmaceuticals.

(11) Pharmaceutical Care Services. In addition to the pharmaceutical care requirements for the pharmacy's specific license classification, the following requirements for sterile preparations compounded pursuant to

prescription drug orders must be met. This paragraph does not apply to the preparation of radiopharmaceuticals.

- (A) Primary provider. There shall be a designated physician primarily responsible for the patient's medical care. There shall be a clear understanding among the physician, the patient, and the pharmacy of the responsibilities of each in the areas of the delivery of care and the monitoring of the patient. This shall be documented in the patient medication record (PMR).
- (B) Patient training. The pharmacist-in-charge shall develop policies to ensure that the patient and/or patient's caregiver receives information regarding drugs and their safe and appropriate use, including instruction when applicable, regarding:
  - (i) Appropriate disposition of hazardous solutions and ancillary supplies;
  - (ii) Proper disposition of controlled substances in the home;
  - (iii) Self-administration of drugs where appropriate;
  - (iv) Emergency procedures including how to contact an appropriate individual in the event of problems or emergencies related to drug therapy; and
  - (v) If the patient or patient's caregiver prepares sterile preparations in the home, the following additional information shall be provided:
    - (I) Safeguards against microbial contamination, including aseptic techniques for compounding intravenous admixtures and aseptic techniques for injecting additives to premixed intravenous solutions;
    - (II) Appropriate storage methods, including storage durations for sterile pharmaceuticals and expirations of self-mixed solutions;
    - (III) Handling and disposition of premixed and self-mixed intravenous admixtures; and
    - (IV) Proper disposition of intravenous admixture compounding supplies such as syringes, vials, ampules, and intravenous solution containers.
- (C) Pharmacist-patient relationship. It is imperative that a pharmacist-patient relationship be established and maintained throughout the patient's course of therapy. This relationship shall be documented in the patient's medication record (PMR).
- (D) Patient monitoring. The pharmacist-in-charge shall develop policies to ensure that:
  - (i) The patient's response to drug therapy is monitored and conveyed to the appropriate healthcare provider;
  - (ii) The first dose of any new drug therapy is administered in the presence of an individual qualified to monitor for and respond to adverse drug reactions; and
  - (iii) Reports of adverse events with a compounded sterile preparation are reviewed promptly and thoroughly to correct and prevent future occurrences.

(12) Drugs, Components, and Materials Used in Sterile Compounding.
- (A) Drugs used in sterile compounding shall be USP/NF grade substances manufactured in an FDA-registered facility.
- (B) If USP/NF grade substances are not available, drugs shall be of a chemical grade in one of the following categories:

(i) Chemically Pure (CP);
(ii) Analytical Reagent (AR);
(iii) American Chemical Society (ACS); or
(iv) Food Chemical Codex.
(C) If a drug, component, or material is not purchased from an FDA-registered facility, the pharmacist shall establish purity and stability by obtaining a Certificate of Analysis from the supplier, and the pharmacist shall compare the monograph of drugs in a similar class to the Certificate of Analysis.
(D) All components shall:
(i) Be manufactured in an FDA-registered facility; or
(ii) In the professional judgment of the pharmacist, be of high quality and obtained from acceptable and reliable alternative sources; and
(iii) Stored in properly labeled containers in a clean, dry area under proper temperatures.
(E) Drug preparation containers and closures shall not be reactive, additive, or absorptive so as to alter the safety, identity, strength, quality, or purity of the compounded drug preparation beyond the desired result.
(F) Components, drug preparation containers, and closures shall be rotated so that the oldest stock is used first.
(G) Container closure systems shall provide adequate protection against foreseeable external factors in storage and use that can cause deterioration or contamination of the compounded drug preparation.
(H) A pharmacy may not compound a preparation that contains ingredients appearing on a federal Food and Drug Administration list of drug products withdrawn or removed from the market for safety reasons.
(13) Compounding Process.
(A) Standard operating procedures (SOPs). All significant procedures performed in the compounding area shall be covered by written SOPs designed to ensure accountability, accuracy, quality, safety, and uniformity in the compounding process. At a minimum, SOPs shall be developed and implemented for:
(i) The facility;
(ii) Equipment;
(iii) Personnel;
(iv) Preparation evaluation;
(v) Quality assurance;
(vi) Preparation recall;
(vii) Packaging; and
(viii) Storage of compounded sterile preparations.
(B) USP/NF. Any compounded formulation with an official monograph in the USP/NF shall be compounded, labeled, and packaged in conformity with the USP/NF monograph for the drug.
(C) Personnel cleansing and garbing.
(i) Any person with an apparent illness or open lesion, including rashes, sunburn, weeping sores, conjunctivitis, and active respiratory infection, that may adversely affect the safety or quality of a drug preparation being compounded shall be excluded from working in ISO Class 5, ISO Class 7, and ISO Class 8 compounding areas until the condition is remedied.

(ii) Before entering the buffer area, compounding personnel must remove the following:
  (I) Personal outer garments (e.g., bandanas, coats, hats, jackets, scarves, sweaters, and vests);
  (II) All cosmetics because they shed flakes and particles; and
  (III) All hand, wrist, and other body jewelry or piercings (e.g., earrings and lip or eyebrow piercings) that can interfere with the effectiveness of personal protective equipment (e.g., fit of gloves and cuffs of sleeves).
(iii) The wearing of artificial nails or extenders is prohibited while working in the sterile compounding environment. Natural nails shall be kept neat and trimmed.
(iv) Personnel shall don personal protective equipment and perform hand hygiene in an order that proceeds from the dirtiest to the cleanest activities as follows:
  (I) Activities considered the dirtiest include donning of dedicated shoes or shoe covers, head and facial hair covers (e.g., beard covers in addition to face masks), and face masks/eye shields. Eye shields are optional unless working with irritants like germicidal disinfecting agents or when preparing hazardous drugs.
  (II) After donning dedicated shoes or shoe covers, head and facial hair covers, and face masks, personnel shall perform a hand hygiene procedure by removing debris from underneath fingernails using a nail cleaner under running warm water followed by vigorous hand washing. Personnel shall begin washing arms at the hands and continue washing to elbows for at least 30 seconds with either a plain (non-antimicrobial) soap or antimicrobial soap and water while in the ante-area. Hands and forearms to the elbows shall be completely dried using lint-free disposable towels, an electronic hands-free hand dryer, or a HEPA filtered hand dryer.
  (III) After completion of hand washing, personnel shall don clean nonshedding gowns enclosed at the neck with sleeves that fit snugly around the wrists.
  (IV) Once inside the buffer area or segregated compounding area and prior to donning sterile powder-free gloves, antiseptic hand cleansing shall be performed using a waterless alcohol-based surgical hand scrub with persistent activity following manufacturer's recommendations. Hands shall be allowed to dry thoroughly before donning sterile gloves.
  (V) Sterile gloves that form a continuous barrier with the gown shall be the last item donned before compounding begins. Sterile gloves shall be donned using proper technique to ensure the sterility of the glove is not compromised while donning. The cuff of the sterile glove shall cover the cuff of the gown at the wrist. When preparing hazardous preparations, the compounder shall use a double glove or shall use single gloves ensuring that the gloves are sterile powder-free chemotherapy-rated gloves. Routine application of sterile 70% IPA shall occur

throughout the compounding day and whenever non-sterile surfaces are touched.

Note: To summarize the order of gowning and garbing, the compounder should follow this order to completion (Steps 1 and 2 may be interchanged.):
1. Don shoe covers.
2. Don hair cover, face mask, and beard cover (if necessary)—no specific order.
3. Perform aseptic handwashing.
4. Dry hands correctly.
5. Don sterile clean room gown.
6. Apply alcohol-based surgical scrub to hands and allow to dry.
7. After entering buffer area, don sterile gloves with cuffs over sleeve of gown.
8. Place compounding supplies in PEC.
9. Apply sterile IPA to gloves before beginning to compound.

(v) When compounding personnel temporarily exit the buffer area environment during a work shift, the exterior gown, if not visibly soiled, may be removed and retained in the ante-area and be re-donned during that same work shift only. However, shoe covers, hair and facial hair covers, face mask/eye shield, and gloves shall be replaced with new ones before reentering the buffer area along with performing proper hand hygiene.

(vi) During high-risk compounding activities that precede terminal sterilization, such as weighing and mixing of nonsterile ingredients, compounding personnel shall be garbed and gloved the same as when performing compounding in an ISO Class 5 environment. Properly garbed and gloved compounding personnel who are exposed to air quality that is either known or suspected to be worse than ISO Class 7 shall re-garb personal protective equipment along with washing their hands properly, performing antiseptic hand cleansing with a sterile 70% IPA-based or another suitable sterile alcohol-based surgical hand scrub, and donning sterile gloves upon reentering the ISO Class 7 buffer area.

(vii) When compounding aseptic isolators or compounding aseptic containment isolators are the source of the ISO Class 5 environment, at the start of each new compounding procedure a new pair of sterile gloves shall be donned within the CAI or CACI. In addition, the compounding personnel should follow the requirements as specified in this rule, unless the isolator manufacturer can provide written documentation based on validated environmental testing that any components of personal protective equipment or cleansing are not required.

(14) Quality Assurance.
  (A) Initial formula validation. Prior to routine compounding of a sterile preparation, a pharmacy shall conduct an evaluation that shows that the pharmacy is capable of compounding a preparation that is sterile and that contains the stated amount of active ingredient(s).
    (i) Low-risk preparations.
      (I) Quality assurance practices include but are not limited to the following:

(-a-) Routine disinfection and air quality testing of the direct compounding environment to minimize microbial surface contamination and maintain ISO Class 5 air quality.

(-b-) Visual confirmation that compounding personnel are properly donning and wearing appropriate items and types of protective garments and goggles.

(-c-) Review of all orders and packages of ingredients to ensure that the correct identity and amounts of ingredients were compounded.

(-d-) Visual inspection of compounded sterile preparations, except for sterile radiopharmaceuticals, to ensure the absence of particulate matter in solutions, the absence of leakage from vials and bags, and the accuracy and thoroughness of labeling.

(II) Example of a media-fill test procedure. This test or an equivalent test is performed at least annually by each person authorized to compound in a low-risk level under conditions that closely simulate the most challenging or stressful conditions encountered during compounding of low-risk level sterile preparations. Once begun, this test is completed without interruption within an ISO Class 5 air quality environment. Three sets of four 5-milliliter aliquots of sterile fluid culture media are transferred with the same sterile 10-milliliter syringe and vented needle combination into separate sealed, empty, sterile 30-milliliter clear vials (i.e., four 5-milliliter aliquots into each of three 30-milliliter vials). Sterile adhesive seals are aseptically affixed to the rubber closures on the three filled vials. The vials are incubated within a range of 20–35 degrees Celsius for a minimum of 14 days. Failure is indicated by visible turbidity in the medium on or before 14 days. The media-fill test must include a positive-control sample.

(ii) Medium-risk preparations.

(I) Quality assurance procedures for medium-risk level compounded sterile preparations include all those for low-risk level compounded sterile preparations as well as a more challenging media-fill test passed annually or more frequently.

(II) Example of a media-fill test procedure. This test or an equivalent test is performed at least annually under conditions that closely simulate the most challenging or stressful conditions encountered during compounding. This test is completed without interruption within an ISO Class 5 air quality environment. Six 100-milliliter aliquots of sterile fluid culture media are aseptically transferred by gravity through separate tubing sets into separate evacuated sterile containers. The six containers are then arranged as three pairs, and a sterile 10-milliliter syringe and 18-gauge needle combination is used to exchange two 5-milliliter aliquots of medium from one container to the other container in the pair. For example, after a 5-milliliter aliquot from the first container is added to the second container in the pair, the second container is agitated for 10 seconds, and then a 5-milliliter aliquot is removed and returned to the first container in the pair. The first container is then agitated for 10 seconds, and the next 5-milliliter aliquot is transferred back to the second container in the pair. Following the two 5-milliliter aliquot exchanges in each pair of containers, a 5-milliliter aliquot of medium from each container is aseptically injected into a sealed, empty, sterile 10-milliliter clear vial using a sterile 10-milliliter syringe and vented needle. Sterile adhesive seals are aseptically affixed to the rubber closures on the three filled vials. The vials are incubated within a range of 20–35 degrees Celsius for a minimum of 14 days. Failure is indicated by visible turbidity in the medium on or before 14 days. The media-fill test must include a positive-control sample.

(iii) High-risk preparations.
 (I) Procedures for high-risk level compounded sterile preparations include all those for low-risk level compounded sterile preparations. In addition, a media-fill test that represents high-risk level compounding is performed twice a year by each person authorized to compound high-risk level compounded sterile preparations.
 (II) Example of a media-fill test procedure for compounded sterile preparations sterilized by filtration. This test or an equivalent test is performed under conditions that closely simulate the most challenging or stressful conditions encountered when compounding high-risk level compounded sterile preparations. (Sterility tests for autoclaved compounded sterile preparations are not required unless they are prepared in batches of more than 25 units.) This test is completed without interruption in the following sequence:
  (-a-) Dissolve 3 grams of nonsterile commercially available fluid culture media in 100 milliliters of non-bacteriostatic water to make a 3% nonsterile solution.
  (-b-) Draw 25 milliliters of the medium into each of three 30-milliliter sterile syringes. Transfer 5 milliliters from each syringe into separate sterile 10-milliliter vials. These vials are the positive controls to generate exponential microbial growth, which is indicated by visible turbidity upon incubation.
  (-c-) Under aseptic conditions and using aseptic techniques, affix a sterile 0.2-micron porosity filter unit and a 20-gauge needle to each syringe. Inject the next 10 milliliters from each syringe into three separate 10-milliliter sterile vials. Repeat the process for three more vials. Label all vials, affix sterile adhesive seals to the closure of the nine vials, and incubate them at 20 to 35 degrees Celsius for a minimum of 14 days. Inspect for microbial growth over 14 days

as described in Chapter 797, Pharmaceutical Compounding— Sterile Preparations, of the USP/NF.

(III) Filter integrity testing. Filters need to undergo testing to evaluate the integrity of filters used to sterilize high-risk preparations such as Bubble Point Testing or comparable filter integrity testing. Such testing is not a replacement for sterility testing and shall not be interpreted as such. Such test shall be performed after a sterilization procedure on all filters used to sterilize each high-risk preparation or batch preparation and the results documented. The results should be compared with the filter manufacturer's specification for the specific filter used. If a filter fails the integrity test, the preparation or batch must be sterilized again using new unused filters.

(B) Finished preparation release checks and tests.
(i) All high-risk level compounded sterile preparations that are prepared in groups of more than 25 identical individual single-dose packages (such as ampuls, bags, syringes, and vials) or in multiple-dose vials for administration to multiple patients or are exposed longer than 12 hours at 2–8 degrees Celsius and longer than six hours at warmer than 8 degrees Celsius before they are sterilized shall be tested to ensure they are sterile and do not contain excessive bacterial endotoxins as specified in Chapter 71, Sterility Tests, of the USP/NF, before being dispensed or administered.
(ii) All compounded sterile preparations, except for sterile radiopharmaceuticals, that are intended to be solutions must be visually examined for the presence of particulate matter and not administered or dispensed when such matter is observed.
(iii) The prescription drug and medication orders, written compounding procedures, preparation records, and expended materials used to make compounded sterile preparations at all contamination risk levels shall be inspected for accuracy of correct identities and amounts of ingredients, aseptic mixing and sterilization, packaging, labeling, and expected physical appearance before they are dispensed or administered.
(iv) Written procedures for checking compounding accuracy shall be followed for every compounded sterile preparation during preparation in accordance with the pharmacy's policies and procedures and immediately prior to release, including label accuracy and the accuracy of the addition of all drug products or ingredients used to prepare the finished preparation and their volumes or quantities. A pharmacist shall ensure that components used in compounding are accurately weighed, measured, or subdivided as appropriate to conform to the formula being prepared.

(C) Environmental testing.
(i) Viable and nonviable environmental sampling testing. Environmental sampling shall occur at a minimum every six months as part of a comprehensive quality management program and under any of the following conditions:
(I) As part of the commissioning and certification of new facilities and equipment;

- (II) Following any servicing of facilities and equipment;
- (III) As part of the recertification of facilities and equipment;
- (IV) In response to identified problems with end products or staff technique; or
- (V) In response to issues with compounded sterile preparations, observed compounding personnel work practices, or patient-related infections (where the compounded sterile preparation is being considered as a potential source of the infection).

(ii) Total particle counts. Certification that each ISO classified area (e.g., ISO Class 5, 7, and 8) is within established guidelines shall be performed no less than every six months and whenever the equipment is relocated or the physical structure of the buffer area or ante-area has been altered. All certification records shall be maintained and reviewed to ensure that the controlled environments comply with the proper air cleanliness, room pressures, and air changes per hour. These certification records must include acceptance criteria and be made available upon inspection by the Board. Testing shall be performed by qualified operators using current state-of-the-art equipment with results of the following:
- (I) ISO Class 5—Not more than 3520 particles 0.5 micrometer and larger size per cubic meter of air;
- (II) ISO Class 7—Not more than 352,000 particles of 0.5 micrometer and larger size per cubic meter of air for any buffer area; and
- (III) ISO Class 8—Not more than 3,520,000 particles of 0.5 micrometer and larger size per cubic meter of air for any ante-area.

(iii) Pressure differential monitoring. A pressure gauge or velocity meter shall be installed to monitor the pressure differential or airflow between the buffer area and the ante-area and between the ante-area and the general environment outside the compounding area. The results shall be reviewed and documented on a log at least every work shift (minimum frequency shall be at least daily) or by a continuous recording device. The pressure between the ISO Class 7 or ISO Class 8 and the general pharmacy area shall not be less than 0.02 inch water column.

(iv) Sampling plan. An appropriate environmental sampling plan shall be developed for airborne viable particles based on a risk assessment of compounding activities performed. Selected sampling sites shall include locations within each ISO Class 5 environment, in the ISO Class 7 and 8 areas, and in the segregated compounding areas at greatest risk of contamination. The plan shall include sample location, method of collection, frequency of sampling, volume of air sampled, and time of day as related to activity in the compounding area and action levels.

(v) Viable air sampling. Evaluation of airborne microorganisms using volumetric collection methods in the controlled air environments shall be performed by properly trained individuals for all compounding risk levels. For low-risk, medium-risk, and high-risk level compounding, air sampling shall be performed at locations that are prone to contamination during compounding activities and during other activities such as staging, labeling, gowning, and cleaning. Locations shall include zones of air backwash turbulence within the laminar airflow workbench and other areas where air backwash turbulence may enter the compounding area. For low-risk level compounded sterile preparations within 12-hour or less beyond-use date prepared in a primary engineering control that maintains an ISO Class 5, air sampling shall be performed at locations inside the ISO Class 5 environment and other areas that are in close proximity to the ISO Class 5 environment during the certification of the primary engineering control.

(vi) Air sampling frequency and process. Air sampling shall be performed at least every six months as a part of the recertification of facilities and equipment. A sufficient volume of air shall be sampled and the manufacturer's guidelines for use of the electronic air sampling equipment followed. At the end of the designated sampling or exposure period for air sampling activities, the microbial growth media plates are recovered and their covers secured and are inverted and incubated at a temperature and for a time period conducive to multiplication of microorganisms. Sampling data shall be collected and reviewed on a periodic basis as a means of evaluating the overall control of the compounding environment. If an activity consistently shows elevated levels of microbial growth, competent microbiology or infection control personnel shall be consulted. A colony forming unit (cfu) count greater than 1 cfu per cubic meter of air for ISO Class 5, greater than 10 cfu per cubic meter of air for ISO Class 7, and greater than 100 cfu per 422 cubic meter of air for ISO Class 8 or worse should prompt a re-evaluation of the adequacy of personnel work practices, cleaning procedures, operational procedures, and air filtration efficiency within the aseptic compounding location. An investigation into the source of the contamination shall be conducted. The source of the problem shall be eliminated, the affected area cleaned, and resampling performed. Counts of cfu are to be used as an approximate measure of the environmental microbial bioburden. Action levels are determined on the basis of cfu data gathered at each sampling location and trended over time. Regardless of the number of cfu identified in the pharmacy, further corrective actions will be dictated by the identification of microorganisms recovered by an appropriate credentialed laboratory of any microbial bioburden captured as a cfu using an impaction air sampler. Highly pathogenic microorganisms (e.g., gram-negative rods, coagulase positive staphylococcus, molds, and yeasts) can be potentially fatal to patients receiving compounded sterile preparations. They must be immediately remedied, regardless of colony forming unit count, with the assistance, if needed, of a competent microbiologist, infection control professional, or industrial hygienist.

(vii) Compounding accuracy checks. Written procedures for double-checking compounding accuracy shall be followed for every compounded sterile preparation during preparation and immediately prior to release, including label accuracy and the accuracy of the addition of all drug products or ingredients used to prepare the finished preparation and their volumes or quantities. At each step of the compounding process, the pharmacist shall ensure that components used in compounding are accurately weighed, measured, or subdivided as appropriate to conform to the formula being prepared.

(15) Quality Control.
    (A) Quality control procedures. The pharmacy shall follow established quality control procedures to monitor the compounding environment and quality of compounded drug preparations for conformity with the quality indicators established for the preparation. When developing these procedures, pharmacy personnel shall consider the provisions of USP Chapter 71, Sterility Tests; USP Chapter 85, Bacterial Endotoxins Test; USP Chapter 795, Pharmaceutical Compounding—Nonsterile Preparations; USP Chapter 797, Pharmaceutical Compounding—Sterile Preparations; USP Chapter 800, Hazardous Drugs—Handling in Healthcare Settings; USP Chapter 823, Positron Emission Tomography Drugs for Compounding, Investigational, and Research Uses; USP Chapter 1160, Pharmaceutical Calculations in Prescription Compounding; and USP Chapter 1163, Quality Assurance in Pharmaceutical Compounding, of the current USP/NF. Such procedures shall be documented and be available for inspection.

    (B) Verification of compounding accuracy and sterility.
        (i) The accuracy of identities, concentrations, amounts, and purities of ingredients in compounded sterile preparations shall be confirmed by reviewing labels on packages, observing and documenting correct measurements with approved and correctly standardized devices, and reviewing information in labeling and certificates of analysis provided by suppliers.
        (ii) If the correct identity, purity, strength, and sterility of ingredients and components of compounded sterile preparations cannot be confirmed, such ingredients and components shall be discarded immediately. Any compounded sterile preparation that fails sterility testing following sterilization by one method (e.g., filtration) is to be discarded and not subjected to a second method of sterilization.
        (iii) If individual ingredients such as bulk drug substances are not labeled with expiration dates when the drug substances are stable indefinitely in their commercial packages under labeled storage conditions, such ingredients may gain or lose moisture during storage and use and shall require testing to determine the correct amount to weigh for accurate content of active chemical moieties in compounded sterile preparations.

Note: As was the case with nonsterile compounding, (14) Quality Assurance and (15) Quality Control above represent the minimum requirements as set forth by TSBP rules. Many pharmacies compounding sterile preparations will have more detailed policies and procedures. Pharmacists working in any pharmacy compounding sterile preparations must become familiar with the policies and procedures of the pharmacy for compounding CSPs.

(e) Records. Any testing or cleaning procedures or other activities required in this subsection shall be documented, and such documentation shall be maintained by the pharmacy.

(1) Maintenance of Records. Every record required under this section must be:
   (A) Kept by the pharmacy and be available for at least two years for inspecting and copying by the Board or its representative and to other authorized local, state, or federal law enforcement agencies and
   (B) Supplied by the pharmacy within 72 hours if requested by an authorized agent of the Board. If the pharmacy maintains the records in an electronic format, the requested records must be provided in an electronic format. Failure to provide the records set out in this section, either on-site or within 72 hours, constitutes prima facie evidence of failure to keep and maintain records in violation of the Act.
(2) Compounding Records.
   (A) Compounding pursuant to patient specific prescription drug orders or medication orders. Compounding records for all compounded preparations shall be maintained by the pharmacy and shall include:
      (i) The date and time of preparation;
      (ii) A complete formula including methodology and necessary equipment which includes the brand name(s) of the raw materials or, if no brand name, the generic name(s) or official name and name(s) of the manufacturer(s) or distributor of the raw materials and the quantities of each. However, if the sterile preparation is compounded according to the manufacturer's labeling instructions, then documentation of the formula is not required;
      (iii) Written or electronic signature or initials of the pharmacist or pharmacy technician or pharmacy technician trainee performing the compounding;
      (iv) Written or electronic signature or initials of the pharmacist responsible for supervising pharmacy technicians or pharmacy technician trainees and conducting in-process and final checks of compounded pharmaceuticals if pharmacy technicians or pharmacy technician trainees perform the compounding function;
      (v) The container used and the number of units of finished preparations prepared; and
      (vi) A reference to the location of the following documentation which may be maintained with other records such as quality control records:
         (I) The criteria used to determine the beyond-use date and
         (II) Documentation of the performance of quality control procedures.
   (B) Compounding records when batch compounding or compounding in anticipation of future prescription drug or medication orders.
      (i) Master work sheet. A master work sheet shall be developed and approved by a pharmacist for preparations prepared in batch. Once approved, a duplicate of the master work sheet shall be used as the preparation work sheet from which each batch is prepared and on which all documentation for that batch occurs. The master work sheet shall contain at a minimum:
         (I) The formula;
         (II) The components;
         (III) The compounding directions;
         (IV) A sample label;
         (V) Evaluation and testing requirements;
         (VI) Specific equipment used during preparation; and
         (VII) Storage requirements.

(ii) Preparation work sheet. The preparation work sheet for each batch of preparations shall document the following:
  (I) Identity of all solutions and ingredients and their corresponding amounts, concentrations, or volumes;
  (II) Lot number for each component;
  (III) Component manufacturer/distributor or suitable identifying number;
  (IV) Container specifications (e.g., syringe or pump cassette);
  (V) Unique lot or control number assigned to batch;
  (VI) Expiration date of batch-prepared preparations;
  (VII) Date of preparation;
  (VIII) Name, initials, or electronic signature of the person(s) involved in the preparation;
  (IX) Name, initials, or electronic signature of the responsible pharmacist;
  (X) Finished preparation evaluation and testing specifications if applicable; and
  (XI) Comparison of actual yield to anticipated or theoretical yield when appropriate.

(f) Office Use Compounding and Distribution of Sterile Compounded Preparations. *Note: Recall that Office Use Compounding may be in violation of the Federal Food, Drug, and Cosmetic Act unless the pharmacy is also registered with FDA as an outsourcing facility under Section 503B of the FDCA. In addition, DEA does not allow pharmacies to provide compounded controlled substances to practitioners for "office use." The pharmacy must have a valid prescription for an individual patient for the compounded controlled substance.*

  (1) General.
    (A) A pharmacy may compound, dispense, deliver, and distribute a compounded sterile preparation as specified in Chapter 562.151–562.156 of the Act.
    (B) A Class A-S pharmacy is not required to register or be licensed under the Texas Food, Drug, and Cosmetic Act to distribute sterile compounded preparations to a Class C or Class C-S pharmacy.
    (C) A Class C-S pharmacy is not required to register or be licensed under the Texas Food, Drug, and Cosmetic Act to distribute sterile compounded preparations that the Class C-S pharmacy has compounded for other Class C or Class C-S pharmacies under common ownership.
    (D) To compound and deliver a compounded preparation under this rule, a pharmacy must:
      (i) Verify the source of the raw materials to be used in a compounded drug;
      (ii) Comply with applicable United States Pharmacopeia guidelines, including the testing requirements and HIPAA;
      (iii) Enter into a written agreement with a practitioner for the practitioner's office use of a compounded preparation;
      (iv) Comply with all applicable competency and accrediting standards as determined by the Board; and
      (v) Comply with the provisions of this rule.
    (E) This rule does not apply to Class B pharmacies compounding sterile radiopharmaceuticals that are furnished for departmental use (e.g., nuclear medicine department) or a physician's use if such authorized users maintain a TDSHS radioactive materials license.
  (2) Written agreement. A pharmacy that provides sterile compounded preparations to practitioners for office use or to another pharmacy shall enter

into a written agreement with the practitioner or pharmacy. The written agreement shall:
- (A) Address acceptable standards of practice for a compounding pharmacy and a practitioner and receiving pharmacy that enter into the agreement, including a statement that the compounded drugs may only be administered to the patient and may not be dispensed to the patient or sold to any other person or entity except to a veterinarian as authorized by Section 563.054 of the Act;
- (B) State that the practitioner or receiving pharmacy should include on a separate log or in a patient's chart, medication order, or medication administration record the lot number and beyond-use date of a compounded preparation administered to a patient;
- (C) Describe the scope of services to be performed by the pharmacy and practitioner or receiving pharmacy, including a statement of the process for:
  - (i) A patient to report an adverse reaction or submit a complaint and
  - (ii) The pharmacy to recall batches of compounded preparations.

(3) Recordkeeping.
- (A) Maintenance of records.
  - (i) Records of orders and distribution of sterile compounded preparations to a practitioner for office use or to an institutional pharmacy for administration to a patient shall be:
    - (I) Kept by the pharmacy and be available for at least two years from the date of the record for inspecting and copying by the Board or its representative and to other authorized local, state, or federal law enforcement agencies;
    - (II) Maintained separately from the records of preparations dispensed pursuant to a prescription or medication order; and
    - (III) Supplied by the pharmacy within 72 hours if requested by an authorized agent of the Board or its representative. If the pharmacy maintains the records in an electronic format, the requested records must be provided in an electronic format. Failure to provide the records set out in this subsection, either on-site or within 72 hours for whatever reason, constitutes prima facie evidence of failure to keep and maintain records.
  - (ii) Records may be maintained in an alternative data retention system, such as a data processing system or direct imaging system, provided the data processing system is capable of producing a hard copy of the record upon the request of the Board, its representative, or other authorized local, state, or federal law enforcement or regulatory agencies.
- (B) Orders. The pharmacy shall maintain a record of all sterile compounded preparations ordered by a practitioner for office use or by an institutional pharmacy for administration to a patient. The record shall include the following information:
  - (i) Date of the order;
  - (ii) Name, address, and phone number of the practitioner who ordered the preparation and, if applicable, the name, address, and phone number of the institutional pharmacy ordering the preparation; and
  - (iii) Name, strength, and quantity of the preparation ordered.

(C) Distributions. The pharmacy shall maintain a record of all sterile compounded preparations distributed pursuant to an order to a practitioner for office use or by an institutional pharmacy for administration to a patient. The record shall include the following information:
  (i) Date the preparation was compounded;
  (ii) Date the preparation was distributed;
  (iii) Name, strength, and quantity in each container of the preparation;
  (iv) Pharmacy's lot number;
  (v) Quantity of containers shipped; and
  (vi) Name, address, and phone number of the practitioner or institutional pharmacy to whom the preparation is distributed.
(D) Audit trail.
  (i) The pharmacy shall store the order and distribution records of preparations for all sterile compounded preparations ordered by and or distributed to a practitioner for office use or by a pharmacy licensed to compound sterile preparations for administration to a patient in such a manner as to be able to provide an audit trail for all orders and distributions of any of the following during a specified time period:
    (I) Any strength and dosage form of a preparation (by either brand or generic name or both);
    (II) Any ingredient;
    (III) Any lot number;
    (IV) Any practitioner;
    (V) Any facility; and
    (VI) Any pharmacy, if applicable.
  (ii) The audit trail shall contain the following information:
    (I) Date of the order and date of the distribution;
    (II) Practitioner's name and address and the name of the institutional pharmacy, if applicable;
    (III) Name, strength, and quantity of the preparation in each container of the preparation;
    (IV) Name and quantity of each active ingredient;
    (V) Quantity of containers distributed; and
    (VI) Pharmacy's lot number.
(4) Labeling. The pharmacy shall affix a label to the preparation containing the following information:
  (A) Name, address, and phone number of the compounding pharmacy;
  (B) The statement: "For Institutional or Office Use Only—Not for Resale" or if the preparation is distributed to a veterinarian the statement: "Compounded Preparation";
  (C) Name and strength of the preparation or a list of the active ingredients and strengths;
  (D) Pharmacy's lot number;
  (E) Beyond-use date as determined by the pharmacist using appropriate documented criteria;
  (F) Quantity or amount in the container;
  (G) Appropriate ancillary instructions such as storage instructions or cautionary statements, including hazardous drug warning labels where appropriate; and
  (H) Device-specific instructions where appropriate.

(g) Recall Procedures.
   (1) The pharmacy shall have written procedures for the recall of any compounded sterile preparation provided to a patient, to a practitioner for office use, or a pharmacy for administration. Written procedures shall include but not be limited to the requirements as specified in (3) below of this rule.
   (2) The pharmacy shall immediately initiate a recall of any sterile preparation compounded by the pharmacy upon identification of a potential or confirmed harm to a patient.
   (3) In the event of a recall, the pharmacist-in-charge shall ensure that:
      (A) Each practitioner, facility, and/or pharmacy to which the preparation was distributed is notified in writing of the recall;
      (B) Each patient to whom the preparation was dispensed is notified in writing of the recall;
      (C) The Board is notified of the recall in writing no later than 24 hours after the recall is issued;
      (D) If the preparation is distributed for office use, the Texas Department of State Health Services, Drugs and Medical Devices Group, is notified of the recall in writing;
      (E) The preparation is quarantined; and
      (F) The pharmacy keeps a written record of the recall including all actions taken to notify all parties and steps taken to ensure corrective measures.
   (4) If a pharmacy fails to initiate a recall, the Board may require a pharmacy to initiate a recall if there is potential for or confirmed harm to a patient.
   (5) A pharmacy that compounds sterile preparations shall notify the Board immediately of any adverse effects reported to the pharmacy or that are known by the pharmacy to be potentially attributable to a sterile preparation compounded by the pharmacy.

V. **USP Chapter 800 Hazardous Drugs—Handling in Healthcare Settings (Review and Summary)**

USP Chapter 800 is listed as an officially approved new chapter in the United States Pharmacopeia 39—National Formulary 34 published on February 1, 2016. Because pharmacies, pharmacists, physicians, nurses, veterinarians, and other healthcare workers and healthcare facilities need time to understand the standard and to prepare for its implementation, USP chose to make Chapter 800 effective on December 1, 2019. The following is a review and summary of USP Chapter 800.

A. Introduction and Scope.
   1. Chapter 800 details practice and quality standards for handling hazardous drugs (HDs) in various healthcare settings. The chapter discusses the handling of HDs from receipt to storage, compounding, dispensing, administration, and disposal of both nonsterile and sterile preparations. Included in the chapter is information on proper engineering controls and quality standards, personnel training, labeling, packaging, and transport and disposal of HDs, along with required measures for spill control, documentation of all aspects of the handling of HDs, and medical surveillance (when applicable).
   2. Chapter 800 applies to all healthcare personnel and all entities who handle hazardous drugs. These personnel and entities include, but are not limited to, pharmacists, pharmacy technicians, pharmacies, physicians, nurses, hospital physician assistants, home healthcare workers, physician practice

facilities, veterinarians, veterinary technicians, and veterinary hospitals and facilities. Entities that handle HDs must incorporate Chapter 800 standards into occupational safety standards.

B. List of Hazardous Drugs.
1. The National Institute of Occupational Safety and Health (NIOSH) maintains a list of hazardous drugs (HDs) and antineoplastic agents used in health care. This list is updated approximately every two years. Chapter 800 requires any entity that stores, compounds, prepares, transports, or administers hazardous drugs to maintain a list of HDs used in the entity along with a copy of the current NIOSH list and to review the list at least every 12 months and update whenever a new agent or dosage form is used. Newly marketed HDs or dosage forms should be reviewed against the entity's list.
2. Some dosage forms of drugs defined as hazardous drugs may not pose a substantial risk of direct occupational exposure to healthcare workers. However, particulate matter from tablets, capsules, and/or packaging materials could present an exposure risk if it contacts skin or mucous membranes. Facilities using hazardous drugs should perform a risk assessment at least annually to determine if new or alternate containment strategies need to be employed to mitigate risks for exposure from HDs.
3. Unintentional exposures to hazardous drugs have been documented. These include transdermal and transmucosal absorption, injection, and ingestion. Containers of HDs have been shown to be contaminated upon arrival to their intended destination. Accidental exposure is also possible for individuals handling body fluids; deactivating, decontaminating, or disinfecting areas contaminated with HDs; and/or contacting HD residue on drug containers, work surfaces, etc.
4. To help minimize the risk of exposure in a pharmacy compounding sterile preparations, the pharmacist-in-charge should develop detailed SOPs and training requirements. Workers must wear personal protective equipment designed to be resistant to cleaning agents and two pairs of chemo gloves. Eye protection and face shields should be worn if splashing is possible, and respiratory protection should be worn if the HD is volatile or if particulate matter can become airborne.

C. Types of Exposure.
1. Chapter 800 provides a detailed list of potential opportunities of exposure at each stage in the handling of HDs from receipt at the facility to disposal of hazardous waste materials.
2. Routes of entry of HDs into the body include transdermal and transmucosal absorption, inhalation, injection, or ingestion through foods and other materials that are contacted by contaminated hands or clothing.

D. Responsibilities of Personnel Handling Hazardous Drugs.
1. The chapter requires that each entity have a designated person to be responsible for developing and implementing HD handling procedures. This individual must be properly trained and qualified to oversee entity compliance with the chapter and applicable state and federal laws and regulations and to ensure competency of all individuals who may come into contact with HDs.
2. All persons involved in the handling of HDs must have a fundamental understanding of practices and precautions and of the evaluation of procedures to ensure the safety and quality of the final HD product or preparation to minimize the risk of harm to the intended patient.

E. Facilities and Engineering Controls.
1. At each stage of the handling of HDs there must be conditions and policies in place to promote safety for patients, workers, and the environment.

2. Before HDs can enter a specific area of a facility, signs must be placed in all locations where the HDs might be found.
3. Access to these areas of a facility should be limited only to properly trained and authorized personnel.
4. The chapter requires that there be designated areas for receiving and unpacking HDs, for storing HDs, and for compounding of nonsterile and sterile preparations.
5. Certain areas must have a negative pressure gradient with respect to surrounding areas of the facilities to reduce the risk of contaminating areas where non-HD-authorized individuals work. These negative-pressure areas must have an uninterrupted power source in the event of a loss of power to the facility.

F. Receipt of HDs.
1. According to Chapter 800, all HDs and all hazardous drug active pharmaceutical ingredients (HD-APIs) must be removed from shipping containers in an area that is negative pressure or neutral pressure relative to the surrounding areas.
2. If HDs or HD-APIs are delivered to a receiving dock or area, the exterior doors should be closed before opening the shipping cartons to prevent external air from blowing into (creating positive pressure into) the receiving area.
3. In addition, shipping cartons containing HDs and/or HD-APIs must not be opened in sterile compounding or positive pressure areas.

G. Storage of HDs.
1. HDs must be stored in areas that can prevent or contain spillage or breakage of a container if it falls. However, HDs must not be stored on the floor.
2. Antineoplastic HDs that are to be counted or compounded to make the final preparation must be stored in an area away from non-HDs in a manner to prevent contamination or personnel exposure.
3. The room for storage of HDs must be vented to the exterior of the facility and must have at least 12 air changes per hour (ACPH).
4. Non-antineoplastic agents with reproductive risk only and final dosage forms of antineoplastic HDs may be stored with non-HD drug inventory if permitted by entity policy.

H. Compounding With HDs.
1. Containment engineering controls to protect a preparation from microbial (if final preparation is to be sterile) and cross-contamination are required throughout the compounding procedures.
2. Containment engineering controls are divided into three types:
   a. Containment Primary Engineering Control (C-PEC);
   b. Containment Secondary Engineering Control (C-SEC); and
   c. Containment supplementary levels of control.
3. A C-PEC is a ventilated device designed to minimize the risk of exposure to the compounder and to the environment when HDs are handled directly.
4. A C-SEC is the room in which the C-PEC is located.
5. Containment supplemental engineering controls, such as closed-system drug-transfer devices (CSTDs), provide additional protection from exposure of the compounder to one or more HDs.
6. C-PECs must be used for compounding both nonsterile and sterile preparations and must:
   a. Be vented to the exterior of the facility through high-efficiency particulate air (HEPA) filters;
   b. Be physically separated from other preparation areas;

      c. Have appropriate air exchange (ACPH);
      d. Have a negative pressure gradient of 0.01–0.03 inches of water column with respect to adjacent areas; and
      e. Operate continuously if they supply any or all of the negative pressure in the C-SEC.
  7. An eyewash station and other applicable emergency safety equipment (e.g., safety showers, fire blankets, etc.) meeting applicable laws and regulations must be readily available, and a sink must be available for handwashing. However, all water sources and drains must be located at least one meter from the C-PEC.
  8. For entities where compounding of both sterile and nonsterile HDs is performed, the C-PECs must be located in separate rooms, unless the C-PECs used for nonsterile compounding can effectively maintain ISO 7 air quality in the room. If the C-PECs for nonsterile and sterile compounding are located in the same room, they must be placed at least one meter apart. If the C-PECs are in the same room, any nonsterile compounding that generates particulate matter may not be performed when sterile compounding is being performed.

I. Nonsterile Compounding with HDs.
  1. In addition to following the regulations set forth in this chapter, entities involved in compounding nonsterile preparation, regardless of whether the compounding involves HDs or not, must also comply with the requirements of USP Chapter 795, Pharmaceutical Compounding—Nonsterile Preparations.
  2. A C-PEC is not required if the entity compounds only nonsterile, non-HD drugs or if the entity is not manipulating HDs in any form except handling the final dosage forms (e.g., counting or repackaging tablets or capsules).

Requirements for C-PECs and C-SECs for compounding nonsterile HDs are summarized in the following table:

Engineering Controls for Nonsterile HD Compounding

C-PEC	C-SEC
Externally vented (preferred) or redundant-HEPA filtered with HEPA filters in series	Externally vented
	12 ACPH
	Negative pressure (0.01–0.03 in water column) relative to adjacent areas

J. Sterile Compounding with HDs.
  1. In addition to following the regulations set forth in this chapter, entities involved in compounding sterile preparation, regardless of whether the compounding involves HDs or not, must also comply with the requirements of USP Chapter 797, Pharmaceutical Compounding—Sterile Preparations.
  2. All containment primary engineering controls used for the purpose of compounding hazardous drugs must be vented to the outside.
  3. As is the case with PECs used in the compounding of sterile non-HD preparations, C-PECs must maintain an ISO Class 5 or better air quality.
  4. Laminar airflow workbenches or Compounding Aseptic Isolators (CAIs) are not acceptable for compounding antineoplastic HDs.

Requirements for C-PECs and C-SECs for compounding sterile HDs are summarized in the following table:

Engineering Controls for Sterile HD Compounding

C-SEC Configuration	C-PEC Requirements	C-SEC Requirements
ISO Class 7 buffer room with ISO Class 7 ante-room	• Vented Externally • Examples: ◦ Class II BSC or CACI	• Vented Externally • 30 ACPH • Negative pressure as described previously
Unclassified C-SCA	• Vented Externally • Examples: ◦ Class II BSC or CACI	• Vented Externally • 12 ACPH • Negative pressure as described previously

K. Environmental Quality and Control.
   1. While there are no currently accepted limits for HD surface contamination, Chapter 800 states that surface sampling should be performed routinely to ensure that cleaning procedures are effective in removing remaining HD residues after handling or compounding.
   2. Surface sampling should include, but not necessarily be limited to, the inside surface of the C-PEC and any equipment contained in it, pass-through chambers, staging surfaces, areas adjacent to the C-PEC, area immediately outside the buffer room or C-SEC, and patient administration areas.
   3. The chapter continues by saying that if any measurable HD residue is found, the designated person should consider taking actions such as reevaluating work practices, retraining personnel, etc.
L. Personal Protective Equipment.
   1. The NIOSH list of antineoplastic agents and other HDs provides some guidance on personal protective equipment (PPE) such as not reusing disposable PPE and decontaminating reusable PPE.
   2. Chapter 800 requires gowns, head and hair covers, shoe covers, and two pairs of powderless chemotherapy gloves when compounding either non-sterile or sterile antineoplastic agents. Two pairs of chemotherapy gloves and gowns resistant to permeability by HDs are also required when administering injectable HDs.
   3. For other activities, the facility's SOPs must describe appropriate PPE to be worn. SOPs must be based on risk of exposure and activities.
   4. At all stages of the handling of HDs from receiving to waste disposal, PPE must be worn.
   5. Chemotherapy gloves must meet the American Society of Testing Materials (ASTM) standard D6978 and should be worn when handling any HD, including non-antineoplastic agents and HDs with reproductive risks. Chapter 800 states that chemotherapy gloves should be changed every 30 minutes unless the manufacturer recommends different intervals.
   6. Chapter 800 states that gowns must close in the back, be disposable, and resist permeability of HDs. Gowns must be changed per the manufacturer's information for permeation of the gown. If there is no information from the manufacturer, then Chapter 800 states gowns are to be changed every 2–3 hours or immediately after a splash or spill. Personnel are not to wear in other areas of a facility the same gown that was worn in HD handling areas.

7. A second pair of shoe covers and sleeve protectors providing protection from HD residue must be donned before entering the C-SEC and must be removed before leaving the HD handling areas and entering other areas of the facility.
8. Appropriate face and eye protection is to be worn when there is a risk of spills or splashes of HDs. Safety eyeglasses with side shields do not provide adequate protection.
9. When unpacking HDs not contained in plastic, personnel should wear elastomeric half-face masks which have been fit-tested with a P100 filter and a multi-gas cartridge.
10. All worn PPE should be considered contaminated and placed in an appropriate waste container to be disposed of properly. PPE used in compounding HDs should be discarded in proper containers before leaving the C-SEC.

M. Personnel Training.
All personnel who handle HDs must be properly trained based on job function. The training must be documented.

N. Receiving, Labeling, Packaging, Transport, and Disposal.
1. A facility must establish SOPs for the receiving, labeling, packaging, transport, and disposal of HDs.
2. Transport of HDs must be labeled, stored, and handled in accordance with applicable federal, state, and local regulations.
3. HDs must be transported in containers that minimize the risk of breakage and leakage,

O. Documentation and Standard Operating Procedures.
1. Any entity handling HDs must maintain SOPs for safe handling of HDs at all stages and locations where HDs are found in the facility.
2. These SOPs are to be reviewed at least annually and should include a hazard communication program, occupational safety program, designation of HD areas, and items discussed above.

P. Medical Surveillance.
1. As part of a comprehensive exposure control program, medical surveillance complements all other attempts by Chapter 800 to minimize risks to healthcare workers.
2. Elements of an appropriate medical surveillance program must be consistent with an entity's policies, and medical records should be consistent with regulations set forth by the Occupational Safety and Health Administration (OSHA).
3. Chapter 800 outlines elements of a medical surveillance plan that should be included for all healthcare workers who may come into contact with hazardous drugs. The chapter also describes elements that should be included in a follow-up plan should HD exposure-related health changes occur. Again, the elements in the recommended medical surveillance and follow-up plans are not exhaustive but provide a good basis for the development of an appropriate program. Once again, however, any medical surveillance plan should follow entity policies.

Chapter H Highlights
Compounding Laws and Rules
Nonsterile Compounding—Board Rule 291.131

1. Nonsterile preparations may be compounded upon presentation of a practitioner's prescription drug or medication order based on a valid pharmacist/patient/prescriber relationship; in anticipation of future prescription drug or medication orders based on routine, regularly observed prescribing patterns; as an incident to research, teaching, or chemical analysis and not for sale or dispensing; or in reasonable quantities for office use by a practitioner and for use by a veterinarian.
2. Pharmacists compounding nonsterile preparations must obtain continuing education appropriate for the type of compounding done by the pharmacist; inspect and approve all components, drug product containers, closures, labeling, and any other materials involved in the compounding process; review all compounding records for accuracy and conduct in-process and final checks to ensure that errors have not occurred in the compounding process; and be responsible for the proper maintenance, cleanliness, and use of all equipment used in the compounding process.
3. Commercially available products and products that are essentially copies of commercially available products may be compounded only under very specific conditions.
4. Compounding pharmacies must have a Class A prescription balance or analytical balance and weights which are subject to inspection by the Texas State Board of Pharmacy.
5. In addition to normal labeling requirements, a compounded prescription label must include the name(s) of the principal active ingredient(s) of the compounded preparation and a statement that the preparation has been compounded by the pharmacy.
6. All significant procedures performed in the compounding area shall be covered by written SOPs designed to ensure accountability, accuracy, quality, safety, and uniformity in the compounding process.
7. All compounding pharmacies must have a documented quality assurance and quality control program.
8. A pharmacy providing compounded preparations to practitioners for office use or to another pharmacy must meet very specific requirements. These include having a written agreement with the practitioner or pharmacy; labeling such products "For Institutional or Office Use Only—Not for Resale" or if the preparation is distributed to a veterinarian the statement: "Compounded Preparation"; maintaining an audit trail of all distributions; and establishing recall procedures. The legality of compounding for office use for nonsterile preparations is currently uncertain under federal law.
9. DEA generally allows pharmacists to compound narcotic controlled substances in Schedules II–V so long as the concentration of the final solution, compound, or mixture is not greater than 20%. DEA does not permit pharmacies to compound controlled substances for "office use." There must be a valid prescription for an individual patient for the compounded controlled substance.

Sterile Compounding—Board Rule 291.132
(Also see Drug Compounding Quality Act in Chapter A)

1. The Texas rules for compounding sterile preparations are substantially similar to the United States Pharmacopeia's Chapter 797.
2. Sterile preparations may be compounded:
    a. Pursuant to a prescription or medication order for a patient from a practitioner;
    b. In anticipation of prescription drug or medication orders based on routine, regularly observed prescribing patterns;
    c. As an incident to research, teaching, or chemical analysis and not for sale or dispensing;
    d. In reasonable quantities for a practitioner's office for office use by the practitioner;
    e. By a Class A-S pharmacy for a Class C-S pharmacy; or

  f. By a Class C-S pharmacy for distribution to other Class C or Class C-S pharmacies under common ownership.
3. Pharmacists compounding sterile preparations are responsible for ensuring that compounded sterile preparations are accurately identified, measured, diluted, and mixed; are correctly purified, sterilized, packaged, sealed, labeled, stored, dispensed, and distributed; and for ensuring the proper maintenance, cleanliness, and use of all equipment used in the compounding process.
4. A pharmacist must inspect and approve all components, drug preparation containers, closures, labeling, and any other materials involved in the compounding process; conduct periodic in-process checks as defined in the pharmacy's policies and procedures; review all compounding records for accuracy; and conduct a final check.
5. A pharmacist shall be accessible at all times 24 hours a day to respond to patients' and other health professionals' questions and needs.
6. Training and Education
  a. Pharmacists' initial training—All pharmacists who compound sterile preparations or who supervise technicians who compound sterile preparations must complete a 20-hour course covering specific areas from an accredited college of pharmacy or a course sponsored by an ACPE accredited provider. In addition, all pharmacists must complete a structured on-the-job didactic and experiential training program at the pharmacy which provides sufficient hours of instruction and experience.
  b. Pharmacy technicians' initial training—All technicians who compound sterile preparations must complete either a single 40-hour ACPE accredited course or a training program accredited by the American Society of Health-System Pharmacists. In addition, all technicians must complete a structured on-the-job didactic and experiential training program at the pharmacy which provides sufficient hours of instruction and experience in the facility's compounding policies and procedures.
  c. Continuing education (CE)—To renew a pharmacist license or renew a pharmacy technician registration, all compounding personnel must obtain two hours of CE covering specific compounding topics if engaged in compounding low-risk and medium-risk sterile preparations or four hours of CE covering specific compounding topics if they engage in compounding high-risk sterile preparations.
  d. Training—The pharmacist-in-charge shall ensure continuing competency of pharmacy personnel through in-service education, training, and media-fill tests to supplement initial training. Personnel competency shall be evaluated during orientation and training prior to the regular performance of those tasks; whenever the quality assurance program yields an unacceptable result; whenever unacceptable techniques are observed; and at least on an annual basis for low-risk and medium-risk level compounding and every six months for high-risk level compounding.
7. Sterile compounding in anticipation of future prescription drug or medication orders and compounding of commercially available products may be done if certain specific requirements are met.
8. Risk levels for sterile compounded preparations are outlined in Chapter 797, Pharmacy Compounding— Sterile Preparations, of the USP/NF (low risk, medium risk, and high risk).
9. Environment
  a. Low risk and medium risk—Must have a clean room meeting specific requirements including having an ante-area and a buffer area.
  b. High risk—In addition to the requirements for low-risk and medium-risk compounding, when high-risk preparations are compounded, the primary engineering control shall be located in a buffer area that provides a physical separation through the use of walls, doors, and pass-throughs and has a minimum differential positive pressure of 0.02 to 0.05 inches water column. Presterilization procedures for high-risk level compounded sterile preparations, such as weighing and mixing, shall be completed in no worse than an ISO Class 8 environment.
10. Cleaning and disinfecting of the sterile compounding area must meet detailed requirements as outlined by Board rule.
11. Primary engineering control device. The pharmacy shall prepare sterile preparations in a primary engineering control device (PEC), such as a laminar air flow hood, biological safety cabinet, compounding aseptic isolator

(CAI), or compounding aseptic containment isolator (CACI), which is capable of maintaining at least ISO Class 5 conditions for 0.5 micrometer particles while compounding sterile preparations.
12. Labeling—In addition to regular prescription labeling requirements, the label of a compounded sterile preparation must include the name(s) of the principal active ingredient(s) and for outpatient prescriptions a statement that the product has been compounded by the pharmacy.
13. Standard Operating Procedures (SOPs)—All significant procedures performed in the compounding area shall be covered by written SOPs designed to ensure accountability, accuracy, quality, safety, and uniformity in the compounding process.
14. Quality Assurance Program—Must have a quality assurance program that includes media-fill test procedures, filter integrity testing, finished preparation release and checks, and environmental testing.
15. Quality Control Procedures—Must follow established quality control procedures to monitor the compounding environment and quality of compounded drug preparations for conformity with the quality indicators including verification of compounding accuracy and sterility.
16. A pharmacy providing compounded sterile preparations to practitioners for office use or to another pharmacy must meet very specific requirements. These include having a written agreement with the practitioner or pharmacy; labeling such products "For Institutional or Office Use Only—Not for Resale" or if the preparation is distributed to a veterinarian the statement: "Compounded Preparation"; maintaining an audit trail of all distributions; and establishing recall procedures. In addition, a pharmacy compounding sterile preparations that are not patient specific would need to be registered as an outsourcing facility with the FDA and meet all requirements of the Drug Compounding Quality Act. (*See Chapter A.*)

CHAPTER I

Institutional Pharmacy (Class C) Rules

CHAPTER I

Institutional Pharmacy (Class C) Rules

Definition from Pharmacy Practice Act

A Class C pharmacy license or an institutional pharmacy license may be issued to:
1. A pharmacy located in an inpatient facility, including a hospital licensed under Chapter 241 or 577, Health and Safety Code, or a hospital maintained by the state;
2. A hospice inpatient facility licensed under Chapter 142, Health and Safety Code; and
3. An ambulatory surgical center licensed under Chapter 243, Health and Safety Code.

Board of Pharmacy Rule 291.71
Purpose

The purpose of these sections is to provide standards in the conduct, practice activities, and operation of a pharmacy located in a hospital or other inpatient facility that is licensed under the Texas Hospital Licensing Law (Chapter 241 of the Health and Safety Code) or the Texas Mental Health Code (Chapter 577); a hospice inpatient facility licensed under Chapter 142, Health and Safety Code; or a pharmacy located in a hospital maintained or operated by the state. The intent of these standards is to establish a minimum acceptable level of pharmaceutical care to the patient so that the patient's health is protected while contributing to positive patient outcomes.

Note: A Class C pharmacy operating an outpatient pharmacy under the same legal entity and at the same address must abide with Class A pharmacy rules but is not required to obtain a Class A pharmacy license.

Board of Pharmacy Rule 291.72
Definitions

A. **Automated compounding or counting device**—An automated device that compounds, measures, counts, and/or prepackages a specified quantity of dosage units of a designated drug product.
B. **Automated medication supply system**—A mechanical device system that performs operations or activities relative to the storage and distribution of medications for administration and which collects, controls, and maintains all transaction information. An automated medication supply system includes both storage systems such as Pyxis™ and robotic dispensing systems such as Robot Rx®.
C. **Clinical pharmacy program**—An ongoing program in which pharmacists are on duty during the time the pharmacy is open for pharmacy services and pharmacists provide direct, focused, and medication-related care for the purpose of optimizing patients' medication therapy and achieving definite outcomes. A clinical pharmacy program includes the following activities:
  1. Prospective medication therapy consultation, selection, and adjustment;
  2. Monitoring laboratory values and therapeutic drug monitoring;
  3. Identifying and resolving medication-related problems; and
  4. Disease state management.
D. **Consultant pharmacist**—A pharmacist retained by a facility on a routine basis to consult with the facility in areas that pertain to the practice of pharmacy.

E. **Direct copy**—Electronic copy or carbonized copy of a medication order, including a facsimile (fax) or digital image.
F. **Distributing pharmacist**—The pharmacist who checks the medication order prior to distribution.
G. **Electronic signature**—A unique security code or other identifier which specifically identifies the person entering information into a data processing system. A facility which uses electronic signatures must:
   1. Maintain a permanent list of the unique security codes assigned to persons authorized to use the system and
   2. Have an ongoing security program capable of identifying misuse and/or unauthorized use of electronic signatures.
H. **Facility**—
   1. A hospital or other patient facility that is licensed under Chapter 241 (Hospitals) of the Texas Health and Safety Code or Chapter 577 (Mental Health Facilities);
   2. A hospice patient facility that is licensed under the Texas Health and Safety Code, Chapter 142;
   3. An ambulatory surgical center licensed under the Texas Health and Safety Code, Chapter 243; or
   4. A hospital maintained by the state.
I. **Floor stock**—Prescription drugs or devices not labeled for a specific patient and maintained at a nursing station or other hospital department (excluding the pharmacy) for the purpose of administration to a patient of the facility.
J. **Formulary**—List of drugs approved for use in the facility by the committee which performs the pharmacy and therapeutics function for the facility.
K. **Full-time pharmacist**—A pharmacist who works in a pharmacy from 30 to 40 hours per week or, if the pharmacy is open fewer than 60 hours per week, one-half of the time the pharmacy is open.
L. **Inpatient**—A person who is duly admitted to the licensed hospital or other hospital facility maintained or operated by the State of Texas or who is receiving long-term care services or Medicare extended care services in a swing bed on the hospital premise or an adjacent, readily accessible facility which is under the authority of the hospital's governing body. For the purpose of this definition, "long term care services" means those services received in a skilled nursing facility which is a distinct part of the hospital and the distinct part is not licensed separately or formally approved as a nursing home by the state, even though it is designated or certified as a skilled nursing facility. An inpatient includes a person confined in any correctional institution operated by the State of Texas.
M. **Institutional pharmacy**—Area or areas in a facility where drugs are stored, bulk compounded, delivered, compounded, dispensed, and distributed to other areas or departments of the facility or dispensed to an ultimate user or his or her agent.
N. **Investigational new drug**—A new drug intended for investigational use by experts qualified to evaluate the safety and effectiveness of the drug as authorized by the Food and Drug Administration.
O. **Medication order**—A written order from a practitioner or a verbal order from a practitioner or his or her authorized agent for the administration of a drug or device usually to an inpatient.
P. **Number of beds**—The total number of beds is determined by the number of beds for which the hospital is licensed by the Texas Department of State Health Services or average daily census as calculated by dividing the total number of inpatients admitted during the previous calendar year by 365 (or 366 if the previous calendar year is a leap year).

Q. **Part-time pharmacist**—A pharmacist either employed or under contract who routinely works less than full time.
R. **Patient**—A person who is receiving services at the facility (including patients receiving ambulatory procedures and patients conditionally admitted as observation patients) or who is receiving long term care services or Medicare extended care services in a swing bed on the hospital premise or an adjacent, readily accessible facility that is under the authority of the hospital's governing body. For the purpose of this definition, the term "long term care services" means those services received in a skilled nursing facility which is a distinct part of the hospital and the distinct part is not licensed separately or formally approved as a nursing home by the state, even though it is designated or certified as a skilled nursing facility. A patient includes a person confined in any correctional institution operated by the State of Texas.
S. **Perpetual inventory**—An inventory which documents all receipts and distributions of a drug product such that an accurate, current balance of the amount of the drug product present in the pharmacy is indicated.
T. **Pharmacist-in-charge**—A pharmacist designated on a pharmacy license as the pharmacist who has the authority or responsibility for a pharmacy's compliance with laws and rules pertaining to the practice of pharmacy.
U. **Pharmacy and therapeutics function**—A committee of the medical staff in the facility which assists in the formulation of broad professional policies regarding the evaluation, selection, distribution, handling, use, and administration and all other matters relating to the use of drugs and devices in the facility.
V. **Pharmacy technician**—An individual who is registered with the Board as a pharmacy technician whose responsibility in a pharmacy is to provide technical services that do not require professional judgment regarding preparing and distributing drugs and who works under the direct supervision of and is responsible to a pharmacist.
W. **Pharmacy technician trainee**—An individual who is registered with the Board as a pharmacy technician trainee and is authorized to participate in a pharmacy's technician training program.
X. **Rural hospital**—A licensed hospital with 75 beds or fewer that:
  1. Is located in a county with a population of 50,000 or less as defined by the United States Census Bureau in the most recent U.S. census or
  2. Has been designated by the Centers for Medicare and Medicaid Services as a critical access hospital, rural referral center, or sole community hospital.
Y. **Supervision**—
  1. Physically present supervision—In a Class C pharmacy, a pharmacist shall be physically present to directly supervise pharmacy technicians or pharmacy technician trainees.
  2. Electronic supervision—In a Class C pharmacy in a facility licensed for 100 beds or fewer, a pharmacist licensed in Texas may electronically supervise pharmacy technicians or pharmacy technician trainees to perform the duties specified in Board Rule 291.73E.2. (Personnel) provided:
    a. The pharmacy uses a system that monitors the data entry of medication orders and the filling of such orders by an electronic method that shall include the use of one or more of the following types of technology:
      (1) Digital interactive video, audio, or data transmission;
      (2) Data transmission using computer imaging by way of still-image capture and store and forward; and
      (3) Other technology that facilitates access to pharmacy services;
    b. The pharmacy establishes controls to protect the privacy and security of confidential records;

c. The pharmacist responsible for the duties performed by a pharmacy technician or pharmacy technician trainee verifies:
   (1) The data entry and
   (2) The accuracy of the filled orders prior to release of the order; and
d. The pharmacy keeps permanent digital records of duties electronically supervised and data transmissions associated with electronically supervised duties for a period of two years.
3. If the conditions of Board Rule 291.73B. below are met, electronic supervision shall be considered the equivalent of direct supervision for the purposes of the Act.

Z. **Tech-check-tech**—Allowing a pharmacy technician to verify the accuracy of work performed by another pharmacy technician relating to the filling of floor stock and unit-dose distribution systems for a patient admitted to the hospital if the patient's orders have previously been reviewed and approved by a pharmacist.

AA. **Unit-dose packaging**—The ordered amount of a drug in a dosage form ready for administration to a particular patient by the prescribed route at the prescribed time and properly labeled with name, strength, and expiration date of the drug.

BB. **Unusable drugs**—Drugs or devices that are unusable for reasons such as they are adulterated, misbranded, expired, defective, or recalled.

CC. **Written protocol**—A physician's order, standing medical order, standing delegation order, or other order or protocol as defined by rule of the Texas State Board of Medical Examiners under the Texas Medical Practice Act.

Board of Pharmacy Rule 291.73
Personnel

A. Requirements for Pharmacist Services.
   1. A facility with 101 beds or more shall be under the continuous on-site supervision of a pharmacist during the time it is open for pharmacy services. Pharmacy technicians may distribute prepackaged and prelabeled drugs from a drug storage area of the facility (e.g., a surgery suite) in the absence of physical supervision of a pharmacist if:
      a. The distribution is under the control of a pharmacist and
      b. A pharmacist is on duty in the facility.
   2. A facility with 100 beds or fewer shall have the services of a pharmacist at least on a part-time or consulting basis according to the needs of the facility except that a pharmacist must be on-site at least once every seven days.
   3. A pharmacist shall be accessible at all times to respond to another health professional's questions and needs. Such access may be through a telephone which is answered 24 hours a day (e.g., an answering or paging service, a list of phone numbers where the pharmacist may be reached, or any other system which accomplishes this purpose).

   Note: If the institution operates an outpatient pharmacy, there must be a full-time pharmacist on-site when the outpatient pharmacy is open, no matter how many beds the hospital is licensed for.

B. Pharmacist-in-Charge (PIC).
   1. General.
      a. A facility licensed for 101 beds or more shall have one full-time pharmacist-in-charge who may be the pharmacist-in-charge for only one such facility except as provided in c. below.
      b. A facility licensed for 100 beds or fewer shall have one pharmacist-in-charge employed or under contract, who is at least on a consulting or part-time basis, but may be employed on a full-time basis if desired, who may be pharmacist-in-charge for no more than 3 facilities or 150 beds.

c. A pharmacist-in-charge may be in charge of one facility with 101 beds or more and one facility with 100 beds or fewer, including a rural hospital, provided the total number of beds does not exceed 150 beds.
d. The pharmacist-in-charge shall be assisted by additional pharmacists, pharmacy technicians, and pharmacy technician trainees commensurate with the scope of services provided.
e. If the pharmacist-in-charge is employed on a part-time consulting basis, a written agreement shall exist between the facility and the pharmacist. A copy shall be made available to the Board on request.
f. The pharmacist-in-charge of a Class C pharmacy with 101 beds or more may not serve as the pharmacist-in-charge of a Class A pharmacy or a Class B pharmacy.

2. Responsibilities. The pharmacist-in-charge shall have the responsibility for, at a minimum, the following:
   a. Providing the appropriate level of pharmaceutical care services to patients of the facility;
   b. Ensuring that drugs and/or devices are prepared for distribution safely and accurately as prescribed;
   c. Supervising a system to ensure maintenance of effective controls against the theft or diversion of prescription drugs and records for such drugs;
   d. Providing written guidelines and approval of the procedure to assure that all pharmaceutical requirements are met when any part of preparing, sterilizing, and labeling of sterile pharmaceuticals is not performed under direct pharmacy supervision;
   e. Participating in the development of a formulary for the facility, subject to approval of the appropriate committee of the facility;
   f. Developing a system to assure that drugs to be administered to patients are distributed pursuant to an original or direct copy of the practitioner's medication order;
   g. Developing a system for the filling and labeling of all containers from which drugs are to be distributed or dispensed;
   h. Assuring that the pharmacy maintains and makes available a sufficient inventory of antidotes and other emergency drugs as well as current antidote information, telephone numbers of regional poison control centers and other emergency assistance organizations, and such other materials and information as may be deemed necessary by the appropriate committee of the facility;
   i. Maintaining records of all transactions of the institutional pharmacy as may be required by applicable state and federal law and as may be necessary to maintain accurate control over and accountability for all pharmaceutical materials including pharmaceuticals and components used in the compounding of preparations. In addition, the pharmacist-in-charge shall participate in policy decisions regarding prescription drug delivery devices;
   j. Participating in those aspects of the facility's patient care evaluation program which relate to pharmaceutical utilization and effectiveness;
   k. Participating in teaching and/or research programs in the facility;
   l. Implementing the policies and decisions of the appropriate committee(s) relating to pharmaceutical services of the facility;
   m. Providing effective and efficient messenger or delivery service to connect the institutional pharmacy with appropriate areas of the facility on a regular basis throughout the normal workday of the facility;
   n. Developing a system for the labeling, storage, and distribution of investigational new drugs, including access to related drug information for

healthcare personnel where such drugs are being administered and concerning the dosage form, route of administration, strength, actions, uses, side effects, adverse effects, interactions, and symptoms of toxicity of investigational new drugs;

o. Assuring that records in a data processing system are maintained so that the data processing system is in compliance with Class C (Institutional) pharmacy requirements;

p. Assuring that a reasonable effort is made to obtain, record, and maintain patient medication records;

q. Assuring the legal operation of the pharmacy, including meeting all inspection and other requirements of all state and federal laws or rules governing the practice of pharmacy; and

r. If the pharmacy uses an automated medication supply system, being responsible for the following:

(1) Reviewing and approving all policies and procedures for system operation, safety, security, accuracy and access, patient confidentiality, prevention of unauthorized access, and malfunction;

(2) Inspecting medications in the automated medication supply system at least monthly for expiration date, misbranding, physical integrity, security, and accountability, except that inspection of medication in the automated medication supply system may be performed quarterly if:

(a) The facility uses automated medication supply systems that monitor expiration dates of prescription drugs and

(b) The security of the system is checked at regularly defined intervals (e.g., daily or weekly);

(3) Assigning, discontinuing, or changing personnel access to the automated medication supply system;

(4) Ensuring that pharmacy technicians, pharmacy technician trainees, and licensed healthcare professionals performing any services in connection with an automated medication supply system have been properly trained on the use of the system and can demonstrate comprehensive knowledge of the written policies and procedures for operation of the system; and

(5) Ensuring that the automated medication supply system is stocked accurately and an accountability record is maintained in accordance with the written policies and procedures of operation.

C. Consultant Pharmacist.
1. A consultant pharmacist may be a pharmacist-in-charge of no more than 3 facilities or 150 beds.
2. A written agreement must exist between the facility and the pharmacist and must be available to the Board upon request.

D. Pharmacists.
1. General.
   a. The pharmacist-in-charge shall be assisted by a sufficient number of staff pharmacists as may be required to operate the pharmacy competently, safely, and adequately to meet the needs of the patients of the facility.
   b. Staff pharmacists shall assist the pharmacist-in-charge in meeting his or her responsibilities listed above.
   c. Pharmacists are responsible for any delegated act performed by pharmacy technicians and pharmacy technician trainees under his or her supervision.
   d. All pharmacists on duty shall be responsible for complying with all state and federal laws or rules governing the practice of pharmacy.

e. A distributing pharmacist shall be responsible for and ensure that the drug is prepared for distribution safely and accurately as prescribed unless the pharmacy's data processing system can record the identity of each pharmacist involved in a specific portion of the preparation of medication orders for distribution. In this case, each pharmacist involved in the preparation of medication orders shall be responsible for and ensure that the portion of the process the pharmacist is performing results in the safe and accurate distribution and delivery of the drug as ordered. The preparation and distribution process for medication orders shall include, but not be limited to, drug regimen review and verification of accurate medication order data entry, preparation, distribution, and performance of the final check of the prepared medication.
2. Duties.
Duties of all pharmacists shall include:
a. Providing those acts or services necessary to provide pharmaceutical care;
b. Receiving, interpreting, and evaluating prescription drug orders and reducing verbal medication orders to writing either manually or electronically;
c. Participating in drug and/or device selection as authorized by law, drug and/or device supplier selection, drug administration, drug regimen review, or drug or drug-related research;
d. Performing a specific act of drug therapy management for a patient delegated to a pharmacist by a written protocol from a physician licensed in this state in compliance with the Medical Practice Act;
e. Accepting the responsibility for:
(1) Distributing prescription drugs and devices with drug components pursuant to medication orders;
(2) Compounding and labeling of prescription drugs and devices with drug components;
(3) Properly and safely storing prescription drugs and devices with drug components; and
(4) Maintaining proper records for prescription drugs and devices with drug components.
3. Special Requirements for Compounding. All pharmacists engaged in compounding nonsterile preparations shall meet the training requirements specified in Board Rule 291.131 (Pharmacies Compounding Nonsterile Preparations). (*See Chapter H in this book.*)
E. Pharmacy Technicians and Pharmacy Technician Trainees.
1. General.
a. All pharmacy technicians and pharmacy technician trainees shall meet the training requirements specified in Board Rule 297.6 (Pharmacy Technician and Pharmacy Technician Trainee Training).
b. A pharmacy technician performing the duties specified in 2.c. below shall complete training regarding:
(1) Procedures for one pharmacy technician to verify the accuracy of actions performed by another pharmacy technician including required documentation and
(2) The duties that may be performed by one pharmacy technician and checked by another pharmacy technician.
c. In addition to the training requirements specified in a. above, pharmacy technicians working in a rural hospital and performing the duties specified in 2.d.(2) below shall complete training on the:
(1) Procedures for verifying the accuracy of actions performed by pharmacy technicians including required documentation;

(2) Duties which may and may not be performed by pharmacy technicians in the absence of a pharmacist; and

(3) The pharmacy technician's role in preventing dispensing and distribution errors.

2. Duties.

   a. Facilities with 101 beds or more. The following functions must be performed under the physically present supervision of a pharmacist:

      (1) Prepacking and labeling unit-dose and multiple-dose packages provided a pharmacist supervises and conducts a final check and affixes his or her name, initials, or electronic signature to the appropriate quality control records prior to distribution;

      (2) Preparing, packaging, compounding, or labeling prescription drugs pursuant to medication orders provided a pharmacist supervises and checks the preparation;

      (3) Bulk compounding or batch preparation provided a pharmacist supervises and conducts in-process and final checks and affixes his or her name, initials, or electronic signature to the appropriate quality control records prior to distribution;

      (4) Distributing routine orders for stock supplies to patient care areas;

      (5) Entering medication order and drug distribution information into a data processing system provided judgmental decisions are not required and a pharmacist checks the accuracy of the information entered into the system prior to releasing the order;

      (6) Loading unlabeled drugs into an automated compounding or counting device provided a pharmacist supervises, verifies that the system was properly loaded prior to use, and affixes his or her name, initials, or electronic signature to the appropriate quality control records;

      (7) Accessing automated medication supply systems after proper training on the use of the automated medication supply system and the demonstration of comprehensive knowledge of the written policies and procedures for its operation; and

      (8) Compounding nonsterile preparations pursuant to medication orders provided the pharmacy technicians or pharmacy technician trainees have completed the training specified in Board Rule 291.131.

   b. Facilities with 100 beds or fewer.

      (1) Physically present supervision. The following functions must be performed under the physically present supervision of a pharmacist unless the pharmacy meets the requirements for a rural hospital and has been approved by the Board to allow pharmacy technicians to perform the duties specified in Section 552.1011 of the Act and d.(2) below:

         (a) Prepacking and labeling unit-dose and multiple-dose packages provided a pharmacist supervises and conducts a final check and affixes his or her name, initials, or electronic signature to the appropriate quality control records prior to distribution;

         (b) Bulk compounding or batch preparation provided a pharmacist supervises and conducts in-process and final checks and affixes his or her name, initials, or electronic signature to the appropriate quality control records prior to distribution;

         (c) Loading unlabeled drugs into an automated compounding or counting device provided a pharmacist supervises, verifies that the system was properly loaded prior to use, and affixes his or her name, initials, or electronic signature to the appropriate quality control records; and

(d) Compounding medium-risk and high-risk sterile preparations pursuant to medication orders provided the pharmacy technicians or pharmacy technician trainees:
    (i) Have completed the training specified in Board Rule 291.133 of this rule and
    (ii) Are supervised by a pharmacist who has completed the training specified in Board Rule 291.133 and who conducts in-process and final checks and affixes his or her name, initials, or electronic signature to the label or, if batch prepared, to the appropriate quality control records. (The name, initials, or electronic signature are not required on the label if it is maintained in a permanent record of the pharmacy.)

(2) Electronic supervision or physically present supervision. The following functions may be performed under the electronic supervision or physically present supervision of a pharmacist:
    (a) Preparing, packaging, or labeling prescription drugs pursuant to medication orders provided a pharmacist checks the preparation prior to distribution;
    (b) Distributing routine orders for stock supplies to patient care areas;
    (c) Entering medication order and drug distribution information into a data processing system provided judgmental decisions are not required and a pharmacist checks the accuracy of the information entered into the system prior to releasing the order;
    (d) Accessing automated medication supply systems after proper training on the use of the automated medication supply system and the demonstration of comprehensive knowledge of the written policies and procedures for its operation;
    (e) Compounding nonsterile preparations pursuant to medication orders provided the pharmacy technicians or pharmacy technician trainees have completed the training specified in Board Rule 291.131; and
    (f) Compounding low-risk sterile preparations pursuant to medication orders provided the pharmacy technicians or pharmacy technician trainees:
        (i) Have completed the training specified in Board Rule 291.133 and
        (ii) Are supervised by a pharmacist who has completed the training specified in Board Rule 291.133 and who conducts in-process and final checks and affixes his or her name, initials, or electronic signature to the label or, if batch prepared, to the appropriate quality control records. (The name, initials, or electronic signature are not required on the label if it is maintained in a permanent record of the pharmacy.)

c. Tech-check-tech. A Class C pharmacy with an ongoing clinical pharmacy program may allow a pharmacy technician to verify the accuracy of the duties specified in (2) below when performed by another pharmacy technician under the following conditions:
    (1) The pharmacy technician:
        (a) Is a registered pharmacy technician and not a pharmacy technician trainee and
        (b) Meets the training requirements specified in Board Rule 297.6 and the training requirements specified in E.1. above;

(2) If the requirements of (1) above are met, a pharmacy technician may verify the accuracy of the following duties performed by another pharmacy technician:
    (a) Filling medication carts;
    (b) Distributing routine orders for stock supplies to patient care areas; and
    (c) Accessing and restocking automated medication supply systems after proper training on the use of the automated medication supply system and the demonstration of comprehensive knowledge of the written policies and procedures for its operation;
(3) The patient's orders have previously been reviewed and approved by a pharmacist; and
(4) A pharmacist is on duty in the facility at all times that the pharmacy is open for pharmacy services.

d. Rural hospitals.
   (1) A rural hospital may allow a pharmacy technician to perform the duties specified in (2) below when a pharmacist is not on duty if:
      (a) The pharmacy technician:
         (i) Is a registered pharmacy technician and not a pharmacy technician trainee and
         (ii) Meets the training requirements specified in Board Rule 297.6 and those specified in E.1. (General) above;
      (b) A pharmacist is accessible at all times to respond to any questions and needs of the pharmacy technician or other hospital employees by telephone, answering or paging service, e-mail, or any other system that makes a pharmacist immediately accessible;
      (c) The pharmacy is appropriately staffed to meet the needs of the pharmacy; and
      (d) A nurse or practitioner at the rural hospital or a pharmacist through electronic supervision as specified in E.2.b.(2) (Electronic Supervision) above verifies the accuracy of the actions of the pharmacy technician.
   (2) If the requirements of (1) above are met, the pharmacy technician may, during the hours that the institutional pharmacy in the hospital is open, perform the following duties in the pharmacy without the direct supervision of a pharmacist:
      (a) Enter medication order and drug distribution information into a data processing system;
      (b) Prepare, package, or label a prescription drug according to a medication order if a licensed nurse or practitioner verifies the accuracy of the order before administration of the drug to the patient;
      (c) Fill a medication cart used in the rural hospital;
      (d) Distribute routine orders for stock supplies to patient care areas; and
      (e) Access and restock automated medication supply cabinets.

3. Procedures.
   a. Pharmacy technicians and pharmacy technician trainees shall handle medication orders in accordance with standard written procedures and guidelines.
   b. Pharmacy technicians and pharmacy technician trainees shall handle prescription drug orders in the same manner as those working in a Class A pharmacy.

F. Owner.
The owner of a Class C pharmacy shall have responsibility for all administrative and operational functions of the pharmacy. The pharmacist-in-charge may advise the owner on administrative and operational concerns. If the owner is not a Texas licensed pharmacist, the owner shall consult with the pharmacist-in-charge or another Texas licensed pharmacist. The owner shall have responsibility for, at a minimum, the following:
1. Establishing policies for procurement of prescription drugs and devices and other products dispensed from the Class C pharmacy;
2. Establishing and maintaining effective controls against the theft or diversion of prescription drugs;
3. If the pharmacy uses an automated pharmacy dispensing system, reviewing and approving all policies and procedures for system operation, safety, security, accuracy and access, patient confidentiality, prevention of unauthorized access, and malfunction;
4. Providing the pharmacy with the necessary equipment and resources commensurate with its level and type of practice; and
5. Establishing policies and procedures regarding maintenance, storage, and retrieval of records in a data processing system so that the system is in compliance with state and federal requirements.

G. Identification of Pharmacy Personnel.
All pharmacy personnel shall wear an identification tag or badge which bears the person's name and identifies him or her by title or function.

H. Ratios.
1. The Board cannot set ratios of pharmacists to pharmacy technicians in Class C pharmacies.
2. Class A rules and ratios do apply to Class C pharmacies in the operation of an outpatient pharmacy (i.e., dispensing prescriptions).

Class C (Institutional) Pharmacy Technician/Trainee Duties

Pharmacy technicians and pharmacy technician trainees are those individuals used in pharmacies whose responsibility is to provide nonjudgmental technical services concerned with the preparation and distribution of drugs under the direct supervision of and responsible to a pharmacist.

Class C pharmacies operating an outpatient pharmacy must comply with all requirements and restrictions for Class A pharmacies with regard to ratios and the duties of pharmacy technicians/trainees. For requirements concerning Class A pharmacies, see Board Rules 291.31 through 291.36. (*See Chapter G of this book.*)

Pharmacy technicians and pharmacy technician trainees involved with inpatient medications in a hospital setting must comply with all requirements and restrictions for Class C pharmacies. The following addresses pharmacy technicians and pharmacy technician trainees in Class C pharmacies.

Under the Texas Pharmacy Act, the Board may not set pharmacist/pharmacy technician ratios in institutional pharmacies. However, a pharmacist must supervise and check the work of pharmacy technicians and pharmacy technician trainees and is responsible for any delegated act performed by pharmacy technicians under his or her supervision. Therefore, the ratio of pharmacists to pharmacy technicians may be limited by the ability of a pharmacist to perform these duties.

Pharmacist Supervision
Pharmacy technicians and pharmacy technician trainees must be under the direct supervision of and be directly responsible to a pharmacist. Electronic supervision may be

Notes

permitted in facilities licensed for 100 beds or fewer if all conditions listed in the definition of "electronic supervision" found in Board Rule 291.72 are met. A pharmacist must conduct a final check of the duties performed by pharmacy technicians and pharmacy technician trainees. Some duties such as bulk compounding, batch preparation, and sterile compounding also require in-process checking by a pharmacist. Pharmacy technicians and pharmacy technician trainees may distribute prepackaged and prelabeled drugs from a satellite pharmacy in the absence of on-site supervision of a pharmacist under the following conditions:

- The distribution is under the control of a pharmacist and
- A pharmacist is on duty in the facility.

Tasks Pharmacy Technicians/Trainees MAY NOT Perform

- Receiving and interpreting prescription drug orders and oral medication orders and reducing these orders to writing either manually or electronically;
- Selecting prescription drugs and/or devices and/or suppliers;
- Interpreting patient profiles and conducting drug regimen reviews; and
- Verifying receipt of controlled substances by initialing and dating invoices of controlled substances received in the pharmacy.

Tasks Pharmacy Technicians MAY Perform But NOT Pharmacy Technician Trainees

Tech-Check-Tech—In facilities with a clinical pharmacy program, a pharmacy technician may check the work of another technician if the pharmacy technician has been properly trained and patient orders have been previously reviewed and approved by a pharmacist. This includes checking of:

- Filling medication carts;
- Distributing routine orders for floor stock supplies to patient care areas; and
- Accessing and restocking automated medication supply systems after proper training on the use of the automated medication supply system and demonstration of comprehensive knowledge of the written policies and procedures for its operation.

Tasks Pharmacy Technicians/Trainees MAY Perform

With proper training and under pharmacist supervision, pharmacy technicians and pharmacy technician trainees MAY perform nonjudgmental technical duties associated with the preparation of a medication order. Medication orders must be handled by pharmacy technicians/trainees in accordance with standard written procedures and guidelines. These duties may include:

- Prepackaging and labeling unit-dose and multiple-dose packages;
- Preparing, packaging, compounding, or labeling prescription drugs pursuant to medication orders;
- Compounding sterile pharmaceuticals for inpatients only (provided proper training has occurred);
- Bulk compounding;
- Distributing routine orders from stock supplies to patient care areas;
- Labeling prescription drugs pursuant to a medication order;
- Preparing the finished product for inspection and final check by pharmacists;
- Entering medication order and drug distribution information into a computer system (provided a pharmacist verifies the accuracy prior to releasing the order);
- Loading bulk unlabeled drugs into an automated compounding or counting device (provided a pharmacist verifies proper loading); and
- Accessing and restocking automated medication supply systems after proper training.

Other Pharmacy Personnel

Any duty that is not required to be performed by pharmacists or by persons designated, trained, and supervised as pharmacy technicians or pharmacy technician trainees may

be performed by other employees of the pharmacy. Examples of duties that may be performed by persons other than pharmacists or pharmacy technicians/trainees include:
- Stocking or cleaning pharmacy shelves and
- Ordering pharmacy stock.

Board of Pharmacy Rule 291.74
Operational Standards

A. Licensing Requirements.
   1. The pharmacy shall be licensed as indicated by the procedures specified in Board Rule 291.1 (Pharmacy License Application). A Class C pharmacy which changes ownership shall notify the Board within 10 days of the change of ownership and apply for a new and separate license as specified in Board Rule 291.3 (Required Notifications).
   2. A Class C pharmacy engaged in the provision of remote pharmacy services, including storage and dispensing of prescription drugs, shall comply with the provisions of Board Rule 291.121.
      Note: This includes remote pharmacy services using automated systems and provision of emergency medication kits and telepharmacy services.
   3. A Class C pharmacy that changes location and/or name shall notify the Board of the change as specified by Board Rule 291.3.
      Note: This rule requires notification no later than 30 days prior to the date for a change in location and within 10 days for a change of name.
   4. A Class C pharmacy owned by a partnership or corporation which changes managing officers shall notify the Board in writing of the names of the new managing officers within 10 days of the change following the procedures in Board Rule 291.3.
   5. A Class C pharmacy shall notify the Board in writing within 10 days of closing following the procedures in Board Rule 291.5 (Closing a Pharmacy).
   6. A fee as specified in Board Rule 291.6 (Pharmacy License Fees) will be charged for the issuance and renewal of a license and the issuance of an amended license.
   7. A separate license is required for each principal place of business, and only one pharmacy license may be issued to a specific location.
   8. Need for Other Class(es) of License(s).
      a. A Class C pharmacy which operates a Class A pharmacy at the same location is not required to obtain a Class A license. However, the Class C pharmacy shall comply with Board Rule 291.31 (Definitions), Board Rule 291.32 (Personnel), Board Rule 291.33 (Operational Standards), Board Rule 291.34 (Records), and Board Rule 291.35 (Official Prescription Records) contained in Class A rules to the extent such rules are applicable to the operation of the pharmacy.
      b. A Class C pharmacy which operates a Class B pharmacy is not required to obtain a Class B license. However, the Class C pharmacy shall comply with Board Rule 291.51 (Definitions), Board Rule 291.52 (Personnel), Board Rule 291.53 (Operational Standards), and Board Rule 291.54 (Records) contained in Class B pharmacy rules to the extent such rules are applicable to the operation of the pharmacy.
   9. A Class C pharmacy engaged in nonsterile compounding shall comply with the provisions of Board Rule 291.131 (Nonsterile Compounding).
   10. Class C pharmacy personnel shall not compound sterile preparations unless the pharmacy has applied for and obtained a Class C-S pharmacy.

11. A Class C pharmacy engaged in the provision of remote pharmacy services, including the storage and dispensing of prescription drugs, shall comply with the provisions of Board Rule 291.121 (Remote Pharmacy Services).
12. A Class C pharmacy engaged in the provision of centralized prescription dispensing and/or centralized prescription drug or medication order processing shall comply with the provisions of Board Rule 291.123 (Centralized Prescription Drug or Medication Order Processing) and/or Board Rule 291.125 (Centralized Prescription Drug Order Dispensing).
13. A Class C pharmacy with an ongoing clinical pharmacy program that proposes to allow a pharmacy technician to verify the accuracy of work performed by another pharmacy technician relating to the filling of floor stock and unit-dose distribution systems for a patient admitted to the hospital if the patient's orders have previously been reviewed and approved by a pharmacist shall make application to the Board as follows.
    a. The pharmacist-in-charge must submit an application on a form provided by the Board containing the following information:
        (1) Name, address, and pharmacy license number;
        (2) Name and license number of the pharmacist-in-charge;
        (3) Name and registration numbers of the pharmacy technicians;
        (4) Anticipated date the pharmacy plans to begin allowing a pharmacy technician to verify the accuracy of work performed by another pharmacy technician;
        (5) Documentation that the pharmacy has an ongoing clinical pharmacy program; and
        (6) Any other information specified on the application.
    b. The pharmacy may not allow a pharmacy technician to check the work of another pharmacy technician until the Board has reviewed and approved the application and issued an amended license to the pharmacy.
    c. Every two years in connection with the application for renewal of the pharmacy license, the pharmacy shall provide updated documentation that the pharmacy continues to have an ongoing clinical pharmacy program as specified in a.(5) above.
14. A rural hospital that wishes to allow a pharmacy technician to perform the duties specified in Board Rule 291.73E.2.d. (Personnel) shall make application to the Board as follows.
    a. Prior to allowing a pharmacy technician to perform the duties specified in Board Rule 291.73E.2.d., the pharmacist-in-charge must submit an application on a form provided by the Board containing the following information:
        (1) Name, address, and pharmacy license number;
        (2) Name and license number of the pharmacist-in-charge;
        (3) Name and registration number of the pharmacy technicians;
        (4) Proposed date the pharmacy wishes to start allowing pharmacy technicians to perform the duties specified in Board Rule 291.73E.2.d.;
        (5) Documentation that the hospital is a rural hospital with 75 or fewer beds and that the rural hospital is either:
            (a) Located in a county with a population of 50,000 or fewer as defined by the United States Census Bureau in the most recent U.S. census or
            (b) Designated by the Centers for Medicare and Medicaid Services as a critical access hospital, rural referral center, or sole community hospital; and
        (6) Any other information specified on the application.

b. A rural hospital may not allow a pharmacy technician to perform the duties specified in Board Rule 291.73E.2.d. until the Board has reviewed and approved the application and issued an amended license to the pharmacy.
c. Every two years when applying for the renewal of the pharmacy license, the pharmacist-in-charge shall update the application for pharmacy technicians to perform the duties specified in Board Rule 291.73E.2.d.

B. Environment.
  1. General Requirements.
     a. Adequate space for proper operation.
     b. Clean and orderly with all equipment in good operating condition.
     c. Sink with hot and cold running water exclusive of restroom facilities and maintained in a sanitary condition.
     d. Proper lighting and ventilation.
     e. Proper temperature for storage of drugs (including drugs in refrigerator).
     f. If pharmacy has flammable materials, there must be a designated area for the storage of flammable materials which meets the requirements set by local and state fire laws.
     g. The institutional pharmacy shall store antiseptics, other drugs for external use, and disinfectants separately from internal and injectable medications.
  2. Security.
     a. The institutional pharmacy shall be enclosed and capable of being locked by key, combination, or other mechanical or electronic means so as to prohibit access by unauthorized individuals. Only individuals authorized by the pharmacist-in-charge shall enter the pharmacy.
     b. Each pharmacist on duty shall be responsible for the security of the institutional pharmacy, including provisions for adequate safeguards against theft or diversion of dangerous drugs, controlled substances, and records for such drugs.
     c. The institutional pharmacy shall have locked storage for Schedule II controlled substances and other drugs requiring additional security.

C. Equipment and Supplies.
Institutional pharmacies distributing medication orders shall have the following equipment:
  1. Data processing system (computer) including a printer or comparable equipment and
  2. Refrigerator and/or freezer and a system or device (e.g., thermometer) to monitor the temperature and humidity to ensure that proper storage requirements are met.

D. Library. (The hard copy or electronic format of the library must be accessible to pharmacy personnel at all times.)
  1. Current copies of pharmacy laws and rules (as in Class A pharmacy requirements);
  2. At least one current or updated reference from each of the following categories:
     a. Drug interactions.
        A reference text on drug interactions such as *Drug Interaction Facts* is required unless other references maintained by the pharmacy contain drug information including information needed to determine severity or significance of the interaction and appropriate recommendations or actions to be taken and
     b. General information reference text;

3. A current or updated reference on injectable drug products;
4. Basic antidote information and the telephone number of the nearest regional poison control center; and
5. Metric/apothecary weight and measure conversion charts.

E. Absence of a Pharmacist.
 1. Medication Orders.
    a. In facilities with a full-time pharmacist, when the pharmacy is closed and a practitioner orders a drug for administration to a bona fide patient of the facility:
       (1) Only sufficient quantities of drugs and devices may be removed from the pharmacy for immediate therapeutic needs.
       (2) Only a designated licensed nurse or practitioner may remove the drugs and devices.
       (3) A record containing the following shall be made: name of patient; name of device or drug; strength and dosage form; dose prescribed; quantity taken; time and date; and signature (first initial and last name or full signature) or electronic signature of the person making the withdrawal.
       (4) Original or direct copy of the medication order may substitute for the record in (3) if all requirements of (3) are met.
       (5) A pharmacist shall verify the withdrawal of the drugs from the pharmacy and perform a drug regimen review as soon as practical as required by G.1.b.(2) below but no more than 72 hours from the time of the withdrawal.
    b. In facilities with a part-time or consultant pharmacist when the pharmacist is not on duty or when the pharmacy is closed:
       (1) Drugs and devices only in sufficient therapeutic quantities may be removed.
       (2) Only a designated licensed nurse or practitioner may remove the drugs and devices.
       (3) Record must be made as required in 1.a.(3) and (4) above.
       (4) A pharmacist shall verify the withdrawal of the drugs from the pharmacy after a reasonable interval but in no event may the interval exceed 7 days.
       (5) A pharmacist shall perform a drug regimen review as specified in G.1.b.(2) below as follows:
          (a) If the facility has an average daily inpatient census of ten or fewer, the pharmacist shall perform the drug review after a reasonable interval but in no event may such interval exceed seven days or
          (b) If the facility has an average inpatient daily census above ten, the pharmacist shall perform the drug review after a reasonable interval but in no event may such interval exceed 96 hours.
          (c) The average daily inpatient census shall be calculated by hospitals annually immediately following the submission of the hospital's Medicare Cost Report, and the number used for these purposes shall be the average of the inpatient daily census in the report and the previous two reports for a three-year period.
 2. Floor Stock.
    In facilities using a floor stock method of drug distribution in the absence of a pharmacist, the following apply:
    a. Drugs and devices may be removed from the pharmacy only in the original manufacturer's container or prepackaged container.

b. Only a designated licensed nurse or practitioner may remove the drugs and devices.
c. A record containing the following shall be made: name of drug or device; strength and dosage form; quantity removed; location of floor stock; date and time; and signature (first initial and last name or full signature) or electronic signature of person making the withdrawal.
d. A pharmacist shall verify the withdrawal of the drugs from the pharmacy after a reasonable interval but no later than 7 days.

3. Rural Hospitals. In rural hospitals when a pharmacy technician performs the duties listed in Board Rule 291.73E.2.d., the following is applicable:
   a. The pharmacy technician shall make a record of all drugs distributed from the pharmacy. The record shall be maintained in the pharmacy for two years and contain the following information:
      (1) Name of patient or location where floor stock is distributed;
      (2) Name of device or drug, strength, and dosage form;
      (3) Dose prescribed or ordered;
      (4) Quantity distributed;
      (5) Time and date of the distribution; and
      (6) Signature (first initial and last name or full signature) or electronic signature of nurse or practitioner that verified the actions of the pharmacy technician.
   b. The original or direct copy of the medication order may substitute for the record specified in a. above provided the medication order meets all of the requirements of a. above.
   c. The pharmacist shall:
      (1) Verify and document the verification of all distributions made from the pharmacy in the absence of a pharmacist as soon as practical but no more than seven days from the time of such distribution;
      (2) Perform a drug regimen review for all medication orders and document such verification including any discrepancies noted by the pharmacist as follows:
         (a) If the facility has an average daily inpatient census of ten or fewer, the pharmacist shall perform the drug review as soon as practical but in no event more than seven days from the time of such distribution or
         (b) If the facility has an average daily inpatient census above ten, the pharmacist shall perform the drug review after a reasonable interval but in no event may such interval exceed 96 hours.
         (c) The average daily inpatient census shall be calculated by hospitals annually immediately following the submission of the hospital's Medicare Cost Report, and the number used for these purposes shall be the average of the inpatient daily census in the report and the previous two reports for a three-year period.
      (3) Review any discrepancy noted by the pharmacist with the pharmacy technician(s) and make any change in procedures or processes necessary to prevent future problems; and
      (4) Report any adverse events that have the potential to harm a patient to the appropriate committee of the hospital that reviews adverse events.

F. Drugs.
   1. Procurement, Preparation, and Storage.
      a. The pharmacist-in-charge is responsible for but may receive input from staff of the facility.

b. The pharmacist-in-charge is responsible for determining specifications of all drugs procured.
c. Institutional pharmacies may not sell, purchase, trade, or possess prescription drug samples unless the pharmacy meets the requirements as specified in Board Rule 291.16 (Samples).
d. All drugs shall be stored at the proper temperatures as defined in the USP/NF and in Board Rule 291.15 (Storage of Drugs).
e. Any drug bearing an expiration date may not be distributed beyond the expiration date of the drug.
f. Outdated and other unusable drugs shall be removed from stock and shall be quarantined together until such drugs are disposed of properly.

2. Formulary.
    a. A formulary shall be developed by the facility committee performing the pharmacy and therapeutics function for the facility. For the purpose of this section, a formulary is a compilation of pharmaceuticals that reflects the current clinical judgment of a facility's medical staff.
    b. The pharmacist-in-charge or pharmacist designated by the pharmacist-in-charge shall be a full voting member of the committee performing the pharmacy and therapeutics function for the facility when such committee is performing the pharmacy and therapeutics function.
    c. A practitioner may grant approval for pharmacists at the facility to interchange in accordance with the facility's formulary for the prescribed drugs on the practitioner's medication orders provided:
        (1) The pharmacy and therapeutics committee has developed a formulary;
        (2) The formulary has been approved by the medical staff committee of the facility;
        (3) There is a reasonable method for the practitioner to override any interchange; and
        (4) The practitioner authorizes pharmacists in the facility to interchange on his or her medication orders in accordance with the facility's formulary through his or her written agreement to abide by the policies and procedures of the medical staff and facility.

3. Prepackaging of Drugs.
    a. Distribution within a facility.
        (1) Drugs may be prepackaged in quantities suitable for internal distribution by a pharmacist or by pharmacy technicians or pharmacy technician trainees under the direction and direct supervision of a pharmacist.
        (2) The label of a prepackaged unit shall indicate:
            (a) Brand name and strength of the drug; if no brand name, then the generic name, strength, and name of the manufacturer or distributor;
            (b) Facility's unique lot number;
            (c) Expiration date based on currently available literature; and
            (d) Quantity of the drug if the quantity is greater than one.
        (3) Records of prepackaging shall be maintained to show:
            (a) Name of the drug, strength, and dosage form;
            (b) Facility's unique lot number;
            (c) Manufacturer or distributor;
            (d) Manufacturer's lot number;
            (e) Expiration date;
            (f) Quantity per prepackaged unit;
            (g) Number of prepackaged units;

(h) Date packaged;
(i) Name, initials, or electronic signature of the prepacker; and
(j) Name, initials, or electronic signature of the responsible pharmacist.
(4) Stock packages, prepackaged units, and control records shall be quarantined together until checked/released by the pharmacist.
b. Distribution to other Class C (Institutional) pharmacies under common ownership.
(1) Drugs may be prepackaged in quantities suitable for distribution to other Class C (Institutional) pharmacies under common ownership by a pharmacist or by pharmacy technicians or pharmacy technician trainees under the direction and direct supervision of a pharmacist.
(2) The label of a prepackaged unit shall indicate:
(a) Brand name and strength of the drug; if no brand name, then the generic name, strength, and name of the manufacturer or distributor;
(b) Facility's unique lot number;
(c) Expiration date based on currently available literature;
(d) Quantity of the drug if the quantity is greater than one; and
(e) Name of the facility responsible for prepackaging the drug.
(3) Records of prepackaging shall be maintained to show:
(a) Name of the drug, strength, and dosage form;
(b) Facility's unique lot number;
(c) Manufacturer or distributor;
(d) Manufacturer's lot number;
(e) Expiration date;
(f) Quantity per prepackaged unit;
(g) Number of prepackaged units;
(h) Date packaged;
(i) Name, initials, or electronic signature of the prepacker;
(j) Name, initials, or electronic signature of the responsible pharmacist; and
(k) Name of the facility receiving the prepackaged drug.
(4) Stock packages, prepackaged units, and control records shall be quarantined together until checked/released by the pharmacist.
(5) The pharmacy shall have a written procedure for the recall of any drug prepackaged for another Class C pharmacy under common ownership. The recall procedures shall require:
(a) Notification to the pharmacy to which the prepackaged drug was distributed;
(b) Quarantine of the product if there is a suspicion of harm to a patient;
(c) A mandatory recall if there is confirmed or probable harm to a patient; and
(d) Notification to the Board if a mandatory recall is instituted.
4. Sterile Preparations Prepared in a Location Other Than the Pharmacy.
A distinctive supplementary label shall be affixed to the container of any admixture. The label shall bear at a minimum:
a. Patient's name and location if not immediately administered;
b. Name and amount of drug(s) added;
c. Name of the basic solution;
d. Name or identifying code of the person who prepared the admixture; and
e. Expiration date of solution.

5. Distribution.
   a. Medication orders.
      (1) Drugs may be given to patients in facilities only on the order of a practitioner. No change in the order for drugs may be made without the approval of a practitioner except as authorized by the practitioner through the practitioner's written approval of the facility's formulary in compliance with F.2.c. (Formulary) above.
      (2) Drugs may be distributed only from the original or direct copy of the medication order.
      (3) Only a pharmacist or intern can receive verbal medication orders or verbal prescription drug orders (i.e., Class A rules apply).
      (4) Pharmacy technicians may not receive verbal medication orders.
      (5) Medication orders are exempt from patient notification and labeling provisions relative to product selection of the Act (Generic Substitution).
   b. Procedures.
      (1) Written policies and procedures for a drug distribution system (best suited for the particular institutional pharmacy) shall be developed and implemented by the pharmacist-in-charge with the advice of the committee performing the pharmacy and therapeutics function for the facility.
      (2) The written policies and procedures for the drug distribution system shall include, but not be limited to, procedures regarding the following:
         (a) Pharmaceutical care services;
         (b) Handling, storage, and disposal of cytotoxic drugs and waste;
         (c) Disposal of unusable drugs and supplies;
         (d) Security;
         (e) Equipment;
         (f) Sanitation;
         (g) Reference materials;
         (h) Drug selection and procurement;
         (i) Drug storage;
         (j) Controlled substances;
         (k) Investigational drugs including the obtaining of protocols from the principal investigator;
         (l) Prepackaging and manufacturing;
         (m) Stop orders;
         (n) Reporting of medication errors, adverse drug reactions/events, and drug product defects;
         (o) Physician orders;
         (p) Floor stocks;
         (q) Drugs brought into the facility;
         (r) Furlough medications;
         (s) Self-administration;
         (t) Emergency drug supply;
         (u) Formulary;
         (v) Monthly inspections of nursing stations and other areas where drugs are stored, distributed, administered, or dispensed;
         (w) Control of drug samples;
         (x) Outdated and other unusable drugs;
         (y) Routine distribution of patient medications;
         (z) Preparation and distribution of sterile preparations;

- (aa) Handling of medication orders when a pharmacist is not on duty;
- (bb) Use of automated compounding or drug dispensing systems;
- (cc) Use of data processing and direct imaging systems;
- (dd) Drug administration to include infusion devices and drug delivery systems;
- (ee) Drug labeling;
- (ff) Recordkeeping;
- (gg) Quality assurance/quality control;
- (hh) Duties, education, and training of professional and nonprofessional staff;
- (ii) Procedures for a pharmacy technician to verify the accuracy of work performed by another pharmacy technician if applicable;
- (jj) Operation of the pharmacy when a pharmacist in not on-site; and
- (kk) Emergency preparedness plan to include continuity of patient therapy and public safety.

6. Discharge Prescriptions. Discharge prescriptions must be dispensed and labeled in accordance with Board Rule 291.33 (Operational Standards) except that certain medications packaged in unit-of-use containers, such as metered-dose inhalers, insulin pens, topical creams or ointments, or ophthalmic or otic preparations that are administered to the patient during the time the patient was a patient in the hospital, are exempt from the labeling requirements in Board Rule 291.33. These may be provided to the patient upon discharge provided the pharmacy receives a discharge order and the product bears a label containing the following information:
   a. Name of the patient;
   b. Name and strength of the medication;
   c. Name of the prescribing or attending practitioner;
   d. Directions for use;
   e. Duration of therapy (if applicable); and
   f. Name and telephone number of the pharmacy.

G. Pharmaceutical Care Services.
   1. The pharmacist-in-charge shall assure that at least the following pharmaceutical care services are provided to patients of the facility.
      a. Drug utilization review.
         A systematic ongoing process of drug utilization review shall be developed with the medical staff to increase the probability of desired patient outcomes and decrease the probability of undesired outcomes from drug therapy.
      b. Drug regimen review.
         (1) For the purpose of promoting therapeutic appropriateness, a pharmacist shall evaluate medication orders and patient medication records for:
             (a) Known allergies;
             (b) Rational therapy-contraindications;
             (c) Reasonable dose and route of administration;
             (d) Reasonable directions for use;
             (e) Duplication of therapy;
             (f) Drug-drug interactions;
             (g) Drug-food interactions;
             (h) Drug-disease interactions;
             (i) Adverse drug reactions;

(j) Proper utilization including overutilization or underutilization; and
(k) Clinical laboratory or clinical monitoring methods to monitor and evaluate drug effectiveness, side effects, toxicity, adverse effects, and appropriateness to continued use of the drug in its current regimen.
(2) The drug regimen review shall be conducted on a prospective basis when a pharmacist is on duty, except for an emergency order, and on a retrospective basis when a pharmacist is not on duty.
(3) In facilities with a part-time pharmacist when a pharmacist is not on duty or when the pharmacy is closed, the drug regimen review shall be conducted after a reasonable interval, not exceeding 7 days if the hospital has an average daily census of ten or fewer or not exceeding 96 hours if the hospital has an average daily census of more than ten.
(4) Any questions regarding the order must be resolved with the prescriber and a written notation of these discussions must be made and maintained.
(5) The drug regimen review may be conducted by remotely accessing the pharmacy's electronic data base from outside the pharmacy by a Texas licensed pharmacist employee of the pharmacy, provided the pharmacy establishes controls to protect the privacy of the patient and the security of confidential records.
  c. Education.
  The pharmacist-in-charge in cooperation with appropriate multidisciplinary staff of the facility shall develop policies that assure:
    (1) The patient and/or patient's caregiver receives information regarding drugs and their safe and appropriate use and
    (2) Healthcare providers are provided with patient specific drug information.
  d. Patient monitoring.
  The pharmacist-in-charge in cooperation with the appropriate multidisciplinary staff of the facility shall develop policies to ensure that the patient's response to drug therapy is monitored and conveyed to the appropriate healthcare provider.
  e. Other pharmaceutical care services which may be provided by pharmacists in the facility include, but are not limited to, the following:
    (1) Managing drug therapy as delegated by a practitioner as allowed under the provisions of the Medical Practice Act;
    (2) Administering immunizations and vaccinations under the written protocol of a physician;
    (3) Managing patient compliance programs;
    (4) Providing preventative healthcare services; and
    (5) Providing case management of patients who are being treated with high-risk or high-cost drugs or who are considered "high risk" due to their age, medical condition, family history, or related concern.
H. Emergency Rooms (ER).
  1. When a pharmacist is on duty in the facility, any prescription drugs supplied to an outpatient, including emergency room patients, may only be dispensed by a pharmacist.
  2. When a pharmacist is not on duty in the facility, the following procedures shall be observed in supplying prescription drugs from the emergency room to be taken home by the patient for self-administration. If a patient has been admitted to the emergency room and assessed by a practitioner at the

hospital, the following procedures shall be observed in supplying prescription drugs from the emergency room.
- a. Drugs may only be supplied in accordance with a system for accountability and control of drugs administered or supplied for the emergency room patients. The system shall be developed by the pharmacist-in-charge.
- b. Only drugs on the emergency room drug list may be supplied. They consist of drugs to meet the immediate needs of emergency room patients.
- c. Drugs must be supplied only in prepackaged quantities not to exceed a 72-hour supply and must be in suitable containers properly prelabeled by the pharmacy department including necessary ancillary labels.
- d. At the time of delivery of the drugs, the practitioner or licensed nurse under the supervision of a practitioner shall complete the label with:
  - (1) Name, address, and telephone number of the facility;
  - (2) Date supplied;
  - (3) Name of practitioner;
  - (4) Name of patient;
  - (5) Directions for use;
  - (6) Unique identification number;
  - (7) Brand name or generic name (with manufacturer) and strength of the drug; and
  - (8) Quantity supplied.
- e. A practitioner or licensed nurse under supervision of the practitioner shall give the medication to the patient and explain its use (patient counseling).
- f. A perpetual record of drugs dispensed in the emergency room shall be maintained with the following:
  - (1) Date dispensed;
  - (2) Practitioner's name;
  - (3) Patient's name;
  - (4) Brand name and strength of the prescription drug or, if no brand name, the generic name, strength, and the name of the manufacturer or distributor of the prescription drug;
  - (5) Quantity dispensed; and
  - (6) Unique identification number.
- g. The pharmacist-in-charge or staff pharmacist shall verify the correctness of the record at least once every seven days.

I. Radiology Departments. (Similar as Board rules for Emergency Rooms)
J. Automated Devices and Systems.
  1. Automated Compounding or Counting Devices. If a pharmacy uses automated compounding or counting devices:
     - a. The pharmacy shall have a method to calibrate and verify the accuracy of the automated compounding or counting device and document the calibration and verification on a routine basis;
     - b. The devices may be loaded with bulk or unlabeled drugs only by a pharmacist or by pharmacy technicians or pharmacy technician trainees under the direction and direct supervision of a pharmacist;
     - c. The label of an automated compounding or counting device container shall indicate the brand name and strength of the drug. If no brand name, the label shall indicate the generic name, strength, and name of the manufacturer or distributor;
     - d. Records of loading bulk or unlabeled drugs into an automated compounding or counting device shall be maintained to show:
       - (1) Name of the drug, strength, and dosage form;
       - (2) Manufacturer or distributor;

(3) Manufacturer's lot number;
(4) Expiration date;
(5) Date of loading;
(6) Name, initials, or electronic signature of the person loading the automated compounding or counting device; and
(7) Signature or electronic signature of the responsible pharmacist; and

e. The automated compounding or counting device shall not be used until a pharmacist verifies that the system is properly loaded and affixes his or her signature to the record specified in d. above.

2. Automated Medication Supply Systems.
   a. Authority to use automated medication supply systems.
   A pharmacy may use an automated medication supply system to fill medication orders provided that:
   (1) The pharmacist-in-charge is responsible for the supervision of the operation of the system;
   (2) The automated medication supply system has been tested by the pharmacy and found to dispense accurately. The pharmacy shall make the results of such testing available to the Board upon request; and
   (3) The pharmacy will make the automated medication supply system available for inspection by the Board for the purpose of validating the accuracy of the system.

   b. Quality assurance program.
   A pharmacy which uses an automated medication supply system to fill medication orders shall operate according to a written program for quality assurance of the automated medication supply system which:
   (1) Requires continuous monitoring of the automated medication supply system and
   (2) Establishes mechanisms and procedures to test the accuracy of the automated medication supply system at least every six months and whenever any upgrade or change is made to the system and documents each such activity.

   c. Policies and procedures of operation.
   (1) When an automated medication supply system is used to store or distribute medications for administration pursuant to medication orders, it shall be operated according to written policies and procedures of operation. The policies and procedures of operation shall establish requirements for operation of the automated medication supply system and shall describe policies and procedures that:
   (a) Include a description of the policies and procedures of operation;
   (b) Provide for a pharmacist's review and approval of each original or new medication order prior to withdrawal from the automated medication supply system:
   (i) Before the order is filled when a pharmacist is on duty except for an emergency order;
   (ii) Retrospectively within 72 hours in a facility with a full-time pharmacist when a pharmacist is not on duty at the time the order is made; or
   (iii) Retrospectively within 7 days in a facility with a part-time or consultant pharmacist when a pharmacist is not on duty at the time the order is made;
   (c) Provide for access to the automated medication supply system for stocking and retrieval of medications which is limited to licensed healthcare professionals, pharmacy technicians, or

pharmacy technician trainees acting under the supervision of a pharmacist;

(d) Provide that all medication to be restocked in the automated medication supply system has been checked by a pharmacist prior to restocking. The actual restocking may be performed by a pharmacy technician after being checked by a pharmacist;

(e) Provide for an accountability record to be maintained which documents all transactions relative to stocking and removing medications from the automated medication supply system;

(f) Require a prospective or retrospective drug regimen review is conducted as specified in G. above; and

(g) Establish and make provisions for documentation of a preventative maintenance program for the automated medication supply system.

(2) A pharmacy which uses an automated medication supply system to fill medication orders shall at least annually review its written policies and procedures, revise them if necessary, and document the review.

d. Automated medication supply systems used for storage and recordkeeping of medications located outside of the pharmacy department (e.g., Pyxis). A pharmacy technician or pharmacy technician trainee may restock an automated medication supply system located outside of the pharmacy department with prescription drugs provided:

(1) Prior to distribution of the prescription drugs, a pharmacist verifies that the prescription drugs pulled to stock the automated supply system match the list of prescription drugs generated by the automated medication supply system except as specified in Board Rule 291.73 (Tech-check-tech rules) or

(2) All of the following occur:

(a) The prescription drugs to restock the system are labeled and verified with a machine-readable product identifier such as a barcode;

(b) Either the drugs are in tamper-evident product packaging (packaged by an FDA registered repackager or manufacturer) that is shipped to the pharmacy or, if any previous manipulation of the product occurs in the pharmacy prior to restocking such as repackaging or extemporaneous compounding, the product must be checked by a pharmacist; and

(c) Quality assurance audits are conducted according to established policies and procedures to ensure accuracy of the process.

e. Recovery plan.

A pharmacy which uses an automated medication supply system to store or distribute medications for administration pursuant to medication orders shall maintain a written plan for recovery from a disaster or any other situation which interrupts the ability of the automated medication supply system to provide services necessary for the operation of the pharmacy. The written plan for recovery shall include:

(1) Planning and preparation for maintaining pharmacy services when an automated medication supply system is experiencing downtime;

(2) Procedures for response when an automated medication supply system is experiencing downtime;

(3) Procedures for the maintenance and testing of the written plan for recovery; and

(4) Procedures for notification of the Board and other appropriate agencies whenever an automated medication supply system experiences downtime for more than two days of operation or a period of time which significantly limits the pharmacy's ability to provide pharmacy services.
3. Verification of Medication Orders Prepared by the Pharmacy Department Through the Use of an Automated Medication Supply System. For the purpose of Board Rule 291.73 (Personnel), a pharmacist must check drugs prepared pursuant to medication orders to ensure that the drug is accurately prepared for distribution as prescribed. This paragraph does not apply to automated medication supply systems used for storage and recordkeeping of medications located outside of the pharmacy department.
   a. This final check shall be considered accomplished if:
      (1) A check of the final product is conducted by a pharmacist after the automated medication supply system has completed preparation of the medication order and prior to delivery to the patient or
      (2) The following checks are conducted by a pharmacist:
         (a) If the automated medication supply system contains unlabeled stock drugs, a pharmacist verifies that those drugs have been accurately stocked and
         (b) A pharmacist checks the accuracy of the data entry of each original or new medication order entered into the automated medication supply system before the order is filled.
   b. If the final check is accomplished as specified in a.(2) above, the following additional requirements must be met.
      (1) The medication order preparation process must be fully automated from the time the pharmacist releases the medication order to the automated system until a completed medication order ready for delivery to the patient is produced.
      (2) The pharmacy has conducted initial testing and has a continuous quality assurance program which documents that the automated medication supply system dispenses accurately as prescribed.
      (3) The automated medication supply system documents and maintains:
         (a) The name(s), initials, or identification code(s) of each pharmacist responsible for the checks outlined in a.(2) above and
         (b) The name(s), initials, or identification code(s) and specific activity(ies) of each pharmacist, pharmacy technician, or pharmacy technician trainee who performs any other portion of the medication order preparation process.
      (4) The pharmacy establishes mechanisms and procedures to test the accuracy of the automated medication supply system at least every month rather than every six months.
4. Automated Checking Device.
   a. An automated checking device is a fully automated device which confirms after a drug is prepared for distribution but prior to delivery to the patient that the correct drug and strength have been labeled with the correct label for the correct patient.
   b. The final check of a drug prepared pursuant to a medication order shall be considered accomplished using an automated checking device provided:
      (1) A check of the final product is conducted by a pharmacist prior to delivery to the patient or the following checks are performed by a pharmacist:

(a) The prepackaged drug used to fill the order is checked by a pharmacist who verifies that the drug is labeled and packaged accurately and
(b) A pharmacist checks the accuracy of each original or new medication order;
(2) The medication order is prepared, labeled, and made ready for delivery to the patient in compliance with Class C (Institutional) pharmacy rules; and
(3) Prior to delivery to the patient:
(a) The automated checking device confirms that the correct drug and strength have been labeled with the correct label for the correct patient and
(b) A pharmacist performs all other duties required to ensure that the medication order has been prepared safely and accurately as prescribed.
c. If the final check is accomplished as specified using an automated checking device, the following additional requirements must be met.
(1) The pharmacy has conducted initial testing of the automated checking device and has a continuous quality assurance program which documents that the automated checking device accurately confirms that the correct drug and strength have been labeled with the correct label for the correct patient.
(2) The pharmacy documents and maintains:
(a) The name(s), initials, or identification code(s) of each pharmacist responsible for the checks outlined in b.(1) above and
(b) The name(s), initials, or identification code(s) and specific activity(ies) of each pharmacist, pharmacy technician, or pharmacy technician trainee who performs any other portion of the medication order preparation process.
(3) The pharmacy establishes mechanisms and procedures to test the accuracy of the automated checking device at least monthly.

Automation in Class C (Institutional) Pharmacies

Q1. What automated devices are recognized in the rules for Class C Pharmacies?
Answer: Basically, there are three types of automated devices:
1. Automated compounding or counting devices;
2. Automated medication supply systems; and
3. Automated checking devices.

Q2. How are the three devices defined?
Answer:
A. **Automated compounding or counting device**—An automated device that compounds, measures, counts, and/or packages a specified quantity of dosage units of a designated drug product.
Note—These devices contain bulk drugs which are counted or compounded. A common example used in a Class C pharmacy is an automated IV compounding device.
B. **Automated medication supply system**—A mechanical system that performs operations or activities relative to the storage and distribution of medication for administration and which collects, controls, and maintains all transaction information.

Note—A common example in Class C pharmacies includes the automated medication carts such as those made by Pyxis, SureMed, or similar dispensing carts located on nursing units.

C. **Automated checking device**—A fully automated device which confirms, after a drug is prepared for distribution but prior to delivery to the patient, that the correct drug and strength have been labeled with the correct label for the correct patient.

Note—These devices use technology to check a final drug order after it has been prepared for delivery to the patient.

Q3. What about automated storage and delivery devices such as kiosks for patients to pick up dispensed prescriptions?

Answer: A Class C pharmacy may use an automated storage and delivery device to deliver dispensed prescriptions to patients at a remote site with Board approval. However, since these devices are located outside of the pharmacy, the rules for these systems can be found in Rule 291.121 in Chapter D.

Automated Compounding or Counting Devices

Q4. Can an automated compounding or counting device be loaded by a pharmacy technician or pharmacy technician trainee?

Answer: Yes. These devices must be loaded by a pharmacist or by a pharmacy technician or trainee under the direction and direct supervision of a pharmacist. In addition, the device has to be labeled with the brand name of the drug and the strength. If there is no brand name, it must be labeled with the generic name of the drug, strength, and the manufacturer or distributor. A record of loading the device must be made which contains the:

1. Name of the drug, strength, and dosage form;
2. Manufacturer or distributor;
3. Manufacturer's lot number;
4. Expiration date;
5. Date of loading;
6. Name, initials, or electronic signature of the person loading the automated compounding or counting device; and
7. Signature or electronic signature of the responsible pharmacist.

Q5. Once the automated compounding or counting device has been loaded and labeled by a technician and a proper record made, is the device ready for use?

Answer: Not yet. A pharmacist must verify that the system was properly loaded and affix his or her signature to the record indicated in the answer to Q4. Once these steps are completed, the device is ready for use to fill medication orders.

Automated Medication Supply Systems

Q6. Under what conditions can an automated medication supply system be used?

Answer: An automated medication supply system may only be used if the pharmacist-in-charge is responsible for the supervision of the operation of the system. Before the first medication order is prepared by the system, the device has to be thoroughly tested and found to dispense accurately. There must also be an ongoing quality assurance program that continuously monitors the system and tests the accuracy of the system at least every six months and whenever an upgrade to the system is made.

Q7. Should an automated medication supply system be operated according to formalized policies and procedures?

Answer: Yes. Board rules require the pharmacy to establish written requirements for the operation of these devices and describe policies and procedures that:

1. Include a description of the policies and procedures of operation;
2. Provide for a pharmacist's review and approval of each original or new medication order filled through the use of the automated medication supply system:
   a. Before the order is filled when a pharmacist is on duty except for an emergency order;
   b. Retrospectively within 72 hours in a facility with a full-time pharmacist when a pharmacist is not on duty at the time the order is made; or
   c. Retrospectively within 7 days in a facility with a part-time or consultant pharmacist when a pharmacist is not on duty at the time the order is made;
3. Provide for access to the automated medication supply system for stocking and retrieval of medications which is limited to licensed healthcare professionals or pharmacy technicians/trainees acting under the supervision of a pharmacist;
4. Provide that a pharmacist is responsible for the accuracy of the restocking of the system. The actual restocking may be performed by a pharmacy technician or pharmacy technician trainee;
5. Provide for an accountability record to be maintained which documents all transactions relative to stocking and removing medications from the automated medication supply system; and
6. Require a prospective or retrospective drug regimen review and establish and make provisions for documentation of a preventative maintenance program for the automated medication supply system.

In addition, the policies and procedures must be reviewed annually and updated if needed.

Q8. Since a properly tested and maintained automated medication supply system is so accurate, is a pharmacist required to conduct a final check of a prescription dispensed by the device?

Answer: The answer depends on where the automated medication supply system is located in the hospital.
1. The answer is "no" if the automated medication supply system is used for storage and recordkeeping of medications located outside of the pharmacy department.
2. The answer is "yes" if the automated medication supply system is located in the pharmacy department. A pharmacist must check drugs prepared pursuant to medication orders to ensure that the drugs are prepared for distribution accurately as prescribed. This check shall be considered accomplished if:
   a. A check of the final product is conducted by a pharmacist after the automated system has completed preparation of the medication order and prior to delivery to the patient or
   b. The following checks are conducted by a pharmacist:
      (1) If the automated medication supply system contains bulk stock drugs, a pharmacist verifies that those drugs have been accurately stocked and
      (2) A pharmacist checks the accuracy of the data entry of each original or new medication order entered into the automated medication supply system before the order is filled.
   c. If the check is performed in the manner indicated in b. above, the following additional requirements must be met:
      (1) The medication order preparation process must be fully automated from the time the pharmacist releases the medication order to the automated system until a completed medication order, ready for delivery to the patient, is produced.
      (2) The pharmacy has conducted initial testing and has a continuous quality assurance program which documents that the automated medication supply system dispenses accurately.
      (3) The automated medication supply system documents and maintains:

Notes

> (a) The name(s), initials, or identification code(s) of each pharmacist responsible for verifying the drugs were accurately stocked in the device and for checking the accuracy of the data entry of each original or new medication order entered into the system and
> (b) The name(s), initials, or identification code(s) and specific activity(ies) of each pharmacist, pharmacy technician, or pharmacy technician trainee who performs any other portion of the medication order preparation process.
>
> (4) The pharmacy establishes mechanisms and procedures to test the accuracy of the automated medication supply system at least every month rather than every six months.

Automated Checking Devices

Q9. Since an automated checking device and an automated medication supply system can both be used to conduct a final check of a completed medication order prior to delivery to a patient, what is the difference between the two systems?

Answer: In an automated medication supply system, the device is actually filling medication orders while checking for accuracy. With the automated checking device, completed medication orders are checked for accuracy using technology such as barcoding.

Q10. Can an automated checking device be used to complete the final check of a dispensed prescription?

Answer: Yes. However, because of the difference described in Q9, the requirements are slightly different. If using an automated checking device, the final check shall be considered accomplished if:

1. A check of the final product is conducted by a pharmacist prior to delivery to the patient or the following checks are performed by a pharmacist:
   a. The prepackaged drug used to fill the order is checked by a pharmacist who verifies that the drug is labeled and packaged accurately and
   b. A pharmacist checks the accuracy of each original or new medication order;
2. The medication order is prepared, labeled, and made ready for delivery to the patient in compliance with Class C pharmacy rules; and
3. Prior to delivery to the patient:
   a. The automated checking device confirms that the correct drug and strength have been labeled with the correct label for the correct patient and
   b. A pharmacist performs all other duties required to ensure that the medication order has been prepared safely and accurately as prescribed.

If the final check is performed by the automated checking device, the following additional requirements must be met.

1. The pharmacy has conducted initial testing of the automated checking device and has a continuous quality assurance program which documents that the automated checking device accurately confirms that the correct drug and strength have been labeled with the correct label for the correct patient.
2. The pharmacy documents and maintains:
   a. The name(s), initials, or identification code(s) of each pharmacist responsible for verifying that the prepackaged drug was labeled and packaged accurately and for checking the accuracy of each original or new medication order and
   b. The name(s), initials, or identification code(s) and specific activity(ies) of each pharmacist, pharmacy technician, or pharmacy technician trainee who performs any other portion of the medication order preparation process.
3. The pharmacy establishes mechanisms and procedures to test the accuracy of the automated checking device at least monthly rather than every six months.

Board of Pharmacy Rule 291.75
Records

A. Maintenance of Records.
  1. Every inventory or other record required to be kept by Board Rules 291.71–291.75 shall be:
     a. Kept by the institutional pharmacy and be available for at least two years from the date of such inventory or record for inspecting and copying by the Board or its representatives and to other authorized local, state, or federal law enforcement agencies and
     b. Supplied by the pharmacy within 72 hours if requested by an authorized agent of the Board. If the pharmacy maintains the records in an electronic format, the requested records must be provided in a mutually agreeable electronic format if specifically requested by the Board or its representative. Failure to provide the records set out in this subsection, either on-site or within 72 hours, constitutes prima facie evidence of failure to keep and maintain records in violation of the Act.
  2. CI and II records shall be maintained separately from all other records.
  3. CIII-V records shall be maintained separately or readily retrievable from all other records of the pharmacy. Readily retrievable means that the controlled substances shall be asterisked, redlined, or in some other manner readily identifiable apart from all other items appearing on the record.
  4. Records, except when specifically required to be maintained in original or hardcopy form, may be maintained in a data processing or direct imaging system provided:
     a. The records in the alternative data retention system contain all of the information required on the manual record and
     b. The alternative data retention system is capable of producing a hard copy of the record upon the request of the Board or other authorized agencies.
B. Outpatient Records.
  1. Outpatient records must be maintained as in Class A pharmacy rules.
  2. Outpatient prescriptions including furlough and discharge prescriptions must meet the requirements of a prescription drug order. Inpatient medication order forms (or copies) do not generally meet the requirements for outpatient prescription drug orders.
  3. A seven-day supply of a Schedule II drug may be dispensed by a pharmacy without an Official Prescription Form if:
     a. The prescription is manually signed by the practitioner and dispensed by the hospital pharmacy before the patient is discharged.
     b. The patient has been "admitted to the hospital" (i.e., hospital inpatient, emergency room patient, or clinic patient).
     c. The quantity does not exceed a seven-day supply.
     d. The prescription is filed in outpatient records with other Schedule II prescriptions.
C. Patient Records.
  1. Original Medication Orders.
     a. Each original medication order or set of orders issued together must bear:
        (1) Patient name and room number or identification number;
        (2) Drug name, strength, and dosage form;
        (3) Directions for use;
        (4) Date; and
        (5) Signature or electronic signature of the practitioner or that of his or her authorized agent.

b. The original medication order shall be maintained with the medication administration records of the patients.
2. Patient Medication Records (PMR).
A patient medication record for each patient shall contain:
   a. Patient information:
      (1) Patient name and room number or ID number;
      (2) Gender and date of birth or age;
      (3) Weight and height;
      (4) Known drug sensitivities and allergies to drugs and/or food;
      (5) Primary diagnoses and chronic conditions;
      (6) Primary physician; and
      (7) Other drugs the patient is receiving.
   b. Medication order information:
      (1) Date of distribution;
      (2) Drug name, strength, and dosage form; and
      (3) Directions for use.
3. Controlled substances records shall be maintained:
   a. In a readily retrievable manner and
   b. In a manner to establish receipt and distribution of all controlled substances.
4. C-II Records.
   a. Must be kept separately from C-III-V and all other records.
   b. Pharmacy shall maintain a perpetual inventory of all C-IIs.
   c. Distribution records of C-IIs shall include:
      (1) Patient name;
      (2) Prescribing or attending practitioner;
      (3) Drug name, dosage form, and strength;
      (4) Time and date administered to the patient and the quantity administered;
      (5) Name, initials, or electronic signature of the individual administering the drug;
      (6) Returns to the pharmacy; and
      (7) Drug waste (witnessed and cosigned electronically or manually by another individual).
5. Floor Stock Records.
   a. Distribution records of C-II-V floor stocks shall include the same as in 4.c.(1)-(7) above.
   b. Floor stock records must be maintained separately from patient records.
   c. The pharmacist must review at least every 30 days to verify proper usage.
6. General Requirements for Records Maintained in a Data Processing System.
   a. If a hospital pharmacy's data processing system is not in compliance with these rules, the pharmacy must maintain a manual recordkeeping system.
   b. Requirements for backup systems.
   Maintain a backup copy of information stored in the data processing system using disk, tape, or another electronic backup system and update this backup copy.
   c. Change or discontinuance of a data processing system.
      (1) Records of distribution and return for all controlled substances. A pharmacy that changes or discontinues use of a data processing system must:
         (a) Transfer the records to the new data processing system or
         (b) Purge the records to a printout which contains the same information as required on the audit trail printout as specified in

7.b. below. The information on this printout shall be sorted and printed by drug name and list all distributions/returns chronologically.

      (2) Other records.
      A pharmacy that changes or discontinues use of a data processing system must:
        (a) Transfer the records to the new data processing system or
        (b) Purge the records to a printout which contains all of the information required on the original document.

      (3) Maintenance of purged records.
      Information purged from a data processing system must be maintained by the pharmacy for two years from the date of initial entry into the data processing system.

   d. Loss of data.
   The PIC shall report to the Board in writing any significant loss of information from the data processing system within 10 days of the discovery of the loss.

7. Data Processing System Maintenance of Records for the Distribution and Return of All Controlled Substances.
   a. Each time a controlled substance is distributed from or returned to the pharmacy, a record of such distribution or return shall be entered into the data processing system.
   b. The system shall have the capacity to produce a hardcopy printout of an audit trail of drug distribution and return for any strength and dosage form of a drug (by either brand or generic name or both) during a specified time period. This printout shall contain:
      (1) Patient's name and room number or patient's facility identification number;
      (2) Prescribing or attending practitioner's name;
      (3) Name, strength, and dosage form of the drug product actually distributed;
      (4) Total quantity distributed from and returned to the pharmacy; and
      (5) If not immediately retrievable via electronic image, the following shall also be included on the printout:
         (a) Prescribing or attending practitioner's address and
         (b) Practitioner's DEA registration number if the medication order is for a controlled substance.
   c. An audit trail printout for each strength and dosage form of the drugs distributed during the preceding month shall be produced at least monthly and be maintained in a separate file at the facility unless the pharmacy complies with d. below. The information on this printout shall be sorted chronologically by drug name and list all distributions/returns for that drug.
   d. The pharmacy may elect not to produce the monthly audit trail printout if the system has a workable (electronic) data retention system which can produce an audit trail of drug distributions and returns for the preceding two years. This audit trail shall be supplied by the pharmacy within 72 hours if requested by an authorized agent of the Board or other authorized agencies.
8. Failure to provide records either on-site or within 72 hours constitutes prima facie evidence of failure to keep and maintain records.
9. For system downtime, auxiliary procedures shall ensure that all data is retained for online data entry as soon as the system is available for use again.

10. Tech-Check-Tech. If a pharmacy has an ongoing clinical pharmacy program and allows pharmacy technicians to verify the accuracy of work performed by other pharmacy technicians, the pharmacy must have a record of the pharmacy technicians and the duties performed.
D. Distribution of Controlled Substances to Another Registrant.
See Chapter B in this book.
E. Other Records to Be Maintained by a Pharmacy.
1. Inventories.
A hard copy of controlled substances inventories is required by Board Rule 291.17. However, the required perpetual inventory of Schedule II controlled substances may be kept in a data processing system if the data processing system is capable of producing a hard copy of the perpetual inventory on-site.
Note: The perpetual inventory is an additional requirement for Class C pharmacies.
2. Other records to be maintained are the same as Board Rule 291.34 (Class A pharmacies).
F. Permission to Maintain Central Records.
See Board Rule 291.34J. (Class A pharmacies).

Records That Pharmacists Should Be Able to Locate in a Class C Pharmacy

A pharmacist-in-charge of a pharmacy or a pharmacist on duty during a compliance inspection or investigation audit in a Class C pharmacy should be able to locate the following records for the previous two years:
1. Annual inventories;
2. Perpetual inventory of Schedule II controlled substances;
3. Controlled substance invoices;
4. Theft and loss reports;
5. Drug destruction reports;
6. Inpatient distribution records for controlled substances;
7. All prescriptions (if the hospital operates an outpatient pharmacy);
8. Daily dispensing printouts or dispensing logs (if the hospital operates an outpatient pharmacy);
9. Prepackaging records if applicable;
10. Pharmacy technician training manual and documentation of technician training;
11. Policy and procedure manual;
12. Records of training for all pharmacists who compound or who supervise preparation of sterile pharmaceuticals;
13. Records of training for all technicians who compound sterile pharmaceuticals; and
14. Documentation of process validation for all pharmacists and technicians who prepare sterile pharmaceuticals.

Board of Pharmacy Rule 291.77
Pharmacies Compounding Sterile Preparations (Class C-S)

Note: This rule requires all Class C pharmacies that are engaged in compounding sterile preparations to obtain a Class C-S license. This provides the Board with information on which pharmacies are performing sterile compounding, but Class C-S pharmacies are still subject to all other Class C rules.

Licensing Requirements. An institutional or ASC pharmacy engaged in the compounding of sterile preparations shall be designated as a Class C-S pharmacy.
1. A Class C-S pharmacy shall register annually or biennially with the Board on a pharmacy license application provided by the Board following the procedures specified in Board Rule 291.1 (Pharmacy License Application). A Class C-S license may not be issued unless the pharmacy has been inspected by the Board to ensure the pharmacy meets the requirements as specified in Board Rule 291.133 (Pharmacies Compounding Sterile Preparations).
2. A Class C-S pharmacy may not renew a pharmacy license unless the pharmacy has been inspected by the Board within the last renewal period.
3. A Class C-S pharmacy which changes ownership shall notify the Board within 10 days of the change of ownership and apply for a new and separate license as specified in Board Rule 291.3 (Required Notifications).
4. A Class C-S pharmacy which changes location and/or name shall notify the Board within 10 days of the change and file for an amended license as specified in Board Rule 291.3.
5. A Class C-S pharmacy owned by a partnership or corporation which changes managing officers shall notify the Board in writing of the names of the new managing officers within 10 days of the change following the procedures in Board Rule 291.3.
6. A Class C-S pharmacy shall notify the Board in writing within 10 days of closing following the procedures in Board Rule 291.5 (Closing a Pharmacy).
7. A fee as specified in Board Rule 291.6 (Pharmacy License Fees) will be charged for the issuance and renewal of a license and the issuance of an amended license.
8. A separate license is required for each principal place of business, and only one pharmacy license may be issued to a specific location.
9. A Class C-S pharmacy licensed under Section 560.051A.3. of the Act, which also operates another type of pharmacy which would otherwise be required to be licensed under the Act, is not required to secure a license for the Class A or B pharmacy. However, such licensee is required to comply with the requirements of Class A or B pharmacy rules to the extent such sections are applicable to the operation of the pharmacy.
10. A Class C-S pharmacy engaged in the compounding of nonsterile preparations shall comply with the provisions of Board Rule 291.131 (Pharmacies Compounding Nonsterile Preparations).
11. A Class C-S pharmacy engaged in the provision of remote pharmacy services including storage and dispensing of prescription drugs shall comply with the provisions of Board Rule 291.121 (Remote Pharmacy Services).
12. A Class C-S pharmacy engaged in centralized prescription dispensing and/or prescription drug or medication order processing shall comply with the provisions of Board Rule 291.123 (Central Prescription Drug or Medication Order Processing) and/or Board Rule 291.125 (Centralized Prescription Dispensing).
13. A Class C-S pharmacy with an ongoing clinical pharmacy program that proposes to allow a pharmacy technician to verify the accuracy of work performed by another pharmacy technician (tech-check-tech) relating to the filling of floor stock and unit-dose distribution systems for a patient admitted to the hospital if the patient's orders have previously been reviewed and approved by a pharmacist shall make application to the Board as follows.
    a. The pharmacist-in-charge must submit an application on a form provided by the Board containing the following information:
        (1) Name, address, and pharmacy license number;
        (2) Name and license number of the pharmacist-in-charge;
        (3) Name and registration numbers of the pharmacy technicians;

Notes

(4) Anticipated date the pharmacy plans to begin allowing a pharmacy technician to verify the accuracy of work performed by another pharmacy technician;
(5) Documentation that the pharmacy has an ongoing clinical pharmacy program; and
(6) Any other information specified on the application.
   b. The pharmacy may not allow a pharmacy technician to check the work of another pharmacy technician until the Board has reviewed and approved the application and issued an amended license to the pharmacy.
   c. Every two years, in connection with the application for renewal of the pharmacy license, the pharmacy shall provide updated documentation that the pharmacy continues to have an ongoing clinical pharmacy program as specified in a.(5) above.
14. A rural hospital that wishes to allow a pharmacy technician to perform the duties specified in Board Rule 291.73E.2.d. (Personnel) shall make application to the Board as follows.
   a. Prior to allowing a pharmacy technician to perform the duties specified in Board Rule 291.73E.2.d., the pharmacist-in-charge must submit an application on a form provided by the Board containing the following information:
      (1) Name, address, and pharmacy license number;
      (2) Name and license number of the pharmacist-in-charge;
      (3) Name and registration number of the pharmacy technicians;
      (4) Proposed date the pharmacy wishes to start allowing pharmacy technicians to perform the duties specified in Board Rule 291.73E.2.d.;
      (5) Documentation that the hospital is a rural hospital with 75 or fewer beds and that the rural hospital is either:
         (a) Located in a county with a population of 50,000 or less as defined by the United States Census Bureau in the most recent U.S. census or
         (b) Designated by the Centers for Medicare and Medicaid Services as a critical access hospital, rural referral center, or sole community hospital; and
      (6) Any other information specified on the application.
   b. A rural hospital may not allow a pharmacy technician to perform the duties specified in Board Rule 291.73E.2.d. until the Board has reviewed and approved the application and issued an amended license to the pharmacy.
   c. Every two years when applying for renewal of the pharmacy license, the pharmacist-in-charge shall update the application for pharmacy technicians to perform the duties specified in Board Rule 291.73E.2.d.

Rules for Class C Pharmacies Located in a Freestanding Ambulatory Surgical Center

Board of Pharmacy Rule 291.76
Class C Pharmacies Located in a
Freestanding Ambulatory Surgical Center (ASC)

A. Introduction.
   1. An Ambulatory Surgical Center is a freestanding facility that is licensed by the Texas Department of State Health Services that primarily provides surgical services to patients who do not require overnight hospitalization or extensive recovery, convalescent time, or observation. The planned total length of stay for an ASC patient shall not exceed 23 hours. Patient stays of greater than 23 hours shall be the result of an unanticipated medical

condition and shall occur infrequently. The 23-hour period begins with the induction of anesthesia.
2. Rules governing ASC pharmacies are substantively similar as for Class C pharmacy rules and some rules for Freestanding Emergency Medical Facility (Class F) rules. For complete details, the actual rule should be consulted, but a summary of the rules is provided below.

B. Personnel and Licensing.
  1. Pharmacist-in-charge. Each ASC pharmacy shall have one pharmacist-in-charge who is employed or under contract at least on a consulting or part-time basis but may be employed on a full-time basis.
  2. Consultant. A written contract shall exist between the ASC and any consultant pharmacist, and a copy of the written contract shall be made available to the Board upon request. The consultant pharmacist may be the pharmacist-in-charge.
  3. An ASC pharmacy shall not compound sterile preparations unless it has applied for and obtained a Class C-S pharmacy license.

C. Environment.
  1. General Requirements.
     a. Each ambulatory surgical center shall have a designated work area separate from patient areas (different from Class C rules), shall have space adequate for the size and scope of pharmaceutical services, and shall have adequate space and security for the storage of drugs.
     b. The ASC pharmacy shall be arranged in an orderly fashion and shall be kept clean. All required equipment shall be clean and in good operating condition.
  2. Security.
     a. The pharmacy and storage areas for prescription drugs and/or devices shall be enclosed and capable of being locked by key, combination, or other mechanical or electronic means so as to prohibit access by unauthorized individuals.
     b. The pharmacist-in-charge shall consult with ASC personnel with respect to the security of the drug storage areas, including provisions for adequate safeguards against theft or diversion of dangerous drugs and controlled substances and security of records for such drugs.
     c. The pharmacy shall have locked storage for Schedule II controlled substances and other drugs requiring additional security.

D. Library. A reference library shall be maintained which includes:
  1. A current copy of laws and rules and
  2. At least one current or updated general drug information reference which is required to contain drug interaction information. This reference shall include information needed to determine severity or significance of the interaction and appropriate recommendations or actions to be taken, basic antidote information, and the telephone number of the nearest regional poison control center.

E. Policies and Procedures.
Written policies and procedures for a drug distribution system shall be established by the pharmacist-in-charge with the advice of the appropriate committee.

F. Formulary.
  1. A formulary may be developed by an appropriate committee of the ASC.
  2. The pharmacist-in-charge or consultant pharmacist shall be a full voting member of any committee which involves pharmaceutical services.
  3. A practitioner may grant approval for pharmacists at the ASC to interchange drugs in accordance with the facility's formulary for the drugs on the practitioner's medication orders provided:

a. A formulary has been developed;
b. The formulary has been approved by the medical staff of the ASC;
c. There is a reasonable method for the practitioner to override any interchange; and
d. The practitioner authorizes the pharmacist in the ASC to conduct an interchange on his or her medication orders in accordance with the facility's formulary through his or her written agreement to abide by the policies and procedures of the medical staff and facility.

G. Drug Distribution for Medication Orders.

The record made when drugs are withdrawn by a licensed nurse or practitioner during the absence of the pharmacist must be verified as follows:
1. If the facility has a full-time pharmacist, this verification must be done as soon as practical but no later than 72 hours from the time of such withdrawal.
2. If the facility has a part-time or consultant pharmacist, the pharmacist shall conduct an audit of patient charts according to the schedule set out in the policies and procedures at a reasonable interval, but such interval must occur at least once in every calendar week that the pharmacy is open.

H. Records and Inventories.
1. Controlled substance records shall be maintained in a manner to establish receipt and distribution of all controlled substances.
2. An ASC pharmacy shall maintain a perpetual inventory of controlled substances in Schedules II–V which shall be verified for completeness and reconciled at least once in every calendar week that the pharmacy is open.
3. Suppliers' invoices of dangerous drugs and controlled substances must be dated and initialed or signed by the person receiving the drugs. A pharmacist shall verify that the controlled drugs listed on the invoices were added to the pharmacy's perpetual inventory by clearly recording his or her initials and the date of the review of the perpetual inventory.
4. Distribution records for controlled substances listed in Schedules II–V shall include the following information:
   a. Patient's name;
   b. Name of the practitioner who ordered the drug;
   c. Name of drug, dosage form, and strength;
   d. Time and date of administration to the patient and the quantity administered;
   e. Signature or electronic signature of individual administering the controlled substance;
   f. Returns to the pharmacy; and
   g. Drug waste (waste is required to be witnessed and cosigned manually or electronically by another individual).
5. The record required by 4. above shall be maintained separately from patient records.
6. A pharmacist shall conduct an audit by randomly comparing the distribution records required by 4. above with the medication orders in the patient record on a periodic basis to verify proper administration of drugs not to exceed 30 days between such reviews.

I. Policies and Procedures Are Not Required For:
1. Stop orders;
2. Furlough medications;
3. Monthly inspection of nursing station;
4. Routine distribution of inpatient drugs; and
5. Handling of medication orders in the absence of a pharmacist.

J. Drugs Supplied for Postoperative Use.
  1. Drugs may only be supplied to patients who have been admitted to the ASC.
  2. Drugs may only be supplied in accordance with the system of control and accountability for drugs supplied from the ASC.
  3. Only drugs on the approved postoperative drug list may be supplied. Such list shall consist of drugs to meet the immediate postoperative needs of the ASC patient.
  4. Drugs may only be supplied in prepackaged quantities not to exceed a 72-hour supply in suitable containers and appropriately prelabeled (including name, address, phone number of the facility, and necessary auxiliary labels) by the pharmacy. However, topicals and ophthalmics in the original manufacturer's containers may be supplied in a quantity exceeding a 72-hour supply.
  5. At the time of delivery of the drug, the information on the label must be completed by the practitioner.
     Note: A practitioner can legally delegate this task to another individual.
  6. A perpetual record of all drugs supplied from the ASC must be kept (same as for drugs supplied from an emergency room).
  7. A pharmacist-in-charge or other pharmacist must review the records at least once every calendar week the pharmacy is open.

CHAPTER I HIGHLIGHTS
Class C (Institutional) Pharmacy Rules

1. A Class C pharmacy is a pharmacy located in an inpatient facility including hospitals, hospices, and ambulatory surgical centers (ASCs).
2. Requirements for pharmacy services
   a. If the facility has 101 or more beds, it must be under continuous on-site supervision of a pharmacist during the times that the pharmacy department is open.
   b. If the facility has 100 beds or fewer, it may have a part-time or consultant pharmacist according to the needs of the facility, but the pharmacist must be on-site at least once every seven days.
   c. For all facilities, a pharmacist must be available for consultation by telephone 24 hours a day.
   d. Class C pharmacies must meet Class A rules for any outpatient pharmacy located at the facility including ratios of pharmacists to pharmacy technicians.
3. Pharmacist-in-Charge (PIC)
   a. Facilities licensed for 101 or more beds must have a full-time PIC. With a few exceptions, that pharmacist cannot serve as PIC for more than one facility.
   b. Facilities licensed for 100 beds or fewer may choose to have a full-time PIC or may have a part-time or consulting PIC who may be PIC for no more than 3 facilities not to exceed a total of 150 beds.
   c. The PIC is responsible for all aspects of the operation of a Class C pharmacy including:
      (1) Participating in the development of a formulary for the facility;
      (2) Participating in those aspects of the facility's patient care evaluation program which relate to pharmaceutical utilization and effectiveness;
      (3) Implementing the policies and decisions of the appropriate committee(s) relating to pharmaceutical services of the facility; and
      (4) Assuring the legal operation of the pharmacy.
4. Pharmacists
   a. Pharmacists are responsible for, among other things, any delegated act performed by pharmacy technicians and pharmacy technician trainees under his or her supervision, ensuring drugs are prepared safely and accurately as prescribed, and complying with all state and federal laws or rules governing the practice of pharmacy.
   b. Only pharmacists (not technicians) may perform the following duties:
      (1) Receiving oral prescription drug orders and oral medication orders and interpreting all orders;
      (2) Selecting prescription drugs and/or devices and/or suppliers;
      (3) Interpreting patient profiles; and
      (4) Verifying receipt of controlled substances by initialing and dating invoices of controlled substances received. However, this can be done by other personnel in a Class C-ASC pharmacy.
5. Pharmacy technicians
   a. There is no ratio of pharmacists to pharmacy technicians in a Class C pharmacy.
   b. Supervision of pharmacy technicians—Except in rural hospitals, most functions of pharmacy technicians must be supervised by physically present pharmacist supervision. However, in facilities with 101 beds or fewer, the following functions may be supervised by electronic supervision:
      (1) Preparing, packaging, or labeling prescription drugs pursuant to medication orders;
      (2) Distributing routine stock supplies to patient care areas;
      (3) Entering medication order and drug distribution information into the computer system;
      (4) Accessing automated medication supply systems;
      (5) Compounding nonsterile preparations pursuant to medication orders; and
      (6) Compounding low-risk sterile preparations pursuant to medication orders.
   c. Tech-check-tech—In facilities with an ongoing clinical pharmacy program, a pharmacy technician (not a trainee) may verify the accuracy of the following duties performed by another pharmacy technician:

(1) Filling medication carts;
(2) Distributing stock supplies to patient care areas; and
(3) Accessing and restocking automated medication supply systems.
6. Rural hospitals—Special rules apply to rural hospitals that allow pharmacy technicians to perform certain tasks in the pharmacy without the direct supervision of a pharmacist.
7. Class C pharmacies must have locked storage for Schedule II controlled substances.
8. Absence of pharmacist (pharmacy is closed)
    a. In facilities with a full-time pharmacist, a designated nurse or physician may remove drugs from the pharmacy to meet patient needs, and a pharmacist shall verify withdrawal of drugs from the pharmacy and perform a drug regimen review no more than 72 hours from the time of withdrawal.
    b. In facilities with a part-time pharmacist, a pharmacist shall verify removal of drugs from the pharmacy within seven days.
9. Drugs may be prepackaged in the pharmacy in quantities suitable for internal distribution and under certain conditions for distribution to hospitals under common ownership.
10. Class C pharmacies must have a systematic ongoing process of drug utilization review (DUR) and perform drug regimen review (DRR) on all medication orders.
    a. In facilities with a full-time pharmacist, DRR must be performed prospectively when a pharmacist is on duty and within 72 hours if a pharmacist is not on duty.
    b. In facilities with a part-time pharmacist, DRR must be performed within seven days if the hospital has an average daily census of ten or fewer patients or within 96 hours if the hospital has an average daily census of more than ten patients.
11. When a pharmacist is not on duty, drugs may be supplied for a patient to take home from the Emergency Room or the Radiology Department in prepackaged quantities not to exceed a 72-hour supply following specific procedures and recordkeeping requirements.
12. Three types of automated systems may be used in a Class C pharmacy:
    a. Automated compounding or counting device—An automated device that compounds, measures, counts, and/or packages a specified quantity of dosage units of a designated drug product.
    b. Automated medication supply system—A mechanical system such as a Pyxis machine that performs operations or activities relative to the storage and distribution of medication for administration and which collects, controls, and maintains all transaction information.
    c. Automated checking device—A fully automated device which confirms, after a drug is prepared for distribution but prior to delivery to the patient, that the correct drug and strength have been labeled with the correct label for the correct patient.
    Note: A Class C pharmacy may also use an automated storage and delivery system to deliver dispensed prescriptions at a remote site with Board approval.
13. Records
    a. A Class C pharmacy must maintain a Patient Medication Record with specific information for each patient.
    b. A perpetual inventory of Schedule II drugs is required in Class C pharmacies and for all controlled substances in a Class C-ASC pharmacy.
    c. A Class C pharmacy's computer system must be able to record the distribution and return of all controlled substances and produce an audit trail within 72 hours.
14. All Class C pharmacies that are engaged in compounding sterile preparations must obtain a Class C-S license.
15. Class C-Ambulatory Surgical Center (ASC) Pharmacies
    a. Class C-ASC pharmacy rules are similar to Class C and some Class F pharmacy rules with some modifications.
    b. Post-operative drugs may be supplied to patients to take home only in prepackaged quantities not to exceed a 72-hour supply.
    c. If the Class C-ASC pharmacy has a full-time pharmacist, records of drugs withdrawn during the absence of the pharmacist must be reviewed by a pharmacist within 72 hours.

d. If the Class C-ASC pharmacy has a part-time or consultant pharmacist, the pharmacist must conduct an audit of patient charts at least every calendar week that the pharmacy is open.
e. Class C-ASC pharmacies must maintain a perpetual inventory of all controlled substances which is verified for completeness and reconciled at least once in every calendar week that the pharmacy is open.
f. Invoices of dangerous drugs and controlled substances must be dated and initialed or signed by the person receiving the drugs. A pharmacist must verify that the controlled drugs listed on the invoices were added to the pharmacy's perpetual inventory.
g. A pharmacist must conduct an audit of distribution records with the medication orders in patient records at least every 30 days.

CHAPTER J

Other Classes of Pharmacies

CHAPTER J

Other Classes of Pharmacies

Nuclear Pharmacy (Class B) Rules

Board of Pharmacy Rule 291.51
Purpose

The purpose of this subchapter is to provide standards for the preparation, labeling, and distribution of radiopharmaceuticals by licensed nuclear pharmacies, pursuant to a radioactive prescription drug order. The intent of this subchapter is to establish a minimum acceptable level of pharmaceutical care to the patient so that the patient's health is protected while contributing to positive patient outcomes. The Board has determined that this subchapter is necessary to protect the health and welfare of the citizens of this state.

Board of Pharmacy Rule 291.52
Definitions

A. **Authorized nuclear pharmacist**—A pharmacist who has completed the specialized training requirements for the preparation and distribution of radiopharmaceuticals and is named on a Texas radioactive material license issued by the Texas Department of State Health Services, Radiation Control Program.
B. **Authorized user**—Any individual or institution named on a radioactive material license issued by the Texas Department of State Health Services, Radiation Control Program.
C. **Diagnostic prescription drug order**—A radioactive prescription drug order issued for a diagnostic purpose.
D. **Dispense**—Preparing, packaging, compounding, or labeling for delivery of a prescription drug or device or a radiopharmaceutical in the course of professional practice to an ultimate user or his or her agent by or pursuant to the lawful order of a practitioner.
E. **Nuclear pharmacy technique**—The mechanical ability required to perform the non-judgmental, technical aspects of preparing and dispensing radiopharmaceuticals.
F. **Radiopharmaceutical**—A drug and/or radioactive drug or device that exhibits spontaneous disintegration of unstable nuclei with the emission of a nuclear particle(s) or photon(s), including any nonradioactive reagent kit or nuclide generator that is intended to be used in the preparation of any such substance.
G. **Radioactive drug service**—The act of distributing radiopharmaceuticals, the participation in radiopharmaceutical selection, and the performance of radiopharmaceutical drug reviews.
H. **Ultimate user**—A person who has obtained and possesses a prescription drug or radiopharmaceutical for administration to a patient by a practitioner.

Board of Pharmacy Rule 291.53
Personnel

A. Pharmacist-in-Charge.
   1. General.
      a. Every nuclear pharmacy shall have an authorized nuclear pharmacist designated on the nuclear pharmacy license as the pharmacist-in-charge

who shall be responsible for a nuclear pharmacy's compliance with state and federal laws and regulations pertaining to the practice of nuclear pharmacy.
- b. The nuclear pharmacy pharmacist-in-charge shall see that directives from the Board are communicated to the owner(s), management, other pharmacists, and interns of the nuclear pharmacy.
- c. Each Class B pharmacy shall have one pharmacist-in-charge who is employed on a full-time basis and who may be the pharmacist-in-charge for only one such pharmacy. However, such pharmacist-in-charge may be the pharmacist-in-charge of:
  - (1) More than one Class B pharmacy if the additional Class B pharmacies are not open to provide pharmacy services simultaneously or
  - (2) During an emergency, up to two Class B pharmacies open simultaneously if the pharmacist-in-charge works at least 10 hours per week in each pharmacy for no more than 30 consecutive days.
- d. The pharmacist-in-charge of a Class B pharmacy may not serve as the pharmacist-in-charge of a Class A pharmacy or a Class C pharmacy with 101 beds or more.

2. Responsibilities.
   - a. Ensuring that radiopharmaceuticals are dispensed and delivered safely and accurately as prescribed;
   - b. Developing a system to assure that all pharmacy personnel responsible for compounding and/or supervising the compounding of radiopharmaceuticals within the pharmacy receive appropriate education and training and competency evaluation;
   - c. Determining that all pharmacists involved in compounding sterile radiopharmaceuticals obtain continuing education appropriate for the type of compounding done by the pharmacist;
   - d. Supervising a system to assure appropriate procurement of drugs and devices and storage of all pharmaceutical materials including radiopharmaceuticals, components used in the compounding of radiopharmaceuticals, and drug delivery devices;
   - e. Assuring that the equipment used in compounding is properly maintained;
   - f. Developing a system for the disposal and distribution of drugs from the Class B pharmacy;
   - g. Developing a system for bulk compounding or batch preparation of radiopharmaceuticals;
   - h. Developing a system for the compounding, sterility assurance, and quality control of sterile radiopharmaceuticals;
   - i. Maintaining records of all transactions of the Class B pharmacy necessary to have accurate control over and accountability for all pharmaceutical materials including radiopharmaceuticals as required by applicable state and federal laws and rules;
   - j. Developing a system to assure the maintenance of effective controls against the theft or diversion of prescription drugs and records for such drugs;
   - k. Assuring that the pharmacy has a system to dispose of radioactive and cytotoxic waste in a manner so as not to endanger the public health; and
   - l. Legally operating the pharmacy including meeting all inspection and other requirements of all state and federal laws or rules governing the practice of pharmacy.

B. Owner. The owner of a Class B pharmacy shall have responsibility for all administrative and operational functions of the pharmacy. The pharmacist-in-charge

may advise the owner on administrative and operational concerns. If the owner is not a Texas licensed pharmacist, the owner shall consult with the pharmacist-in-charge or another Texas licensed pharmacist. The owner shall have responsibility for, at a minimum, the following:
1. Establishing policies for procurement of prescription drugs and devices and other products dispensed from the Class B pharmacy;
2. Establishing policies and procedures for the security of the prescription department including the maintenance of effective controls against the theft or diversion of prescription drugs;
3. If the pharmacy uses an automated pharmacy dispensing system, reviewing and approving all policies and procedures for system operation, safety, security, accuracy and access, patient confidentiality, prevention of unauthorized access, and malfunction;
4. Providing the pharmacy with the necessary equipment and resources commensurate with its level and type of practice; and
5. Establishing policies and procedures regarding maintenance, storage, and retrieval of records in a data processing system such that the system is in compliance with state and federal requirements.

C. Authorized Nuclear Pharmacist.
  1. General.
     a. The pharmacist-in-charge shall be assisted by a sufficient number of additional authorized nuclear pharmacists as may be required to operate the pharmacy competently, safely, and adequately to meet the needs of the patients of the pharmacy.
     b. All personnel performing tasks in the preparation and distribution of radiopharmaceuticals shall be under the direct supervision of an authorized nuclear pharmacist. General qualifications for an authorized nuclear pharmacist are the following. A pharmacist shall:
        (1) Meet minimal standards of training and experience in the handling of radioactive materials in accordance with the requirements of the Texas Regulations for Control of Radiation of the Texas Department of State Health Services, Radiation Control Program;
        (2) Be a pharmacist licensed by the Board to practice pharmacy in Texas; and
        (3) Submit to the Board either:
           (a) Written certification that he or she has current Board certification as a nuclear pharmacist by the Board of Pharmaceutical Specialties or
           (b) Written certification signed by a preceptor authorized nuclear pharmacist that he or she has achieved a level of competency sufficient to independently operate as an authorized nuclear pharmacist and has satisfactorily completed 700 hours in a structured educational program consisting of both:
              (i) 200 hours of didactic training in a program approved by the Radiation Control Program, Texas Department of State Health Services involving the following:
                 (I) Radiation physics and instrumentation;
                 (II) Radiation protection;
                 (III) Mathematics pertaining to the use and measurement of radioactivity;
                 (IV) Radiation biology; and
                 (V) Chemistry of radioactive material for medical use and
              (ii) 500 hours of supervised practical experience in a nuclear pharmacy involving the following:

(I) Shipping, receiving, and performing related radiation surveys;
(II) Using and performing checks for proper operation of instruments used to determine the activity of dosages, survey meters, and, if appropriate, instruments used to measure alpha- or beta-emitting radionuclides;
(III) Calculating, assaying, and safely preparing dosages for patients or human research subjects;
(IV) Using administrative controls to avoid adverse medical events in the administration of radioactive material; and
(V) Using procedures to prevent or minimize contamination.
c. Authorized nuclear pharmacists are solely responsible for the direct supervision of pharmacy technicians and pharmacy technician trainees and for delegating nuclear pharmacy techniques and additional duties, other than those listed in 3. below, to pharmacy technicians and pharmacy technician trainees. Each authorized nuclear pharmacist shall:
   (1) Verify the accuracy of all acts, tasks, or functions performed by pharmacy technicians and pharmacy technician trainees and
   (2) Be responsible for any delegated act performed by pharmacy technicians and pharmacy technician trainees under his or her supervision.
d. All authorized nuclear pharmacists while on duty shall be responsible for complying with all state and federal laws or rules governing the practice of pharmacy.
e. The dispensing pharmacist shall ensure that the drug is dispensed and delivered safely and accurately as prescribed.

2. Special Requirements for Compounding.
   a. Nonsterile preparations. All pharmacists engaged in compounding nonsterile preparations, including radioactive preparations, shall meet the training requirements specified in Board Rule 291.131 (Pharmacies Compounding Nonsterile Preparations).
   b. Sterile preparations. All pharmacists engaged in compounding sterile preparations, including radioactive preparations, shall meet the training requirements specified in Board Rule 291.133 (Pharmacies Compounding Sterile Preparations).

3. Duties.
   Duties which may only be performed by an authorized nuclear pharmacist are as follows:
   a. Receiving verbal therapeutic prescription drug orders and reducing these orders to writing, either manually or electronically;
   b. Receiving verbal diagnostic prescription drug orders in instances where patient specificity is required for patient safety (e.g., radiolabeled blood products or radiolabeled antibodies) and reducing these orders to writing, either manually or electronically;
   c. Interpreting and evaluating radioactive prescription drug orders;
   d. Selecting drug products; and
   e. Performing the final check of the dispensed prescription before delivery to the patient to ensure that the radioactive prescription drug order has been dispensed accurately as prescribed.

D. Pharmacy Technicians and Pharmacy Technician Trainees.
   1. General.
   All pharmacy technicians and pharmacy technician trainees shall meet the training requirements specified in Board Rule 297.6 (Pharmacy Technician and Pharmacy Technician Trainee Training).

2. Special Requirements for Compounding.
   a. Nonsterile preparations. All pharmacy technicians and pharmacy technician trainees engaged in compounding nonsterile preparations, including radioactive preparations, shall meet the training requirements specified in Board Rule 291.131 (Pharmacies Compounding Nonsterile Preparations).
   b. Sterile preparations. All pharmacy technicians and pharmacy technician trainees engaged in compounding sterile preparations, including radioactive preparations, shall meet the training requirements specified in Board Rule 291.133 (Pharmacies Compounding Sterile Preparations).
3. Duties.
   a. Pharmacy technicians and pharmacy technician trainees may not perform any of the duties listed as duties that may only be performed by an authorized nuclear pharmacist.
   b. An authorized nuclear pharmacist may delegate to pharmacy technicians and pharmacy technician trainees any nuclear pharmacy technique which is associated with the preparation and distribution of radiopharmaceuticals provided:
      (1) An authorized nuclear pharmacist verifies the accuracy of all acts, tasks, and functions performed by pharmacy technicians and pharmacy technician trainees and
      (2) Pharmacy technicians and pharmacy technician trainees are under the direct supervision of and responsible to a pharmacist.
4. Ratio of Authorized Nuclear Pharmacists to Pharmacy Technicians and Pharmacy Technician Trainees.
   a. The ratio of authorized nuclear pharmacists to pharmacy technicians and pharmacy technician trainees may be 1:4 provided at least one of the four technicians is a pharmacy technician and is trained in the handling of radioactive materials.
   b. The ratio of authorized nuclear pharmacists to pharmacy technician trainees may not exceed 1:3.

Board of Pharmacy Rule 291.54
Operational Standards

A. Licensing Requirements.
   1. A Class B pharmacy must provide evidence to the Board of the possession of a Texas Department of State Health Services radioactive material license or proof of application for a radioactive material license.
   2. It is unlawful for a person to provide radioactive drug services unless such provision is performed by a person licensed to act as an authorized nuclear pharmacist as defined by the Board or is a person acting under the direct supervision of an authorized nuclear pharmacist acting in accordance with the Act and rules and the rules of the Texas Department of State Health Services, Radiation Control Program. This rule does not apply to:
      a. Licensed practitioners or designated agents for administration to his or her patient in accordance with the requirements of the Texas Department of State Health Services, Radiation Control Program and
      b. Institutions or facilities with nuclear medicine services operated by a practitioner licensed by the Texas Department of State Health Services, Radiation Control Program.
   3. A Class B pharmacy engaged in the compounding of nonsterile preparations including radioactive preparations shall comply with the provisions of Board Rule 291.131 (Pharmacies Compounding Nonsterile Preparations).

4. A Class B pharmacy engaged in the compounding of sterile preparations including radioactive preparations shall comply with the provisions of Board Rule 291.133 (Pharmacies Compounding Sterile Preparations) using only radiopharmaceuticals from FDA-approved drug products.
5. A Class B pharmacy may not renew a pharmacy license unless the pharmacy has been inspected by the Board within the last renewal period.

B. Environment.
1. The pharmacy shall be arranged in an orderly fashion and kept clean. All required equipment shall be clean and in good operating condition.
2. The pharmacy shall have a sink with hot and cold running water within the pharmacy, exclusive of restroom facilities, available to all pharmacy personnel and maintained in a sanitary condition.
3. The pharmacy shall be properly lighted and ventilated.
4. The temperature of the pharmacy shall be maintained within a range compatible with the proper storage of drugs. The temperature of the refrigerator shall be maintained within a range compatible with the proper storage of drugs requiring refrigeration.
5. If the pharmacy has flammable materials, the pharmacy shall have a designated area for the storage of flammable materials. Such area shall meet the requirements set by local and state fire laws.

C. Prescription Dispensing and Delivery.
1. Generic Substitution. A pharmacist may substitute on a prescription drug order issued for a brand name product provided the substitution is authorized and performed in compliance with Chapter 309 of the Act (Substitution of Drug Products).
2. Prescription Containers (immediate inner containers).
   a. A drug dispensed pursuant to a radioactive prescription drug order shall be dispensed in an appropriate immediate inner container as follows.
      (1) If a drug is susceptible to light, the drug shall be dispensed in a light-resistant container.
      (2) If a drug is susceptible to moisture, the drug shall be dispensed in a tight container.
      (3) The container should not interact physically or chemically with the drug product placed in it so as to alter the strength, quality, or purity of the drug beyond the official requirements.
   b. Immediate inner prescription containers or closures shall not be reused.
3. Delivery Containers (outer containers).
   a. Prescription containers may be placed in suitable containers for delivery which will transport the radiopharmaceutical safely in compliance with all applicable laws and regulations.
   b. Delivery containers may be reused provided they are maintained in a manner to prevent cross contamination.
4. Labeling.
   a. The immediate inner container of a radiopharmaceutical shall be labeled with:
      (1) The standard radiation symbol;
      (2) The words "caution—radioactive material" or "danger—radioactive material";
      (3) The name of the radiopharmaceutical or its abbreviation; and
      (4) The unique identification number of the prescription.
   b. The outer container of a radiopharmaceutical shall be labeled with:
      (1) The name, address, and phone number of the pharmacy;
      (2) The date dispensed;

(3) The directions for use if applicable;
(4) The unique identification number of the prescription;
(5) The name of the patient if known or the statement "for physician use" if the patient is unknown;
(6) The standard radiation symbol;
(7) The words "caution—radioactive material" or "danger—radioactive material";
(8) The name of the radiopharmaceutical or its abbreviation;
(9) The amount of radioactive material contained in millicuries (mCi), microcuries (uCi), or bequerels (Bq) and the corresponding time that applies to this activity if different from the requested calibration date and time;
(10) The initials or identification codes of the person preparing the product and the authorized nuclear pharmacist who checked and released the final product unless recorded in the pharmacy's data processing system. The record of the identity of these individuals shall not be altered in the pharmacy's data processing system;
(11) If a liquid, the volume in milliliters;
(12) The requested calibration date and time; and
(13) The expiration date and/or time.
c. The amount of radioactivity shall be determined by radiometric methods for each individual preparation immediately at the time of dispensing. Calculations shall be made to determine the amount of activity that will be present at the requested calibration date and time due to radioactive decay in the intervening period, and this activity and time shall be placed on the label as required in 4.b above.

D. Equipment.
1. Vertical laminar flow hood;
2. Dose calibrator;
3. A calibrated system or device (i.e., thermometer) to monitor the temperature to ensure that proper storage requirements are met if preparations are stored in the refrigerator;
4. Class A prescription balance or analytical balance;
5. Scintillation analyzer;
6. Microscope and hemocytometer;
7. Equipment and utensils necessary for the proper compounding of prescription drug or medication orders;
8. Appropriate disposal containers for used needles, syringes, etc., and, if applicable, cytotoxic waste from the preparation of chemotherapeutic agents and/or biohazardous waste;
9. All necessary supplies;
10. Adequate glassware, utensils, gloves, syringe shields, remote handling devices, and adequate equipment for product quality control;
11. Adequate shielding material;
12. Data processing system including a printer or comparable equipment;
13. Radiation dosimeters for visitors and personnel and log entry book;
14. Exhaust/fume hood with monitor; and
15. Adequate radiation monitor(s).

E. Library (current or updated versions in hard copy or electronic format).
1. Texas Pharmacy Act and Rules;
2. Texas Dangerous Drug Act and Rules;
3. Texas Controlled Substances Act and Rules;
4. Federal Controlled Substances Act and Rules; and
5. A minimum of one text dealing with nuclear medicine science.

F. Radiopharmaceuticals and/or Radioactive Materials.
1. Radiopharmaceuticals may only be dispensed pursuant to a radioactive prescription drug order.
2. An authorized nuclear pharmacist may distribute radiopharmaceuticals to authorized users for patient use. A nuclear pharmacy may also furnish radiopharmaceuticals for departmental or physician's use if such authorized users maintain a Texas radioactive materials license.
3. An authorized nuclear pharmacist may transfer to authorized users radioactive materials not intended for drug use in accordance with the requirements of the Texas Department of State Health Services, Radiation Control Program.
4. Transportation of radioactive materials from the nuclear pharmacy must be in accordance with current state and federal transportation regulations.
5. Procurement and Storage.
    a. The pharmacist-in-charge shall have the responsibility for the procurement and storage of drugs but may receive input from other appropriate staff relative to such responsibility.
    b. Prescription drugs and devices shall be stored within the prescription department or a locked storage area.
    c. All drugs shall be stored at the proper temperature as defined in the USP/NF and Board Rule 291.15 (Storage of Drugs).
    d. The pharmacy's generator(s) shall be stored and eluted in an ISO Class 7 or ISO Class 8 environment as specified in Board Rule 291.133.

Board of Pharmacy Rule 291.55
Records

A. Policy and Procedure Manual.
1. A Class B pharmacy must maintain a policy and procedure manual that is a compilation of written policy and procedure statements for the operation of the pharmacy.
2. A technical operations manual of nuclear pharmacy functions must be prepared which reflects current changes in techniques and organization. All pharmacy personnel must be familiar with the contents.
3. The pharmacist-in-charge prepares the policy and procedure manual with input from the affected personnel and other involved staff and committees to govern procurement, preparation, distribution, storage, disposal, and procedures relative to procurement of multisource items, inventory, investigational drugs, and new drug applications.
B. Prescriptions (radioactive prescription drug orders).
Note: Radioactive prescription drug orders may not be refilled (Board Rule 291.55(b)(8)).
1. Prescription drug order information shall include:
    a. Name of the patient, if applicable, at the time of the order;
    b. Name of institution;
    c. Name and, if for a controlled substance, address and DEA registration number of the practitioner;
    d. Name of the radiopharmaceutical;
    e. Amount of radioactive material contained in millicuries (mCi), microcuries (uCi), or bequerels (Bq) and the corresponding time that applies to this activity if different than the requested calibration date and time;
    f. Date and time of calibration; and
    g. Date of issuance.

2. At the time of dispensing, a pharmacist is responsible for adding the following information to the original prescription:
   a. Unique identification number of the prescription drug order;
   b. Initials or identification code of the person who compounded the sterile radiopharmaceutical and the pharmacist who checked and released the product unless maintained in a readily retrievable format;
   c. Name, quantity, lot number, and expiration date of each product used in compounding the sterile radiopharmaceutical; and
   d. Date of dispensing if different from the date of issuance.

Clinic Pharmacy (Class D) Rules

Board of Pharmacy Rule 291.91
Definitions

A. **Clinic**—A facility/location other than a physician's office where limited types of dangerous drugs or devices restricted to those listed in and approved for the clinic's formulary are stored, administered, provided, or dispensed to outpatients.
B. **Consultant pharmacist**—A pharmacist retained by a clinic on a routine basis to consult with the clinic in areas that pertain to the practice of pharmacy.
C. **Continuous supervision**—Supervision provided by the pharmacist-in-charge, consultant pharmacist, and/or staff pharmacist that consists of on-site and telephone supervision, routine inspection, and a policy and procedure manual.
D. **Indigent**—Person who meets or falls below 185% of the federal poverty income guidelines as established from time to time by the U.S. Department of Health and Human Services.
E. **Limited type of device**—An instrument, apparatus, implement, machine, contrivance, implant, in vitro reagent, or other similar or related article, including any component part or accessory, that is required under federal or state law to be ordered or prescribed by a practitioner that is contained in the clinic formulary and that is to be administered, dispensed, or provided according to the objectives of the clinic.
F. **Limited type of drug**—A dangerous drug contained in the clinic formulary that is to be administered, dispensed, or provided according to the objectives of the clinic.
G. **Outpatient**—An ambulatory patient who comes to a clinic to receive services related to the objectives of the clinic and departs the same day.
H. **Pharmacist**—A person licensed by the Board to practice pharmacy.
I. **Pharmacist-in-charge**—The pharmacist designated on a pharmacy license as the pharmacist who is responsible for a pharmacy's compliance with laws and rules pertaining to the practice of pharmacy.
J. **Prepackaging**—A method of packaging a drug product into a single container which contains more than one dosage unit and usually contains sufficient quantity of medication for one normal course of therapy.
K. **Provide**—To supply one or more unit doses of a nonprescription drug or dangerous drug to a patient.
L. **Standing delegation order**—A written order from a physician and designed for a patient population with specific diseases, disorders, health problems, or sets of symptoms which provides authority for and a plan for use with patients presenting themselves prior to being examined or evaluated by a physician to assure that such acts are carried out correctly and are distinct from specific orders written for a particular patient. (Physician does not examine the patient first.)

M. **Standing medical order**—A written order from a physician or the medical staff of an institution for patients who have been examined or evaluated by a physician and where such an order is used as a guide in preparing and carrying out medical and/or surgical procedures. (Physician examines the patient first.)
N. **Supportive personnel**—Individuals under the supervision of a pharmacist-in-charge, designated by the pharmacist-in-charge, and for whom the pharmacist-in-charge assumes legal responsibility and who function and perform under the instructions of the pharmacist-in-charge.
O. **Unit of use**—A sufficient quantity of a drug product for one normal course of therapy.

Board of Pharmacy Rule 291.92
Personnel

A. Pharmacist-in-Charge—There is no limit on the number of Class D pharmacies he or she can supervise.
   1. General.
      a. A pharmacist-in-charge is employed or under written agreement at least on a consulting or part-time basis and may be a pharmacist-in-charge of more than one Class D pharmacy.
      b. A written agreement shall exist between the clinic and the pharmacist-in-charge, and a copy of the agreement must be available to the Board (i.e., during compliance inspections).
   2. Responsibilities.
      a. Continuous supervision of registered nurses, licensed vocational nurses, physician assistants, pharmacy technicians, pharmacy technician trainees, and assistants carrying out the pharmacy-related aspects of provision;
      b. Documented periodic on-site visits;
      c. Development of a formulary for the clinic with the clinic's pharmacy and therapeutics committee;
      d. Procurement and storage of drugs and/or devices;
      e. Determining specifications of all drugs and/or devices;
      f. Maintenance of records to maintain accurate control and accountability for all drugs and/or devices;
      g. Development and at least annual review of a policy and procedure manual with the clinic's pharmacy and therapeutics committee;
      h. Meeting inspection and other applicable requirements of the Texas Pharmacy Act including Class D rules;
      i. Dispensing prescription drug orders; and
      j. Conducting in-service training at least annually for supportive personnel who provide drugs related to actions, contraindications, adverse reactions, and pharmacology of drugs contained in the formulary.
B. Consultant Pharmacist.
   1. May be the pharmacist-in-charge.
   2. May be retained by more than one clinic.
C. Staff Pharmacists.
   1. The pharmacist-in-charge may be assisted by a sufficient number of additional pharmacists.
   2. A staff and/or consultant pharmacist shall assist the pharmacist-in-charge in meeting the responsibilities of the pharmacist-in-charge.
   3. A staff and/or consultant pharmacist shall be responsible for any delegated act performed by supportive personnel under his or her supervision.

D. Supportive Personnel.
1. Qualifications.
   a. Shall possess education and training necessary to carry out their responsibilities. (May be a nurse supervised by a physician and pharmacists.)
   b. Shall be qualified to perform the pharmacy tasks assigned to them.
2. Duties.
   a. Prepackaging and labeling unit-of-use packages under the direct supervision of a pharmacist. The pharmacist conducts in-process and final checks and affixes his or her signature to quality control records;
   b. Maintaining inventories of drugs and/or devices; and
   c. Maintaining pharmacy records.
3. Absence of the Pharmacist. The pharmacist-in-charge shall designate from among the supportive personnel a person to supervise the day-to-day pharmacy-related operations of the clinic.
4. There is no pharmacist to supportive personnel ratio.

E. Owner. The owner of a Class D pharmacy shall have responsibility for all administrative and operational functions of the pharmacy. The pharmacist-in-charge may advise the owner on administrative and operational concerns. If the owner is not a Texas licensed pharmacist, the owner shall consult with the pharmacist-in-charge or another Texas licensed pharmacist. The owner shall have responsibility for, at a minimum, the following:
1. Establishing policies for procurement of prescription drugs and devices and other products provided or dispensed from the Class D pharmacy;
2. Establishing and maintaining effective controls against the theft or diversion of prescription drugs;
3. Providing the pharmacy with the necessary equipment and resources commensurate with its level and type of practice; and
4. Establishing policies and procedures regarding maintenance, storage, and retrieval of records in a data processing system such that the system is in compliance with state and federal requirements.

Board of Pharmacy Rule 291.93
Operational Standards

A. Registration.
1. General Requirements.
   a. A Class D pharmacy shall obtain a license from the Board following the procedures specified in Board Rule 291.1 (Pharmacy License Application).
   b. A copy of the policy and procedure manual which includes the formulary shall be provided to the Board with the initial license application.
   c. Fees.
      (1) A fee as specified in Board Rule 291.6 will be charged for licensure.
      (2) A pharmacy operated by the state or a local government is not required to pay a license fee.
   d. Change of ownership. A Class D pharmacy that changes ownership must notify the Board within 10 days of the change in ownership and apply for a new and separate license as specified in Board Rule 291.3.
   e. Change in name or location. A Class D pharmacy shall notify the Board of any change in name or location as specified in Board Rule 291.3.
   Note: The Board requires notification no later than 30 days prior to the date for a change in location and within 10 days for a change of name.
   f. A separate license is required for each principal place of business. Only one pharmacy license may be issued to a specific location.

g. A Class D pharmacy shall notify the Board in writing within 10 days of a change of the pharmacist-in-charge or staff pharmacist or consultant pharmacist.
h. A Class D pharmacy shall notify the Board in writing within 10 days of closing following the procedures specified in Board Rule 291.5.
2. Registration Requirements for Facilities That Operate at Temporary Clinic Sites. A facility that operates a clinic at one or more temporary locations may be licensed as a Class D Pharmacy and provide dangerous drugs from the temporary locations provided:
a. The pharmacy complies with the registration requirements in A. (Registration) above;
b. The pharmacy has a permanent location where all dangerous drugs and records are stored within the Class D pharmacy or within the pharmacy's mobile unit. This is allowed provided the mobile clinic vehicle is parked at the location of the Class D pharmacy in a secure area with adequate measures to prevent unauthorized access and the drugs are maintained at proper temperatures;
c. No dangerous drugs are stored or left for later pick up by the patient at a temporary location. All drugs must be returned to the permanent location each day;
d. The permanent location is the address of record for the pharmacy;
e. The facility has no more than six temporary locations in operation simultaneously;
f. The pharmacy notifies the Board of the locations of the temporary locations where drugs will be provided and the schedule for operation of such clinics; and
g. The pharmacy notifies the Board within 10 days of a change in address, the closing of a temporary location, or a change in the schedule of operation of a clinic.

B. Environment.
1. General Requirements.
a. There must be a designated area(s) for the storage of dangerous drugs and/or devices.
b. The pharmacy shall not be unclean, unsanitary, or under any condition which endangers the health, safety, or welfare of the public.
c. The Class D pharmacy shall comply with all federal, state, and local health laws and ordinances.
d. A sink with hot and cold running water shall be available to all pharmacy personnel and be maintained in a sanitary condition.
2. Security.
a. Only authorized personnel may have access to storage areas for dangerous drugs and/or devices.
b. Storage areas for dangerous drugs and/or devices shall be locked by key, combination, or other mechanical or electronic means so as to prohibit access by unauthorized individuals.
c. The pharmacist-in-charge is responsible for the security of all storage areas for dangerous drugs and/or devices.
d. The pharmacist-in-charge shall consult with clinic personnel with respect to the security of the pharmacy.
e. Housekeeping and maintenance duties shall be carried out in the pharmacy while the pharmacist-in-charge, consultant pharmacist, staff pharmacist, or supportive personnel are on the premises.

C. Equipment. Each Class D pharmacy shall maintain the following equipment and supplies.
 1. If the Class D pharmacy prepackages drugs for provision:
    a. A typewriter or comparable equipment and
    b. An adequate supply of child-resistant, moisture-proof, and light-proof containers and prescription, poison, and other applicable identification labels used in dispensing and providing of drugs.
 2. If the Class D pharmacy maintains dangerous drugs requiring refrigeration and/or freezing, a refrigerator and/or freezer.
 3. If the Class D pharmacy compounds prescriptions, a properly maintained Class A prescription balance (with weights) or equivalent analytical balance which shall be inspected at least every three years.
D. Library. A reference library shall be maintained which includes the following:
 1. Current topics of the following laws:
    a. Texas Pharmacy Act and Rules and
    b. Texas Dangerous Drug Act.
 2. Current copies of at least two of the following references:
    a. "Facts and Comparisons" with current supplements;
    b. "American Hospital Formulary Service" with current supplements;
    c. "United States Pharmacopeia Dispensing Information" (USP DI);
    d. "Physician's Desk Reference" (PDR);
    e. "American Drug Index";
    f. A reference text on drug interactions such as *Drug Interaction Facts*. A separate reference is not required if other references maintained by the pharmacy contain drug interaction information including information needed to determine the severity or significance of the interaction and appropriate recommendations or actions to be taken;
    g. Reference texts in any of the following subjects: toxicology, pharmacology, or drug interactions; or
    h. Reference texts pertinent to the major function(s) of the clinic.
E. Drugs and Devices.
 1. Formulary.
    a. Each Class D pharmacy shall have a formulary which lists all drugs and devices that are administered, dispensed, or provided by the Class D pharmacy.
    b. The formulary shall be limited to the following types of drugs and devices, exclusive of injectable drugs for administration in the clinic and nonprescription drugs, except as provided in d. below.
       (1) Anti-infective drugs;
       (2) Musculoskeletal drugs;
       (3) Vitamins;
       (4) Obstetrical and gynecological drugs and devices;
       (5) Topical drugs; and
       (6) Serums, toxoids, and vaccines.
    c. The formulary shall not contain the following drugs or types of drugs:
       (1) Nalbuphine (Nubain®);
       (2) Drugs to treat erectile dysfunction; and
       (3) Schedule I–V controlled substances.
    d. Expanded formulary. Clinics with a patient population which consists of at least 80% indigent patients may petition the Board to operate with a formulary which includes types of dangerous drugs and/or devices, other than those listed in E.1.b. above, based upon documented

objectives of the clinic under the following conditions. However, controlled substances and other drugs prohibited in E.1.c. above are not allowed under any circumstances.

(1) Such petition shall contain an affidavit with the notarized signature of the medical director, the pharmacist-in-charge, and the owner/chief executive officer of the clinic and include the following documentation:
   (a) The objectives of the clinic;
   (b) The total number of patients served by the clinic during the previous fiscal year or calendar year;
   (c) The total number of indigent patients served by the clinic during the previous fiscal year or calendar year;
   (d) The percentage of clinic patients who are indigent based upon the patient population during the previous fiscal year or calendar year;
   (e) The proposed formulary and the need for additional types of drugs based upon objectives of the clinic; and
   (f) If the provision of any drugs on the proposed formulary requires special monitoring, the Class D pharmacy shall submit relevant sections of the clinic's policy and procedure manual regarding the provision of drugs that require special monitoring.

(2) The petition shall be resubmitted every two years with the application for the renewal of the pharmacy license.
   (a) Such renewal petition shall contain the documentation required in d.(1) above.
   (b) If at the time of the renewal of the pharmacy license the patient population for the previous fiscal year or calendar year is below 80% indigent patients, the clinic shall be required to submit an application for a Class A pharmacy license or shall limit the clinic formulary to those types of drugs and/or devices listed in 1.b. and c. above.

(3) If a Class D pharmacy wishes to add additional drugs to the expanded formulary, the pharmacy shall petition the Board in writing prior to adding such drugs to the formulary. The petition shall identify drugs to be added and the need for the additional drugs based upon objectives of the clinic as specified in d.(1) above.

(4) The following additional requirements shall be satisfied for clinic pharmacies with expanded formularies.
   (a) Supportive personnel who are providing drugs shall be licensed nurses or practitioners.
   (b) If the pharmacy provides drugs which require special monitoring (i.e., drugs which require follow-up laboratory work or drugs which should not be discontinued abruptly), the pharmacy shall have policies and procedures for the provision of prescription drugs to patients and the monitoring of patients who receive such drugs.
   (c) The pharmacist-in-charge, consultant pharmacists, or staff pharmacists shall conduct retrospective drug regimen reviews of a random sample of patients of the clinic on at least a quarterly basis. The pharmacist-in-charge shall be responsible for ensuring that a report regarding the drug regimen review, including the number of patients reviewed, is submitted to the clinic's medical director and the pharmacy and therapeutics committee of the clinic.

            (d) If a pharmacy provides antipsychotic drugs:
                (i) A practitioner of the clinic shall initiate the therapy;
                (ii) A practitioner shall monitor and order ongoing therapy; and
                (iii) The patient shall be physically examined by the practitioner at least on a yearly basis.
        (5) The Board may consider the following items in approving or disapproving a petition for an expanded formulary:
            (a) Degree of compliance on past compliance inspections;
            (b) Size of the patient population of the clinic;
            (c) Number and types of drugs contained in the formulary; and
            (d) Objectives of the clinic.
2. Storage.
    a. Drugs and/or devices which bear the words "Caution: Federal Law Prohibits Dispensing Without Prescription" or "Rx only" shall be stored in secured storage areas.
    b. All drugs shall be stored at the proper temperatures as defined in Board Rule 291.15 (Storage of Drugs).
    c. Any drug or device bearing an expiration date may not be provided, dispensed, or administered beyond the expiration date of the drug and/or device.
    d. Outdated drugs or devices shall be removed from stock and shall be quarantined together until such drugs or devices are disposed.
    e. Controlled substances may not be stored at the Class D pharmacy.
3. Drug Samples.
    a. Drug samples of drugs listed on the clinic's formulary and supplied to physicians by manufacturers shall be properly stored, labeled, provided, or dispensed by the Class D pharmacy in the same manner as prescribed by these rules for dangerous drugs.
    b. Samples of controlled substances may not be stored, provided, or dispensed in the Class D pharmacy.
4. Prepackaging and Labeling for Provision.
    a. Drugs may be prepackaged and labeled for provision in the Class D pharmacy. Such prepackaging shall be performed by a pharmacist or supportive personnel under the direct supervision of a pharmacist in the Class D pharmacy and shall be for the internal use of the clinic (i.e., cannot be used by another clinic) unless additional registration (as a distributor) is obtained from the Texas Department of Health.
    b. Drugs must be prepackaged in suitable containers.
    c. The label of the prepackaged unit shall bear:
        (1) The name, address, and telephone number of the clinic;
        (2) Directions for use which may include incomplete directions for use provided:
            (a) Labeling with incomplete directions for use has been authorized by the pharmacy and therapeutics committee;
            (b) Precise requirements for completion of the directions for use are developed by the pharmacy and therapeutics committee and maintained in the pharmacy policy and procedure manual; and
            (c) The directions for use are completed by practitioners, pharmacists, or licensed nurses;
        (3) Name and strength of the drug; if a generic name, the name of the manufacturer or distributor of the drug;
        (4) Quantity;
        (5) Lot number and expiration date; and
        (6) Appropriate ancillary label(s).

d. Records of prepackaging shall be maintained according to Board Rule 291.94C (Records).
5. Labeling for Provision of Drugs and/or Devices in an Original Manufacturer's Container.
   a. Drugs and/or devices in an original manufacturer's container shall be labeled prior to provision with the information set out in 4.c. above.
   b. Drugs and/or devices in an original manufacturer's container may be labeled by:
      (1) A pharmacist in a pharmacy licensed by the Board or
      (2) Supportive personnel in a Class D pharmacy provided the drugs and/or devices and control records required by Board Rule 291.94D (Records) are quarantined together until checked and released by a pharmacist.
   c. Records of labeling for provision of drugs and/or devices in an original manufacturer's container shall be maintained according to Board Rule 291.94E (Records).
6. Provision (providing drugs).
   a. Drugs and devices may only be provided to patients of the clinic.
   b. At the time of the initial provision, a licensed nurse or practitioner shall provide verbal and written information on side effects, interactions, and precautions concerning the drug or device provided (patient counseling). If the provision of subsequent drugs is delivered to the patient at the patient's residence or another designated location, the following is applicable:
      (1) Written information as specified in b. above shall be delivered with the medication.
      (2) The pharmacy shall maintain and use adequate storage or shipment containers and use shipping processes to ensure drug stability and potency. Such shipping processes shall include the use of appropriate packaging material and/or devices to ensure that the drug is maintained at an appropriate temperature range to maintain the integrity of the medication throughout the delivery process.
      (3) The pharmacy shall use a delivery system which is designed to ensure that the drugs are delivered to the appropriate patient.
   c. The provision of drugs or devices shall be under the continuous supervision of a pharmacist according to standing delegation orders or standing medical orders and in accordance with written policies and procedures and completion of the label as specified in g. below.
   d. Drugs and/or devices may only be provided in accordance with the system of control and accountability for drugs and/or devices provided by the clinic. Such a system shall be developed and supervised by the pharmacist-in-charge.
   e. Only drugs and/or devices listed in the clinic formulary may be provided.
   f. Drugs and/or devices may only be provided in prepackaged quantities in suitable containers and/or original manufacturer's containers which are appropriately labeled as set out in E.4. and E.5. above.
   g. Such drugs and/or devices shall be labeled by a pharmacist licensed by the Board. However, when drugs and/or devices are provided under the supervision of a physician according to standing delegation orders or standing medical orders, designated supportive personnel may at the time of provision affix an ancillary label or print on the label the following information:
      (1) Patient's name; however, the name of the patient's partner or family member is not required to be on the label of a drug prescribed for

a partner for a sexually transmitted disease or for a patient's family members if the patient has an illness determined to be pandemic by the Centers for Disease Control and Prevention, the World Health Organization, or the Governor's office;
(2) Any information necessary to complete the directions for use;
(3) Date of provision; and
(4) Practitioner's name.
    h. Records of provision shall be maintained according to Board Rule 291.94E (Records).
    i. Controlled substances may not be provided or dispensed.
    j. Nonsterile compounded preparations may only be provided by the Class D pharmacy in accordance with Board Rule 291.131 (Pharmacies Compounding Nonsterile Preparations).
7. Dispensing. Dangerous drugs may only be dispensed by a pharmacist pursuant to a prescription drug order in accordance with Board Rules 291.31–291.35 (Class A pharmacy rules).

F. Pharmacy and Therapeutics Committee.
1. The Class D pharmacy shall have a pharmacy and therapeutics committee which shall be composed of at least three persons and shall include the pharmacist-in-charge, the medical director of the clinic, and a person who is responsible for provision of drugs and devices.
2. The pharmacy and therapeutics committee shall develop the policy and procedure manual.
3. The pharmacy and therapeutics committee shall meet at least annually to:
    a. Review and update the policy and procedure manual and
    b. Review the retrospective drug utilization review reports submitted by the pharmacist-in-charge if the Class D pharmacy has an expanded formulary.

G. Policies and Procedures.
1. Written policies and procedures shall be developed by the pharmacy and therapeutics committee and implemented by the pharmacist-in-charge.
2. The policy and procedure manual shall include but not be limited to the following:
    a. A current list of the names of the pharmacist-in-charge, consultant pharmacist, staff pharmacist(s), supportive personnel designated to provide drugs and/or devices, and the supportive personnel designated to supervise the day-to-day pharmacy-related operations of the clinic in the absence of the pharmacist;
    b. Functions of the pharmacist-in-charge, consultant pharmacist, staff pharmacist(s), and supportive personnel;
    c. Objectives of the clinic;
    d. Formulary;
    e. A copy of the written agreement between the pharmacist-in-charge and the clinic;
    f. Date of last review/revision of the policy and procedure manual; and
    g. Policies and procedures for:
(1) Security;
(2) Equipment;
(3) Sanitation;
(4) Licensing;
(5) Reference materials;
(6) Storage;
(7) Packaging-repackaging;
(8) Dispensing;

(9) Provision;
(10) Retrospective drug regimen review;
(11) Supervision;
(12) Labeling-relabeling;
(13) Samples;
(14) Drug destruction and returns;
(15) Drug and/or device procuring;
(16) Receiving of drugs and/or devices;
(17) Delivery of drugs and/or devices;
(18) Recordkeeping; and
(19) Inspection.

H. Supervision. The pharmacist-in-charge, consultant pharmacist, or staff pharmacist shall personally visit the clinic on at least a monthly basis to ensure that the clinic is following established policies and procedures. However, clinics operated by state or local governments and funded by local, state, or federal government sources may petition the Board for an alternative visitation schedule under the following conditions:
1. Such petition shall contain an affidavit with the notarized signatures of the medical director, the pharmacist-in-charge, and the owner/chief executive officer of the clinic which states that the clinic has a current policy and procedure manual on file, has adequate security to prevent diversion of dangerous drugs, and is in compliance with all rules governing Class D pharmacies.
2. The Board may consider the following items in determining an alternative schedule:
   a. The degree of compliance on past compliance inspections;
   b. The size of the patient population of the clinic;
   c. The number and types of drugs contained in the formulary; and
   d. The objectives of the clinic.
3. Such petition shall be resubmitted every two years with the application for renewal of the pharmacy license.

Board of Pharmacy Rule 291.94
Records

A. Maintenance of Records.
1. Every inventory or other record required to be kept under the provisions of Board Rule 291.91 (Definitions), Board Rule 291.92 (Personnel), Board Rule 291.93 (Operational Standards), and Board Rule 291.94 (Records) in a Class D pharmacy shall be:
   a. Kept by the pharmacy and be available for at least two years from the date of such inventory or record for inspecting and copying by the Board or its representative and to other authorized local, state, or federal law enforcement agencies and
   b. Supplied by the pharmacy within 72 hours if requested by an authorized agent of the Board. If the pharmacy maintains the records in an electronic format, the requested records must be provided in a mutually agreeable electronic format if specifically requested by the Board or its representative. Failure to provide the records set out in this rule, either on-site or within 72 hours, constitutes prima facie evidence of failure to keep and maintain records in violation of the Act.
2. Records, except when specifically required to be maintained in original or hardcopy form, may be maintained in an alternative data retention system such as a data processing system or direct imaging system provided:

a. The records maintained in the alternative system contain all of the information required on the manual record and
b. The data processing system is capable of producing a hard copy of the record upon the request of the Board, its representative, or other authorized local, state, or federal law enforcement or regulatory agencies.
3. Invoices and records of receipt may be kept at a location other than the pharmacy. Any such records not kept at the pharmacy shall be supplied by the pharmacy within 72 hours if requested by an authorized agent of the Board.

B. On-Site Visits. A record of on-site visits by the pharmacist-in-charge, consultant pharmacist, or staff pharmacist shall be maintained and include the following information:
1. Date of the visit;
2. Pharmacist's evaluation of findings; and
3. Signature of the visiting pharmacist.

C. Prepackaging. Records of prepackaging shall include the following:
1. Name, strength, and dosage form of the drug;
2. Name of the manufacturer;
3. Manufacturer's lot number;
4. Expiration date;
5. Facility's lot number;
6. Quantity per package and number of packages;
7. Date packaged;
8. Name(s), signatures, or electronic signatures of the supportive personnel who prepackage the drug under direct supervision of a pharmacist; and
9. Name, signature, or electronic signature of the pharmacist who prepackages the drug or supervises the prepackaging and checks and releases the drug.

D. Labeling. Records of the labeling of drugs or devices in the original manufacturer's containers shall include the following:
1. Name and strength of the drug or device labeled;
2. Name of the manufacturer;
3. Manufacturer's lot number;
4. Manufacturer's expiration date;
5. Quantity per package and number of packages;
6. Date labeled;
7. Name of the supportive personnel affixing the label; and
8. The signature of the pharmacist who checks and releases the drug.

E. Provision. Records of drugs or devices provided shall include logs, patient records, or other acceptable methods for documentation. Documentation shall include:
1. Patient name;
2. Name, signature, or electronic signature of the person who provided the drug or device;
3. Date provided; and
4. The name of the drug or device and quantity provided.

F. Dispensing. Recordkeeping requirements for a dangerous drug dispensed by a pharmacist are the same as for a Class A pharmacy as set out in Board Rule 291.34 (Records).

Notes

Nonresident Pharmacies (Class E) Statutes and Rules

(Primarily Out-of-State Mail Service Pharmacies or Out-of-State Internet Pharmacies)

A Class E pharmacy license or nonresident pharmacy license may be issued to a pharmacy located in another state whose primary business is to:
1. Dispense a prescription drug or device under a prescription drug order and deliver the drug or device to a patient, including a patient in this state, by United States mail, common carrier, or delivery service;
2. Process a prescription drug order for a patient including a patient in this state; or
3. Perform another pharmaceutical service as defined by Board rule.

Section 556.0551 Inspection of a Licensed Nonresident Pharmacy
A. The Board may inspect a nonresident pharmacy licensed by the Board that compounds sterile preparations as necessary to ensure compliance with the safety standards or other requirements of the Act and Board rules.
B. A nonresident pharmacy shall reimburse the Board for all expenses including travel incurred by the Board in inspecting the pharmacy as provided in A. above.

Section 560.052 Qualifications
A. The Board by rule shall establish the standards that each pharmacy and the pharmacy's employees involved in the practice of pharmacy must meet to qualify for licensing as a pharmacy in each classification.
B. To qualify for a pharmacy license, an applicant must submit to the Board:
   1. A license fee set by the Board except as provided by D. below and
   2. A completed application that:
      a. Is on a form prescribed by the Board;
      b. Is given under oath;
      c. Includes proof that:
         (1) A pharmacy license held by the applicant in this state or another state, if applicable, has not been restricted, suspended, revoked, or surrendered for any reason and
         (2) No owner of the pharmacy for which the application is made has held a pharmacist license in this state or another state, if applicable, that has been restricted, suspended, revoked, or surrendered for any reason; and
      d. Includes a statement of:
         (1) The ownership;
         (2) The location of the pharmacy;
         (3) The license number of each pharmacist who is employed by the pharmacy, if the pharmacy is located in this state, or who is licensed to practice pharmacy in this state, if the pharmacy is located in another state;
         (4) The pharmacist license number of the pharmacist-in-charge; and
            Note: Since "pharmacist" is defined in the Act as a person licensed by TSBP, this means that Class E pharmacies must have a Texas licensed PIC.
         (5) Any other information the Board determines necessary.
C. A pharmacy located in another state that applies for a license, in addition to satisfying the requirements of this chapter, must provide to the Board:

1. Evidence that the applicant holds a pharmacy license, registration, or permit in good standing issued by the state in which the pharmacy is located;
2. The name of the owner and pharmacist-in-charge of the pharmacy for service of process;
3. Evidence of the pharmacy's ability to provide the Board a record of a prescription drug order dispensed or delivered by the pharmacy to a resident of or practitioner in this state no later than 72 hours after the time the Board requests the record as authorized by Chapter 562 of the Act (compounded and prepackaged drugs including compounded products for office use);
4. An affidavit by the pharmacist-in-charge that states that the pharmacist has read and understands the laws and rules relating to the applicable license;
5. Proof of creditworthiness; and
6. An inspection report issued:
   a. No more than two years before the date the license application is received and
   b. By the pharmacy licensing board in the state of the pharmacy's physical location, except as provided by F. below.
D. This section of the Act is not related to Class E pharmacies.
E. This section of the Act is not related to Class E pharmacies.
F. A Class E pharmacy may submit an inspection report issued by an entity other than the pharmacy licensing board of the state in which the pharmacy is physically located if:
  1. The state's licensing board does not conduct inspections;
  2. The inspection is substantively equivalent to an inspection conducted by the Board as determined by Board rule; and
  3. The inspecting entity meets specifications adopted by the Board for inspecting entities.
G. A license may not be issued to a pharmacy that compounds sterile preparations unless the pharmacy has been inspected by the Board to ensure that the pharmacy meets the safety standards and other requirements of this Act and Board rules.
H. The Board may accept, as satisfying the inspection requirement in G. above for a pharmacy located in another state, an inspection report issued by the pharmacy licensing board in the state in which the pharmacy is located if:
  1. The Board determines that the other state has comparable standards and regulations applicable to pharmacies, including standards and regulations related to health and safety and
  2. The pharmacy provides to the Board any requested documentation related to the inspection.

Section 561.0031 Additional Renewal Requirement for a Class E Pharmacy

A. In addition to the renewal requirements under Section 561.003 of the Act, the Board shall require that a Class E pharmacy have on file with the Board an inspection report issued:
  1. No more than three years before the date the renewal application is received and
  2. By the pharmacy licensing board in the state of the pharmacy's physical location, except as provided by B. below.
B. A Class E pharmacy may have on file with the Board an inspection report issued by an entity other than the pharmacy licensing board of the state in which the pharmacy is physically located if the requirements of Section 560.052F. of the Act are met.

Board of Pharmacy Rule 291.14
Pharmacy License Renewal

A. In addition to the renewal requirements in Board Rule 291.14.A., a Class E pharmacy shall have on file with the Board an inspection report issued:
  1. No more than three years before the date the renewal application is received and
  2. By the pharmacy licensing board in the state of the pharmacy's physical location except as provided in Board Rule 291.104 (Operational Standards).

Section 565.003 Additional Grounds for Discipline Regarding an Applicant for or a Holder of a Nonresident Pharmacy License

Note: These are the only grounds for discipline of a Class E pharmacy.

Unless compliance would violate the pharmacy or drug statutes or rules in the state in which the pharmacy is located, the Board may discipline an applicant for or the holder of a nonresident pharmacy license if the Board finds that the applicant or license holder has failed to comply with:
  1. Section 481.074, 481.075, 481.0755, 481.0756, 481.0761, 481.0762, 481.0763, 481.07635, 481.0764, 481.0765, or 481.0766, Health and Safety Code (Texas Controlled Substances Act);
  2. Texas substitution requirements regarding:
     a. The practitioner's directions concerning generic substitution;
     b. The patient's right to refuse generic substitution; or
     c. Notification to the patient of the patient's right to refuse substitution;
  3. Any Board rule relating to providing drug information to the patient or the patient's agent in written form or by telephone; or
  4. Any Board rule adopted under Section 554.051(a) of the Act and determined by the Board to be applicable under Section 554.051(b) of the Act.

Note: A Class E pharmacy also must comply with Board Rule 291.101.

Section 565.053 Discipline of a Nonresident Pharmacy; Notice to Resident State

The Board shall give notice of a disciplinary action by the Board against a license holder located in another state to the regulatory or licensing agency of the state in which the pharmacy is located.

Section 565.054 Service of Process on a Nonresident Pharmacy

A. Service of process on a nonresident pharmacy under Section 565.058 or 566.051 of the Act or for disciplinary action taken by the Board under Section 565.061 of the Act shall be on the owner and pharmacist-in-charge of the pharmacy as designated on the pharmacy's license application.
B. The complaining party shall mail by certified mail, return receipt requested, and postage prepaid a copy of the process served to the license holder at the address of the license holder designated on the license application.

Board of Pharmacy Rule 291.101
Purpose

A. The purpose of these rules is to provide standards for the operation of Class E (Nonresident) pharmacies which dispense a prescription drug or device under a prescription drug order and deliver the drug or device to a patient in this state by the United States mail, a common carrier, or a delivery service.
B. These rules are in accordance with Section 554.051(a) and (b) of the Act which permit the Board to make rules concerning the operation of licensed pharmacies in this state applicable to pharmacies licensed by the Board that are located in another state. The Board has determined that these rules are necessary to protect the health and welfare of the citizens of this state.

C. Unless compliance would violate the pharmacy or drug laws or rules in the state in which the pharmacy is located, Class E pharmacies are required to comply with the provisions of Board Rules 291.101–291.105 (Purpose, Definitions, Personnel, Operational Standards, and Records).

Board of Pharmacy Rule 291.102
Definitions

The following words and terms shall have the following meanings unless the context clearly indicates otherwise.
  A. **Act**—The Texas Pharmacy Act, Chapters 551–566, Occupations Code, as amended.
  B. **Accurately as prescribed**—Dispensing, delivering, and/or distributing a prescription drug order:
     1. To the correct patient (or agent of the patient) for whom the drug or device was prescribed;
     2. With the correct drug in the correct strength, quantity, and dosage form ordered by the practitioner; and
     3. With correct labeling (including directions for use) as ordered by the practitioner provided, however, that nothing herein shall prohibit pharmacist substitution if substitution is conducted in strict accordance with applicable laws and rules, including Subchapter A of Chapter 562 of the Texas Pharmacy Act relating to Prescription and Substitution Requirements.
  C. **Board**—Texas State Board of Pharmacy.
  D. **Class E pharmacy license or nonresident pharmacy license**—A license issued to a pharmacy located in another state whose primary business is to:
     1. Dispense a prescription drug or device under a prescription drug order and
     2. Deliver the drug or device to a patient including a patient in this state by the United States mail, common carrier, or delivery service.
  E. **Confidential record**—Any health-related record, including a patient medication record, prescription drug order, or medication order that:
     1. Contains information that identifies an individual and
     2. Is maintained by a pharmacy or pharmacist.
  F. **Deliver or delivery**—The actual, constructive, or attempted transfer of a prescription drug or device or controlled substance from one person to another whether or not for a consideration.
  G. **Dispense**—Preparing, packaging, compounding, or labeling, in the course of professional practice, a prescription drug or device for delivery to an ultimate user or the user's agent under a practitioner's lawful order.
  H. **Distribute**—To deliver a prescription drug or device other than by administering or dispensing.
  I. **Generically equivalent**—A drug that is "pharmaceutically equivalent" and "therapeutically equivalent" to the drug prescribed.
  J. **New prescription drug order**—A prescription drug order that:
     1. Has not been dispensed to the patient in the same strength and dosage form by this pharmacy within the last year;
     2. Is transferred from another pharmacy; and/or
     3. Is a discharge prescription drug order.
     Note: Furlough prescription drug orders are not considered new prescription drug orders.
  K. **Pharmaceutically equivalent**—Drug products which have identical amounts of the same active chemical ingredients in the same dosage form and which meet the identical compendial or other applicable standards of strength, quality, and

purity according to the United States Pharmacopeia or other nationally recognized compendium.
- L. **Pharmacist**—For the purpose of this subchapter, a person licensed to practice pharmacy in the state where the Class E pharmacy is located.
- M. **Pharmacist-in-charge**—The pharmacist designated on a pharmacy license as the pharmacist who has the authority or responsibility for a pharmacy's compliance with statutes and rules pertaining to the practice of pharmacy.
- N. **Practitioner**—
  1. A person licensed or registered to prescribe, distribute, administer, or dispense a prescription drug or device in the course of professional practice in this state, including a physician, dentist, podiatrist, or veterinarian but excluding a person licensed under the Act;
  2. A person licensed by another state, Canada, or the United Mexican States in a health field in which, under the law of this state, a license holder in this state may legally prescribe a dangerous drug; or
  3. A person practicing in another state and licensed by another state as a physician, dentist, veterinarian, or podiatrist, who has a current federal Drug Enforcement Administration registration number, and who may legally prescribe a Schedule II, III, IV, or V controlled substance as specified under Chapter 481, Health and Safety Code, in that other state.
- O. **Prescription drug order**—An order from a practitioner or a practitioner's designated agent to a pharmacist for a drug or device to be dispensed.
- P. **Therapeutically equivalent**—Pharmaceutically equivalent drug products which when administered in the same amounts will provide the same therapeutic effect, identical in duration and intensity.

Board of Pharmacy Rule 291.103
Personnel

As specified in Section 562.101(f) of the Act (Supervision of Pharmacy), a Class E pharmacy shall be under the continuous on-site supervision of a pharmacist and shall designate one pharmacist licensed to practice pharmacy by the regulatory or licensing agency of the state in which the Class E pharmacy is located and who is licensed as a pharmacist in Texas to serve as the pharmacist-in-charge of the Class E pharmacy license.

Board of Pharmacy Rule 291.104
Operational Standards

- A. Licensing Requirements.
  1. A Class E pharmacy shall register with the Board on a pharmacy license application provided by the Board following the procedures specified in Board Rule 291.1.
  2. On the initial application, the pharmacy shall follow the procedures specified in Board Rule 291.1 (Pharmacy License Application) and provide the following additional information specified in Section 560.052(c) and (f) of the Act (Qualifications):
     a. Evidence that the applicant holds a pharmacy license, registration, or permit issued by the state in which the pharmacy is located;
     b. The name of the owner and pharmacist-in-charge of the pharmacy for service of process;
     c. Evidence of the applicant's ability to provide to the Board a record of a prescription drug order dispensed by the applicant to a resident of this state no later than 72 hours after the time the Board requests the record;

- d. An affidavit by the pharmacist-in-charge which states that the pharmacist has read and understands the laws and rules relating to a Class E pharmacy;
- e. Proof of creditworthiness; and
- f. An inspection report issued no more than two years before the date the license application is received and conducted by the pharmacy licensing board in the state of the pharmacy's physical location.

3. On renewal of a license, the pharmacy shall complete the renewal application provided by the Board and, as specified in Section 561.0031 of the Act, provide an inspection report issued no more than three years before the date the renewal application is received and conducted by the pharmacy licensing board in the state of the pharmacy's physical location. A Class E pharmacy may submit an inspection report issued by the Board or its designee if the state's licensing board does not conduct inspections.
4. A Class E pharmacy which changes ownership shall notify the Board within ten days of the change of ownership and apply for a new and separate license as specified in Board Rule 291.3 (Required Notifications).
5. A Class E pharmacy which changes location shall notify the Board no later than 30 days before the date of the change and file for an amended license as specified in Board Rule 291.3 (Required Notifications).
6. A Class E pharmacy owned by a partnership or corporation which changes managing officers shall notify the Board in writing of the names of the new managing officers within ten days of the change following the procedures in Board Rule 291.3 (Required Notifications).
7. A Class E pharmacy shall notify the Board in writing within ten days of closing.
8. A separate license is required for each principal place of business, and only one pharmacy license may be issued to a specific location.
9. A fee as specified in Board Rule 291.6 (Pharmacy License Fees) will be charged for the issuance and renewal of a license and the issuance of an amended license.
10. The Board may grant an exemption from the licensing requirements of this Act on the application of a pharmacy located in a state of the United States other than this state that restricts its dispensing of prescription drugs or devices to residents of this state to isolated transactions.
11. A Class E pharmacy engaged in the centralized dispensing of prescription drug or medication orders shall comply with the provisions of Board Rule 291.125 (Centralized Prescription Dispensing).
12. A Class E pharmacy engaged in central processing of prescription drug or medication orders shall comply with the provisions of Board Rule 291.123 (Central Prescription or Medication Order Processing).
13. A Class E pharmacy engaged in the compounding of nonsterile preparations shall comply with the provisions of Board Rule 291.131 (Pharmacies Compounding Nonsterile Preparations).
14. A Class E pharmacy shall not compound sterile preparations unless the pharmacy has applied for and obtained a Class E-S pharmacy license and complies with Board Rule 291.133 (Pharmacies Compounding Sterile Preparations).
15. A Class E pharmacy which operates as a community type of pharmacy which would otherwise be required to be licensed under Section 560.051(a)(1) (Community Pharmacy (Class A)) of the Act shall comply with the provisions of Board Rule 291.31 (Definitions), Board Rule 291.32 (Personnel), Board Rule 291.33 (Operational Standards), Board Rule 291.34 (Records), and Board Rule 291.35 (Official Prescription Requirements). A Class E pharmacy

which operates as a nuclear pharmacy which would otherwise be required to be licensed under Section 560.051(a)(2) (Nuclear Pharmacy (Class B)) of the Act shall comply with the provisions of Board Rule 291.51 (Purpose), Board Rule 291.52 (Definitions), Board Rule 291.53 (Personnel), Board Rule 291.54 (Operational Standards), and Board Rule 291.55 (Records) contained in Nuclear Pharmacy (Class B) to the extent such sections of the Act and Board rules are applicable to the operation of the pharmacy.

B. Prescription Dispensing and Delivery.
  1. General.
     a. All prescription drugs and/or devices shall be dispensed and delivered safely and accurately as prescribed.
     b. The pharmacy shall maintain adequate storage or shipment containers and use shipping processes to ensure drug stability and potency. Such shipping processes shall include the use of packaging material and devices to ensure that the drug is maintained at an appropriate temperature range to maintain the integrity of the medication throughout the delivery process.
     c. The pharmacy shall use a delivery system which is designed to assure that the drugs are delivered to the appropriate patient.
     d. All pharmacists shall exercise sound professional judgment with respect to the accuracy and authenticity of any prescription drug order they dispense. If the pharmacist questions the accuracy or authenticity of any prescription drug order, he or she shall verify the order with the practitioner prior to dispensing.
     e. Prior to dispensing a prescription, pharmacists shall determine in the exercise of sound professional judgment that the prescription is a valid prescription. A pharmacist may not dispense a prescription drug if the pharmacist knows or should have known that the prescription was issued on the basis of an Internet-based or telephone consultation without a valid patient-practitioner relationship.
     Note: While e. above is in the Act and Board rule, the practice of telemedicine/telehealth is now a "legal" practice in Texas. This practice also includes an Internet-based or telephone consultation with a practitioner.
     f. Rule B.1.e. above does not prohibit a pharmacist from dispensing a prescription when a valid patient-practitioner relationship is not present in an emergency situation (e.g., a practitioner taking calls for the patient's regular practitioner).
  2. Drug Regimen Review.
     a. For the purpose of promoting therapeutic appropriateness, a pharmacist prior to or at the time of dispensing a prescription drug order shall review the patient's medication record. Such review shall at a minimum identify clinically significant:
        (1) Inappropriate drug utilization;
        (2) Therapeutic duplication;
        (3) Drug-disease contraindications;
        (4) Drug-drug interactions;
        (5) Incorrect drug dosage or duration of drug treatment;
        (6) Drug-allergy interactions; and
        (7) Clinical abuse/misuse.
     b. Upon identifying any clinically significant conditions, situations, or items listed in a. above, the pharmacist shall take appropriate steps to avoid or resolve the problem including consultation with the prescribing practitioner. The pharmacist shall document such occurrences.

3. Patient Counseling and Provision of Drug Information.
   a. To optimize drug therapy, a pharmacist shall communicate to the patient or the patient's agent information about the prescription drug or device which, in the exercise of the pharmacist's professional judgment, the pharmacist deems significant such as the following:
      (1) The name and description of the drug or device;
      (2) Dosage form, dosage, route of administration, and duration of drug therapy;
      (3) Special directions and precautions for preparation, administration, and use by the patient;
      (4) Common severe side effects or adverse effects or interactions and therapeutic contraindications that may be encountered, including their avoidance, and the action required if they occur;
      (5) Techniques for self-monitoring of drug therapy;
      (6) Proper storage;
      (7) Refill information; and
      (8) Action to be taken in the event of a missed dose.
   b. Such communication shall be:
      (1) Provided to new and existing patients of a pharmacy with each new prescription drug order. A new prescription drug order is one that has not been dispensed by the pharmacy to the patient in the same dosage and strength within the last year;
      (2) Provided for any prescription drug order dispensed by the pharmacy on the request of the patient or patient's agent;
      (3) Communicated orally in person unless the patient or patient's agent is not at the pharmacy or a specific communication barrier prohibits such oral communication; and
      (4) Reinforced with written information. The following is applicable concerning this written information.
         (a) Written information must be in plain language designed for the patient and printed in an easily readable font comparable to but no smaller than 10-point Times Roman. This information may be provided to the patient in an electronic format such as e-mail if the patient or patient's agent requests the information in an electronic format and the pharmacy documents the request.
         (b) When a compounded product is dispensed, information shall be provided for the major active ingredient(s) if available.
         (c) For new drug entities, if no written information is initially available, the pharmacist is not required to provide information until such information is available provided:
            (i) The pharmacist informs the patient or the patient's agent that the product is a new drug entity and written information is not available;
            (ii) The pharmacist documents the fact that no written information was provided; and
            (iii) If the prescription is refilled after written information is available, such information is provided to the patient or patient's agent.
         (d) The written information accompanying the prescription or the prescription label shall contain the statement "Do not flush unused medications or pour down a sink or drain." A drug product on a list of medicines developed by FDA which recommends disposal by flushing is not required to bear this statement.

c. Only a pharmacist may orally provide drug information to a patient or patient's agent and answer questions concerning prescription drugs. Nonpharmacist personnel may not ask questions of a patient or patient's agent which are intended to screen and/or limit interaction with the pharmacist.
d. If prescriptions are routinely delivered outside the area covered by the pharmacy's local telephone service, the pharmacy shall provide a toll-free telephone line which is answered during normal business hours to enable communication between the patient and a pharmacist.
e. The pharmacist shall place on the prescription container or on a separate sheet delivered with the prescription container in both English and Spanish the local and toll-free telephone number of the pharmacy and the statement: "Written information about this prescription has been provided for you. Please read this information before you take the medication. If you have questions concerning this prescription, a pharmacist is available during normal business hours to answer these questions at (insert the pharmacy's local and toll-free telephone numbers)."
f. The provisions of this paragraph do not apply to patients in facilities where drugs are administered to patients by a person required to do so by the laws of the state (i.e., nursing homes).
g. Nothing in this subparagraph shall be construed as requiring a pharmacist to provide consultation when a patient or patient's agent refuses such consultation. The pharmacist shall document such refusal for consultation.
4. Labeling. At the time of delivery, the dispensing container shall bear a label that contains the following information:
   a. The name, physical address, and phone number of the pharmacy;
   b. If the drug is dispensed in a container other than the manufacturer's original container, the date after which the prescription should not be used or beyond-use date. Unless otherwise specified by the manufacturer, the beyond-use date shall be one year from the date the drug is dispensed or the manufacturer's expiration date, whichever is earlier. The beyond-use date may be placed on the prescription label or on a flag label attached to the bottle. A beyond-use date is not required on the label of a prescription dispensed to a person at the time of his or her release from prison or jail if the prescription is for no more than a 10-day supply of medication;
   c. The prescription label or the written information accompanying the prescription shall contain the statement "Do not flush unused medications or pour down a sink or drain." A drug product on a list of medicines developed by FDA which recommends disposal by flushing is not required to bear this statement; and
   d. Any other information that is required by the pharmacy or drug laws or rules in the state in which the pharmacy is located.
C. Generic Substitution. Unless compliance would violate the pharmacy or drug laws or rules in the state in which the pharmacy is located, a pharmacist in a Class E pharmacy may dispense a generically equivalent drug product and shall comply with the provisions of Board Rule 309.3 (Generic Substitution) and Board Rule 309.7 (Dispensing Responsibilities).
D. Therapeutic Drug Interchange. A switch to a drug providing a similar therapeutic response to the one prescribed shall not be made without prior approval of the prescribing practitioner. This does not apply to generic substitution. For generic substitution, see the requirements of C. above.

1. The patient shall be notified of the therapeutic drug interchange prior to or upon delivery of the dispensed prescription to the patient. Such notification shall include:
   a. A description of the change;
   b. The reason for the change;
   c. Whom to notify with questions concerning the change; and
   d. Instructions for return of the drug if not wanted by the patient.
2. The pharmacy shall maintain the documentation of patient notification of therapeutic drug interchange which shall include:
   a. The date of the notification;
   b. The method of notification;
   c. A description of the change; and
   d. The reason for the change.

E. Transfer of Prescription Drug Order Information. Unless compliance would violate the pharmacy or drug laws or rules in the state in which the pharmacy is located, a pharmacist in a Class E pharmacy may not refuse to transfer prescriptions to another pharmacy that is making the transfer request on behalf of the patient.

F. Prescriptions for Schedule II–V Controlled Substances. Unless compliance would violate the pharmacy or drug laws or rules in the state in which the pharmacy is located, a pharmacist in a Class E pharmacy who dispenses a prescription for a Schedule II–V controlled substance for a resident of Texas shall electronically send the prescription information to the Board no later than the next business day after the prescription is dispensed as specified in Board Rule 315.6 (Electronic Reporting).

Board of Pharmacy Rule 291.105
Records

A. Maintenance of Records.
   1. Every record required to be retained under Class E rules shall be:
      a. Kept by the pharmacy and be available for at least two years from the date of such inventory or record for inspecting and copying by the Board or its representatives and to other authorized local, state, or federal law enforcement or regulatory agencies and
      b. Supplied by the pharmacy within 72 hours if requested by an authorized agent of the Board. If the pharmacy maintains the records in an electronic format, the requested records must be provided in a mutually agreeable electronic format if specifically requested by the Board or its representative. Failure to provide the records set out in this rule, either on-site or within 72 hours, constitutes prima facie evidence of failure to keep and maintain records in violation of the Act.
   2. Records, except when specifically required to be maintained in original or hardcopy form, may be maintained in an alternative data retention system such as a data processing system or direct imaging system provided:
      a. The records maintained in the alternative system contain all of the information required on the manual record and
      b. The data processing system is capable of producing a hard copy of the record upon the request of the Board or its representative or other authorized local, state, or federal law enforcement or regulatory agencies.

B. Auto-Refill Programs.
   A pharmacy may use a program that automatically refills prescriptions that have existing refills available to improve patient compliance with and adherence to

prescribed medication therapy. The following is applicable to enroll patients into an auto-refill program:
1. Notice of availability of an auto-refill program shall be given to the patient or the patient's agent, the patient or the patient's agent must affirmatively indicate that he or she wishes to enroll in such a program, and the pharmacy shall document such indication.
2. The patient or patient's agent shall have the option to withdraw from such a program at any time.
3. Auto-refill programs may be used for refills of dangerous drugs and Schedule IV and V controlled substances. Schedule II and III controlled substances may not be dispensed by an auto-refill program.
Note: Schedule II prescriptions do not have refills.
4. As is required for all prescriptions, a drug regimen review shall be completed on all prescriptions filled as a result of an auto-refill program. Special attention shall be noted for drug regimen review warnings of duplication of therapy, and all such conflicts shall be resolved with the prescribing practitioner prior to refilling the prescription.

C. Civil Litigation and Complaint Records. A Class E pharmacy shall keep a permanent record of:
1. Any civil litigation commenced against the pharmacy by a Texas resident and
2. Complaints that arise out of a prescription for a Texas resident lost during delivery.

Board of Pharmacy Rule 291.106
Pharmacies Compounding Sterile Preparations (Class E-S)

Licensing Requirements. A nonresident pharmacy engaged in the compounding of sterile preparations shall be licensed as a Class E-S pharmacy.
1. A Class E-S pharmacy shall register with the Board on a pharmacy license application provided by the Board following the procedures specified in Board Rule 291.1 (Pharmacy License Application).
2. A Class E-S license may not be issued unless the pharmacy has been inspected by the Board or its designee to ensure the pharmacy meets the requirements as specified in Board Rule 291.133 (Pharmacies Compounding Sterile Preparations). A Class E-S pharmacy shall reimburse the Board for all expenses including travel related to the inspection of the Class E-S pharmacy.
3. On the initial application, the pharmacy shall follow the procedures specified in Board Rule 291.1 and then provide the following additional information specified in Section 560.052(c) and (f) of the Act (Qualifications):
   a. Evidence that the applicant holds a pharmacy license, registration, or permit issued by the state in which the pharmacy is located;
   b. The name of the owner and pharmacist-in-charge of the pharmacy for service of process;
   c. Evidence of the applicant's ability to provide to the Board a record of a prescription drug order dispensed by the applicant to a resident of this state no later than 72 hours after the time the Board requests the record;
   d. An affidavit by the pharmacist-in-charge which states that the pharmacist has read and understands the laws and rules relating to a Class E pharmacy; and
   e. Proof of creditworthiness.
4. A Class E-S pharmacy may not renew a pharmacy license unless the pharmacy has been inspected by the Board or its designee within the last renewal period.

5. A Class E-S pharmacy which changes ownership shall notify the Board within ten days of the change of ownership and apply for a new and separate license as specified in Board Rule 291.3 (Required Notifications).
6. A Class E-S pharmacy which changes location and/or name shall notify the Board as specified in Board Rule 291.3.
   Note: This requires notification no later than 30 days prior to the date for a change in location and within 10 days for a change of name.
7. A Class E-S pharmacy owned by a partnership or corporation which changes managing officers shall notify the Board in writing of the names of the new managing officers within ten days of the change as specified in Board Rule 291.3.
8. A Class E-S pharmacy shall notify the Board in writing within ten days of closing.
9. A separate license is required for each principal place of business, and only one pharmacy license may be issued to a specific location.
10. A fee as specified in Board Rule 291.6 (Pharmacy License Fees) will be charged for the issuance and renewal of a license and the issuance of an amended license.
11. The Board may grant an exemption from the licensing requirements of this Act on the application of a pharmacy located in a state of the United States other than this state that restricts its dispensing of prescription drugs or devices to residents of this state to isolated transactions.
12. A Class E-S pharmacy engaged in the centralized dispensing of prescription drug or medication orders shall comply with the provisions of Board Rule 291.125 (Centralized Prescription Dispensing).
13. A Class E-S pharmacy engaged in central processing of prescription drug or medication orders shall comply with the provisions of Board Rule 291.123 (Central Prescription Drug or Medication Order Processing).
14. A Class E-S pharmacy engaged in the compounding of nonsterile preparations shall comply with the provisions of Board Rule 291.131 (Pharmacies Compounding Nonsterile Preparations).
15. A Class E-S pharmacy engaged in the compounding of sterile preparations shall comply with the provisions of Board Rule 291.133.
16. A Class E-S pharmacy, which would otherwise be required to be licensed under Section 560.051(a)(5) of the Act concerning Class E pharmacies, is required to comply with the provisions of Board Rule 291.101 (Purpose), Board Rule 291.102 (Definitions), Board Rule 291.103 (Personnel), Board Rule 291.104 (Operational Standards), and Board Rule 291.105 (Records).

Freestanding Emergency Medical Care Facility Pharmacy (Class F) Rules (FEMCF)

Board of Pharmacy Rule 291.151
Pharmacies Located in a Freestanding Emergency Medical Care Facility (Class F)

A. Purpose. The purpose of this rule is to provide standards in the conduct, practice activities, and operation of a pharmacy located in a freestanding emergency medical care facility (FEMCF) that is licensed by the Texas Department of State Health Services or in a freestanding emergency medical care facility operated by a hospital that is exempt from registration as provided by 254.052, Health and Safety Code. Class F pharmacies located in a freestanding emergency medical care facility shall comply with this rule.

B. Definitions. The following words and terms shall have the following meanings unless the context clearly indicates otherwise.
1. **Act**—The Texas Pharmacy Act.
2. **Administer**—The direct application of a prescription drug by injection, inhalation, ingestion, or any other means to the body of a patient by: (A) a practitioner, an authorized agent under his or her supervision, or other person authorized by law or (B) the patient at the direction of a practitioner.
3. **Automated medication supply system**—A mechanical system that performs operations or activities relative to the storage and distribution of medications for administration and which collects, controls, and maintains all transaction information.
4. **Board**—Texas State Board of Pharmacy.
5. **Consultant pharmacist**—A pharmacist retained by a facility on a routine basis to consult with the FEMCF in areas that pertain to the practice of pharmacy.
6. **Controlled substance**—A drug, immediate precursor, or other substance listed in Schedules I–V or Penalty Groups 1–4 of the Texas Controlled Substances Act, as amended, or a drug, immediate precursor, or other substance included in Schedules I–V of the Federal Comprehensive Drug Abuse Prevention and Control Act of 1970, as amended (Public Law 91-513).
7. **Dispense**—Preparing, packaging, compounding, or labeling for delivery a prescription drug or device in the course of professional practice to an ultimate user or his or her agent by or pursuant to the lawful order of a practitioner.
8. **Distribute**—The delivery of a prescription drug or device other than by administering or dispensing.
9. **Downtime**—Period of time during which a data processing system is not operable.
10. **Electronic signature**—A unique security code or other identifier which specifically identifies the person entering information into a data processing system. A facility which uses electronic signatures must:
    a. Maintain a permanent list of the unique security codes assigned to persons authorized to use the data processing system and
    b. Have an ongoing security program which is capable of identifying misuse and/or the unauthorized use of electronic signatures.
11. **Floor stock**—Prescription drugs or devices not labeled for a specific patient and maintained at a nursing station or other FEMCF department (excluding the pharmacy) for the purpose of administration to a patient of the FEMCF.
12. **Formulary**—A list of drugs approved for use in the FEMCF by an appropriate committee of the freestanding emergency medical care facility.
13. **Freestanding emergency medical care facility (FEMCF)**—A freestanding facility that is licensed by the Texas Department of State Health Services pursuant to Chapter 254, Health and Safety Code, to provide emergency care to patients.
14. **Hard copy**—A physical document that is readable without the use of a special device (i.e., data processing system, computer, etc.).
15. **Investigational new drug**—A new drug intended for investigational use by experts qualified to evaluate the safety and effectiveness of the drug as authorized by FDA.
16. **Medication order**—An order from a practitioner or his or her authorized agent for administration of a drug or device.
17. **Pharmacist-in-charge**—A pharmacist designated on a pharmacy license as the pharmacist who has the authority or responsibility for a pharmacy's compliance with laws and rules pertaining to the practice of pharmacy.

18. **Pharmacy**—An area or areas in a facility, separate from patient care areas, where drugs are stored, bulk compounded, delivered, compounded, dispensed, and/or distributed to other areas or departments of the FEMCF or dispensed to an ultimate user or his or her agent.
19. **Prescription drug**—
    a. A substance for which federal or state law requires a prescription before it may be legally dispensed to the public;
    b. A drug or device that under federal law is required, prior to being dispensed or delivered, to be labeled with either of the following statements:
        (1) "Caution: federal law prohibits dispensing without prescription" or "Rx only" or another legend that complies with federal law or
        (2) "Caution: federal law restricts this drug to use by or on order of a licensed veterinarian"; or
    c. A drug or device that is required by any applicable federal or state law or regulation to be dispensed on prescription only or is restricted to use by a practitioner only.
20. **Prescription drug order**—
    a. An order from a practitioner or his or her authorized agent to a pharmacist for a drug or device to be dispensed or
    b. An order pursuant to Chapter 157 (Texas Medical Practice Act).
21. **Full-time pharmacist**—A pharmacist who works in a pharmacy from 30 to 40 hours per week or, if the pharmacy is open fewer than 60 hours per week, one-half of the time the pharmacy is open.
22. **Part-time pharmacist**—A pharmacist who works less than full time.
23. **Pharmacy technician**—An individual who is registered with the Board as a pharmacy technician and whose responsibility in a pharmacy is to provide technical services that do not require professional judgment regarding preparing and distributing drugs and who works under the direct supervision of and is responsible to a pharmacist.
24. **Pharmacy technician trainee**—An individual who is registered with the Board as a pharmacy technician trainee and is authorized to participate in a pharmacy's technician training program.
25. **Texas Controlled Substances Act**—The Texas Controlled Substances Act (Chapter 481, Health and Safety Code).

C. Personnel.
   1. Pharmacist-in-Charge.
      a. General. Each freestanding emergency medical care center shall have one pharmacist-in-charge who is employed or under contract at least on a consulting or part-time basis but may be employed on a full-time basis.
      b. Responsibilities. The pharmacist-in-charge shall have the responsibility for, at a minimum, the following:
         (1) Establishing specifications for procurement and storage of all materials including drugs, chemicals, and biologicals;
         (2) Participating in the development of a formulary for the FEMCF subject to approval of the appropriate committee of the FEMCF;
         (3) Distributing drugs to be administered to patients pursuant to an original or direct copy of the practitioner's medication order;
         (4) Filling and labeling all containers from which drugs are to be distributed or dispensed;
         (5) Maintaining and making available a sufficient inventory of antidotes and other emergency drugs both in the pharmacy and patient care areas, as well as current antidote information, telephone numbers of regional poison control centers and other emergency assistance

organizations, and such other materials and information as may be deemed necessary by the appropriate committee of the FEMCF;

(6) Maintaining records of all transactions of the FEMCF pharmacy as may be required by applicable state and federal law and as may be necessary to maintain accurate control over and accountability for all pharmaceutical materials;

(7) Participating in those aspects of the FEMCF patient care evaluation program which relate to pharmaceutical material utilization and effectiveness;

(8) Participating in teaching and/or research programs in the FEMCF;

(9) Implementing the policies and decisions of the appropriate committee(s) relating to pharmaceutical services of the FEMCF;

(10) Providing effective and efficient messenger and delivery service to connect the FEMCF pharmacy with appropriate areas of the FEMCF on a regular basis throughout the normal workday of the FEMCF;

(11) Labeling, storing, and distributing investigational new drugs, including maintaining information in the pharmacy and nursing station where such drugs are being administered concerning the dosage form, route of administration, strength, actions, uses, side effects, adverse effects, interactions, and symptoms of toxicity of investigational new drugs;

(12) Meeting all inspection and other requirements of the Texas Pharmacy Act and this rule;

(13) Maintaining records in a data processing system such that the data processing system is in compliance with the requirements for the FEMCF; and

(14) Ensuring that a pharmacist visits the FEMCF at least once each calendar week that the facility is open.

2. Consultant Pharmacist.
   a. The consultant pharmacist may be the pharmacist-in-charge.
   b. A written contract shall exist between the FEMCF and any consultant pharmacist, and a copy of the written contract shall be made available to the Board upon request.
3. Pharmacists.
   a. General.
      (1) The pharmacist-in-charge shall be assisted by a sufficient number of additional licensed pharmacists as may be required to operate the FEMCF pharmacy competently, safely, and adequately to meet the needs of the patients of the facility.
      (2) All pharmacists shall assist the pharmacist-in-charge in meeting the responsibilities as outlined in C.1.b. above and in ordering, administering, and accounting for pharmaceutical materials.
      (3) All pharmacists shall be responsible for any delegated act performed by pharmacy technicians or pharmacy technician trainees under his or her supervision.
      (4) All pharmacists while on duty shall be responsible for complying with all state and federal laws or rules governing the practice of pharmacy.
   b. Duties. Duties of the pharmacist-in-charge and all other pharmacists shall include, but need not be limited to, the following:
      (1) Receiving and interpreting prescription drug orders and oral medication orders and reducing these orders to writing either manually or electronically;

(2) Selecting prescription drugs and/or devices and/or suppliers; and
(3) Interpreting patient profiles.
  c. Special requirements for compounding nonsterile preparations. All pharmacists engaged in compounding nonsterile preparations shall meet the training requirements specified in Board Rule 291.131 (Pharmacies Compounding Nonsterile Preparations).
4. Pharmacy Technicians and Pharmacy Technician Trainees.
  a. General. All pharmacy technicians and pharmacy technician trainees shall meet the training requirements specified in Board Rule 297.6 (Pharmacy Technician and Pharmacy Technician Trainee Training).
  b. Duties. Pharmacy technicians and pharmacy technician trainees may not perform any of the duties listed in 3.b. above. Duties may include, but need not be limited to, the following functions under the direct supervision of a pharmacist:
    (1) Prepacking and labeling unit-dose and multiple-dose packages provided a pharmacist supervises and conducts a final check and affixes his or her name, initials, or electronic signature to the appropriate quality control records prior to distribution;
    (2) Preparing, packaging, compounding, or labeling prescription drugs pursuant to medication orders provided a pharmacist supervises and checks the preparation;
    (3) Compounding nonsterile preparations pursuant to medication orders provided the pharmacy technicians or pharmacy technician trainees have completed the training specified in Board Rule 291.131;
    (4) Bulk compounding provided a pharmacist supervises and conducts in-process and final checks and affixes his or her name, initials, or electronic signature to the appropriate quality control records prior to distribution;
    (5) Distributing routine orders for stock supplies to patient care areas;
    (6) Entering medication order and drug distribution information into a data processing system provided judgmental decisions are not required and a pharmacist checks the accuracy of the information entered into the system prior to releasing the order or in compliance with the absence of pharmacist requirements contained in D.6.d. and D.6.e. below;
    (7) Maintaining inventories of drug supplies;
    (8) Maintaining pharmacy records; and
    (9) Loading drugs into an automated medication supply system. For the purpose of this clause, direct supervision may be accomplished by physically present supervision or electronic monitoring by a pharmacist.
  c. Procedures.
    (1) Pharmacy technicians and pharmacy technician trainees shall handle medication orders in accordance with standard written procedures and guidelines.
    (2) Pharmacy technicians and pharmacy technician trainees shall handle prescription drug orders in the same manner as pharmacy technicians or pharmacy technician trainees working in a Class A pharmacy.
  d. Special requirements for nonsterile compounding. All pharmacy technicians and pharmacy technician trainees engaged in compounding nonsterile preparations shall meet the training requirements specified in Board Rule 291.131.
5. Owner. The owner of an FEMCF pharmacy shall have responsibility for all administrative and operational functions of the pharmacy. The

pharmacist-in-charge may advise the owner on administrative and operational concerns. If the owner is not a Texas licensed pharmacist, the owner shall consult with the pharmacist-in-charge or another Texas licensed pharmacist. The owner shall have responsibility for, at a minimum, the following:
   a. Establishing policies for procurement of prescription drugs and devices and other products dispensed from the FEMCF pharmacy;
   b. Establishing and maintaining effective controls against the theft or diversion of prescription drugs;
   c. If the pharmacy uses an automated medication supply system, reviewing and approving all policies and procedures for system operation, safety, security, accuracy and access, patient confidentiality, prevention of unauthorized access, and malfunction;
   d. Providing the pharmacy with the necessary equipment and resources commensurate with its level and type of practice; and
   e. Establishing policies and procedures regarding maintenance, storage, and retrieval of records in a data processing system such that the system is in compliance with state and federal requirements.
6. Identification of Pharmacy Personnel. All pharmacy personnel shall be identified as follows.
   a. Pharmacy technicians. All pharmacy technicians shall wear an identification tag or badge that bears the person's name and identifies him or her as a pharmacy technician.
   b. Pharmacy technician trainees. All pharmacy technician trainees shall wear an identification tag or badge that bears the person's name and identifies him or her as a pharmacy technician trainee.
   c. Pharmacist interns. All pharmacist interns shall wear an identification tag or badge that bears the person's name and identifies him or her as a pharmacist intern.
   d. Pharmacists. All pharmacists shall wear an identification tag or badge that bears the person's name and identifies him or her as a pharmacist.

D. Operational Standards.
   1. Licensing Requirements.
      a. An FEMCF pharmacy shall register annually or biennially with the Board on a pharmacy license application provided by the Board following the procedures specified in Board Rule 291.1 (Pharmacy License Application).
      b. An FEMCF pharmacy which changes ownership shall notify the Board within 10 days of the change of ownership and apply for a new and separate license as specified in Board Rule 291.3 (Required Notifications).
      c. An FEMCF pharmacy which changes its name shall notify the Board of the change within 10 days and file for an amended license as specified in Board Rule 291.3.
      d. When an FEMCF pharmacy changes location, a new completed application must be filed no later than 30 days before the date of the change of location.
      e. An FEMCF pharmacy owned by a partnership or corporation which changes managing officers shall notify the Board in writing of the names of the new managing officers within 10 days of the change following the procedures in Board Rule 291.3.
      f. An FEMCF pharmacy shall notify the Board in writing within 10 days of closing following the procedures in Board Rule 291.5 (Closing a Pharmacy).
      g. A fee as specified in Board Rule 291.6 (Pharmacy License Fees) will be charged for issuance and renewal of a license and the issuance of an amended license.

h. A separate license is required for each principal place of business, and only one pharmacy license may be issued to a specific location.
i. An FEMCF pharmacy which also operates another type of pharmacy which would otherwise be required to be licensed under Section 560.051(a)(1) of the Act concerning Class A pharmacies is not required to secure a license for the other type of pharmacy provided, however, such license is required to comply with the provisions of Board Rule 291.31 (Definitions), Board Rule 291.32 (Personnel), Board Rule 291.33 (Operational Standards), Board Rule 291.34 (Records), and Board Rule 291.35 (Official Prescription Requirements) to the extent such sections of the Act and Board rules are applicable to the operation of the pharmacy.
j. An FEMCF pharmacy engaged in the compounding of nonsterile preparations shall comply with the provisions of Board Rule 291.131.
2. Environment.
   a. General requirements.
      (1) Each freestanding emergency medical care center shall have a designated work area separate from patient areas, shall have space adequate for the size and scope of pharmaceutical services, and shall have adequate space and security for the storage of drugs.
      (2) The FEMCF pharmacy shall be arranged in an orderly fashion and shall be kept clean. All required equipment shall be clean and in good operating condition.
   b. Special requirements.
      (1) The FEMCF pharmacy shall have locked storage for Schedule II controlled substances and other controlled drugs requiring additional security.
      (2) The FEMCF pharmacy shall have a designated area for the storage of poisons and externals separate from drug storage areas.
   c. Security.
      (1) The pharmacy and storage areas for prescription drugs and/or devices shall be enclosed and capable of being locked by key, combination, or other mechanical or electronic means so as to prohibit access by unauthorized individuals. Only individuals authorized by the pharmacist-in-charge may enter the pharmacy or have access to storage areas for prescription drugs and/or devices.
      (2) The pharmacist-in-charge shall consult with FEMCF personnel with respect to the security of the drug storage areas including provisions for adequate safeguards against theft or diversion of dangerous drugs, controlled substances, and records for such drugs.
      (3) The pharmacy shall have locked storage for Schedule II controlled substances and other drugs requiring additional security.
3. Equipment and Supplies. Freestanding emergency medical care centers supplying drugs for outpatient use shall have the following equipment and supplies:
   a. Data processing system including a printer or comparable equipment;
   b. Adequate supply of child-resistant, moisture-proof, and light-proof containers; and
   c. Adequate supply of prescription labels and other applicable identification labels.
4. Library. A reference library shall be maintained that includes the following in hard copy or electronic format and that pharmacy personnel shall be capable of accessing at all times:
   a. Current copies of the following:
      (1) Texas Pharmacy Act and rules;
      (2) Texas Dangerous Drug Act and rules;

(3) Texas Controlled Substances Act and rules; and
(4) Federal Controlled Substances Act and rules or an official publication describing the requirements of the Federal Controlled Substances Act and rules.
  b. At least one current or updated general drug information reference which is required to contain drug interaction information. This includes information needed to determine severity or significance of the interaction and appropriate recommendations or actions to be taken, basic antidote information, and the telephone number of the nearest regional poison control center.
5. Drugs.
  a. Procurement, preparation, and storage.
    (1) The pharmacist-in-charge shall have the responsibility for the procurement and storage of drugs but may receive input from other appropriate staff of the facility relative to such responsibility.
    (2) The pharmacist-in-charge shall have the responsibility for determining specifications of all drugs procured by the facility.
    (3) FEMCF pharmacies may not sell, purchase, trade, or possess prescription drug samples unless the pharmacy meets all of the following conditions:
      (a) The pharmacy is owned by a charitable organization described in the Internal Revenue Code of 1986 or by a city, state or county government;
      (b) The pharmacy is a part of a healthcare entity which provides health care primarily to indigent or low-income patients at no or reduced cost;
      (c) The samples are for dispensing or provision at no charge to patients of such a healthcare entity;
      (d) The samples are possessed in compliance with the Prescription Drug Marketing Act of 1986;
      (e) All drugs shall be stored at the proper temperatures as defined in the USP/NF and in Board Rule 291.15 (Storage of Drugs);
      (f) Any drug bearing an expiration date may not be dispensed or distributed beyond the expiration date of the drug; and
      (g) Outdated drugs shall be removed from dispensing stock and shall be quarantined together until such drugs are disposed of.
  b. Formulary.
    (1) A formulary may be developed by an appropriate committee of the FEMCF.
    (2) The pharmacist-in-charge, consultant pharmacist, or designee shall be a full voting member of any committee that involves pharmaceutical services.
    (3) A practitioner may grant approval for pharmacists at the FEMCF to interchange drugs in accordance with the facility's formulary for the drugs on the practitioner's medication orders provided:
      (a) A formulary has been developed;
      (b) The formulary has been approved by the medical staff of the FEMCF;
      (c) There is a reasonable method for the practitioner to override any interchange; and
      (d) The practitioner authorizes a pharmacist in the FEMCF to interchange on his or her medication orders in accordance with the facility's formulary through the pharmacist's written agreement

to abide by the policies and procedures of the medical staff and facility.
   c. Prepackaging and loading drugs into an automated medication supply system.
      (1) Prepackaging of drugs.
         (a) Drugs may be prepackaged in quantities suitable for internal distribution only by a pharmacist or by pharmacy technicians or pharmacy technician trainees under the direction and direct supervision of a pharmacist.
         (b) The label of a prepackaged unit shall indicate:
            (i) Brand name and strength of the drug; if no brand name, the generic name, strength, and name of the manufacturer or distributor;
            (ii) Facility's lot number;
            (iii) Expiration date; and
            (iv) Quantity of the drug if quantity is greater than one.
         (c) Records of prepackaging shall be maintained to show:
            (i) The name of the drug, strength, and dosage form;
            (ii) Facility's lot number;
            (iii) Manufacturer or distributor;
            (iv) Manufacturer's lot number;
            (v) Expiration date;
            (vi) Quantity per prepackaged unit;
            (vii) Number of prepackaged units;
            (viii) Date packaged;
            (ix) Name, initials, or electronic signature of the prepacker; and
            (x) Signature or electronic signature of the responsible pharmacist.
         (d) Stock packages, repackaged units, and control records shall be quarantined together until they are checked and released by the pharmacist.
      (2) Loading unit-of-use drugs into automated medication supply systems.

Automated medication supply systems may be loaded with unit-of-use drugs only by a pharmacist or by pharmacy technicians or pharmacy technician trainees under the direction and direct supervision of a pharmacist. Direct supervision may be accomplished by physically present supervision or electronic monitoring by a pharmacist. For the pharmacist to electronically monitor, the medication supply system must allow for barcode scanning to verify the loading of drugs, and a record of the loading must be maintained by the system and accessible for electronic review by the pharmacist.

6. Medication Orders.
   a. Drugs may be administered to patients in FEMCFs only on the order of a practitioner. No change in the order for drugs may be made without the approval of a practitioner except as authorized by the practitioner in compliance with 5.b. above.
   b. Drugs may be distributed only pursuant to the practitioner's medication order.
   c. FEMCF pharmacies shall be exempt from the labeling provisions and patient notification requirements of Sections 562.006 and 562.009 of the Act as they apply to drugs distributed pursuant to medication orders.

d. In FEMCFs with a full-time pharmacist, if a practitioner orders a drug for administration to a bona fide patient of the facility when the pharmacy is closed, the following is applicable.
   (1) Prescription drugs and devices only in sufficient quantities for immediate therapeutic needs of a patient may be removed from the FEMCF pharmacy.
   (2) Only a designated licensed nurse or practitioner may remove such drugs and devices.
   (3) A record shall be made at the time of the withdrawal by the authorized person removing the drugs and devices. The record shall contain the following information:
      (a) Name of the patient;
      (b) Name of device or drug, strength, and dosage form;
      (c) Dose prescribed;
      (d) Quantity taken;
      (e) Time and date; and
      (f) Signature or electronic signature of the person making the withdrawal.
   (4) The medication order in the patient's chart may substitute for such a record provided the medication order meets all the requirements of (3) above.
   (5) The pharmacist shall verify the withdrawal as soon as practical but in no event more than 72 hours from the time of such withdrawal.
e. In FEMCFs with a part-time or consultant pharmacist, if a practitioner orders a drug for administration to a bona fide patient of the FEMCF when the pharmacist is not on duty or when the pharmacy is closed, the following is applicable.
   (1) Prescription drugs and devices only in sufficient quantities for therapeutic needs may be removed from the FEMCF pharmacy.
   (2) Only a designated licensed nurse or practitioner may remove such drugs and devices.
   (3) A record shall be made at the time of the withdrawal by the authorized person removing the drugs and devices. The record shall meet the same requirements as specified in 6.d. above.
   (4) The pharmacist shall conduct an audit of the patient's medical record at a reasonable interval according to the schedule described in the policies and procedures, but such interval must occur at least once in every calendar week that the pharmacy is open.

7. Floor Stock. In facilities using a floor stock method of drug distribution, the following is applicable for removing drugs or devices in the absence of a pharmacist.
   a. Prescription drugs and devices may be removed from the pharmacy only in the original manufacturer's container or prepackaged container.
   b. Only a designated licensed nurse or practitioner may remove such drugs and devices.
   c. A record shall be made at the time of the withdrawal by the authorized person removing the drug or device. The record shall contain the following information:
      (1) Name of the drug, strength, and dosage form;
      (2) Quantity removed;
      (3) Location of floor stock;
      (4) Date and time; and
      (5) Signature or electronic signature of the person making the withdrawal.

d. A pharmacist shall verify the withdrawal according to the following schedule.
   (1) In facilities with a full-time pharmacist, the withdrawal shall be verified as soon as practical but in no event more than 72 hours from the time of such withdrawal.
   (2) In facilities with a part-time or consultant pharmacist, the withdrawal shall be verified after a reasonable interval. The interval must occur at least once in every calendar week that the pharmacy is open.
   (3) The medication order in the patient's chart may substitute for the record required in 7.c. above provided the medication order meets all the requirements of 7.c. above.
8. Policies and Procedures. Written policies and procedures for a drug distribution system appropriate for the freestanding emergency medical center shall be developed and implemented by the pharmacist-in-charge with the advice of the appropriate committee. The written policies and procedures for the drug distribution system shall include, but not be limited to, procedures regarding the following:
   a. Controlled substances;
   b. Investigational drugs;
   c. Prepackaging and manufacturing;
   d. Medication errors;
   e. Orders of a physician or other practitioner;
   f. Floor stock;
   g. Adverse drug reactions;
   h. Drugs brought into the facility by the patient;
   i. Self-administration;
   j. Emergency drug tray;
   k. Formulary if applicable;
   l. Drug storage areas;
   m. Drug samples;
   n. Drug product defect reports;
   o. Drug recalls;
   p. Outdated drugs;
   q. Preparation and distribution of IV admixtures;
   r. Procedures for supplying drugs for postoperative use if applicable;
   s. Use of automated medication supply systems;
   t. Use of data processing systems; and
   u. Drug regimen review.
9. Drugs Supplied for Outpatient Use. Drugs supplied to patients for outpatient use shall be supplied according to the following procedures.
   a. Drugs may only be supplied to patients who have been admitted to the FEMCF.
   b. Drugs may only be supplied in accordance with the system of control and accountability established for drugs supplied from the FEMCF. This system shall be developed and supervised by the pharmacist-in-charge or staff pharmacist designated by the pharmacist-in-charge.
   c. Only drugs listed on the approved outpatient drug list may be supplied. This list shall be developed by the pharmacist-in-charge and the medical staff and shall consist of drugs of the nature and type to meet the immediate postoperative needs of the freestanding emergency medical center patient.
   d. Drugs may only be supplied in prepackaged quantities not to exceed a 72-hour supply in suitable containers and appropriately prelabeled (including name, address, phone number of the facility, and necessary

auxiliary labels) by the pharmacy. However, topicals and ophthalmics in the original manufacturer's containers may be supplied in a quantity exceeding a 72-hour supply.

e. At the time of the delivery of the drug, the practitioner shall complete the label so that the prescription container bears a label with at least the following information:
(1) Date supplied;
(2) Name of practitioner;
(3) Name of patient;
(4) Directions for use;
(5) Brand name and strength of the drug; if no brand name, then the generic name of the drug dispensed, strength, and the name of the manufacturer or distributor of the drug; and
(6) Unique identification number.

Note: A practitioner can legally delegate this task to another individual.

f. After the drug has been labeled, the practitioner or a licensed nurse under the supervision of the practitioner shall give the appropriately labeled, prepackaged medication to the patient.

g. A perpetual record of all drugs which are supplied from the FEMCF shall be maintained which includes:
(1) Name, address, and phone number of the facility;
(2) Date supplied;
(3) Name of practitioner;
(4) Name of patient;
(5) Directions for use;
(6) Brand name and strength of the drug; if no brand name, then the generic name of the drug dispensed, strength, and the name of the manufacturer or distributor of the drug; and
(7) Unique identification number.

h. The pharmacist-in-charge or a pharmacist designated by the pharmacist-in-charge shall review the records at least once in every calendar week the pharmacy is open.

10. Drug Regimen Review.
    a. A pharmacist shall evaluate medication orders and patient medication records for:
    (1) Known allergies;
    (2) Rational therapy including contraindications;
    (3) Reasonable dose and route of administration;
    (4) Reasonable directions for use;
    (5) Duplication of therapy;
    (6) Drug-drug interactions;
    (7) Drug-food interactions;
    (8) Drug-disease interactions;
    (9) Adverse drug reactions;
    (10) Proper utilization including overutilization or underutilization; and
    (11) Clinical laboratory or clinical monitoring methods to monitor and evaluate drug effectiveness, side effects, toxicity or adverse effects, and appropriateness to continued use of the drug in its current regimen.
    b. A retrospective, random drug regimen review as specified in the pharmacy's policies and procedures shall be conducted to verify proper usage of drugs on a periodic basis not to exceed 31 days between such reviews.
    c. Any questions regarding the order must be resolved with the prescriber and a written notation of these discussions made and maintained.

E. Records.
  1. Maintenance of Records.
     a. Every inventory or other record required to be retained under the provisions of this rule (FEMCF pharmacy) shall be:
        (1) Kept by the pharmacy and be available for at least two years from the date of such inventory or record for inspecting and copying by the Board or its representative and other authorized local, state, or federal law enforcement agencies and
        (2) Supplied by the pharmacy within 72 hours if requested by an authorized agent of the Board. If the pharmacy maintains the records in an electronic format, the requested records must be provided in a mutually agreeable electronic format if specifically requested by the Board or its representative. Failure to provide these records, either on-site or within 72 hours, constitutes prima facie evidence of failure to keep and maintain records in violation of the Act.
     b. Records of controlled substances listed in Schedule II shall be maintained separately and readily retrievable from all other records of the pharmacy.
     c. Records of controlled substances listed in Schedules III–V shall be maintained separately or readily retrievable from all other records of the pharmacy. Readily retrievable means that the controlled substances shall be asterisked, redlined, or in some other manner readily identifiable apart from all other items appearing on the record.
     d. Records, except when specifically required to be maintained in original or hardcopy form, may be maintained in an alternative data retention system such as a data processing or direct imaging system provided:
        (1) The records in the alternative data retention system contain all of the information required on the manual record and
        (2) The alternative data retention system is capable of producing a hard copy of the record upon the request of the Board, its representative, or other authorized local, state, or federal law enforcement or regulatory agencies.
     e. Controlled substance records shall be maintained in a manner to establish receipt and distribution of all controlled substances.
     f. An FEMCF pharmacy shall maintain a perpetual inventory of controlled substances listed in Schedules II–V which shall be verified for completeness and reconciled at least once in every calendar week that the pharmacy is open.
     g. Distribution records for controlled substances listed in Schedules II–V shall include the following information:
        (1) Patient's name;
        (2) Practitioner's name who ordered the drug;
        (3) Name of the drug, dosage form, and strength;
        (4) Time and date of administration to patient and quantity administered;
        (5) Signature or electronic signature of individual administering the controlled substance;
        (6) Returns to the pharmacy; and
        (7) Drug waste (waste is required to be witnessed and cosigned manually or electronically by another individual).
     h. The record required by g. above shall be maintained separately from patient records.
     i. A pharmacist shall conduct an audit on a periodic basis not to exceed 30 days by randomly comparing the distribution records required by g. above with the medication orders in the patient record to verify proper administration of drugs.

2. Patient Records.
   a. Each medication order or set of orders issued together shall bear the following information:
      (1) Patient name;
      (2) Drug name, strength, and dosage form;
      (3) Directions for use;
      (4) Date; and
      (5) Signature or electronic signature of the practitioner or that of his or her authorized agent defined as a licensed nurse employee or full-time, part-time, or consultant pharmacist of the FEMCF.
   b. Medication orders shall be maintained with the medication administration record in the medical records of the patient.
3. General Requirements for Records Maintained in a Data Processing System.
   a. If an FEMCF pharmacy's data processing system is not in compliance with the Board's requirements, the pharmacy must maintain a manual recordkeeping system.
   b. The facility shall maintain a backup copy of information stored in the data processing system using disk, tape, or another electronic backup system and update this backup copy on a regular basis to assure that data is not lost due to a system failure.
   c. A pharmacy that changes or discontinues the use of a data processing system must:
      (1) Transfer the records to the new data processing system or
      (2) Purge the records to a printout which contains:
         (a) All of the information required on the original document or
         (b) For records of distribution and return for all controlled substances, the same information as required on the audit trail printout as specified in f. below. The information on the printout shall be sorted and printed by drug name and list chronologically all distributions and returns.
   d. Maintenance of purged records. Information purged from a data processing system must be maintained by the pharmacy for two years from the date of initial entry into the data processing system.
   e. The pharmacist-in-charge shall report to the Board in writing any significant loss of information from the data processing system within 10 days of the discovery of the loss.
   f. The data processing system shall have the capacity to produce a hard-copy printout of an audit trail of drug distribution and return for any strength and dosage form of a drug (by either brand or generic name or both) during a specified time period. This printout shall contain the following information:
      (1) Patient's name and room number or patient's facility identification number;
      (2) Prescribing or attending practitioner's name;
      (3) Name, strength, and dosage form of the drug product distributed;
      (4) Total quantity distributed from and returned to the pharmacy; and
      (5) If not immediately retrievable by electronic image, the following shall also be included on the printout:
         (a) Prescribing or attending practitioner's address and
         (b) Practitioner's DEA registration number if the medication order is for a controlled substance.
   g. An audit trail printout for each strength and dosage form of the drugs distributed during the preceding month shall be produced at least monthly and shall be maintained in a separate file at the facility. The information

on this printout shall be sorted by drug name and list chronologically all distributions and returns for that drug.

    h. The pharmacy may elect not to produce the monthly audit trail printout if the data processing system has a workable (electronic) data retention system which can produce an audit trail of drug distribution and returns for the preceding two years. The audit trail required shall be supplied by the pharmacy within 72 hours if requested by an authorized agent of the Board or other authorized local, state, or federal law enforcement or regulatory agencies.

    i. In the event that an FEMCF pharmacy which uses a data processing system experiences system downtime, the pharmacy must have an auxiliary procedure which will ensure that all data is retained for online data entry as soon as the system is available for use again.

4. Distribution of Controlled Substances to Another Registrant. A pharmacy may distribute controlled substances to a practitioner, another pharmacy, or another registrant without being registered to distribute under the following conditions.

    a. The registrant to whom the controlled substance is to be distributed is registered under the Federal Controlled Substances Act to possess that controlled substance.

    b. The total number of dosage units of controlled substances distributed to other registrants by a pharmacy may not exceed 5.0% of all controlled substances dispensed and distributed by the pharmacy during the 12-month period in which the pharmacy is registered. If at any time the pharmacy exceeds 5.0%, the pharmacy is required to obtain an additional DEA registration to distribute controlled substances.

    c. If the distribution is for a Schedule III, IV, or V controlled substance, a record shall be maintained which indicates:

        (1) The actual date of distribution;

        (2) The name, strength, and quantity of controlled substances distributed;

        (3) The name, address, and DEA registration number of the distributing pharmacy; and

        (4) The name, address, and DEA registration number of the pharmacy, practitioner, or other registrant to whom the controlled substances are distributed.

    d. If the distribution is for a Schedule I or II controlled substance, the following is applicable.

        (1) The pharmacy, practitioner, or other registrant who is receiving the controlled substances shall issue Copy 1 and Copy 2 of DEA Form 222.

        (2) The distributing pharmacy shall:

            (a) Complete the area on DEA Form 222 titled "To Be Filled in by Supplier";

            (b) Maintain Copy 1 of DEA Form 222 at the pharmacy for two years; and

            (c) Forward Copy 2 of DEA Form 222 to the divisional office of DEA.

5. Other Records. Other records to be maintained by the pharmacy include:

    a. A permanent log of the initials or identification codes which identifies each pharmacist by name. The initials or identification code shall be unique to ensure that each pharmacist can be identified (i.e., identical initials or identification codes cannot be used);

    b. Copy 3 of DEA Form 222 which has been properly dated, initialed, and filed and all copies of each unaccepted or defective order form and any

attached statements or other documents. For each order filled using the DEA Controlled Substance Ordering System (CSOS), the original signed order and all linked records for that order shall be maintained;
   c. A copy of the power of attorney to sign DEA Forms 222 (if applicable);
   d. Suppliers' invoices of dangerous drugs and controlled substances dated and initialed or signed by the person receiving the drugs. A pharmacist shall verify that the controlled drugs listed on the invoices were added to the pharmacy's perpetual inventory by clearly recording his or her initials and the date of the review of the perpetual inventory;
   e. Suppliers' credit memos for controlled substances and dangerous drugs;
   f. A copy of inventories required by Board Rule 291.17 (Inventory Requirements) except that a perpetual inventory of controlled substances listed in Schedule II may be kept in a data processing system if the data processing system is capable of producing a hard copy of the perpetual inventory on-site;
   g. Reports of surrender or destruction of controlled substances and/or dangerous drugs to an appropriate state or federal agency;
   h. Records of distribution of controlled substances and/or dangerous drugs to other pharmacies, practitioners, or registrants; and
   i. A copy of any notification required by the Act or these rules including, but not limited to, the following:
      (1) Reports of theft or significant loss of controlled substances to DEA and the Board;
      (2) Notification of a change in pharmacist-in-charge of a pharmacy; and
      (3) Reports of a fire or other disaster which may affect the strength, purity, or labeling of drugs, medications, devices, or other materials used in the diagnosis or treatment of injury, illness, and disease.
6. Permission to Maintain Central Records. Any pharmacy that uses a centralized recordkeeping system for invoices and financial data shall comply with the following procedures.
   a. Controlled substance records. Invoices and financial data for controlled substances may be maintained at a central location provided the following conditions are met.
      (1) Prior to the initiation of central recordkeeping, the pharmacy submits written notification by registered or certified mail to the divisional director of DEA and submits a copy of this written notification to the Board. Unless the registrant is informed by the divisional director of DEA that permission to keep central records is denied, the pharmacy may maintain central records commencing 14 days after receipt of notification by the divisional director.
      (2) The pharmacy maintains a copy of the notification required in a.(1) above, and
      (3) The records to be maintained at the central record location shall not include executed DEA order forms, prescription drug orders, or controlled substance inventories which shall be maintained at the pharmacy.
   b. Dangerous drug records. Invoices and financial data for dangerous drugs may be maintained at a central location.
   c. Access to records. If the records are kept on microfilm, computer media, or in any form requiring special equipment to render the records easily readable, the pharmacy shall provide access to such equipment with the records.

d. Delivery of records. The pharmacy agrees to deliver all or any part of such records to the pharmacy location within two business days of written request of a Board agent or any other authorized official.

Central Prescription Drug or Medication Order Processing Pharmacy (Class G) Rule

> **Board of Pharmacy Rule 291.153**
> **Central Prescription Drug or**
> **Medication Order Processing Pharmacy (Class G)**

A. Purpose.
   1. The purpose of this rule is to provide standards for a centralized prescription drug or medication order processing pharmacy.
   2. Any facility established for the primary purpose of processing prescription drug or medication drug orders shall be licensed as a Class G pharmacy under the Act. A Class G pharmacy shall not store bulk drugs or dispense prescription drug orders. Nothing in this rule shall prohibit an individual pharmacist employee, individual pharmacy technician employee, or individual pharmacy technician trainee employee who is licensed or registered in Texas from remotely accessing the pharmacy's electronic database from a location other than a licensed pharmacy to process prescription or medication drug orders, provided the pharmacy establishes controls to protect the privacy and security of confidential records. Furthermore, the Texas licensed pharmacist or the registered pharmacy technician or pharmacy technician trainee may not engage in the receiving of written prescription or medication orders or the maintenance of prescription or medication drug orders at the non-licensed remote location.
B. Definitions. The following words and terms shall have the following meanings unless the context clearly indicates otherwise. Any term not defined in this rule shall have the definition set out in the Act.
   1. **Centralized prescription drug or medication order processing**—The processing of a prescription drug or medication order by a Class G pharmacy on behalf of another pharmacy, a healthcare provider, or a payor. Centralized prescription drug or medication order processing does not include the dispensing of a prescription drug but includes any of the following:
      a. Receiving, interpreting, or clarifying prescription drug or medication drug orders;
      b. Data entering and transferring of prescription drug or medication order information;
      c. Performing drug regimen review;
      d. Obtaining refill and substitution authorizations;
      e. Verifying accurate prescription data entry;
      f. Interpreting clinical data for prior authorization for dispensing;
      g. Performing therapeutic interventions; and
      h. Providing drug information concerning a patient's prescription.
   2. **Full-time pharmacist**—A pharmacist who works in a pharmacy from 30 to 40 hours per week or, if the pharmacy is open fewer than 60 hours per week, one-half of the time the pharmacy is open.

C. Personnel.
 1. Pharmacist-in-Charge.
    a. General. Each Class G pharmacy shall have one pharmacist-in-charge who is employed on a full-time basis and who may be the pharmacist-in-charge for only one such pharmacy.
    b. Responsibilities. The pharmacist-in-charge shall have responsibility for the practice of pharmacy at the pharmacy for which he or she is the pharmacist-in-charge. The pharmacist-in-charge may advise the owner on administrative or operational concerns. The pharmacist-in-charge shall have, at a minimum, the following responsibilities:
       (1) Educating and training pharmacy technicians and pharmacy technician trainees;
       (2) Maintaining records of all transactions of the Class G pharmacy required by applicable state and federal laws and rules/regulations;
       (3) Adhering to policies and procedures regarding the maintenance of records in a data processing system so that the data processing system is in compliance with Class G pharmacy requirements; and
       (4) Legally operating the pharmacy including meeting all inspection and other requirements of all state and federal laws or rules/regulations governing the practice of pharmacy.
 2. Owner. The owner of a Class G pharmacy shall have responsibility for all administrative and operational functions of the pharmacy. The pharmacist-in-charge may advise the owner on administrative and operational concerns. If the owner is not a Texas licensed pharmacist, the owner shall consult with the pharmacist-in-charge or another Texas licensed pharmacist. The owner shall have responsibility for, at a minimum, the following:
    a. Providing the pharmacy with the necessary equipment and resources commensurate with its level and type of practice and
    b. Establishing policies and procedures regarding maintenance, storage, and retrieval of records in a data processing system so that the system is in compliance with state and federal laws and rules/regulations.
 3. Pharmacists.
    a. General.
       (1) The pharmacist-in-charge shall be assisted by a sufficient number of additional licensed pharmacists as may be required to operate the Class G pharmacy competently, safely, and adequately to meet the needs of the patients of the pharmacy.
       (2) All pharmacists shall assist the pharmacist-in-charge in meeting his or her responsibilities.
       (3) Pharmacists are solely responsible for the direct supervision of pharmacy technicians and pharmacy technician trainees and for designating and delegating duties, other than those listed in b. (Duties) below, to pharmacy technicians and pharmacy technician trainees. Each pharmacist shall be responsible for any delegated act performed by pharmacy technicians and pharmacy technician trainees under his or her supervision.
       (4) Pharmacists shall directly supervise pharmacy technicians and pharmacy technician trainees who are entering prescription data into the pharmacy's data processing system by one of the following methods.
          (a) Physically present supervision. A pharmacist shall be physically present to directly supervise a pharmacy technician or pharmacy technician trainee who is entering prescription order or medication order data into the data processing system. Each

prescription or medication order entered into the data processing system shall be verified at the time of data entry.
- (b) Electronic supervision. A pharmacist may electronically supervise a pharmacy technician or pharmacy technician trainee who is entering prescription order or medication order data into the data processing system provided the pharmacist:
  - (i) Has the ability to immediately communicate directly with the technician/trainee;
  - (ii) Has immediate access to any original document containing prescription or medication order information or other information related to the dispensing of the prescription or medication order. Such access may be through imaging technology provided the pharmacist has the ability to review the original, hardcopy documents if needed for clarification; and
  - (iii) Verifies the accuracy of the data-entered information prior to the release of the information to the system for storage.
- (c) Electronic verification of data entry by pharmacy technicians or pharmacy technician trainees. A pharmacist may electronically verify the data entry of prescription information into a data processing system provided:
  - (i) The pharmacist has the ability to immediately communicate directly with the technician/trainee;
  - (ii) The pharmacist electronically conducting the verification is either a:
    - (I) Texas licensed pharmacist or
    - (II) Pharmacist employed by a Class E pharmacy that has the same owner as the Class G pharmacy where the pharmacy technicians/trainees are located or that has entered into a written contract or agreement with the Class G pharmacy, which outlines the services to be provided and the responsibilities and accountabilities of each pharmacy in compliance with state and federal laws and rules/regulations;
  - (iii) The pharmacy establishes controls to protect the privacy and security of confidential records; and
  - (iv) The pharmacy keeps permanent records of prescriptions electronically verified for a period of two years.
- (5) All pharmacists while on duty shall be responsible for complying with all state and federal laws or rules/regulations governing the practice of pharmacy.

b. Duties. Duties which may be performed only by a pharmacist are as follows:
 (1) Receiving oral prescription drug or medication orders and reducing these orders to writing either manually or electronically;
 (2) Interpreting prescription drug or medication orders;
 (3) Selecting drug products;
 (4) Verifying the data entry of the prescription drug or medication order information at the time of data entry prior to the release of the information to a Class A, Class C, or Class E pharmacy for dispensing;
 (5) Communicating to the patient or patient's agent information about the prescription drug or device which in the exercise of the pharmacist's professional judgment the pharmacist deems significant, as specified in Board Rule 291.33(c) (Operational Standards);

(6) Communicating to the patient or the patient's agent on his or her request for information concerning any prescription drugs dispensed to the patient by the pharmacy;

(7) Assuring that a reasonable effort is made to obtain, record, and maintain patient medication records; and

(8) Interpreting patient medication records and performing drug regimen reviews.

4. Pharmacy Technicians and Pharmacy Technician Trainees.
   a. General. All pharmacy technicians and pharmacy technician trainees shall meet the training requirements specified in Board Rule 297.6 (Pharmacy Technician and Pharmacy Technician Trainee Training).
   b. Duties.
      (1) Pharmacy technicians and pharmacy technician trainees may not perform any of the duties listed in 3.b. above.
      (2) A pharmacist may delegate to pharmacy technicians and pharmacy technician trainees any nonjudgmental technical duty associated with the preparation and distribution of prescription drugs provided:
         (a) A pharmacist verifies the accuracy of all acts, tasks, and functions performed by pharmacy technicians and pharmacy technician trainees and
         (b) Pharmacy technicians and pharmacy technician trainees are under the direct supervision of and responsible to a pharmacist.
      (3) Pharmacy technicians and pharmacy technician trainees may perform only nonjudgmental technical duties associated with the preparation of prescription drugs as follows:
         (a) Initiating and receiving refill authorization requests and
         (b) Entering prescription or medication order data into a data processing system.
   c. Ratio of on-site pharmacists to pharmacy technicians and pharmacy technician trainees. A Class G pharmacy may have a ratio of pharmacists to pharmacy technicians and pharmacy technician trainees of 1:8 provided:
      (1) At least seven are pharmacy technicians and not pharmacy technician trainees and
      (2) The pharmacy has written policies and procedures regarding the supervision of pharmacy technicians and pharmacy technician trainees.

   Note: The ratio for Class G allows only one technician out of the total of eight to be a technician trainee.

5. Identification of Pharmacy Personnel. All pharmacy personnel shall be identified as follows.
   a. Pharmacy technicians. All pharmacy technicians shall wear an identification tag or badge that bears the person's name and identifies him or her as a pharmacy technician or a certified pharmacy technician if the technician maintains a current certification approved by the Board.
   b. Pharmacy technician trainees. All pharmacy technician trainees shall wear an identification tag or badge that bears the person's name and identifies him or her as a pharmacy technician trainee.
   c. Pharmacist interns. All pharmacist interns shall wear an identification tag or badge that bears the person's name and identifies him or her as a pharmacist intern.
   d. Pharmacists. All pharmacists shall wear an identification tag or badge that bears the person's name and identifies him or her as a pharmacist.

D. Operational Standards.
   1. General Requirements.
      a. A Class A, Class C, or Class E Pharmacy may outsource prescription drug or medication order processing to a Class G pharmacy provided the pharmacies:
         (1) Have the same owner or have entered into a written contract or agreement which outlines the services to be provided and the responsibilities and accountabilities of each pharmacy in compliance with state and federal laws and rules/regulations and
         (2) Share a common electronic file or have appropriate technology to allow access to sufficient information necessary or required to perform a non-dispensing function.
      b. A Class G pharmacy shall comply with the provisions applicable to the class of pharmacy contained in either Board Rules 291.3–291.35 (Definitions, Personnel, Operational Standards, Records, and Official Prescription Requirements) in Class A pharmacies or Board Rules 291.72–291.75 (Definitions, Personnel, Operational Standards, and Records) in Class C pharmacies or Board Rules 291.102–291.105 (Definitions, Personnel, Operational Standards, and Records) in Class E pharmacies to the extent applicable for the specific processing activity and this rule including:
         (1) Duties which must be performed by a pharmacist and
         (2) Supervision requirements for pharmacy technicians and pharmacy technician trainees.
   2. Licensing Requirements.
      a. A Class G pharmacy shall register with the Board on a pharmacy license application provided by the Board following the procedures specified in Board Rule 291.1 (Pharmacy License Application).
      b. A Class G pharmacy which changes ownership shall notify the Board within 10 days of the change of ownership and apply for a new and separate license as specified in Board Rule 291.3 (Required Notifications).
      c. A Class G pharmacy which changes its name shall notify the Board of the change within 10 days and file for an amended license as specified in Board Rule 291.3.
      d. When a Class G pharmacy changes location, a new completed application must be filed no later than 30 days before the date of the change of location.
      e. A Class G pharmacy owned by a partnership or corporation which changes managing officers shall notify the Board in writing of the names of the new managing officers within 10 days of the change following the procedures in Board Rule 291.3.
      f. A Class G pharmacy shall notify the Board in writing within 10 days of closing following the procedures in Board Rule 291.5 (Closing a Pharmacy).
      g. A fee as specified in Board Rule 291.6 (Pharmacy License Fees) will be charged for issuance and renewal of a license and the issuance of an amended license.
      h. A separate license is required for each principal place of business, and only one pharmacy license may be issued to a specific location.
   3. Environment.
      a. General requirements.
         (1) The pharmacy shall be arranged in an orderly fashion and kept clean. All required equipment shall be in good operating condition.
         (2) The pharmacy shall be properly lighted and ventilated.

b. Security.
   (1) Each pharmacist while on duty shall be responsible for the security of the prescription department including provisions for effective control against theft or diversion of prescription drug records.
   (2) The pharmacy shall be locked by key, combination, or other mechanical or electronic means to prohibit unauthorized access when a pharmacist is not on-site.
4. Policies and Procedures. A policy and procedure manual shall be maintained by the Class G pharmacy and be available for inspection. The manual shall:
   a. Outline the responsibilities of each of the pharmacies;
   b. Include a list of the names, addresses, telephone numbers, and all license/registration numbers of the pharmacies involved in centralized prescription drug or medication order processing; and
   c. Include policies and procedures for:
      (1) Protecting the confidentiality and integrity of patient information;
      (2) Maintaining appropriate records to identify the name(s), initials, or identification code(s) and specific activity(ies) of each pharmacist or pharmacy technician who performed any processing;
      (3) Complying with state and federal laws and rules/regulations;
      (4) Operating a continuous quality improvement program for pharmacy services designed to objectively and systematically monitor and evaluate the quality and appropriateness of patient care, pursue opportunities to improve patient care, and resolve identified problems; and
      (5) Annually reviewing the written policies and procedures and documenting such review.

E. Records.
   1. Every record required to be retained under the provisions of this rule shall be:
      a. Kept by the pharmacy and be available for at least two years from the date of such inventory or record for inspecting and copying by the Board or its representative and to other authorized local, state, or federal law enforcement agencies and
      b. Supplied by the pharmacy within 72 hours if requested by an authorized agent of the Board. If the pharmacy maintains the records in an electronic format, the requested records must be provided in a mutually agreeable electronic format if specifically requested by the Board or its representative. Failure to provide the records set out in this rule, either on-site or within 72 hours, constitutes prima facie evidence of failure to keep and maintain records in violation of the Act and rules.
   2. The pharmacy shall maintain appropriate records which identify by prescription drug or medication order the name(s), initials, or identification code(s) of each pharmacist, pharmacy technician, or pharmacy technician trainee who performs a processing function for a prescription drug or medication order. Such records may be maintained:
      a. Separately by each pharmacy and pharmacist or
      b. In a common electronic file as long as the records are maintained in such a manner that the data processing system can produce a printout which lists the functions performed by each pharmacy and pharmacist.
   3. In addition, the pharmacy shall comply with the recordkeeping requirements applicable to the class of pharmacy to the extent applicable for the specific processing activity and this rule.

Limited Prescription Delivery Pharmacy (Class H) Rule

Board of Pharmacy Rule 291.155
Limited Prescription Delivery Pharmacy (Class H)

Note: This is a very limited type of pharmacy license since the pharmacy must be owned by a hospital district and must be located in a county without another pharmacy.

A. Purpose.
  1. The purpose of this rule is to provide standards for a limited prescription delivery pharmacy.
  2. Any facility established for the primary purpose of limited prescription delivery by a Class A pharmacy shall be licensed as a Class H pharmacy under the Act. A Class H pharmacy shall not store bulk drugs or dispense a prescription drug order.
  3. A Class H pharmacy may deliver prescription drug orders for dangerous drugs. A Class H pharmacy may not deliver prescription drug orders for controlled substances.
B. Definitions. Any term not defined in this rule shall have the definition set out in Section 551.003 of the Act.
C. Personnel.
  1. Pharmacist-in-Charge.
     a. General. Each Class H pharmacy shall have one pharmacist-in-charge who is employed or under written agreement at least on a part-time basis but may be employed on a full-time basis. The pharmacist-in-charge may be the pharmacist-in-charge for more than one limited prescription delivery pharmacy.
     b. Responsibilities. The pharmacist-in-charge shall have responsibility for the practice of pharmacy at the pharmacy for which he or she is the pharmacist-in-charge. The pharmacist-in-charge may advise the owner on administrative or operational concerns. The pharmacist-in-charge shall have at a minimum the following responsibilities:
        (1) Educating and training pharmacy technicians and pharmacy technician trainees;
        (2) Maintaining records of all transactions of the Class H pharmacy required by applicable state and federal laws and rules/regulations;
        (3) Adhering to policies and procedures regarding the maintenance of records; and
        (4) Legally operating the pharmacy including meeting all inspection and other requirements of all state and federal laws or rules/regulations governing the practice of pharmacy.
  2. Owner. The owner of a Class H pharmacy shall have responsibility for all administrative and operational functions of the pharmacy. The pharmacist-in-charge may advise the owner on administrative and operational concerns. If the owner is not a Texas licensed pharmacist, the owner shall consult with the pharmacist-in-charge or another Texas licensed pharmacist. The owner shall have at a minimum the following responsibilities:
     a. Providing the pharmacy with the necessary equipment and resources commensurate with its level and type of practice and
     b. Establishing policies and procedures regarding maintenance, storage, and retrieval of records in compliance with state and federal laws and rules/regulations.

3. Pharmacists.
    a. The pharmacist-in-charge shall be assisted by a sufficient number of additional licensed pharmacists as may be required to operate the Class H pharmacy competently, safely, and adequately to meet the needs of the patients of the pharmacy.
    b. All pharmacists shall assist the pharmacist-in-charge in meeting his or her responsibilities.
    c. Pharmacists shall be responsible for any delegated act performed by the pharmacy technicians under his or her supervision.
4. Pharmacy Technicians and Pharmacy Technician Trainees.
    a. General. All pharmacy technicians and pharmacy technician trainees shall meet the training requirements specified in Board Rule 297.6 (Pharmacy Technician and Pharmacy Technician Trainee Training).
    b. Duties. Duties include:
        (1) Delivering previously verified prescription drug orders to a patient or patient's agent provided a record of prescriptions delivered is maintained and
        (2) Maintaining pharmacy records.
5. Identification of Pharmacy Personnel. All pharmacy personnel shall be identified as follows.
    a. Pharmacy technicians. All pharmacy technicians shall wear an identification tag or badge that bears the person's name and identifies him or her as a pharmacy technician or a certified pharmacy technician if the technician maintains a current certification approved by the Board.
    b. Pharmacy technician trainees. All pharmacy technician trainees shall wear an identification tag or badge that bears the person's name and identifies him or her as a pharmacy technician trainee.
    c. Pharmacist interns. All pharmacist interns shall wear an identification tag or badge that bears the person's name and identifies him or her as a pharmacist intern.
    d. Pharmacists. All pharmacists shall wear an identification tag or badge that bears the person's name and identifies him or her as a pharmacist.

D. Operational Standards.
    1. General Requirements. A Class A or Class E Pharmacy may outsource limited prescription delivery to a Class H pharmacy provided the pharmacies have entered into a written contract or agreement which outlines the services to be provided and the responsibilities and accountabilities of each pharmacy in compliance with state and federal laws and rules/regulations.
    2. Licensing Requirements.
        a. A Class H pharmacy shall register with the Board on a pharmacy license application provided by the Board following the procedures specified in Board Rule 291.1 (Pharmacy License Application).
        b. A Class H pharmacy must be owned by a hospital district and located in a county without another pharmacy. If a Class A or Class C pharmacy is established in a county in which a Class H pharmacy has been located under this rule, the Class H pharmacy may continue to operate in that county.
        c. A Class H pharmacy which changes ownership shall notify the Board within 10 days of the change of ownership and apply for a new and separate license as specified in Board Rule 291.3 (Required Notifications).
        d. A Class H pharmacy which changes location and/or name shall notify the Board of the change and file for an amended license as specified in Board Rule 291.3.

Note: This requires notification no later than 30 days prior to the date for a change in location and no later than 10 days prior to the date for a change of name.

    e. A Class H pharmacy shall notify the Board in writing within 10 days of closing following the procedures in Board Rule 291.5 (Closing a Pharmacy).

    f. A fee as specified in Board Rule 291.6 (Pharmacy License Fees) will be charged for issuance and renewal of a license and the issuance of an amended license. However, a pharmacy operated by the state or a political subdivision of the state that qualifies for a Class H license is not required to pay a fee to obtain a license.

    g. A separate license is required for each principal place of business, and only one pharmacy license may be issued to a specific location.

3. Environment.
    a. General requirements.
        (1) The pharmacy shall have a designated area for the storage of previously verified prescription drug orders.
        (2) The pharmacy shall be arranged in an orderly fashion and kept clean.
        (3) A sink with hot and cold running water shall be available to all pharmacy personnel and shall be maintained in a sanitary condition at all times.
    b. Security.
        (1) Only authorized personnel may have access to storage areas for dangerous drugs.
        (2) When a pharmacist, pharmacy technician, or pharmacy technician trainee is not present, all storage areas for dangerous drugs and devices shall be locked by key, combination, or other mechanical or electronic means so as to prohibit access by unauthorized individuals.
        (3) The pharmacist-in-charge shall be responsible for the security of all storage areas for dangerous drugs including provisions for adequate safeguards against theft or diversion of dangerous drugs and records for such drugs.
        (4) Housekeeping and maintenance duties shall be carried out in the pharmacy while the pharmacist-in-charge, consultant pharmacist, staff pharmacist, or pharmacy technician/trainee is on the premises.
4. Library. A reference library shall be maintained which includes current copies of the following in hard copy or electronic format:
    a. Texas Pharmacy Act and rules;
    b. Texas Dangerous Drug Act;
    c. At least one current or updated patient information reference such as:
        (1) United States Pharmacopeia Dispensing Information, Volume II (Advice to the Patient) or
        (2) A reference text or information leaflets which provide patient information; and
    d. Basic antidote information and the telephone number of the nearest regional poison control center.
5. Delivery of Drugs.
    a. The pharmacist-in-charge, consultant pharmacist, staff pharmacist, pharmacy technician, or pharmacy technician trainee must be present at the pharmacy to deliver prescriptions.
    b. Prescriptions for controlled substances may not be stored or delivered by the pharmacy.

c. Prescriptions may be stored at the pharmacy for no more than 15 days. If prescriptions are not picked up by the patient, the medications are to be destroyed using a reverse distribution service.
d. The pharmacist-in-charge, consultant pharmacist, or staff pharmacist shall personally visit the pharmacy on at least a weekly basis and conduct monthly audits of prescriptions received and delivered by the pharmacy.

E. Records.
1. Every record required to be retained under the provisions of this rule shall be:
   a. Kept by the pharmacy and be available for at least two years from the date of such inventory or record for inspecting and copying by the Board or its representative and to other authorized local, state, or federal law enforcement agencies and
   b. Supplied by the pharmacy within 72 hours if requested by an authorized agent of the Board. If the pharmacy maintains the records in an electronic format, the requested records must be provided in a mutually agreeable electronic format if specifically requested by the Board or its representative. Failure to provide the records set out in this rule, either on-site or within 72 hours, constitutes prima facie evidence of failure to keep and maintain records in violation of the Act.
2. A record of on-site visits by the pharmacist-in-charge, consultant pharmacist, or staff pharmacist shall be maintained and include the following information:
   a. Date of the visit;
   b. Pharmacist's evaluation of findings; and
   c. Signature of the visiting pharmacist.
3. Records of prescription drug orders delivered to the Class H pharmacy shall include:
   a. Patient name;
   b. Name and quantity of drug delivered;
   c. Name and address of pharmacy delivering the prescription drug order; and
   d. Date received at the Class H pharmacy.
4. Records of drugs delivered to a patient or patient's agent shall include:
   a. Patient name;
   b. Name, signature, or electronic signature of the person who picks up the prescription drug;
   c. Date delivered; and
   d. Name of the drug and quantity delivered.
5. Ownership of pharmacy records. For the purposes of these rules, a pharmacy licensed under the Act is the only entity which may legally own and maintain prescription drug records.

CHAPTER J HIGHLIGHTS
Other Classes of Pharmacies
Class B (Nuclear) Pharmacy

1. Every nuclear pharmacy shall have an authorized nuclear pharmacist as the pharmacist-in-charge who shall be responsible for a nuclear pharmacy's compliance with state and federal laws and regulations pertaining to the practice of nuclear pharmacy.
2. Nuclear pharmacists must either be Board certified or have 200 hours of didactic training in a program approved by the Texas Department of State Health Services, Radiation Control Program, and 500 hours of supervised practical experience in a nuclear pharmacy.
3. The ratio of authorized nuclear pharmacists to pharmacy technicians and pharmacy technician trainees may be 1:4 provided at least one of the four technicians is a pharmacy technician and is trained in the handling of radioactive materials.
4. There are no refills on radiopharmaceutical prescriptions.
5. The immediate inner container of a radiopharmaceutical shall be labeled with:
    a. The standard radiation symbol;
    b. The words "caution—radioactive material" or "danger—radioactive material";
    c. The name of the radiopharmaceutical or its abbreviation; and
    d. The unique identification number of the prescription.
6. The outer container of a radiopharmaceutical must meet specific labeling requirements including the name of the patient if known or the statement "for physician use" if the patient is unknown; the standard radiation symbol; the words "caution—radioactive material" or "danger—radioactive material"; the name of the radiopharmaceutical; the amount of radioactive material; the requested calibration date and time; and the expiration date and/or time.
7. Nuclear pharmacies must have a policy and procedure manual for the operation of the pharmacy.
8. Sterile compounded preparations must be prepared following Board Rule 291.133.

Class D (Clinic) Pharmacy

1. Class D pharmacies are locations other than a physician's office where a limited formulary of dangerous drugs and devices are stored and provided only to patients of the clinic.
2. A Class D formulary may include:
    a. Anti-infective drugs;
    b. Musculoskeletal drugs;
    c. Vitamins;
    d. Obstetrical and gynecological drugs and devices;
    e. Topical drugs; and
    f. Serums, toxoids, and vaccines
3. A Class D formulary may not include:
    a. Nalbuphine (Nubain®);
    b. Drugs used to treat erectile dysfunction; and
    c. Schedule I–V controlled substances.
4. A Class D pharmacy that serves at least 80% indigent patients may petition the Board for an expanded formulary. If the Class D pharmacy uses an expanded formulary, the following additional requirements must be met:
    a. Supportive personnel providing drugs must be licensed nurses or practitioners.
    b. The pharmacy must have policies and procedures for drugs on the formulary that require special monitoring.
    c. Retrospective drug regimen reviews of a random sample of clinic patients must be done on a quarterly basis.

    d. If the pharmacy provides antipsychotic drugs, the therapy must be initiated by a physician of the clinic, a practitioner shall monitor ongoing therapy, and the patient shall be physically examined by a physician at least yearly.
5. Provision of Drugs
    a. Drugs are prepackaged by a pharmacist or supportive personnel (under direct supervision of a pharmacist) and are provided to patients by a clinic employee.
    b. If using an expanded formulary, drugs can only be provided by licensed nurses or practitioners.
    c. Drugs must be provided in accordance with a system of control and accountability established by the clinic and developed and supervised by the pharmacist-in-charge.
    d. Drugs can only be provided to patients of the clinic.
    e. Only drugs on the clinic formulary can be provided.
    f. A licensed nurse or practitioner must provide verbal and written information to the patient on side effects, interactions, and precautions.
6. Any drugs dispensed to patients must be dispensed by a pharmacist subsequent to receiving a prescription from a practitioner.
7. Supervision
    a. The pharmacist-in-charge, consultant pharmacist, or staff pharmacist must personally visit the Class D pharmacy at least monthly.
    b. There is no limit to the number of Class D pharmacies a pharmacist-in-charge can supervise.
8. Pharmacy and Therapeutics Committee
    a. The clinic must have a pharmacy and therapeutics committee which shall develop a policy and procedure manual.
    b. The pharmacy and therapeutics committee shall meet at least annually to review and update the policy and procedure manual and review retrospective drug utilization review reports.
9. Unlike most other classes of pharmacies, a Class D pharmacy may have prescription drug samples but may not have samples of controlled substances.

Class E (Nonresident) Pharmacy

1. Class E pharmacies are licensed as nonresident pharmacies which are located in another state. Their primary business is to dispense a prescription drug or device under a prescription drug order and deliver the drug or device to patients including patients in Texas.
2. Class E pharmacies must have a pharmacist-in-charge who is a licensed Texas pharmacist.
3. Unless compliance would violate the pharmacy or drug laws or rules in the state in which the pharmacy is located, Class E pharmacies are required to comply with the provisions of Board Rules 291.101–291.105 (Purpose, Definitions, Personnel, Operational Standards, and Records).
4. Patient counseling is required for all new prescription drug orders. Prescriptions filled by Class E pharmacies are treated as delivered prescriptions, so a Class E pharmacy may meet the counseling requirements by providing written information regarding the prescription as well as a statement that a pharmacist is available for counseling via a toll-free telephone number.
5. A Class E pharmacy that compounds sterile products must register with the Board as a Class E-S pharmacy and meet all Class E-S rules.

Class F (Freestanding Emergency Medical Care Facility) Pharmacy

1. A Freestanding Emergency Medical Care Facility (FEMCF) is a freestanding facility that is licensed by the Texas Department of State Health Services pursuant to Chapter 254, Health and Safety Code, to provide emergency care to patients.
2. Each freestanding emergency medical care facility shall have one pharmacist-in-charge who is employed or under contract at least on a consulting or part-time basis but may be employed on a full-time basis.

3. The pharmacy and storage areas for prescription drugs and/or devices shall be enclosed and capable of being locked to prohibit access by unauthorized individuals. Only individuals authorized by the pharmacist-in-charge may enter the pharmacy or have access to storage areas for prescription drugs and/or devices.
4. The pharmacy shall have locked storage for Schedule II controlled substances and other drugs requiring additional security.
5. In the absence of a pharmacist, only a designated licensed nurse or practitioner may remove drugs from the pharmacy in sufficient quantities for the immediate therapeutic needs of a patient.
6. In Class F pharmacies with a full-time pharmacist, the pharmacist shall verify the withdrawal of drugs from the pharmacy as soon as practical but in no event more than 72 hours from the time of such withdrawal.
7. In Class F pharmacies with a part-time or consultant pharmacist, the pharmacist shall conduct an audit of the patient's medical record according to the schedule set out in the pharmacy's policies and procedures at least once in every calendar week that the pharmacy is open.
8. A Class F pharmacy must maintain a perpetual inventory of controlled substances which shall be verified for completeness and reconciled at least once in every calendar week that the pharmacy is open.
9. Invoices of dangerous drugs and controlled substances must be dated and initialed or signed by the person receiving the drugs. A pharmacist shall verify that the controlled drugs listed on the invoices were added to the pharmacy's perpetual inventory by clearly recording his or her initials and the date of the review of the perpetual inventory.
10. Drugs may be supplied for outpatient use only in prepackaged quantities not to exceed a 72-hour supply if pre-labeled by the pharmacy. At the time of the delivery of the drug, the practitioner or licensed nurse under the practitioner's supervision must complete the label.
11. A retrospective drug regimen review must be conducted at least every 31 days to verify proper usage of drugs.

Class G (Central Prescription Drug Order or Medication Order Processing) Pharmacy

1. A Class G pharmacy license is issued to a facility established for the primary purpose of processing prescription drug or medication drug orders on behalf of another pharmacy, a healthcare provider, or a payor.
2. A Class G pharmacy does not store or dispense drugs but may perform the following:
    a. Receiving, interpreting, or clarifying prescription drug or medication drug orders;
    b. Data entering and transferring of prescription drug or medication order information;
    c. Performing drug regimen review;
    d. Obtaining refill and substitution authorizations;
    e. Verifying accurate prescription data entry;
    f. Interpreting clinical data for prior authorization for dispensing;
    g. Performing therapeutic interventions; and
    h. Providing drug information concerning a patient's prescription.
3. A Class G pharmacy may have a ratio of pharmacists to pharmacy technicians and pharmacy technician trainees of 1:8. However, only one of those may be a pharmacy technician trainee.
4. Pharmacists, pharmacy technicians, and pharmacy technician trainee employees may work remotely and access the pharmacy's electronic database to process prescription drug orders or medication orders.

Class H (Limited Prescription Delivery) Pharmacy

1. A Class H pharmacy is a unique and limited type of pharmacy that is owned by a hospital district and is located in a county without another pharmacy.
2. A Class H pharmacy provides limited prescription services for a Class A pharmacy.
3. A Class H pharmacy shall not store bulk drugs or dispense prescription drug orders.
4. A Class H pharmacy may only deliver filled prescriptions for dangerous drugs for the Class A pharmacy and may not deliver prescriptions for controlled substances.

INDEX

Index

A

Absence of pharmacist
    Class A (community) pharmacy, G.13–15
    Class C (institutional) pharmacy, I.16–17
Accutane, A.19
Accelerated refills, G.41
Acute pain, prescription limits for opioids, B.40–41
Administration of epinephrine by pharmacist, D.67–69
Administration of medication by pharmacists, D.12–13
Adulteration, A.11
Advanced Practice Registered Nurses (APRNs), C.9–11
Advertising prescription drugs by pharmacists/pharmacies, A.16–17, D.18
Alcohol, A.35–36
Alternative dispute resolution, D.11, F.33–34
Ambulances, distribution of controlled substances to, B.19
Ambulatory surgical center, I.36–39
Anabolic steroids, B.4
Automated devices and systems
    Class A (community) pharmacies, G.27–33
    Class C (institutional) pharmacies, I.23–30
Automatic refills, B.45, G.41
Automated storage and delivery systems (kiosks), D.78–79
Auto refill programs, B.45, G.41

B

Batch compounding
    Nonsterile preparations, H.14
    Sterile preparations, H.20, H.60
Balance, prescription, E.14–15
Beyond-use date for dispensed drugs, G.21–22
Biennial inventory, B.26
Biological products, A.5, A.9
    Substitution of, D.57–68
Biosimilars, A.5, D.63
    Interchangeability of, D.55–58
Bioterrorism, reporting to Texas Department of State Health Services, D.67
Bulk transfers of prescriptions, G.48

C

CARA (Comprehensive Addiction and Recovery Act of 2016), B.51
Canadian practitioners, C.2, C.21, G.35–37
Central fill, E.23–24
Central prescription drug or medication order processing pharmacy (Class G), J.47–52
Central processing, E.24–25
Centralized prescription dispensing, E.23–24
Centralized prescription and medication order processing, E.24–25
Central recordkeeping (DEA), B.28
Certification programs, pharmacists, E.1–2
Changing information on a controlled substance prescription, B.31–32
Charitable drug donations, C.16–20
Class A (community) pharmacy rules, G.1–54
    Absence of pharmacist, G.13–15
    Automated devices and systems, G.27–33
    Computer record system, G.43–46
    Counseling, G.15–18
    Customized patient medication packages, G.25–26
    Data processing record system, G.43–46
    Drug storage, G.24
    Drug regimen review, G.2, G.18–19
    Environment, G.12–15
    Equipment and supplies, G.24
    Label requirements, G.20–23
        Chart of, G.23
    Library requirements, G.24
    Licensing of, D.46–50, G.11–12
    Manual record system, G.43
    Owners, G.6
    Patient counseling, G.15–18
    Patient medication records, G.42–43
    Personnel, G.5–11
    Owner, G.6
    Pharmacist-in-charge (PIC), G.5–6
    Pharmacists, G.6–8
    Pharmacy technicians and trainees, G.8–11
    Pharmaceutical care services, G.18–19
    Prescription containers, G.20
        Label requirements, G.20–23
            Chart of, G.23
    Prescription dispensing and delivery, G.15–20
    Prescription drug order records
        Computer system, G.43–46
        Data processing system, G.43–46
        Manual system, G.43
    Prepackaging of drugs, G.24–25
    Records, G.33–50
    Reference books, G.24
    Security, G.12–13
    Storage of drugs, G.24
Class A-S pharmacy rule, G.50–51
Class B (nuclear) pharmacy rules, J.1–9
    Equipment, J.7
    Label requirements, J.7
    Library requirements, J.7

Class B (nuclear) pharmacy rules (*continued*)
   Licensing of (registration), D.46–50, J.5–6
   Personnel, J.1–5
      Nuclear pharmacists, J.3–4
      Pharmacist-in-charge (PIC), J.1–2
      Pharmacy technicians and trainees, J.4–5
   Policy and procedure manual, J.8
   Records, J.8–9
   Reference books, J.7
Class C (institutional) pharmacy rules, I.1–42
   Absence of pharmacist, I.16–17
   Automated devices and systems, I.23–30
   Computer record system, I.32–34
   Consultant pharmacists, I.6
   Data processing record system, I.32–34
   Discharge prescriptions, I.21
   Drug regimen review, I.21–22
   Emergency rooms, I.22–23
   Equipment and supplies, I.15
   Floor stock
      Distribution system, I.16–17
      Records of, I.32
   Formulary, I.18
   Inventory (perpetual), I.34
   Library requirements, I.15–16
   Licensing, D.46–50, I.13–15
   Owner, I.11
   Patient records, I.31–34
   Perpetual inventory, I.34
   Personnel, I.4–13
      Consultant pharmacist, I.6
      Owner, I.11
      Pharmacist-in-charge, I.4–6
      Pharmacists, I.6–7
      Pharmacy technicians and trainees, I.7–10
   Pharmaceutical care services, I.21–22
   Pharmacist supervision, I.3–4
   Policies and procedures, I.20–21
   Prepackaged drugs, distribution of, I.18–19
   Radiology department, I.23
   Records, I.31–34
   Reference books, I.15–16
   Rural hospitals, I.3, I.10, I.14–17
   Security, I.15
   Sterile preparations, H.19–64, I.13, I.34
   Tech-check-tech, I.4, I.9–10
Class C pharmacy in Free Standing Ambulatory Surgical Center, I.36–39
Class C-S pharmacy, I.34–36
Class D (clinic) pharmacy rules, J.9–19
   Definitions, J.9–10
   Dispensing of drugs, J.17
   Equipment and supplies, J.13
   Formulary and expanded formulary, J.13–15
   Labeling, J.15–17
   Licensing—Registration, D.46–50, J.11–12
   Library requirements, J.13
   Personnel, J.10–11
      Consultant pharmacist, J.10
      Owner, J.11
      Pharmacist-in-charge, J.10
      Pharmacists, J.10
      Supportive personnel, J.11
   Pharmacy and therapeutics committee, J.17
   Policy and procedure manual, J.17–18
   Prepackaging of drugs, J.15–17
   Provision of drugs, J.16–17
   Records, J.18–19
   Reference books, J.13
   Samples, J.15
   Security requirements, J.12
   Storage of drugs and devices, J.12, J.15
   Supervision, J.18
Class E (nonresident) pharmacy statutes and rules, J.20–31
   Discipline of, J.22
   Drug regimen review, J.26
   Generic substitution, J.28
   Grounds for discipline, J.22
   Inspection of, J.20
   Licensing, D.46–50, J.20–21
   Patient counseling, J.27–28
   Personnel, J.24
   Records, J.29–30
   Therapeutic drug interchange, J.28–29
Class E-S pharmacy, J.30–31
Class F (freestanding emergency medical center) pharmacy, J.31–47
Class G (central prescription drug or medication order processing) pharmacy, J.47–52
Class H (limited prescription delivery) pharmacy, J.53–56
Clinic pharmacies (see Class D pharmacy rules)
Clinics, Pain Management, B.41
Closing a pharmacy, E.10–12
Collaborative practice (see Drug therapy management)
Community pharmacy (see Class A pharmacy rules)
Complaints, F.1–6
Compounding, A.5–7, H.1–72
   Compounding rules, H.1–72
   Controlled substances, B.5–7
   FDA Policy on, A.5–7, H.1–3
   Flavoring medication, H.9
   History and status, H.1–3
   Nonsterile preparations, H.5–18
   Office use (physicians, hospitals, other pharmacies), H.2–3, H.15–18, H.61–64
   Policy, FDA, A.5–7, H.1–3
   Sterile preparations, H.19–64, I.3, I.34
   vs. Manufacturing, A.5–7, H.1–3
Compounding Quality Act, A.5–7, H.1–3
Computer systems
   Class A (community) pharmacy, G.43–46
   Class C (institutional) pharmacy, I.32–34
Confidentiality, E.18–20
   Execution of convicts, E.33
   Investigation information, F.22

Confidential records, patient access to, E.19–20
Consultant pharmacist, I.1, I.6, J.9–10
Consumer medication information, A.17–18
Consumer notification—complaints, F.1–6
Continuing education, D.38–44
    Pharmacists, D.38–44
    Pharmacy technicians, D.90–95
Controlled substances
    Ambulances—distribution to, B.18–19
    Biennial inventory, B.26
    Breakage and spillage of, B.21
    Cannabidiol (CBD), B.2
    Changing information on a controlled substance prescription, B.31–32
    Central recordkeeping, B.28
    Corresponding responsibility, B.34–35
    Comparison—Federal law with Texas law, differences, B.55–56
    Compounding of, B.5–7
    Convicted felon rule, B.21–22
    DEA Form 41, B.23–24
    DEA Form 106, B.20–21
    DEA Form 222, B.12–16
        Sample of, B.17
    DEA Form 224, B.10
    DEA number—Confirmation of, B.9
    Destruction and disposal of, B.23–25
    Detoxification (narcotics), B.50–51
    Disposal of, B.23–25
    Distributor rule (DEA), B.16
    Drug schedules, B.3–5
    Electronic prescriptions of, B.32–34
        Mandatory use of, B.29–30
    Employee screening procedures, B.22, B.29–30
    Employee responsibility to report diversion, B.22
    Forms
        DEA Form 41, B.23–24
        DEA Form 106, B.20–21
        DEA Form 222, B.12–16
            Sample of, B.17
        DEA Form 224, B.10
    History of Federal Controlled Substances Act, B.1–2
    Inspections (DEA), B.25–26
    Inventories, B.26–27
    Loss or Theft of, B.20–21
    Mandatory electronic prescriptions, B.29–30
    Methadone, uses of, B.50–51
    Methamphetamine controls, B.51–53
    Multiple Schedule II prescriptions, B.38–39
    Narcotic detoxification, B.50–51
    Narcotic dependence, treatment of, B.50–51
    Ordering controlled substances
        Schedule II, B.12–16
        Schedule III–V, B.16
    Pharmacist's corresponding responsibility, B.34–35
    Power of Attorney, B.13–14
    Prescription Drug Monitoring Program, Texas, B.47–49
    Prescriptions, B.37–47
        Changing information on, B.31–32
        Filing of, B.27–28
    Records of, B.26–28
    Red flags, B.34, B.48, E.20–22
    Registration, B.7–12
        Application for DEA registration, B.10–11
        Confirmation of DEA registration, B.9
        Exemption from DEA registration, B.9–10
        Form 224, B.10–11
        Temporary use of, B.12
        Texas Department of Public Safety (DPS), B.3
    Return of, B.24–25
    Schedule II prescriptions, B.37–44
        Electronic, B.32–34, B.37–38
            Mandatory use of, B.29
        Emergency verbal, B.38
        Faxing of, B.37
        Hospice patients, B.37
        Long term care patients, B.37
        Ordering Schedule IIs, B.12–16
        Multiple prescriptions for, B.38–39
        Partial filling of, B.39–40
        Time limit for filling, B.40
    Schedule III–V prescriptions, B.44–47
        Electronic, B.32–34
            Mandatory use of, B.29
        Ordering, B.16
        OTC sale of C-V products, B.46–47, G.24
        Partial filling of, B.45
        Refills of, B.45
        Transfer of, B.46
    Schedule V products
        OTC sales of, B.46–47, G.24
    Schedules of controlled substances, B.3–5
    Storage and security of, B.19–20
    Take back programs, B.24–25
    Theft or Significant Loss of, B.20–21
    Transfer of controlled substances between registrants, B.16–17
    Texas Prescription Monitoring Program for Controlled Substances, B.47–49
    Treatment of narcotic dependence, B.50–51
Corresponding responsibility, B.34–35, D.67
    For controlled substances (DEA), B.33–37
    For all prescriptions (TSBP), D.67
Counseling, G.15–18
Criminal offenses, F.36–37
Criminal history evaluation, D.19–20
Current Good Manufacturing Practices (CGMPs), A.22
Customized patient medication packages, G.25–27

D

Dangerous drugs, C.1–21, D.2
    Possession of, C.4–5
    Delivery (sale) of, C.5–6

Dangerous Drug Act (Texas), C.1–13
Data processing system
    Class A (community) pharmacy, G.43–46
    Class C (institutional) pharmacy, I.32–33
Dead prescriber, C.3
Deceased prescriber, C.3
Demonstration (Pilot) projects, D.13–15
Designated agent, C.1, D.2, G.2
Destruction and disposal of drugs, B.23–25, E.30–33
Devices, Medical, A.25–29
Detoxification, B.50–51
Dextromethorphan, C.14–15
Dietary supplements, A.23–25
Disaster provisions (pharmacies—pharmacists), D.52–53
Discharge prescriptions, I.21
Disciplinary action, F.8–37
    Alternative Dispute Resolution (ADR), F.33–34
    Confidentiality, F.34
    Default orders, F.31
    Formal disciplinary action, F.34
    Guidelines, F.34–37
    Informal conferences and settlements, F.31–33
    Mediation, F.33–34
    Penalties, F.28–30, F.37
    Pharmacies, F.13–15
    Pharmacists and applicants, F.8–13
    Pharmacy technicians and trainees, F.16–18
    Procedures, Rules of, F.31–37
    Remedial Plan, F.24–25
Dispensed drugs, beyond-use date, G.21
Dispensing
    Disaster provisions, D.52–53
    Out-of-state prescriptions, C.21
    Quick reference guide, C.21
    Rural areas (physicians), D.80–81
    Veterinarians, D.81
Dispensing directive (generic substitution), D.62–63
Dispensing of opioid antagonist, C.7–8
Dispensing errors, records of, G.42
Disposal and destruction of drugs, B.23–25, E.30–33
Distributor 5% rule, B.16, G.53
    DEA, B.16
    TSBP, G.48–49
Dosage form substitution, D.58–59
Drug Addiction Treatment Act (DATA), B.50–51
Drug donation program, C.16–19
Drug Enforcement Administration (DEA)
    DEA Form 41, B.23–24
    DEA Form 106, B.20–21
    DEA Form 222, B.12–16
        Sample of, B.17
    DEA Form 224, B.10
    DEA number—Confirmation of, B.9
    Registration, B.7–12
DEA web site, forms and resources, B.53
Drug Quality and Security Act (DQSA), A.5–9
Drug Price Competition and Patent Restoration Act, A.2
Drug recalls, A.16, E.12

Drug regimen review, G.18–19, I.21–22, J.26
    Remote, G.18–19
Drug samples, A.2–4, E.15–16, I.18, J.15
Drug schedules, B.3–5
Drug storage, E.15
    Class A (community) pharmacy, G.24
    Class D (clinic) pharmacy, J.12, J.15
    Controlled substances, B.19–20
Drug Supply Chain Security Act (DSCSA), A.7–9
Drugs used for execution, E.33
Drug therapy management under protocol, E.2–5
Durham-Humphrey Amendments, A.1–2

E

Electronic prescription drug orders, B.32–34, D.63, G.36–37
Electronic controlled substance prescriptions, B.32–34, G.36
    Mandatory use of, B.29
Electronic supervision and verification of pharmacy technicians, G.7, I.3–4, I.9
Emergency medication kits, D.72–73
Emergency Schedule II prescription, B.30
Emergency verbal prescriptions (Schedule II drugs), B.30
Emergency refills, G.39–41
Emergency remote pharmacy, D.52–53
Emergency rooms, I.22–23
Emergency temporary pharmacist license, D.34
Emergency temporary pharmacy technician registration, D.95–96
Ephedrine controls, B.51–53
Epinephrine
    Administration by Pharmacist, D.12–13
    Prescription for various entities, D.69–70
Examinations, D.20–22
Execution drugs, E.33
Expiration dates for dispensed drugs, G.21–22

F

Facsimiles, B.37, B.44, G.36–37
Faxes (see Facsimiles)
Federal Hazard Communication Standard, A.31
Federal Hazardous Substances Act, A.30
FDA Compounding Quality Act, A.5–7, H.2–3
FDA Modernization Act (FDAMA), A.4, A.28
FDA Safety and Innovation Act, A.5
Fees
    Pharmacist license, D.36
    Pharmacy license, D.50
    Pharmacy technician, D.88
Fines (see Penalties)
Flavoring medication, H.9

Floor stock
    Distribution system, I.16–17
    Records of, I.32
Food, Drug, and Cosmetic Act, A.1–29
    Adulteration, A.11
    Advertising prescription drugs by pharmacists/pharmacies, A.16–17
    Biological products, A.5, A.9
    CGMPs, A.22
    Compounding (vs. manufacturing), A.5–7, H.1–3
    Consumer medication information, A.17–18
    Current Good Manufacturing Practices (CGMPs), A.22
    Dietary supplements, A.23–25
    Drug Quality and Security Act (DQSA), A.5–9
    Drug Price Competition and Patent Protection Act, A.2
    Drug Supply Chain and Security Act (DSCSA), A.7–9
    Durham-Humphrey Amendments, A.1–2
    FDA Modernization Act (FDAMA), A.4, A.28
    Good Manufacturing Practices (GMPs), A.22
    Ipecac syrup—labeling of, A.14
    Kefauver-Harris Amendments, A.2
    Medical devices, A.25–29
    Medical foods, A.25
    Medication guides, A.17–18
    Misbranding, A.11
    National Drug Code (NDC), A.22
    NDC (National Drug Code), A.22
    New drugs, A.25–29
    New drug classification system, A.21
    Off-label use, A.21
    OTC drugs, A.11–16
    Over-the-counter drugs, A.11–16
    Patient package inserts, A.17
    Pregnancy labeling, A.22–23
    Prescription Drug Marketing Act (PDMA), A.2–4
    Recalls, drugs, and devices, A.16, E.12
    Risk Evaluation and Mitigation Strategies (REMS), A.18–20
    Special warning requirements, A.13–15
    Tamper-evident packaging, A.15
    Unapproved use of drugs, A.21
    Unlabeled use of drugs, A.21
    Warning requirements, OTC drugs, A.13–15
Foreign practitioners, C.2, C.21, G.35
Formulary
    Class C (institutional) pharmacy, I.18
    Class D (clinic) pharmacy, J.13–15
Freestanding emergency medical center pharmacy (Class F), J.31–46

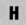

Gases, Medical, C.20
Generic substitution, D.55–66
    Class E (nonresident) pharmacy, J.28
    Dispensing directive, D.62–63
    Orange book (FDA), A.23, D.65
    Purple book (FDA), A.23, D.65
Glaucoma specialists (optometrists), C.11
Good Manufacturing Practices (GMPs), A.22
Grounds for disciplinary action
    Pharmacies, F.13–15
    Pharmacists, F.8–13
    Pharmacy technicians and trainees, F.16–18

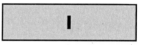

Hazard Communication Standard, Federal, A.31
Hazardous drugs (USP Chapter 800), H.64–69
Hazardous Substances Act, Federal, A.30
Health Information Technology for Economic and Clinical Health Act (see HITECH Act)
Health Insurance Portability and Accountability Act (HIPAA), A.36–41
HITECH Act, A.40–41
HIPAA, A.36–41
HIPAA (Texas), A.41–43
Home health agencies, C.15–16
Hospice drug disposal, B.25
Hospice patients, B.37, B.39–40
Hospital pharmacy (see Class C pharmacy rules)
Hospitals, rural, I.3, I.10, I.14–16

I

Imaging prescription records, G.37
Immunizations and vaccinations, D.15–18
Impaired pharmacists and pharmacy students program, D.82
Inactive license (pharmacists), D.44–46
Informal conferences, F.31–33
Inspections (Board of Pharmacy), F.6–7
Institutional pharmacy (see Class C pharmacy rules)
Internet prescriptions, B.35–36, D.79, E.20, G.34
Internet sites (pharmacies), D.71, F.2–3
Interns
    Definitions, D.23–25
    Duties of, D.30
    Identification of, D.29
Internship program, D.23–31
    Definitions, D.23–25
    Extended internship program, D.28–29
    Goals and objectives, D.25–27
    Hours, D.27
    Intern trainees, D.24
    Preceptor requirements, D.30–31
    Resident intern, D.24
    Student intern, D.25, D.27–28
Intravenous medications (see Compounding sterile preparations)

Inventories, E.16–18
    Annual inventory, E.16–17
    Change of ownership inventory, E.17
    Change of PIC inventory, E.18
    Federal and Texas Controlled Substances Act, B.26–27
    General requirements, E.16
    Initial inventory, E.16–17
    Perpetual inventory, B.27, E.17–18
        Class C pharmacy, I.32, I.34
        Class F Pharmacy, J.43, J.46
    Remote pharmacy sites, D.78, D.79, D.81
    Remote pharmacies, D.73, D.75, D. 76, D.77
Ipecac syrup—labeling of, A.14
iPLEDGE program, A.19
Isotretinoin, A.19

K

Kefauver-Harris Amendments, A.2
Kickbacks from pharmacies, pharmacists, E.1, F.10
Kiosks (see Automated storage and delivery systems)

L

Labeling requirements
    Class A (community) pharmacies, G.20–23
        Chart of, G.23
    Class B (nuclear) pharmacies, J.6–7
    Class D (clinic) pharmacies, J.15–17
Liability claims—reporting requirement, D.96–97
Library requirements
    Class A (community) pharmacies, G.24
    Class B (nuclear) pharmacies, J.7
    Class C pharmacies (institutional), I.15–16
    Class D pharmacies (clinic), J.13
    Class F pharmacies (free standing emergency medical center), J.37–38
Licensing
    Pharmacies (general), D.46–55
        Class A (community), G.11–12
        Class B (nuclear), J.5–6
        Class C (institutional), I.13–15
        Class D (clinic), J.11–12
        Class E (nonresident), J.20–21
        Class F (free standing emergency medical center), J.36–37
        Emergency Remote Pharmacy, D.52–53
        Fees, D.50
    Pharmacists, D.20–46
        Continuing education requirements, D.38–44
        Emergency temporary pharmacist license, D.34
        Examination, D.20–22
        Expiration of license, D.35–38
        Inactive status, D.44–46
        Military service members, veterans, spouses, D.33–34
        Reciprocity, D.32–33
        Renewal of, D.35–38
Limited prescription delivery pharmacy (Class H), J.53–56
Listed chemicals (DEA), B.5, B.51–52
Long term care facilities
    Automated pharmacy systems, use in, D.74–75
    Emergency medication kits, use in, D.72–73
    Labeling requirements, G.21–22
    Partial filling of Schedule II prescriptions, B.39–40
    Schedule II facsimile prescriptions, B.37

M

Mailing and delivering prescription drugs, A.34–35, G.17–18
Mail order nonresident pharmacy (see Class E pharmacy statutes and rules)
Mail order resident (in-state) pharmacy (see Class A pharmacy rules)
Malpractice claims—reporting requirement, D.96–99
Marijuana, B.2
Mediation (alternative dispute resolution), F.33–34
Medical devices, A.25–29
Medical foods, A.25
Medical gases, C.20
Medication guides, A.17–18
Med-Packs, G.25–27
Mental or physical exam
    Pharmacists, interns, and applicants, F.20–21
    Pharmacy technicians, F.18
Methadone, use of, B.50–51
Methamphetamine controls, B.51–53
Mexican practitioners, C.2, C.21, G.35–37
Mid-level practitioners, B.8, B.29, C.9–11
Military service members, veterans, spouses
    Pharmacist license, D.33–34
    Technician registration, D.95
Mineral oil, A.13
Misbranding, A.11
Multiple prescriptions for Schedule II drugs, B.38–39

N

Nalaxone (see Opioid antagonists)
Narcotic detoxification, B.50–51
Narcotic dependence, treatment of, B.50–51
Narrow therapeutic index drugs, D.59
National Drug Code (NDC), A.22
New drugs, A.20
New drug classification system, A.21
Nonresident pharmacy, J.20–31
Nonsterile compounding, H.1–18
Notifications
    Pharmacies, D.71–72, E.6–10

Pharmacists, D.66–D.67
Pharmacy technicians, D.95
Nuclear pharmacists, J.3–4
Nuclear pharmacy (see Class B pharmacy), J.1–9
Nurse practitioners (APRNs), C.9–11
Nursing homes (see Long term care facilities)

O

Office use compounding (physicians, hospitals, other pharmacies), H.2–3, H.15–18, H.61–64
Office use prescription, C.3
Official prescription form, B.42–44
    Exceptions to use of, B.44
Off-label use, A.21
Opioid antagonists, C.7–8
Opioid prescription limits for acute pain, B.40–41
Optometric glaucoma specialists, C.11
Optometrists, C.11–13
Orange Book, A.23, D.65
Out-of-state prescriptions, C.21
Outsourcing facilities—FDA (sterile compounding), A.6–7
Outsourcing pharmacy (central fill), E.23
Over-the-counter drugs, A.11–16

P

Pain management clinics, B.41, E.21
Pain prescriptions for acute pain, limits, B.40–41
Partial filling Schedule II prescriptions, B.38–39
Partial filling Schedule III–V prescriptions, B.45
Patient access to confidential records, E.19–20
Patient counseling, G.15–18
    Class E (nonresident) pharmacy, J.27–28
    Class D (clinic) pharmacy, J.16
Patient medication records
    Class A (community) pharmacy, G.42–43
    Class C (institutional) pharmacy, I.32
Patient package inserts, A.17
Patient-practitioner relationship (Telemedicine), D.79, G.34
Peer review committees, D.83–84
Penalties and sanctions, F.19–20, F.28–30
Perpetual inventory, B.27, E.17–18
    Class C pharmacy, I.32, I.34
    Class F pharmacy, J.43, J.46
    Remote pharmacy sites, D.73, D.75, D.76, D.77
Pharmaceutical care services
    Class A (community) pharmacy, G.18–19
    Class C (institutional) pharmacy, I.21–22
Pharmacies
    Classes of, D.46–48
    Closing, E.10–12
    Licensing of, D.46–55

Notifications to Board, D.71–72, E.6–10
    Supervision of, D.70
Pharmacist-in-charge (PIC)
    Class A (community) pharmacy, G.5–6
    Class B (nuclear) pharmacy, J.1–2
    Class C (institutional) pharmacy, I.4–6
    Class D (clinic) pharmacy, J.10
    Class F (free standing emergency medical center) pharmacy, J.33–34
Pharmacist certification programs, E.1–2
Pharmacists
    Disciplinary action, F.8–13
    Drug Therapy Management, E.2–5
    Emergency temporary pharmacist license, E.34
    Inactive license, D.44–46
    License by examination, D.20–22
    License by reciprocity, D.32–33
    Notifications, D.66–67
    Prescriptive Authority, E.3–5
    Professional responsibility of, E.20–23
    Signing of prescriptions by, E.3–5
Pharmacist interns
    Duties of, D.30
    Internship program, D.23–31
    Extended internship program, D.28–29
    Goals and objectives, D.25–27
    Hours, D.27
    Preceptor requirements, D.30–31
Pharmacy balance (see Balance)
Pharmacy peer review committees, D.83–84
Pharmacy residency programs, D.11–12
Pharmacy technicians/trainees, D.86–96
    Certification of pharmacy technicians, D.87
        Exemption from, D.90
    Continuing education requirements, D.90–95
    Class A (community) pharmacies
        Duties, G.9–11
        Ratio
            General rule, G.9–10
            Special rule, D.85
        Supervision, G.6–7
            Electronic supervision, G.7
    Class B (nuclear) pharmacies, J.5
        Ratio, J.5
    Class C (institutional) pharmacies, I.7–12
        Duties, I.8–12
        Ratio, I.11
    Discipline of, F.16–18
    Electronic supervision of, G.7, I.9
    Notifications to Board, D.95
    Ratios
        Class A (community) pharmacies
            General rule, G.9–10
            Special rule, D.85
        Class B (nuclear) pharmacies, J.5
        Class C (institutional) pharmacies, I.11
    Registration of, D.86–88
        Military service members, veterans, spouses, D.95

Pharmacy technicians/trainees (*continued*)
    Supervision of (Class A), G.6–7
    Tech-check-tech, I.4, I.9–10
    Technician trainees, D.88–90
    Training programs, D.88–90
Physical or mental exam
    Pharmacists, interns, and applicants, F.20–21
    Pharmacy technicians, F.18
Physician assistants (PAs), C.9–10
Physicians (see Practitioners)
Physician dispensing, D.80–81
Physician prescribing for self or family members, C.2–3
Physician self-prescribing, C.2–3
Pick-up locations for prescriptions, E.14
Pilot and demonstration projects, D.13–15
Policy and procedure manual
    Class B (nuclear) pharmacies, J.8
    Class C (institutional) pharmacies, I.20–21
    Class D (clinic) pharmacies, J.17–18
    Class F (free standing emergency medical center) pharmacies, J.41–42
Power of attorney, B.12–14
Practitioners, C.2, D.4, G.4
    Scope of practice, C.2
    Self-prescribing, C.3–4
        Canadian, C.2, C.21, G.35–37
        Mexican, C.2, C.21, G.35–37
Preceptor requirements, D.30–31
Pregnancy labeling, A.22–23
Prepackaging of drugs
    Class A pharmacy, G.24–25
    Class C pharmacy, I.18–19
    Class D pharmacy, J.15, J.19
    Class F pharmacy, J.39
Prescription Drug Marketing Act (PDMA), A.2–3
Prescription Drug Monitoring Program (PMP), Texas, B.47–49
Prescription drug recalls, A.16, E.12
Prescriptions
    Beyond-use date, G.21–22
    Bulk transfer of, G.48
    Chart of legal prescriptions, C.21
    Containers (Class A pharmacies), G.20
    Dispensing and delivery (Class A pharmacies), G.15–20
    Electronic, B.32–34, D.63, G.36–37
    Facsimiles, B.37, B.44, G.36–37
        Schedule II prescriptions, B.37
    Faxes (see Facsimiles)
    Internet prescriptions, B.35–36, D.79, E.20, G.34
    Label requirements, G.20–23
        Chart of, G.23
    Limits for acute pain, B.41
    Pick-up locations, E.14
    Radioactive/Radiopharmaceuticals, J.8–9
    Records of (Class A pharmacies)
        Computer system, G.43–46
        Data processing system, G.43–46
        Manual system, G.43

    Refills, G.39–41
        Accelerated, G.41
        Automatic, B.45, G.45
        Auto refill programs, B.45, G.41
        PRN, G.39
    Return of prescription drugs, B.19, B.24–25, E.12–14
    Return of undelivered prescription drugs to stock, G.22
    Signing of—by pharmacists, E.3–4
    Storage of records, B.27–28, G.37
    Tamper-resistant requirements, A.35
    Transfer of, G.46–48
    Verbal, B.32, G.36
Prescription samples, A.2–4, E.15–16, G.24, J.15
Privacy regulations (see HIPAA)
PRN refills, G.39
Procedures for disciplinary action, F.31–37
Professional responsibility of pharmacist, E.20–23
Professional liability claims/reporting requirement, D.96–99
Provision of drugs (Class D pharmacy), J.16–17
Pseudoephedrine controls, B.51–53
Purple Book (FDA), A.23, D.65

Q

Quick reference guide to dispensing, C.21

R

Radioactive prescriptions, J.8–9
Radiopharmaceutical prescriptions, J.8–9
Ratio—Pharmacy technicians to pharmacist
    Class A (community) pharmacies
        General rule, G.9–10
        Special rule, D.85
    Class B (nuclear) pharmacies, J.5
    Class C (institutional) pharmacies, I.11
Recalls, prescription drugs, A.16, E.12
Reciprocity (pharmacists), D.32–33
Records
    Class A pharmacy, G.33–50
    Class B pharmacy, J.8–9
    Class C pharmacy, I.31–34
    Class D pharmacy, J.18–19
    Class E pharmacy, J.29–30
    Class F pharmacy, J.43–47
    Class G pharmacy, J.52
    Class H pharmacy, J.56
    Dispensing errors, G.42
Red Flags, B.34, B.38, E.20–22
Refills, G.39–41
    Accelerated, G.41
    Automatic, B.45, G.41
    Auto refill programs, B.45, G.41
    Emergency, D.70–71, G.43–45

PRN, G.39
Schedules III–V, B.41
Registered technician (see Pharmacy technicians)
Registration, DEA (controlled substances), B.7–12
Remedial plan, F.24–25
Remote dispensing site, D.77–78
Remote drug regimen review, G.18–19
Remote pharmacist practice (see Central processing)
Remote pharmacy, emergency (see Emergency remote pharmacy)
Remote pharmacy services rules (summary), D.72–79
    Automated pharmacy systems, summary of (LTC, hospice, prisons.), D.74–75
    Automated storage and delivery systems (kiosks), D.78–79
    Emergency medication kits, summary of, D.73
    Telepharmacy, summary of, D.76–78
REMS, A.18–20
Retail pharmacy (see Class A pharmacy rules)
Return of dispensed controlled substances to pharmacy for destruction, B.24–25
Return of prescription drugs, B.24–25, E.12–14
Return to stock of undelivered prescription drugs, G.22
Risk Evaluation and Mitigation Strategies (REMS), A.18–20
Risk levels (sterile preparations), H.33–37
Rural hospitals, I.3, I.10–11, I.14–17
Rural physicians—dispensing, D.80–81

S

Safe disposal notification for Schedule II prescriptions, B.41, G.19–20
Samples, prescription, A.2–4, E.15–16, G.24, J.15
Satellite pharmacies, E.25–30
Schedule II prescriptions, B.37–44
    Electronic, B.32–34, B.37–38
        Mandatory use of, B.29
    Emergency verbal, B.30
    Faxing of, B.37
    Hospice patients, B.37
    Long term care patients, B.37
    Multiple prescriptions for, B.38–39
    Notification of safe disposal, G.19–20
    Partial filling of, B.39–40
    Time limit for filling, B.40
Schedule III–V prescriptions, B.44–46
    Electronic, B.32–34
        Mandatory use of, B.29
    OTC sale of C-V prescriptions, B.46–47, G.24
    Partial filling of, B.45
    Refills of, B.45
    Transfer of, B.46
Schedules of controlled substances, B.3–5
Score transfer, D.22
Scope of practice, C.2
Security requirements
    Class A (community) pharmacies, G.12–13
    Class C (institutional) pharmacies, I.15
    Class D (clinic) pharmacies, J.12
    Class F (free standing emergency medical center) pharmacies, J.37
    Controlled substances, B.19–21
Self-prescribing by practitioners, C.2–3
Signing prescription drug orders—PAs and APNs, C.9–11
Signing prescription drug order—pharmacists, E.3–5
Sterile compounding, H.19–64, I.3, I.34
Sterile pharmaceuticals (compounding sterile preparations), H.19–64, I.3, I.34
Storage of drugs
    Class A (community) pharmacies, G.24
    Class D (clinic) pharmacies, J.12, J.15
    Controlled substances, B.19–20
Storage of prescription records, B.27–28, G.37
Subpoenas, F.22–23
Substitution
    Biologicals, D.55–66
    Generic, D.55–66
        Dosage form, D.58–59
Supervision of pharmacies, D.70
    Class D (clinic) pharmacies, J.18
Supervision of pharmacy technicians, Class A (community), G.6–7
Supportive personnel, Class D (clinic) pharmacies, J.10–11
Sworn disclosure statement, D.49–50

T

Tamper-evident packaging, OTC drugs, A.15
Tamper-resistant prescription requirements, A.35
Tax-free alcohol, A.35–36
Tech-check-tech, I.4, I.9–10
Technicians—see pharmacy technicians
Telemedicine, D.79, G.34
Telepharmacy, summary of rules, D.76–78
Telephone prescriptions (see Verbal prescriptions)
Temporary absence of pharmacist, Class A (community), G.13–15
Temporary suspension or restriction of registration (pharmacy technicians), F.18–19
Temporary suspension or restriction of license (pharmacist or pharmacy), F.23
Texas Dangerous Drug Act, C.1–13
Texas official prescription form (Schedule II drugs), B.42–44
    Exceptions to use of, B.44
Texas Prescription Drug Monitoring Program (PMP), B.47–49
Texas prescription program for controlled substances, B.47–49
Texas State Board of Pharmacy
    Complaints to, F.1–6
    Organization of, D.6–10
Texas triplicate prescription form (see Official prescription form)
Therapeutic drug interchange, G.19
Therapeutic optometrists, C.11–13

Track and Trace, A.7–9
Transfer of controlled substances between registrants, B.16–17
Transfer of prescriptions, G.46–48
    Bulk transfers, G.48
    Schedules III–V, B.46
    Unfilled controlled substance prescriptions, B.46
Treatment of narcotic dependence, B.50–51
Triplicate prescription form (see Official prescription form)

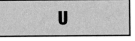

Unapproved use of prescription drugs, A.21
Undelivered prescription medication, returning to stock, G.25
Unlabeled use of prescription drugs, A.21
Unprofessional conduct, F.9–11
USP Chapter 797 (see Sterile compounding)
USP Chapter 800 (see Hazardous drugs)

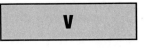

Vaccinations and immunizations, D.15–18
Verbal prescriptions, B.32, G.36
    Emergency Schedule II, B.30
    Schedules III–V, B.32
Veterinarians, administration and provision of drugs, D.81

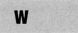

Wintergreen oil, A.13